EPIDEMIOLOGY, CAUSES AND PREVENTION OF SKIN DISEASES

Grob *et al:* Epidemiology, Causes and Prevention of Skin Diseases

ERRATUM

Will readers please note that the correct name of the co-editor of this book is M. A. Weinstock

Epidemiology, Causes and Prevention of Skin Diseases

Edited by J.J. Grob,
R.S. Stern, R.M. MacKie and
W.A. Weinstock

b

**Blackwell
Science**

© 1997 by
Blackwell Science Ltd
Editorial Offices:
Osney Mead, Oxford OX2 0EL
25 John Street, London WC1N 2BL
23 Ainslie Place, Edinburgh EH3 6AJ
350 Main Street, Malden
  MA 02148 5018, USA
54 University Street, Carlton
  Victoria 3053, Australia

Other Editorial Offices:
Blackwell Wissenschafts-Verlag GmbH
Kurfürstendamm 57
10707 Berlin, Germany

Blackwell Science KK
MG Kodenmacho Building
7–10 Kodenmacho Nihombashi
Chuo-ku, Tokyo 104, Japan

First published 1997

Set by Setrite Typesetters, Hong Kong
Printed and bound in Great Britain
at the University Press, Cambridge

The Blackwell Science logo is a
trade mark of Blackwell Science Ltd,
registered at the United Kingdom
Trade Marks Registry

A catalogue record for this title
is available from the British Library

ISBN 0-632-04256-7

DISTRIBUTORS

  Marston Book Services Ltd
  PO Box 269, Abingdon
  Oxon OX14 4YN
  (*Orders*: Tel: 01235 465500
           Fax: 01235 465555)

USA
  Blackwell Science, Inc.
  Commerce Place
  350 Main Street
  Malden, MA 02148 5018
  (*Orders*: Tel: 800 759-6102
           617 388-8250
           Fax: 617 388-8255)

Canada
  Copp Clark Professional
  200 Adelaide Street West, 3rd Floor,
  Toronto, Ontario
  Canada, M5H 1W7
  (*Orders*: Tel: 416-597-1616
           800-815-9417
           Fax: 416-597-1617)

Australia
  Blackwell Science Pty Ltd
  54 University Street
  Carlton, Victoria 3053
  (*Orders*: Tel: 03 9347 0300
           Fax: 03 9349 3016)

Library of Congress
Cataloging-in-Publication Data

Epidemiology, causes, and prevention
  of skin diseases/edited by
  J.J. Grob ... [et al.].
       p.   cm.
  Includes bibliographical references
  and index.
  ISBN 0-632-04256-7
  1. Skin—Diseases—Epidemiology.
  2. Skin—Diseases—Prevention.
  I. Grob, J.J.
  [DNLM: 1. Skin Diseases — prevention & control.
  2. Skin Diseases — epidemiology.
  WR 140 E627 1997]
  RL72.E58 1997
  616.5 — dc21
  DNLM/DLC
  for Library of Congress   96-39073

Contents

List of Contributors

B.K. ARMSTRONG *New South Wales Cancer Council, PO Box 572, Kings Cross 2011, Australia*

P. AUTIER *Division of Epidemiology and Biostatistics, European Institute of Oncology, Via Ripamonti 435, 20141 Milan, Italy*

R. BARAN *Nail Disease Center, 42, rue des Serbes, 06400 Cannes, France*

S. BASTUJI-GARIN *Department of Public Health, Hôpital Henri Mondor, Université Paris XII, 94010 Créteil, France*

M. BINDER *Department of Dermatology, University of Vienna Medical School, Waehringer Guertel 18-20, A-1090 Vienna, Austria*

M. BLETTNER *Department of Epidemiology, German Cancer Research Center, Heidelberg, Germany*

J.J. BONERANDI *Service de Dermatologie, Hôpital Sainte-Marguerite, 270 Boulevard de Ste Marguerite, 13009 Marseille, France*

M.-L. BOUSCARY *INSERM Research Unit 379 'Epidemiology and Social Sciences Applied to Medical Innovation', Paoli-Calmettes Institute, 232, Bd Sainte Marguerite, 13273 Marseille, France*

P. BROUQUI *Unité des Rickettsies, CNRS UPRESA-6020 13385 Marseille, France*

M. CASTELAIN *Department of Dermatology, Hôpital Sainte-Marguerite, 270 Boulevard de Ste Marguerite, BP 29, 13277 Marseille Cedex 9, France*

J.-P. CESARINI *Fondation Ophtalmologique Adolphe de Rothschild, 25, rue Manin, 75019 Paris, France*

O. CHOSIDOW *Service de Médecine Interne, Groupe Hospitalier Pitié-Salpêtrière, 83 boulevard de l'Hôpital, 75013 Paris, France*

A. CLAUDY *Department of Dermatology, Edouard Herriot Hospital, 69374 Lyon, France*

Y.M. CLAYTON *St John's Institute of Dermatology, St. Thomas's Hospital, London SE1 7EH, UK*

B. CRIBIER *Clinique Dermatologique, University Hospital of Strasbourg, 67091 Strasbourg, France*

H. DESPERRIERE *Service de Dermato-Vénéréo-Léprologie, Centre Hospitalier de Cayenne, BP 6006 Rue des Flamboyants, 97306 Cayenne Cedex, French Guiana*

T.L. DIEPGEN *Dermatoepidemiology Unit, Department of Dermatology, University of Erlangen, Hartmannstrasse 14, 91052 Erlangen, Germany*

B.L. DIFFEY *Regional Medical Physics Department, Dryburn Hospital, Durham DH1 5TW, UK*

N. DUPIN *Service de Médecine Interne, Groupe Hospitalier Pitié-Salpêtrière, 83 boulevard de l'Hôpital, 75013 Paris, France*

J.M. ELWOOD *Hugh Adam Cancer Epidemiology Unit, Department of Preventive and Social Medicine, Otago Medical School, PO Box 913, Dunedin, New Zealand*

C. ENERBÄCK *Department of Dermatology, Sahlgrenska University Hospital, S-413 45 Göteborg, Sweden*

F. ENLUND *Department of Clinical Genetics, Ostra Hospital, S-416 85 Göteborg, Sweden*

S. EUVRARD *Department of Dermatology, Edouard Herriot Hospital, 69374 Lyon, France*

J.D. FINE *Department of Dermatology, The University of North Carolina at Chapel Hill, 3100 Thurston Building, CB#7287 and the National Epidermolysis Bullosa Registry, Chapel Hill, NC, USA*

A.Y. FINLAY *Department of Dermatology, University of Wales College of Medicine, Heath Park, Cardiff CF4 4XN, UK*

C. FRANCES *Service de Médecine Interne, Groupe Hospitalier Pitié-Salpêtrière, 83 boulevard de l'Hôpital, 75651 Paris, France*

R.P. GALLAGHER *Cancer Control Research Program, British Columbia Cancer Agency, 600W 10th Avenue, Vancouver BC, Canada V5Z 4E6*

C. GARBE *Department of Dermatology, Eberhard-Karls-University, Liebermeisterstrasse 25, D-72076 Tübingen, Germany*

C.F. GARLAND *Department of Family and Preventive Medicine, University of California, 9500 Gilman Drive, La Jolla, CA 92093-0631, USA*

F.C. GARLAND *Department of Family and Preventive Medicine, University of California, 9500 Gilman Drive, La Jolla, CA 92093-0631, USA*

E.D. GORHAM *Department of Family and Preventive Medicine, University of California, 9500 Gilman Drive, La Jolla, CA 92093-0631, USA*

J. GOUVERNET *DIM Adults, Hôpital de la Timone, 13005 Marseille, France*

J.J. GROB *Service de Dermatologie, Hôpital Sainte-Marguerite, 270 Boulevard de Ste Marguerite, BP 29, 13277 Marseille Cedex 9, France*

G. GUILLET *Chu Morvan-Dermato-Allergologie, 29609 Brest Cedex, France*

M.H. GUILLET *Chu Morvan-Dermato-Allergologie, 29609 Brest Cedex, France*

A.K. GUPTA *Division of Dermatology, Department of Medicine, University of Toronto, Toronto, Ontario, Canada*

M.A. GUPTA *Department of Psychiatry, University of Western Ontario, London, Ontario, Canada*

E.A. HOLLY *Department of Epidemiology and Biostatistics, School of Medicine, University of California, San Francisco, CA 94143 and Department of Health Research and Policy, School of Medicine, Stanford University, Stanford CA 94305, USA*

D. LE THI HUONG *Service de Médecine Interne, Groupe Hospitalier Pitié-Salpêtrière, 83 boulevard de l'Hôpital, 75651 Paris, France*

M. D'INCAN *Department of Dermatology, Hôtel-Dieu, BP 69, F-63003 Clermont-Ferrand Cedex 01, France*

A. INEROT *Department of Dermatology, Sahlgrenska University Hospital, S-413 45 Göteborg, Sweden*

J. JOPSON *Hugh Adam Cancer Epidemiology Unit, Department of Preventive and Social Medicine, Otago Medical School, PO Box 913, Dunedin, New Zealand*

J. KANITAKIS *Department of Dermatology, Edouard Herriot Hospital, 69374 Lyon, France*

H. KITTLER *Department of Dermatology, University of Vienna Medical School, Waehringer Guertel 18-20, A-1090 Vienna, Austria*

J.M. LACHAPELLE *Unit of Dermato-allergology and Dermato-immunology, Louvain University, 30, Clos Chapelle-aux-Champs, UCL 3033, B-1200 Brussels, Belgium*

R.G.B. LANGLEY *Department of Dermatology, Massachusetts General Hospital, Harvard Medical School, Bartlett 410, 40 Blossom Street, Boston, MA 02114, USA*

D.C.W. MABEY *Department of Infectious and Tropical Diseases, London School of Hygiene and Tropical Medicine, London, UK*

R.M. MACKIE *Department of Dermatology, Robertson Building, University of Glasgow, Glasgow G12 8QQ, UK*

T. MARTINSSON *Department of Clinical Genetics, Ostra Hospital, S-416 85 Göteborg, Sweden*

J.-P. MOATTI *Department of Economics, University Aix-Marseille II, and INSERM Research Unit 379 'Epidemiology and Social Sciences Applied to Medical Innovation', Paoli-Calmettes Institute, 232, Bd Sainte Marguerite, 13273 Marseille, France*

L. NALDI *Coordinating Centre of the Italian Group for Epidemiologic Research in Dermatology, and Department of Dermatology, Bergamo General Hospital, Largo Barozzi, 1, 24100 Bergamo, Italy*

K. PALMA-LARGO *Service de Dermato-Vénéréo-Leprologie, Centre Hospitalier de Cayenne, BP 6006 Rue des Flamboyants, 97306 Cayenne Cedex, French Guiana*

H. PEHAMBERGER *Department of Dermatology, University of Vienna Medical School, Waehringer Guertel 18-20, A-1090 Vienna, Austria*

L. PELI *Coordinating Centre of the Italian Group for Epidemiologic Research in Dermatology, and Department of Dermatology, Bergamo General Hospital, Largo Barozzi, 1, 24100 Bergamo, Italy*

M. PIEPKORN *Division of Dermatology, University of Washington, Box 356524, Seattle, WA 98195-6524, USA*

R. PRADINAUD *Service de Dermato-Vénéréo-Léprologie, Centre Hospitalier de Cayenne, BP 6006 Rue des Flamboyants, 97306 Cayenne Cedex, French Guiana*

F.H.J. RAMPEN *Department of Dermatology, Sint Anna Hospital, Joannes Zwijsenlaan 121, 5340 BE Oss, The Netherlands*

D. RAOULT *Unité des Rickettsies, CNRS UPRESA-6020, 13385 Marseille, France*

M.J.M. DE ROOIJ *Department of Dermatology, University Hospital Sint Radboud, PO Box 9101, 6500 HB Nijmegen, The Netherlands*

J.-C. ROUJEAU *Service de Dermatologie, Hôpital Henri Mondor, Université Paris XII, 94010 Créteil, France*

R. SAMBUC *DIM. Hôpital de la Conception, 13005 Marseille, France*

H. SANCHO-GARNIER *EPIDAURE, University of Montpellier, Montpellier, France*

H. SANDOVSKY-LOSICA *Department of Human Microbiology, Tel-Aviv University, Tel-Aviv 69978, Israel*

J.L. SAN MARCO *Laboratoire de Santé Publique, Université de la Mediterranee, Hôpital Timone, 13005 Marseille, France*

E. SEGAL *Department of Human Microbiology, Tel-Aviv University, Tel-Aviv 69978, Israel*

A.J. SOBER *Department of Dermatology, Massachusetts General Hospital, Harvard Medical School, Bartlett 410, 40 Blossom Street, Boston, MA 02114, USA*

P. SOUTEYRAND *Department of Dermatology, Hôtel-Dieu, BP 69, F-63003 Clermont-Ferrand Cedex 01, France*

E. SØYLAND *Department of Dermatology, and Laboratory for Immunohistochemistry and Immunopathology, Rikshospitalet, University of Oslo, Oslo, Norway*

R.S. STERN *Department of Dermatology, Beth Israel Hospital, Harvard Medical School, 330 Brookline Avenue, Boston, MA 02215, USA*

E.L. SVEJGAARD *Department of Dermatology, Bispebjerg Hospital, Bispebjerg Bakke 23, 2400 Copenhagen, Denmark*

G. SWANBECK *Department of Dermatology, Sahlgrenska University Hospital, S-413 45 Göteborg, Sweden*

A. TAÏEB *Unité de Dermatologie Pédiatrique, Hôpital Pellegrin-Enfants, 33076 Bordeaux, France*

V. VINCENT *Centre National de Reference des Mycobacteries, Institut Pasteur, 25, rue du Docteur Roux, 75724 Paris Cedex 15, France*

CH. DE VROEY *Laboratory for Mycology, Prince Leopold Institute of Tropical Medicine, Nationalestraat 155, B-2000 Antwerp, Belgium*

J. WAHLSTRÖM *Department of Clinical Genetics, Ostra Hospital, S-416 85 Göteborg, Sweden*

M.A. WEINSTOCK *Dermatoepidemiology Unit, V A Medical Center — 111D, 830 Chalkstone Avenue, Providence, RI 02908-4799, USA*

H.C. WILLIAMS *Dermatoepidemiology Unit, Queen's Medical Centre, University Hospital, Nottingham NG7 2UH, UK*

K. WOLFF *Department of Dermatology, University of Vienna Medical School, Waehringer Guertel 18-20, A-1090 Vienna, Austria*

M. YHR *Department of Clinical Genetics, Ostra Hospital, S-416 85 Göteborg, Sweden*

Preface

The idea for a comprehensive book on epidemiology and prevention of skin diseases was first proposed in May 1995 in Marseille at the *First International Conference on Epidemiology, Causes and Prevention of Skin Diseases*. This congress brought together the world's foremost specialists in epidemiological studies in dermatology. It is to those contributors that I first wish to express my gratitude.

For dermatologists to whom epidemiology and prevention seem arcane, unrelated to their usual practice, I would suggest that these fields have provided, and will continue to provide, answers to many practical questions they are faced with every day. What is the cause of skin diseases such as melanoma, psoriasis, atopic dermatitis or leg ulcers, in the sense not of their immunological or biochemical mechanisms but rather of the factors that determine their appearance and disappearance? What environmental factors, such as pollution, climate, radiation, life style, stress, infections, food, drugs and toxins, trigger, induce or precipitate these diseases? How can we control these environmental factors and their impact on the incidence or severity of skin diseases? What role does genetic predisposition play in skin diseases such as atopic dermatitis, skin carcinoma, drug-induced eruption or, indeed, any other skin disease? Why do some skin diseases particularly affect the elderly, children or patients with immunodeficiency? Why are some skin diseases common in a particular country or region? How relevant is our impression that the frequency of a given dermatosis tends to increase or decrease in our usual practice? How can we detect a skin disease at an earlier stage, and is this really useful? How can we identify subjects at high risk for a given skin disease, such as skin cancer or eczema, and what information should we give to these people? Is our practice in line with scientific evidence? How can we judge the quality of the information that we read in dermatological journals? How can we show the decision-makers that skin diseases are common, that they have a major impact on the quality of life, and thus that the money spent on treatment and research is justified? Answers to these questions and many others may be found in the fields of epidemiology and prevention. Some answers can be found in this book, designed to be easily used by non-specialists.

For dermatologists who are interested in epidemiology and prevention, and for epidemiologists interested in skin diseases, this book is a basic working document covering the state of the art in this field.

For students training in dermatology, I would emphasize that epidemiology and prevention will be major themes in medicine in the next century. Dermatologists will be called on to manage skin diseases at an earlier, often asymptomatic, stage or even before they occur. They will have to base their decisions on stategies with documented efficacy and take into account cost-benefit and cost-effectiveness. This book was designed to familiarize the reader with these aspects of dermatology.

J.J. Grob

Section 1
Epidemiology and Prevention

1
Introduction to Epidemiology and Prevention in Dermatology

J.J. GROB, R. SAMBUC AND J. GOUVERNET

Unlike clinical medicine, which studies disease as it affects individuals, epidemiology is the study of disease as it affects populations. Originally epidemiology dealt with infectious disease like smallpox, but it has been applied to non-infectious diseases such as melanoma or psoriasis.

The purpose of this short chapter is to highlight the different ways in which epidemiology can be useful to dermatologists, and to define basic epidemiological concepts used in this book.

Descriptive epidemiology of skin disorders

Information on the health of a population is obtained by estimating *morbidity* (diseases) and *mortality* (deaths). The simplest health indicators are frequency of a given disease, the risk that an individual will develop a given disease, mortality due to a given disease, and the characteristics of the groups most exposed to a given disease. Frequency of a disease in a given population can be characterized by its *incidence* (proportion of new cases per day, month or year) and by *point prevalence* (proportion of existing cases of a disease at a given date). Incidence which does not depend on the course of the disease is well suited to the study of causal process, whereas prevalence, which depends on incidence as well as duration of the disease, is better suited to the assessment of the impact of the disease on public health. The risk that a given individual will develop the disease can be calculated by *cumulative incidence* (number of new cases in a given period in a given group) or evaluated from the *incidence rate* or *density* (number of new cases per total person-time of observation, expressed in cases/10^n person-year). The proportion of deaths is assessed by *mortality rate,* which is more or less the incidence of death. All these indicators can be calculated in the general population, or in a subgroup defined on criteria such as age, sex, occupation, etc. It should be stressed that morbidity and mortality are not the only indicators used to assess the health of a population. More complex health indicators can be useful to measure the impact of a disease in a population, such as quality of life or socio-economic indicators.

These descriptive data can be obtained either in the general population or in samples of the population in a variety of ways. They can be recorded on a given date or more continuously monitored through several years. They can be obtained from obligatory notification. They can be collected by systematic examination of patients/or even by questioning patients. They can be compiled from the records of hospitals, medical laboratories or pathologists. They can be supplied through a network of general practitioners or specialists. They can be deduced by studying prescriptions' records in health insurance. The exhaustivity, the quality of the data but also the cost of collection vary greatly from one type of survey to another. Some monitoring systems are looking for both exhaustivity and continuity in a population, as is the case for obligatory notification of deaths or diseases to national or international organizations (WHO), or *registry* recording of a given disease in a given area.

It has to be underlined that the estimation of a disease can be completely biased. A disease can be underestimated or overestimated, depending on the quality of the diagnostic criteria (assessed by their positive and negative predictive value; see below), as well as on the training of physicians. This is particularly true in dermatology, in which diagnosis often depends on an array of findings and not on the results of a sensitive and specific test. Another problem in the field of skin diseases is that many people do not look for medical care and are thus overlooked. This depends on the type of disease, but also on socio-economic characteristics of the population, and on availability of heath-care structures and health insurance. Furthermore, many patients do not look for medical care, simply because they do not even know they are ill. This is again probably true for minor skin disorders.

In comparison with other diseases, skin diseases have a high morbidity, a low mortality (mostly due to skin cancers), and a strong impact on quality of life. They account for a high proportion of all primary medical consultations, and a low proportion of hospitalizations. They have a low cost per case, but due to their high incidence and their high interference with socioprofessional life, the cost for society is probably high. Dermatology includes the study of not only skin diseases but also skin manifestations of a great number of diseases. For this reason, dermatology largely overlaps with a variety of fields including allergology, angiology, gynaecology, internal medicine, oncology, proctology and sexually transmitted diseases. On the basis of descriptive epidemiology, skin diseases can be divided into several groups.

1 Frequent, chronic and debilitating skin diseases (high prevalence, high impact on quality of life) including inflammatory diseases, i.e. psoriasis or atopic dermatitis, leg ulcers, severe long-lasting acne, chronic urticaria, chronic idiopathic pruritus, generalized alopecia areata, extensive vitiligo. In some geographical areas, Hansen's disease belongs to this group. In developed countries where there is a high cosmetic demand, skin-ageing androgenogenetic alopecia may also be recorded in this group.

2 Frequent chronic minor skin disorders (high prevalence) including benign skin tumours (such as naevi in young people and seborrhoeic warts in older people). Keratoses and small carcinomas can probably be classified in this group.

3 Frequent transient benign skin diseases (high incidence, low prevalence except in some defined groups) including common bacterial, viral and fungal infectious diseases, minor adolescent acne, contact dermatitis, acute urticaria and benign drug-induced skin reactions.

4 Rare (or relatively rare) but severe skin diseases (low incidence and prevalence, high mortality or high impact on quality of life) including melanoma, large mutilating carcinomas, cutaneous lymphoma, connective-tissue diseases (systemic sclerosis, systemic lupus erythematosus), severe drug-induced reactions (Lyell), chronic inflammatory bullous diseases and inherited disorders of keratinization or the dermo-epidermal junction.

Investigative epidemiology and skin diseases

Epidemiology can also be used to formulate and test hypotheses about the pathogenesis of skin diseases and to support biological findings. Descriptive epidemiology can provide evidence to suspect a causal relationship between a given environmental factor and a disease. The characteristics (age, sex, race, socio-economic class, occupation, geography, etc.) of the subgroups with highest frequency and/or mortality of a given disease can be suggestive of an exposure to an environmental factor. For example, the very high incidence of skin cancers in Australia as compared to European countries suggested the role of sun exposure. If a given population or a cohort is known to be exposed to a given environmental factor, an excess mortality in this population compared with the expected number (*standardized mortality ratios* (SMR)) also suggests a connection with this environmental factor. *Correlative studies* (which search for a correlation between the incidence of a given disease and descriptive characteristics such as time or season or place) and *cross-sectional surveys* (which search for the presence, at the same time, of a given disease and a potentially causal factor) can also provide aetiological hypotheses. For example, a correlative study of melanoma incidence and latitude can suggest the role of sun exposure on the development of this tumour, and a cross-sectional study of the number of naevi in subjects with marked dermatoheliosis can suggest the role of chronic sun exposure in the disappearance of naevi.

Once causal hypotheses have been formulated, they have to be tested. *Analytical epidemiology* seeks a statistical association between a disease and a factor, which can be environmental or inherited. If this relation is significant, this factor is called a *risk factor*. Investigative epidemiology can be prospective or retrospective. There are two main types of *retrospective studies*, namely case-control studies and exposed–non-exposed studies or *cohort studies*. A *case-control study* is a retrospective comparison of the exposure to a factor in a group of patients and in a group of disease-free individuals. For example, to assess the role of smoking in skin cancers, one could use a questionnaire to compare number of cigarettes smoked per year during the last 20 years in a group of patients with skin cancer and a control group. *Retrospective cohort studies* compare the incidence of a given disease in a population known to be highly exposed to a given factor with its incidence in a non-exposed group. To evaluate the role of chronic sun exposure on skin ageing, one could compare facial skin ageing in a group of fishermen and a sample of the general population. There are also two types of *prospective studies*, namely cohort studies and experimental studies. Both compare exposed and non-exposed subjects. A *prospective cohort study* compares the incidence of a given disease during a follow-up period in a cohort of individuals known to be exposed to a given factor and in a control cohort. Exposure and disease are measured during the follow-up period. For example, to evaluate the role of diabetes on some skin disorders, one could prospectively evaluate skin disorders and glycaemia during the next 10 years in a cohort on new-onset diabetes and a control cohort. An *experimental study* is basically a prospective cohort study in which the investigator determines, by randomization, who will be exposed and non-exposed. For instance, to evaluate whether or not vitamin E protects the skin from ageing, one could randomize people in two groups, those who will take vitamin E over 10 years and those who will not.

It should be stressed that these study designs are not equivalent as far as application is concerned. Retrospective cohort studies are not always possible. For example, how can we identify a cohort who has regularly consumed a lot of vitamin E? Similarly, retrospective studies can be impossible when the risk factor cannot be measured retrospectively. For example, one cannot measure consumption of selenium in the last 10 years. For rare diseases like melanoma, case-control studies are efficient; cohort studies are impossible since they would require an enormous number of individuals. For instance, it would take

several hundred thousands of people if one wanted to design a cohort study for studying a risk factor for Merkel's tumour. For rare exposure (e.g. exposure to nuclear radiations), retrospective cohorts are efficient. For example, one can follow people living near the nuclear reactor in Chernobyl. On the other hand, to assess the role of nuclear radiation in a given disease, a case-control study would require an enormous number of people to find a few who have been exposed to nuclear radiation. Although they are more relevant than other studies, experimental studies are not always ethical. For example, it would be unacceptable to expose people to nuclear radiation. Finally, from a practical point of view, retrospective studies are easier to realize and far less expensive.

Basically, all these analytical studies compare the rate of development of a disease depending on the presence or absence of exposure to a given factor. This rate is expressed by *relative risks* (RR) (incidence of disease in exposed individuals divided by the incidence in the non-exposed) in cohort studies and *odds ratios* (OR) in case-control studies. OR is a good approximation of RR if the disease is rare. RR is in fact a measure of strength of the association between a given factor and a disease. To be significant, RR must differ from 1, i.e. its confidence interval should not include 1. If RR is >1, the factor is likely to be a risk factor. If RR is <1, the factor may play a protective role.

Studies of the association of only one factor and the probability of occurrence of a disease are oversimplifications which do not take into account *confounding factors*. For instance, if a study shows a higher risk for melanoma in sunscreen users, one could deduce that sunscreen is a causal factor for melanoma. In fact, this could be due to a double association of sun exposure with both skin cancer and sunscreen use. Those who use a sunscreen are also those who are the most sun-exposed. *Multivariate analysis* is a way to evaluate RR after adjustment for potential confounding factors. In our example, multivariate analysis enables assessment of the role of sunscreens taking sun exposure into account.

It must be emphasized that an association between a risk factor and a disease is not necessarily causal. For example, sunburn and red hair are both risk factors for melanoma, but only sunburn may be causal. The probability that a given risk factor is causal depends not only on the strength of the association but also on several criteria such as the clinical and scientific relevance, specificity of the association, chronology (the cause must precede the effect) and existence of a dose–effect relationship.

On the basis of analytical epidemiology, skin diseases can be schematically divided into three main groups:
1 Diseases with demonstrated involvement of an environmental factor, including skin cancers, infectious diseases, skin ageing, drug-induced skin reactions, contact dermatitis, occupational eczemas and photodermatoses.
2 Diseases with probable environmental factors, currently under investigation, including atopic dermatitis and psoriasis.
3 Other diseases with no current hypothesis involving an environmental factor.

Prevention and screening of skin disorders

Schematically, there are two types of prevention: primary and secondary. The target of *primary prevention* is to reduce the incidence of a disease. Campaigns against excessive sun exposure are an example of primary prevention of both naevi and melanoma. *Secondary prevention* aims at decreasing the prevalence of a disease by shortening its duration. If precursors are considered as the first phase of cancers, removing congenital naevi is an example of secondary prevention of melanoma. *Screening* consists in testing apparently healthy people to detect a disease at an early stage. It can be considered as a type of secondary prevention.

Epidemiology helps to evaluate the risk due to exposure to a given factor and to design primary prevention campaigns. Cohort studies enable calculation of *attributable risk*, i.e. the incidence of disease attributable to an exposure in the exposed group, or the *population attributable risk*, i.e. the number of cases in a population that would be eliminated if an exposure to an environmental risk factor was removed. The population attributable risk is a key factor in public health decision-making concerning primary prevention.

Epidemiology also helps to identify *high-risk populations* which can be targeted for prevention and screening. For this purpose, all risk factors identified in case-control and cohort studies can be useful even if they are not potentially causal (for example, colour of the hair for the melanoma), and even if they cannot be modified by any intervention (for example, genetic markers).

Epidemiology provides a basis for screening. A screening programme is useful on condition that its advantages, namely the change in prognosis of the disease in some cases by earlier diagnosis, outweigh its disadvantages, namely high cost and side effects of a test used in a majority of individuals without disease. Therefore, several questions must be taken into account before undertaking a screening programme.
• Does the severity of the disease in terms of mortality, sequelae or cost justify screening?
• Can an early diagnosis of this disease significantly improve prognosis?
• Can a high-risk group be identified to target screening and decrease cost?
• Is this high-risk group accessible (socially or financially)?
• Are there sufficient financial fundings from a health-care system to screen for this disease?
• Is there a high-quality and low-cost screening test available?

A good screening test for a given disease in a given population must meet several requirements. In addition to simplicity, safety and low cost, it must have a very good *positive predictive value* (percentage of true cases in those with a positive test, when this test is used in this given population) and a good *negative predictive value* (percentage of disease-free individuals in those with a negative test, when this test is used in this given population). Positive and negative predictive values depend not only on *sensitivity* (probability of a positive test in an individual with the disease) and *specificity* (probability of a negative test in an individual without the disease) of the test, but also on the prevalence of the disease in this given population. A good screening test has also to be reliable, which means that it has to be precise and to have good *intraobserver* and *interobserver reproducibility*.

The impact of prevention campaigns or any healthcare intervention can be measured in terms of *efficacy* (advantage of the intervention for the individuals), *effectiveness* (goal achievement at a level of a population), *efficiency* (effectiveness as a function of resources allocated), *cost-efficiency* (resources needed to obtain a given effectiveness) and *cost-benefit* (extent to which the expenses have contributed to community well-being, or extent to which the cost of a disease can be reduced at the level of the community). This type of approach may lead to assessing, for instance, the 'cost of a human life', which is something outwith purely medical concerns. Comparison of data before and after a health-care intervention, comparison of two communities where different strategies have been used and comparison of two prospective cohorts in which intervention is or is not implemented are the main study designs to evaluate health-care intervention. However, the evaluation of a prevention policy is always a very difficult challenge because of the delay between prevention strategies and effects, because of the difficulties in evaluating indirect and social costs and because of the major influence of psychosocial criteria.

Epidemiology and the dermatologist

The dermatologist should keep in mind that health-care politics are based on secular trends of major health indicators, cost-economics assessments, identification and measurement of the role of environmental factors and evaluation of health-care interventions. In most countries, there is a clear lack of descriptive data about the frequency of skin disorders, about the impact of skin diseases on quality of life and socio-economic life and the need for skin care. Dermatologists who are looking for recognition of their role in public health can benefit from the availability of accurate data on skin disorders, since their frequency and impact are probably underestimated.

The dermatologist should also keep in mind that epidemiology provides not only major information about frequency, cause, course and impact of dermatological diseases, but is also a tool which is useful in clinical and laboratory research. The basis of epidemiological studies, including proper design of study, clear formulation of objectives and adequate selection of samples, can also be applied to biological and clinical trials. Clinical dermatology, particularly the study of rare skin disorders, can benefit from epidemiological tools such as registries which collect longitudinal data on a great number of cases. Epidemiological methodology can also be used to investigate the links between genotypic alterations and phenotypic features of inherited skin diseases or to study the genetics of populations. Various types of investigations, including the validation of definition criteria for a disease, the assessment of diagnostic and prognostic tests for clinical investigations, the validation of scales for therapeutic trials, the validation of therapeutic interventions at the level of populations, the critical review of the literature and many other major applications, require the same appropriate methodology.

Furthermore, we unconsciously use epidemiological data in our daily clinical practice. We have to realize that when we suspect a diagnosis in a given individual, on the basis of clinical, histological and biological data, we unconsciously evaluate the 'predictive value' of these data. Since 'predictive value' (see above) depends on the prevalence of the disease, the diagnostic assessment depends on how we have subjectively evaluated the prevalence of the suspected disease in the group (age, sex, risk factors, etc.) to which the patient belongs. For example, the criteria which easily enable making a diagnosis of melanoma in a 40-year-old white patient are hardly considered sufficient to establish the diagnosis of melanoma in a 5-year-old black child, since the first patient belongs to a group (white adults) in which the prevalence of melanoma is high, whereas the second belongs to a group in which the prevalence is very low (black children).

Epidemiological investigations are underused in dermatology. The authors would urge dermatologists to learn about epidemiological tools and adopt them in the same way that they have adopted biological tools in the last 20 years.

2
Epidemiological Bases for Dermatologists

P. AUTIER AND H. SANCHO-GARNIER

Introduction

This chapter presents the key elements to be considered when reading a report on an epidemiological investigation aimed at establishing cause–effect relationships between factors (individual, behavioural, environmental) and a disease. Types of epidemiological design are presented, with their ability to demonstrate the existence of a cause–effect relationship. These elements are then put into perspective for interpreting results from cohort and case-control studies on skin cancers. Finally, frequent misinterpretations of epidemiological results are discussed.

Modern epidemiology basically addresses three domains: (i) the disease distribution in populations and their impact on health; (ii) the identification of factors (genetic, environmental, behavioural) related to disease occurrence; and (iii) the impact of interventions (preventive or curative) on disease occurrence. Modern epidemiology is also tending to become an essential part of health economics, disease management, quality assurance and assessment of performance of therapeutic and diagnostic methods (often named 'clinical epidemiology').

Most epidemiological studies examine relationships between so-called *exposures* and *diseases*. Exposures are all factors suspected to play a role in disease occurrence, or exposures to interventions aimed at preventing or healing the disease. A disease is any event of public health importance, e.g. death because of a given disease, a complication of a given disease or a side effect due to a medicine.

Interpretation of clinical or epidemiological studies essentially depends on the *design* of the study. A design can be defined as the ensemble of relationships between the various elements involved in a study: how time from exposure to disease is assessed, how and when laboratory tests are done, the statistical analysis, and so on. It is the design that fundamentally tells which data will be collected and how, and how they will be analysed.

Assessment of the cause–effect relationship

When the study goal is to ascertain a *cause–effect relationship* between an exposure and a disease, three key elements are to be considered in the design: (i) the time relationship between exposure and disease; (ii) the control of biases and confounding factors; and (iii) the existence of a 'control' group.

Time relationship

To be a cause of a disease, an exposure must be present before the disease occurrence. If this principle seems straightforward, it is sometimes difficult in a study to ascertain whether the cause or the disease was present first.

When several exposures are considered together as potential independent risk factors, and when these risk factors may influence each other, it is similarly crucial to ascertain the time sequence when the various factors were active, since the presence of a factor may simply result from the action of a factor that already existed before. For instance, in most epidemiological studies, sunscreen use is slightly more frequent among patients with skin cancer than among subjects free of such cancer. Perhaps this association is due to the fact that other risk factors for skin cancer were present before sunscreen use, for instance, sunburns during childhood. Because having suffered from sunburn fosters sunscreen use, sunscreen use may in turn appear as a risk factor for skin cancer. Disentangling such complex relationships may require elaborate analysis (Autier *et al.*, 1995).

Biases and confounding

A *bias* is a systematic error in the design or conduct of a study that leads to erroneous results (Hennekens & Buring, 1987). Biases may occur during any step of a study, and therefore many types of bias have been described, for instance, inappropriate selection of control subjects ('selection' bias), or different attention paid to subjects suffering from the disease under study than to subjects free of that disease ('observation' and 'interview' biases).

In the study between a given exposure and a disease, *confounding* occurs when a second factor is (i) associated with the exposure under study and (ii) also associated with the disease, and the association with the disease must be independent of the association with the exposure under study (Fig. 2.1).

The following numerical example shows a confounding by age: in this data set, (i) exposure is more frequent before 50 years old, but (ii) when looking at the unexposed groups, disease frequency remains higher at older age (30/80 against 10/40). Hence, the association between disease frequency and age is independent of being exposed or not. The net result of this confounding by age is that the risk calculated for each age stratum is higher than for the whole data set.

Example

All data set

Exposure	Disease present	Disease absent	Total
Yes	140	110	250
No	40	80	120

Risk of disease in exposed group compared with unexposed group: (140/250)/(40/120) = 1.68.

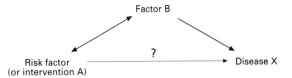

Fig. 2.1 Confounding of factor A–disease X relationship by factor B.

Age < 50 years

Exposure	Disease present	Disease absent	Total
Yes	100	90	190
No	10	30	40

Risk of disease in exposed group compared with unexposed group: (100/190)/(10/40) = 2.10.

Age ⩾ 50 years

Exposure	Disease present	Disease absent	Total
Yes	40	20	60
No	30	50	80

Risk of disease in exposed group compared with unexposed group: (40/60)/(30/80) = 1.78.

Different statistical methods have been developed to *adjust* for confounding factors, such as the Mantel–Haenszel method, the logistic regression (for case-control and cohort designs), the Poisson regression (for cohort designs with incidence data) and the Cox proportional hazard regression (for survival data). In our example, the *age-adjusted risk of disease* in the exposed group compared with the non-exposed group is 1.91, hence slightly higher than the *crude risk* value of 1.68.

Age, gender and other risk factors for the disease under study are the usual potential confounders. Indeed, the appropriate statistical control of confounding effect implies that data on confounders of importance have not been omitted from questionnaires.

Control group

A control group is necessary to evaluate the magnitude of the extra risk (or extra benefit) due to an exposure (or an intervention). According to the study design, the control group will be constituted by subjects free of the disease (case-control studies), or not exposed to the suspected risk factor (cohort studies) or not receiving the intervention (placebo arm in an experiment).

Types of epidemiological design

Classification of study designs has been undertaken on the basis of their aptitude to assess cause–effect relationships and control confounding.

Descriptive designs

Descriptive designs constitute the basic tools for disease surveillance. They are not appropriate to establish cause–effect relationships. However, careful examination of descriptive data may lead to identifying the relevant questions to be addressed by other types of design. Currently, sophisticated statistical methods exist to get maximum benefit from descriptive data (Estève *et al.*, 1994).

Descriptive studies

These studies describe the incidence, prevalence or mortality of a disease. *Prevalence* is the number of subjects suffering from a given disease existing in a population at a given time (e.g. the percentage of the population suffering from psoriasis in 1996). *Incidence* is the number of new cases of the disease in a population per unit of time (e.g. number of new melanoma cases per 100 000 persons per year).

Cross-sectional surveys generally aim at estimating the prevalence of diseases, of their risk factors and of the degree of implementation of eventual preventive or curative methods.

Disease registries (i.e. epidemiological surveillance) gather data on incidence and mortality. Registries provide invaluable information on the public health weight of a disease, of its progress and of the long-term impact of eventual preventive or curative programmes. For instance, to appraise the impact of screening for melanoma, a cancer registry should be able to tell whether screen-detected melanomas display a lower Breslow thickness than melanoma detected in usual clinical practice, which may result in a decrease in mortality due to melanoma.

A particularly useful application of registries is *time–trend analysis*: complete registries about a disease permit examination of the variation of its incidence (or mortality) before and after introduction of new preventive or curative means. For instance, time–trend in mortality related to melanoma has formed the basis for examining the impact of a public education campaign in Scotland (MacKie & Hole, 1992). Caution should be taken with concluding a cause–effect relationship from time–trend analysis since many factors may concur to explain a given change in incidence or mortality, and often the expected change was already observable before the introduction of the new preventive or curative means.

Ecological studies

Typically, ecological analysis plots together frequencies of a disease with frequencies of an exposure, and then looks at whether there is a significant correlation between the two. An example of ecological analysis is the higher incidence of cancers in countries where total fat consumption is, on average, higher, hence suggesting a positive correlation between cancer occurrence and fat intake. One should be prudent with the ecological approach, since it neither informs about the time relationship between exposure and disease, nor allows control for confounding variables, and rarely provides information on the multiple phenomena linking an exposure to a disease (Morgenstern, 1982).

Transversal (cross-sectional) comparisons

This design compares characteristics presented by a group of diseased subjects with a group of subjects free of that disease (Fig. 2.2). An example is the usual finding that cancer patients have lower blood lipid values than subjects free of cancer.

The key problem with this type of observation is that it is impossible to establish whether it was the

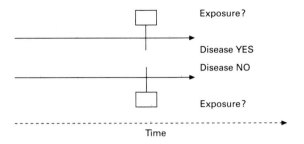

Fig. 2.2 Cross-sectional study.

presence of cancer that led to lower blood lipid values or whether subjects with low blood lipid levels convey a higher risk to develop a cancer.

Analytical designs

These designs allow the assessment of the time relationship between exposure and disease and also allow control of confounders if, of course, adequate data have been collected.

Cohort study

The exposure(s) take(s) place first, then disease

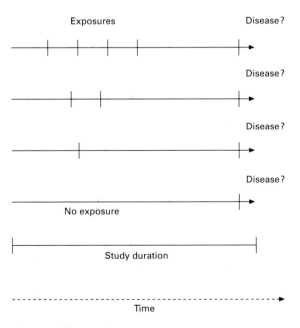

Fig. 2.3 Cohort study.

occurrence is ascertained (Fig. 2.3). At the study's end, disease occurrence (being an incidence, or the presence/absence of the disease) is classified according to various levels of exposure. Risk of disease is then computed by dividing the disease occurrence observed in an exposure category by the disease occurrence in a *referent category*, habitually constituted by the subjects who never experienced the exposure under study (see the example above). Examples of cohort studies are the higher incidence of non-melanoma skin cancers in psoralens and ultraviolet A (PUVA)-treated patients (Stern *et al.*, 1984), or the risk factors for non-melanoma skin cancer in women (Hunter *et al.*, 1990).

Case-control study

Cases are subjects with the disease under study; controls are subjects without the disease under study and coming from the same *source population* as cases. An assessment of exposure is carried out retrospectively (Fig. 2.4). The main difference with the cross-sectional design is that exposure assessment concerns the period of time before the disease occurrence.

Traditionally, *hospital-based case-control studies* incorporate cases detected in hospitals, and controls are other patients present in that hospital but free of the disease of interest. The main problem of hospital-based case-control designs lies in the uncertainties about the respective origin of cases and controls: subjects

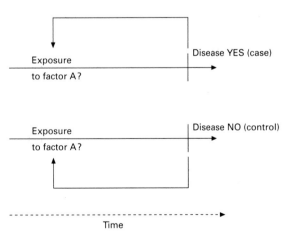

Fig. 2.4 Case-control study.

with (skin) cancers may come from one part of a country, and controls drawn from a surgical ward may come from another part of the country. Anyhow, hospital-based designs are well suited to explore host characteristics; they should be avoided for the exploration of environmental or behavioural risk factors. *Population-based case-control studies* incorporate cases derived from population-based disease registries and controls consist of a sample of the source population of cases.

Although it is more prone to biases and less qualified to accurately assess exposures than the cohort design, the success of the case-control design lies principally in its relatively low cost and shorter duration. Also, it was primarily conceived to explore rare diseases (e.g. melanoma, brain tumours).

Experimental designs

The prospective randomized study is generally regarded as the design providing best evidence of a cause–effect relationship. Randomization allows equivalent distribution of confounding factors between the study arms (even of the unknown confounding factors) and blinding procedures avoid observational and interview biases.

This design is, however, not without weaknesses (Buysse *et al.*, 1991): many exposures cannot be studied in an experimental way. For testing behavioural changes, experimental designs may pose a problem as an experiment does not necessarily reproduce the actual behaviours: for instance, a test of the capacity of sunscreens to prevent solar-induced skin lesions has been undertaken in subjects highly aware of health hazards associated to the sunlight, many of them having a history of skin cancer (Thompson *et al.*, 1993; Naylor *et al.*, 1995). Although these experiments documented the ability of sunscreens to prevent solar-induced skin lesions in humans, their results are not necessarily applicable to subjects using sunscreens as a tool to get a suntan without incurring sunburns (Autier *et al.*, 1995; Stern, 1995).

Interpretation of causality in cohort and case-control studies

The interpretation of analytical epidemiological studies

involves evaluating the likelihood that the results reflect the biases present in the design or study conduct, the possibility of confounding factors, the role of misclassification, the role of chance and the assessment of causality.

Bias

Bias will provide erroneous results. Case-control design suffers from potential inadequacies, either in the selection of cases or controls, or from the manner in which the data are acquired. In case-control studies, information on exposure is normally obtained after disease status is established, and the studied groups are samples (representative or not) from the population. Biased risk estimates will result if the selection processes leading to inclusion of cases and controls in the study are different (*selection bias*), or if exposure information is not obtained in a comparable manner from the two groups, for example because of a systematic difference in the way cases and controls answer a question (*recall bias*). Furthermore, it is often hard to order in a time scale the different environmental or behavioural exposures collected during the study (which exposure could have influenced another exposure?).

In cohort studies, information is obtained on exposures before disease status is determined, and all cases of disease arising in a given time period should be ascertained (e.g. through registries). Information on exposure from cases and controls is therefore comparable (although not always accurate), and unbiased estimates of disease (or mortality) incidence rates can be calculated. In turn, cohort studies are vulnerable to drop-outs due to the exposure or to the disease under study, that is subjects who are lost to follow-up may precisely be those subjects susceptible to provide the needed information about the exposure and/or the disease of interest.

Potential sources of bias must be carefully examined during the protocol building process. From simulations, Edwards *et al.* (1994) have estimated the impact of interview biases on study power and ability to detect disease–exposure associations. Uncorrected interview variability could yield risk estimates biased downward from 1.8 to 1.3. These findings illustrate the importance of interview biases and the necessity to implement quality-control procedures to eliminate them.

Confounding

Confounding will manifest in a similar way in both cohort and case-control studies. It is necessary to know to what extent the risk estimate changes or does not change when the effect of the putative confounding factor(s) is controlled (i.e. after 'adjustment for the confounder'). This change (if any) in the risk estimate is an index of the degree of confounding.

In epidemiological studies on skin cancers, the most important known confounder for sun exposure is the 'skin type' or the skin reaction to sunlight. Persons with sun-sensitive skin will tend to avoid exposure to sunlight and protect themselves against solar radiations. The result will be a 'negative confounding effect' between sensitivity to sunlight and exposure to sunlight: in the absence of adjustment for sensitivity to sunlight, the association between exposure to sunlight and skin cancer may appear smaller than it really is because, on the one hand, high sensitivity to sunlight is associated with restricted exposure to sunlight and, on the other hand, high sensitivity to sunlight is a risk factor for skin cancer.

Misclassification

Misclassification, i.e. errors in classifying disease status and measuring exposure, may occur in both types of study. For instance, in a study on skin cancer, it could happen that a certain proportion of the control subjects may carry the disease at its earliest stage (i.e. *in situ* skin cancer) and should have been diagnosed as cases. One may expect that in most circumstances, control subjects who are in reality cases would be rare, since most diseases are 'rare' (e.g. melanoma). However, when the disease under study is particularly common (e.g. non-melanoma skin cancers), the effect of such misclassification error may become appreciable. The consequences are equivalent when misdiagnosed cases (e.g. benign tumours erroneously classified as malignant tumours) are included in the disease group.

Data gathering on exposures may entail inordinate amounts of random error. Random errors in exposure assessment are often put forward to explain the apparent absence of risk associated to factors acknowledged to be difficult to describe or quantify, such as diet or sun exposure.

Usually, measurement errors lead to underestimating the risks. In this respect, an advantage of cohort studies over case-control studies is that information on exposure is obtained before disease status is ascertained. One can therefore have more confidence that errors in measurement are the same for individuals who become cases (i.e. who develop the disease of interest) and the remainder of the cohort.

Misclassification not only modifies towards lower values the factor–disease relationship, but also alters the quality of this relationship (i.e. the 'dose–response curve') (Doll & Peto, 1978). In studies dealing with sun exposure, the type of measurements used may be summarized under three headings: (i) measurement of potential exposure to sun (e.g. age at arrival in a sunny country like Australia); (ii) measurement of actual exposure to the sun (e.g. depending upon sophistication of questionnaires or use of an ultraviolet radiation dosimeter); and (iii) measurement of biological response to sun exposure (e.g. sunburn, solar-induced chronic skin damage) (Armstrong & English, 1989). A number of sources of error may affect these measurements. For example, place, duration and time of day for outdoor exposure as well as protective behaviour when in the sunlight may substantially misclassify the true exposure of individual subjects. In addition, measures of actual exposure to sunlight generally depend on subjective recall and thus may be totally erroneous: who remembers what type of protective measures against sun exposure his/her mother was using when he/she was a baby or young child, although this period of life seems to play a major role in skin cancer initiation? Most of these errors are likely to be non-differential (i.e. similar in subjects with and without disease) leading to substantial attenuation of any real association (Armstrong, 1988).

Measurement error may also affect the possibility of controlling confounding. If sun sensitivity is ill-measured, it will not be possible to fully control confounding due to this factor, and the *residual* confounding may contribute to masking the association between sun exposure and skin cancer.

Chance

Chance also has a role. When an unconfounded estimate of relative risk is available, data interpretation concentrates on chance. This issue is addressed by classical statistics which estimate the significance level associated with the difference observed between cases and controls in their exposure histories. In a cohort design, the most informative way to describe the role of chance is to estimate the relative risk (see the example above) and its confidence limits (usually the '95% confidence limits'). If the 95% confidence limits incorporate unity (1.0), one generally concludes a non-significant difference between cases and controls, i.e. there is more than a 5% chance that the difference observed between the cases and the controls may be explained by statistical hazard alone. In case-control studies, *odds ratios* are calculated as surrogates for relative risk, often reported as *estimated* relative risks in publications.

Causality

Finally, interpretation moves to seeking whether a causal association could explain the results. The word 'cause' is used here in a probabilistic sense. By saying that a factor is a cause of disease, we mean that the presence of the factor results in an increase in risk. From this viewpoint, a disease may have many causes, some of which may operate synergistically, that is, a factor may need the presence of another to be effective. For instance, ultraviolet radiation 'necessitates' white skin to cause skin cancer. Causality may be judged according to three positive criteria: the strength of the association; its internal and external consistency; and its biological credibility.

• *Strength of association*: relative risks less than 2.0 may simply reflect some unperceived bias or confounding factor; relative risks over 5.0 are unlikely to be the mere result of confounding or bias (Breslow & Day, 1980).

• *Consistency*: is the factor–disease association seen in all subgroups where it is expected to be found, and is there a dose–response relationship? The extent to which the study results are consistent with previous studies is also taken into consideration to support or refute a causal interference.

• *Biological credibility*: if the results can be understood in biological terms, they will be more convincing. However, while pertinent, the response to this question is not especially convincing: it is all too easy to propose credible biological mechanisms relating most exposures to most diseases. On the other hand, the failure to perceive such a mechanism may only reflect our ignorance (Cole, 1980).

Finally, the most cogent type of causal argument is to observe how the frequency of a disease changes when the presumed cause is removed from the environment.

Notes of caution

Common improper tenets guide the development or interpretation of epidemiological studies.

1 Matching diseased and non-diseased subjects on age, gender and, eventually, on other factor(s) is often regarded as an elegant way to control confounding. However, matching techniques should be avoided. Confounding by age and gender is easily controlled by multivariate statistical models. Matching should be reserved for two situations: (i) when a variable is handled with difficulty by statistical methods during analysis (e.g. 'to pertain to a family'); (ii) when the number of diseased subjects (cases) is small (i.e. less than 30), then matching one case with several controls (two to five controls per case) may increase the statistical power of the study.

2 It is often believed that the appropriate control for confounding implies that all potential confounding factors should be included into multiple logistic regression models. However, first controlling for rare confounders is of little relevance (i.e. confounders present in less than 5% of control subjects). Second, factors may pertain to the same causal pathway; for instance:

exposure A ➜ exposure B ➜ disease.

Including exposure B in a logistic model may substantially reduce the actual relationship between exposure A and the disease. For instance, if the risk of melanoma associated with the use of sunscreen preparations containing 5-methoxypsoralen is deemed to be partly due to the aptitude of this molecule to foster the naevi development, then naevi count should not be added to a statistical model estimating the association between melanoma and use of sunscreens containing 5-methoxypsoralen.

3 The absence of statistically significant (i.e. $P < 0.05$) difference between the groups of exposed and non-exposed subjects for a factor does not mean that this factor does not confound the exposure–disease relationship under study.

References

Armstrong, B.K. (1988) Epidemiology of malignant melanoma: intermittent or total accumulated exposure to sun? *Journal of Dermatological and Surgical Oncology*, **14**, 835–849.

Armstrong, B.K. & English, D.R. (1989) Cutaneous malignant melanoma. In: *Cancer Epidemiology and Prevention* (eds D. Schottenfeld & T. Fraumeni), pp. 53–70. Academic Press, London.

Autier, P., Doré, J.F., Schifflers, E. *et al.* for the EORTC Melanoma Cooperative Group (1995) Melanoma and use of sunscreens: an EORTC case-control study in Germany, Belgium and France. *International Journal of Cancer*, **61**, 749–755.

Breslow, N.E. & Day, N. (1980) *Statistical Methods in Cancer Research*, Vol. 1. *The Analysis of Case-Control Studies*. IARC Scientific Publications No. 32. International Agency for Research on Cancer, Lyon.

Buysse, M., Autier, P. & Piedbois, P. (1991) Clinical trials in cancer prevention. In: *Reducing the Risk of Cancer*. Open University, Cambridge.

Cole, P. (1980) The case-control study in cancer epidemiology. In: *Statistical Methods in Cancer Research*, Vol. 1. *The Analysis of Case-Control Studies* (eds N.E. Breslow & N. Day), IARC Scientific Publications No. 32, pp. 14–40. International Agency for Research on Cancer, Lyon.

Doll, R. & Peto, R. (1978) Cigarette smoking and bronchial carcinoma: dose and time relationships among regular smokers and life-long non-smokers. *Journal of Epidemiology and Community Health*, **32**, 303–313.

Edwards, S., Slattery, M.L., Mori, M. *et al.* (1994) Objective system for interviewer performance evaluation for use in epidemiological studies. *American Journal of Epidemiology*. **140**, 1020–1028.

Estève, J., Benhamou, E. & Raymond, L. (1994) Descriptive epidemiology. In: *Statistical Methods in Cancer Research*, Vol. 4. IARC Scientific Publications No. 128. International Agency for Research on Cancer, Lyon.

Hennekens, C.H. & Buring, J.E. (1987) *Epidemiology in Medicine*. Little, Brown and Company, Boston.

Hunter, D.J., Colditz, G.A., Stampfer, M.J., Rosner, B., Willet, W.C. & Speizer, F.E. (1990) Risk factors for basal cell carcinoma in a prospective cohort of women. *Annals of Epidemiology and Public Health*, **1**, 13–23.

Naylor, M.F., Boyd, A., Smith, D.W., Cameron, G.S., Hubbard, D. & Nelder, K.H. (1995) *Archives of Dermatology*, **131**, 170–175.

MacKie, R. & Hole, D. (1992) Audit of public education campaign to encourage earlier detection of malignant melanoma. *British Medical Journal*, **304**, 1012–1015.

Morgenstern, H. (1982) Uses of ecologic analysis in epidemiologic research. *American Journal of Public Health*, **72**, 1336–1344.

Stern, R.S. (1995) Sunscreens for cancer prevention. *Archives of Dermatology*, **131**, 220–221.

Stern, R.S., Laird N., Melski, J., Parrish, J.A., Fitzpatrick, T.B. & Howard, L.B. (1984) Cutaneous squamous-cell carcinoma in patients treated with PUVA. *New England Journal of Medicine*, **310**, 1156–1161.

Thompson, S.C., Jolley, D. & Marks, R. (1993) Reduction of solar keratoses by regular sunscreen use. *New England Journal of Medicine*, **329**, 1147–1151.

3
Prevention

Advantages and Limitations of Screening

J.L. SAN MARCO

When the natural progression of a disease — development, risk and protection factors — passes from the mysterious calamity stage to that of comprehensible problem, when it becomes possible to demonstrate the existence of a preclinical phase before diagnosis, we wish to intervene before the disease reaches the diagnosis phase. We seek to avoid its onset or to block its progression at an early preclinical stage. The aim of this early intervention is to eliminate the risks associated with the onset of the disease or to reduce their gravity and improve the prognosis by early treatment. The most effective solution is undoubtedly to prevent the initial onset of the disease, but this is only possible when we are dealing with a single-factor disease and can intervene against the causal factor; the most obvious example is that of vaccinations, as long as an effective and danger-free vaccine is available.

Except with infectious diseases that meet all these requirements, all we can do is attempt to find evidence for the existence of the disease before it becomes difficult or impossible to cure, once it has been revealed by diagnosis. We attempt to interrupt the progression of the disease at an early, preclinical stage, before any symptoms are complained of and before diagnosis is possible, in the hope that treating the disease early will mean that it can be treated more effectively and at a lower cost in human and financial terms.

This brings us to the essential difference between diagnosis and screening. Diagnosis is made in response to symptoms presented by the patient; their onset has worried the patient who has taken the initiative to seek treatment. Diagnostic examinations and the treatment that ensues are administered only to patients that are affected and at their initiative. There is no guarantee that this initiative is taken at the right time — in fact, it often comes too late. But whether or not patients declare their symptoms at the right moment, only a very small percentage of the population is involved.

This is far from being the case with screening, which is by no means the same thing as early diagnosis. Screening, following the decision taken by an external authority, is administered to the whole population at risk of developing the disease in question, and involves people who consider themselves to be unaffected by the disease. Screening should distinguish, within this population, between those who are really unaffected and those that are affected without being aware of it. Screening reveals the existence of a disease that is still dormant. The purpose is to launch a programme of treatment that will be far more effective than it would have been had it only been initiated following revelation by diagnosis months, or even years, later.

It is perhaps worth reviewing here the requirements that must be met if a screening campaign for a disease is to be usefully undertaken with some chance of success:

• The natural history of the disease must be well enough known to allow comparison between the natural progression of the 'spontaneous' form of the disease and its progression after transformation by screening and early treatment.

• The test administered to the target population should be discriminatory: it should distinguish as clearly as possible between healthy subjects and suspected cases.

- The test should be simple to administer and as unintrusive as possible for the subjects.
- It should be designed to take into account the extent of the spread of the disease among the population.
- A reliable diagnosis should be available to confirm suspected disease in the event of a positive test result, as of course should effective treatment.
- The cost of the campaign should be acceptable in relation to the potential benefit to society.
- Finally, it is important that there should be consensus with regard to the benefits of screening among the population concerned and the medical profession.

Let us now re-examine these requirements in reverse order of difficulty.

The test must be a good test

The purpose of the test is to distinguish, by a positive or negative result, between healthy subjects and those who are suspected of being carriers of the target disease. The capacity to recognize infected subjects is referred to as the *sensitivity* of the test, while the capacity to recognize healthy subjects is known as the *specificity*.

There is no test that allows perfect classification of healthy subjects and suspected cases. There is no net with a sufficiently fine mesh to guarantee a 100% catch. Also, there is always some overlap in the border area between the two groups, where it is not possible to distinguish between healthy and suspected cases. While with a good test this grey area is reduced to a minimum, it can never be totally eliminated.

If we decide that the primary aim is not to allow any suspected case to slip through the net, and therefore give priority to the sensitivity of the test, this will inevitably be at the expense of the specificity: certain healthy subjects will be wrongly classified. The converse is true if priority is given to the specificity and to classifying all the healthy subjects correctly. For example, if we consider as diabetics all subjects whose glycaemia rate is higher than 1.20 g/l, we will be treating some healthy subjects; if, on the other hand, we treat only patients with a rate above 1.40 g/l, some patients who need treatment will go without. No test is ever perfect. It is the clinical practitioner who must choose between these two opposing alternatives, on the basis of what is required from the test results.

The test must be simple and clearly effective

The test will be administered on a vast scale; it is therefore imperative that it should require neither too many medical procedures, nor too much time to administer the test and obtain the results. The test is administered to a large and apparently healthy population who have no expectations from it but rather submit to it, passively in the first instance. The constraints involved should be kept to a minimum if they are to be tolerated. Nor should the diagnostic confirmation procedure involve an excessive burden in terms of time, cost or constraints for the patients.

In due course, once the results of the campaign are known and published, it may be hoped that the population will be convinced of its benefits, will support it and demand the extension of the campaign. This underlines another important difference between screening and medical care: the legal obligation to use all known means that are required for a treatment procedure must here be replaced by the obligation to produce satisfactory results.

The test must be well suited to the target population

If the test is carried out under identical conditions, it will give the same results regardless of the population to which it is administered: the intrinsic conditions are always the same, in the right hands. The rate of error — subjects wrongly classified as positive or negative — is generally low if it is a good test.

If the specificity is high (high percentage of healthy subjects correctly classified) and if it is administered to a population where the target disease is widespread, it will give a number of wrongly classified healthy subjects (false-positives, not confirmed by diagnosis) that is low compared with the number of suspected cases subsequently confirmed (the true-positives).

A positive result in the test will have to be strongly significant: the test is said to have a good *predictive value*. When applied to positive results, this is said to be *positive predictive value*; for negative results, it is referred to as *negative predictive value*.

The same test administered to another population where the disease is rare will have the same rate of false-positives, but the number of these will be high compared with the number of true-positives (which is low since the disease is rare). The good test has thus lost any predictive value.

A test can only be administered to a population where the expected frequency of the target disease is high. To launch a screening campaign when the expected number of true-positives is of the same order as the expected number of false-positives would be scandalously inept. While a screening campaign can obviously only be justified for a serious disease, it should equally be undertaken only if the disease is also widespread.

The test should provide results that are of benefit

This may seem obvious, but it is sometimes necessary to restate the obvious. The test may be of benefit to the patient or to society. For the patient, it must be possible to confirm the diagnosis by a series of appropriate examinations and transform suspicion into certainty. Diagnostic tests are no better than screening tests: they must be designed to suit the target group that will include a high number of affected subjects, since they have been preselected by the screening tests. The screening test had been administered to groups where the affected subjects were proportionally rarer.

Finally, once the diagnosis is confirmed, it is important that treatment be available, all the more so since treatment administered at this early stage in the progression of the disease is appreciably more effective. This point is worth dwelling on, since a well-conducted screening campaign, even if it is quite without real benefit, will always appear to prolong the medical history of an affected patient, and may thus lead to the fallacious conclusion that the patient has a prolonged life expectancy: to the clinical history is added the duration of the preclinical phase between screening and diagnosis. A positively-screened patient is simply ill for a longer period!

A second element further enhances the apparent effectiveness of the screening campaign. Screening attempts to provide evidence for a series of diseases that are still asymptomatic. The future progression of these diseases is highly variable. In some cases it will be explosive, with a brief preclinical phase that can easily escape detection, even by repeated screening. For other slower cases, the more gradual their progression, the greater will be their chance of being detected by screening.

Screening results in overrepresentation of slow diseases, those that kill slowly or not at all. To be screened positive becomes almost a guarantee of longevity, without the natural progression of the disease being altered one iota.

The only way to prove with absolute certainty that screening confers any real benefit is by comparing the life expectancy of two groups, chosen completely at random, of which only one is screened. For breast cancer, this experiment was carried out before it was known whether or not breast cancer screening was of any real benefit. It is, however, easy to see the difficulty of proposing this method, however indispensable it may be, to target populations or to decision-makers who are not used to this kind of reasoning. Random distribution of the beneficiaries of screening is indispensable in order to prove with certainty that they are getting some benefit by comparing them with another group that has also been chosen at random. Once this proof has been obtained, it will be possible to launch a campaign that will be of undoubted benefit to the whole of the population at risk.

If the benefit sought is social — for instance, if the aim is to protect society against the spread of a contagious disease — the advantages of the campaign should be weighed up just as carefully. In the case of a sexually transmissible disease, screening can only be proposed if the disease is sufficiently widespread for the revelation of seropositivity to have a reasonable chance of reflecting actual contamination — if the predictive value of the test in this population is sufficiently high. Then it would be necessary, to ensure the protection of the unaffected population, to see that all the subject's potential sexual partners are informed of his or her serological status. Should this announcement be made as soon as the results of the test are known, before confirmation, in order to gain in effectiveness, or should we wait for confirmation in order to be sure of only giving the alert on the basis of a certainty? In the last case, should the positively-screened subject be locked up between the two stages to eliminate any possible risk? It is easy to understand from this outline of the practical aspects why the unanimous position on this issue of those involved in acquired immune deficiency syndrome (AIDS) is that screening is not the right solution.

We must consider other courses of action that might be expected to be more effective.

The precocity of the treatment must transform the prognosis

The prolongation of life expectancy must be accompanied by a real transformation of the quality of the patient's life. In the case of cancer, the aim of early screening is to reduce the risk of onset of metastases that occur early on and heavily load the prognosis of the disease when it is only detected at the clinical stage. If the group of randomly selected American women presented a better life expectancy than those who, under identical conditions, had not had the benefit of screening, it is because the first group were operated on before the onset of metastases. But in addition, the ablation of a small tumour without any local extension means (or should mean) that the scale of the operation and its sequelae, whether physical (lymphatic circulation, etc.) or psychological (tumorectomy instead of amputation), is reduced.

The cost of the screening campaign must be acceptable for the local authority

Putting things this way enables us to avoid launching into calculations of the price of years of life gained by screening. Much care must be taken when dealing with the cost of screening from the economic point of view. Contrary to the old adage, it is not better to prevent than to cure: firstly, because the cost of a screening campaign does not replace the cost of medical care — it is added to it; secondly, because we have to continue to treat all the patients that have been detected without screening, as well as those who

have been screened positive and confirmed as having the disease; and above all, screening must be administered to the whole population at risk of developing the disease, and ideally there will be more negative than positive results, but they will all have involved expenditure.

Finally, a screening test of perfect efficacy will result in the patients that have been saved by this procedure reappearing later with another disease, which will entail further expenditure.

As for attempting to calculate the cost of the years of life gained, this too involves factors that are very difficult to handle: in what state is the subject one has saved by early treatment from an otherwise fatal issue? In the case of cancers that occur preferentially in the second stage of life, is not one prolonging the existence of subjects who have ceased to be productive, and who in any case are prevented from remaining productive by the disease itself and the treatment?

It is much wiser to analyse the cost of the campaign and determine whether, in view of what it costs and what benefits it confers overall, it is acceptable to society. In any case, this approach is only conceivable in a society that disposes of an efficient health-care system and therefore a high standard of living. All that remains is to establish the priorities between the diseases that are suitable for screening, and to decide which of them should be dealt with first.

The predicted cost-benefit ratio is a major factor in choosing which campaigns to run, in relation with the state of health of the society concerned and the available resources.

Society as a whole must accept the screening campaign and support its findings

To the regret of the organizers, this is not something that goes without saying. The demand for screening does not initially come from the target population. The population undergoes the first phases before forming any opinion. The reasons for a possibly hostile reaction are numerous.

For most of the subjects tested, for whom the absence of disease will be confirmed, this announcement is not felt as reassuring news, since they had not previously thought about the problem, but rather as non-news, spiced with a dash of anxiety during the waiting period for the results. The rarer cases who are informed of their disease and who should, after confirmation of the validity of the campaign, be the ones who most benefit from it, sometimes tend to blame the screening organizers for having 'made them ill'! And then there are those cases — admittedly rare — where the result is misleading, and subjects have been wrongly reassured or wrongly worried. Finally, those who have refused the test go on to become the zealots of refusal, in order to justify with hindsight their negligence or their fear of knowing the truth. It is important to be aware of these difficulties that may persist even when the judicious choice of a campaign makes them seem insignificant. For breast cancer, preclinical screening is the only method that can improve the prognosis, and, what is more, it can do so without the price to pay being an amputation.

This description of screening leads one to reject proposals to make obligatory the various screening campaigns that have been approved. The results of campaigns must be assessed and published among the populations concerned in order to win firstly their support and subsequently a demand on their part for the action that has been started to be continued and extended. The sign of the success of a campaign might be public demand — which must be resisted — to speed up the rhythm of the campaigns, as is the case at present for screening for cancer of the neck of the uterus.

Currently, the sharpest criticism is focused on the proposals of the French medical board (Conférence de Consensus), which recommends a smear every three years. The women who undergo this examination every year or even more frequently, as well as their doctors, consider the proposal to space out this test as unjustifiable backsliding. It is true that screening at regular intervals means that there is a risk of missing out on all the events that have occurred between two tests. But thorough knowledge of the natural history of a disease and a sound analysis of the cost of a campaign provide the basis for responding effectively to this argument. What are the respective costs of a campaign and the benefits it brings in terms of cancers avoided, if screening is carried out every 3 years, every 2 years or every year? With annual

screening, the costs go through the roof for benefits that are insignificant.

But what we are dealing with here is the quest in some quarters for the total eradication of risk, which is a chimera! And this illusion may be reinforced by more dubious motives. Nevertheless, the fact remains that a screening campaign, even if it fulfils all the requirements we have outlined above, can have no chance of being launched or pursued unless it enjoys the participation and active support of the medical profession, and we must therefore be able to convince them of its value.

As for 'opportunistic' screening, carried out daily in doctors' surgeries in the course of routine consultations, it can give good individual results, which suggests that it should be encouraged. But it does present two serious disadvantages. Firstly, it cannot be assessed with certainty, which makes the decision-makers hesitant. Secondly, it can only reach women who are under medical referral and only during the periods when they are under such referral. Young women who generally have frequent smears between 25 and 50 years of age stop being monitored after that age, when the risk is in fact increasing. This is a case of wastage and inefficiency which cannot be tolerated much longer.

For a screening campaign, rigorous assessment is even more vital than in the case of a treatment campaign. Not all diseases can be usefully screened. Not all screening campaigns are fit to be launched. And when a screening campaign is launched, it must only be under conditions that guarantee its success.

Some Economists' Thoughts About Prevention of Skin Cancer

J.-P. MOATTI AND M.-L. BOUSCARY

In a growing number of developed countries, prevention of incidence and mortality from malignant melanoma of the skin tends to be considered as a major public health problem. In the British White Paper *The Health of the Nation* (UK Secretary of State for Health, 1992), one of the main objectives is to reduce ill-health and death caused by skin cancer, with a target to halt the year-on-year increase in the incidence of this cancer by 2005. In the United States, primary prevention of cutaneous melanoma (CM) and non-melanoma skin cancers (NMSC) has focused on health education campaigns encouraging sensible sun-exposure behaviours, while secondary prevention consists of a yearly national campaign jointly sponsored by the American Academy of Dermatology and the American Cancer Society (Koh *et al.*, 1990). In Australia, there has been widespread efforts for systematic preventive programmes since the 1970s (Smith, 1979). In European countries, such as France, Germany and Italy, preventive programmes have not yet been nationally organized but there have been various regional experiments for both early detection screening campaigns and general public media information campaigns (Bonerandi *et al.*, 1992; Cristofolini *et al.*, 1993a; Pehamberger *et al.*, 1993).

Because effectiveness of these health education packages and early detection campaigns has yet to be proved, there has been concern about the cost-effectiveness of these preventive efforts, either for choosing the best alternatives or even for discussing their rationality and interest in comparison with other public health priorities (Austoker, 1994; Melia *et al.*, 1994). In the current context of government policies of all Western countries to control escalation of health-care costs, a first (and most familiar) contribution of the health economist can be to clarify this issue of cost-effectiveness: *what does it mean for a preventive strategy to be cost-effective?* And, how can economic assessment help with choosing between alternative screening and educational preventive strategies? There is, however, a second potential contribution of economists to the current debate about prevention of skin cancer, which is definitely less familiar for health-care professionals but may indeed be more important.

It is a well-established fact in the field of social psychology applied to public health that knowledge and even positive attitudes towards prevention do not necessarily lead to individual adoption of preventive behaviours (Becker, 1974). And, it has been empirically verified that widespread adequate public knowledge of risk factors for CM does not mechanistically mean diffusion of safe ultraviolet radiation (UVR) exposure behaviours (Grob *et al.*, 1993; Jarrett *et al.*, 1993). Because standard microeconomics theory has always

been interested in better understanding and modelling individual behaviours towards risk and uncertainty (Von Neumann & Morgenstern, 1947), it can be a helpful tool to analyse barriers met by health education campaigns for effectively changing sun-related attitudes and behaviours. Economists can suggest useful answers to the following question: *what conditions make it rational for individuals to reduce their lifelong exposure to ultraviolet radiation?*

In this chapter, we will try to deal with these two issues successively in order to present some possible contributions of economists to the prevention of skin cancer.

In search of cost-effectiveness

Cost-effectiveness (CE) analysis in health policy, and its close relatives (cost-utility and cost-benefit analysis) are methods of summarizing information on the relationship between the resources expended on a health intervention and the health outcomes that result from the intervention (Drummond *et al.*, 1987). Suppose that there are N different mutually exclusive health interventions IM_i (Table 3.1), for example alternative screening strategies for early detection and surveillance of CM differing according to their organizational schemes, their target population (general population vs. different 'high-risk' groups) and their frequency. Each intervention is associated with a given cost C_i, which is measured relative to the status quo (no preventive programme is IM_0). Each intervention leads to an aggregate incremental change

Table 3.1 Cost-effectiveness (CE) comparison of mutually exclusive medical strategies.

Alternative strategies	Total costs (in 1000 FF)	Effectiveness (e.g. number of life-years saved)
IM_0 (status quo)	0	0
IM_1	200	40
IM_2	300	20
IM_3	300	30
IM_4	300	50
IM_5	500	75
IM_6	550	70

FF, French francs.

in health of the target population ΔH_i (for example, total number of life-years gained by the intervention). The CE analysis algorithm to choose between the interventions of Table 3.1 will be the following:

1 Rank the health interventions in terms of their cost going from lowest to highest total cost, and remove from the list any health intervention that costs the same (or more than) as a prior intervention on the list but produces lower incremental health benefits (in Table 3.1, IM_2 and IM_3 are totally dominated by IM_4, and IM_6 by IM_5).

2 Compute the incremental (marginal) cost-effectiveness ratios of one intervention in comparison with the previous one on the list $(C_i - C_{i-1})/(\Delta H_i - \Delta H_{i-1})$ (Table 3.2).

3 Eliminate from the list any health intervention with an incremental cost-effectiveness ratio greater than that of the next intervention on the list (in Table 3.2, IM_4 is 'weakly' dominated by IM_5; going directly from IM_1 to IM_5 produces more additional benefit for a lower cost per unit of benefit than going from IM_1 to IM_4.

4 Table 3.3 gives the three most cost-effective strategies selected by the algorithm, but does not allow us to make a final decision.

Of course, if there is a budget constraint, i.e. there is a maximum total amount of health-care resources that can be allocated to this prevention programme, the decision will be straightforward: in Table 3.3, a global budget lower than 200 000 FF (French francs) will lead to the decision that no programme can be implemented; if the budget is $\geq 200\,000$ and $< 500\,000$ FF, IM_1 will be chosen and a budget $\geq 500\,000$ will allow the choice of IM_5. The CE analysis algorithm, however, does not solve the question of whether an investment in health is worth its cost.

The final selection of one strategy among the ones which are cost-effective always requires the specification (explicitly or implicitly through the exogenous definition of a budget constraint) of a *threshold cost-effectiveness ratio* $(R_{Threshold})$, i.e. the maximum additional cost that society is willing to devote to obtaining an additional unit of health benefit. In our example, choosing strategy IM_1 would mean that $R_{Threshold}$ is 5000 FF per year of life gained and that society is willing to pay no more than 5000 FF to gain an additional year of life for its members through prevention of skin cancer; choosing IM_5 will mean that the threshold has increased to 8571 FF per additional life-year gained, etc.

Strategies	Total costs (in 1000 FF)	Effectiveness (life-years saved)	Marginal CE ratio (FF per additional life-year saved)
IM_0	0	0	0
IM_1	200	40	5 000
IM_4	300	50	10 000
IM_5	500	75	8 000

Table 3.2 Cost-effectiveness (CE) comparison of mutually exclusive medical strategies (after elimination of totally dominated strategies).

FF, French francs.

Strategies	Total costs (in 1000 FF)	Effectiveness (life-years saved)	Marginal CE ratio (FF per additional life-year saved)
IM_0	0	0	0
IM_1	200	40	5000
IM_5	500	75	8571

Table 3.3 Final selection of strategies according to cost-effectiveness (CE) criteria.

FF, French francs.

Two important conclusions can be derived from this very simplistic example:

1 To decide if an intervention is (or is not) 'cost-effective' always implies a reference to a 'threshold cost-effectiveness ratio': $R(C_{tot})$ where C_{tot} is the total amount of health-care resources available for a specific programme.

2 *To decide if an intervention is (or is not) 'cost-effective' always implies a societal value judgement*: Are the additional (marginal) benefits worth the additional (marginal) costs?

Unfortunately, there are not very many data in the international literature, on the one hand, about costs for the health-care system as well as patients themselves and, on the other hand, about effectiveness of primary prevention health education campaigns for skin cancers as well as secondary prevention interventions aimed at improving management of suspicious lesions in primary care. The most detailed economic evidence comes from the experience of the health campaign for early diagnosis of CM in the general population carried out in the province of Trentino (Italy) since 1977 (Cristofolini *et al.*, 1993b). The cost per year of lives saved by this campaign during the period 1977–85 in this Italian province was calculated to be $400, which is a fairly acceptable low range in comparison with most usual medical interventions for increasing life expectancy in our health-care systems (Birch & Gafni, 1992).

Decision-makers, however, must legitimately remain cautious before devoting resources for organizing similar health campaigns in other countries to facilitate early diagnosis of CM. First, the calculated CE ratio may be quite sensitive to epidemiological hypotheses about what would have spontaneously happened (expected incidence of deaths due to CM) in the same region in the absence of the preventive screening campaign. Secondly, costs of early diagnosis campaigns may be very sensitive to institutional and organizational aspects in each country such as the effective role of primary-care physicians in each health-care system: for example, in New Zealand, it has been estimated that if general practitioners did a full-skin examination annually, even restricted to adults aged 35–64 years, they would need to commit up to 5% of their clinical work time to this activity alone (Austoker, 1994). Finally, efforts for targeting screening and skin surveillance toward individuals at high risk of CM (age >40 years, family history of melanoma, ethnicity, high number of raised naevi on the arms) may significantly improve the cost-effectiveness ratio of these programmes: experience from Western Australia suggested that more than half of all new patients with CM arose in a subpopulation which constitutes less than one-fifth of the general population and whose identification by physicians seems feasible (English & Armstrong, 1988).

Efforts for *experimenting screening programmes in high-risk groups for CM* should therefore not be discarded on the basis of *a priori* conclusions, such as the idea that targeted prevention will, by definition, not reach all sections of the population. This is, of course, true but the question is whether additional costs of prevention in the general public in comparison with screening in more restricted at-risk groups are really worth the additional benefits. Experimental assessment of alternative early detection and surveillance strategies (using, if feasible, randomized designs) is therefore badly needed, and should include detailed analysis of costs of campaigns.

The highest uncertainties remain about the cost-effectiveness ratios of mass media campaigns for reduction of individual exposures to ultraviolet radiation (Rhodes, 1995). But assessment of effectiveness of such campaigns will always raise very complex methodological issues. There is always a practical difficulty in comparing intervention in a general population with a control group which could be totally free from the intervention. The campaign itself (leading to more aggressive case detection) will modify measurement of incidence, and it has been shown that 'increased' CM incidence can result from public education and intensification of case detection (MacKie & Hole, 1992).

In search of 'rational' avoidance of ultraviolet radiation

Decision scientists such as economists and psychologists have long been interested in how individuals make decisions under conditions of uncertainty, how various risks are perceived and what factors influence choice. Individual subjective judgements of relative risk may differ markedly from 'objective' expert assessments (Slovic, 1987). *Expected utility theory* (EUT), which is the dominant theory in decision sciences since the pioneering work of Von Neumann and Morgenstern (1947), is focused on decisions whose consequences cannot be known with certainty, the range of possible outcomes having probabilities attached to them. The theory postulates that individuals making choices between options should evaluate them in terms of their expected value (or utility), i.e. the relative value attached by the individual to the outcome weighted by its probability of occurrence. EUT also forms the basis for the applied analysis of medical decision-making (Weinstein & Fineberg, 1980).

In the case of UVR and skin cancer, individuals are *de facto* faced with a choice between two lotteries. If they choose not to reduce their exposure to the sun (Lottery 1), they will have a probability P to have a cancer (outcome U1) and nonetheless a $(1-P)$ probability not to have a cancer in the future (U3). If they choose Lottery 2, they will have a reduced probability P' ($<P$) to have a cancer and a $(1-P')$ probability to have an intermediate outcome (U2), which is not having a cancer but having experienced a reduced pleasure and benefit (utility) from sun exposure throughout the period. Individuals will choose the 'preventive' lottery if and only if its expected utility $[P' \cdot U1 + (1-P')U2]$ is superior to that of the alternative lottery implying no reduction of sun exposure $[P \cdot U1 = (1-P')U3]$.

Framing the problem in this way makes it clear that there are many rational reasons for individuals to maintain exposure to the sun which would be considered 'excessive' from a public health point of view. Some of them are related to *lack or misinterpretation of probabilistic information*. A common distinction in the decision theory literature is that between subjective probabilities (π) and 'objective' probabilities (P). If individuals' subjective estimation of their own probability of having a CM due to their sun sensitivity and history of sun exposure is lower than the 'real' probability, because of lack of awareness and information about current epidemiological evidence linking UVR to this cancer, they may decide not to modify their behaviour. Individuals may also have poor information about the consequences (and disutility) of some of the possible outcomes: for example, they may underestimate future costs, for

themselves, their family and society as a whole, of treating maligant melanoma (Creagan, 1989). Inequality between π and P and underestimation of consequences of the disease suggest a role for health education interventions to enhance the information base of the public and specific risk groups.

However, some misinterpretation of probabilistic information by individuals may indeed have some strong and 'rational' basis. Researchers such as Tversky and Kahneman (1974) have suggested that individuals, when faced with complex risky choices, use a variety of cognitive 'rules of thumb', which these authors call *heuristics* in order to simplify the choice problem and to make final decisions. Due to 'availability heuristics', individuals will judge an event to be more likely if instances are easily recalled or imagined. It is the availability of experience and information which influences the perception of likelihood. 'Representativeness heuristics' mean that the probability of an event is evaluated according to the degree to which it is considered representative of, or similar to, some specific major characteristic of the population from which it originates. In practice, the problem stems from a tendency to use a preconceived notion of the average as a reference standard against which to judge likelihood of a risky event: for example, high-risk individuals for CM may underestimate their risk by assimilation to the 'average' (fairly small in that case) they perceive in the general population to which they belong. In 'anchoring heuristics', the estimate of a value is arrived at by adjustment from some arbitrary initial starting point or 'anchor', etc.

All these phenomena in subjective perception of probabilistic risk will lead to individual attitudes and behaviours such as *overconfidence in personal judgement and desire for certainty* which, for example, will incite individuals to assimilate to zero small risks (like increased risk of CM due to one additional UVR exposure) or *denial of risk* ('it won't happen to me'). Determinants of underestimation of personal risk and personal optimism have been investigated in depth in the case of automobile driving and seat-belt behaviour (Slovic *et al.*, 1978), and an interesting parallel may be made with sun-related behaviours. First, hazardous activities for which personal risks are often underestimated tend to be seen as under the individual's control. Second, they tend to be familar hazards whose risks are low enough that the individual's personal experience is overwhelmingly benign: despite frequent exposure to the sun, sun-bathers make exposure after exposure without major mishap. This personal experience demonstrates to them that they have 'nothing to fear' from the sun while their indirect experience via the media shows them that skin cancer does happen — to others. Given such misleading experiences, people may feel quite justified in neglecting risks associated with UVR. In the case of seat belts, it has been shown that inciting individuals to think of the probability of accidents, not on the basis of each individual trip, but from the point of view of life-long risk associated with driving, significantly increases their willingness to systematically use this prevention device.

Another interest of the EUT framework is to point out that decisions under conditions of uncertainty cannot be predicted from probability information alone. *Decision is also a function of a number of values reflecting individual preferences* that may differ among individuals, making it rational for different subjects to adopt different behaviours, even if they have the same level of information about the risk.

Individuals may attach *different values to the outcomes* (getting a skin cancer or not). They may estimate differently the values attached to *process or intermediate outcomes* such as the various benefits (psychological, aesthetic, social prestige of looking good, etc.) they can derive from UVR or from prevention (reduced anxiety due to reduction of UVR exposure). Moreover, individuals may have *different preferences regarding risk per se.*

Risk neutrality means that an individual will be indifferent between the certainty of a 5-year increase of life expectancy and a gamble with a 0.5 chance of a 10-year increase and a 0.5 chance of immediate death, because the mathematical expectation of both choices is the same. It has been empirically proven that when outcomes concern health (probability of life and death), most individuals are strongly risk averse (i.e. they attach a great value to the avoidance of risk taking) (Gafni & Torrance, 1984): they will not exchange the certainty of five more years against a gamble unless the mathematical expectation of the latter is a lot more than 5 (for example, if the probability of death is small and the probability of

gaining ten more years instead of five is close to 1). But, there is also evidence that individuals (even the same ones) may be risk seekers where they are confronted with health risks with small (or very small) probabilities (such as the ones associated with individual UVR exposure) (Hellinger, 1989).

A final element, in the case of skin cancer, is that individuals face a *time trade-off*: exposure to the sun is an immediate short-term source of pleasure and satisfaction while benefits from avoiding CM or NMSC are delayed later at some uncertain moment in the future. To make their decision, individuals have to compare immediate costs with future benefits and they may differ in their individual rate of time preference. To assess the present value of a future benefit derived from a preventive programme, economic assessment traditionally uses a discount rate according to the formula $P_B = B_n(1 + r)^{-n}$ with P_B being the present value of benefit B in year n and r is the annual discount rate (Keeler & Cretin, 1983). The higher the discount rate (corresponding to strong preference in favour of present in comparison to future), the lower the present value of the future benefit: for example, with 5% and 10% discount rates, one year of life gained in 10 years will be, respectively, considered equivalent to immediate gains of 0.61 and 0.39 year.

These developments about EUT, apart from making a plea for more intensive psychological and psycho-social research on individual and collective attitudes and behaviours toward risks of skin cancer, suggest *practical recommendations about inherent limits of mass media primary prevention campaigns.*

1 Increasing information and risk awareness is a necessary condition but is not at all a sufficient condition for changing individual behaviours. Public opinion campaigns, about risks of UVR, should have the limited goal of influencing social norms to make people more conscious of the existence of the risk of skin cancer.

2 Because, at best, UVR avoidance will only prevent a fraction of the CM cases, potential 'unexpected' side effects of mass campaigns for reduction of UVR exposure must be carefully monitored. They may produce false reassurance leading to delayed diagnosis among those who avoid the sun, are darkly pigmented or who have evolving tumours in sun-protected sites. They may also promote unnecessary guilt and negative social sanctions for CM patients. And, finally, they may unintentionally focus public attention away from other more effective interventions aimed at promoting skin awareness and self-assessment as well as acceptability of screening and surveillance to facilitate early diagnosis.

3 Media campaigns must absolutely be considered as one component of structured programmes including health-care professionals' contribution to secondary prevention.

References

Austoker, J. (1994) Melanoma: prevention and early diagnosis. *British Medical Journal*, **308**, 1682–1686.

Becker, M.H. (1974) The health belief model and personal health behavior. *Health Education Monographs*, **2**, 220–243.

Birch, S. & Gafni, A. (1992) Cost-effectiveness/utility analyses: do current decision rules lead us to where we want to be? *Journal of Health Economics*, **11**, 279–296.

Bonerandi, J.J., Grob, J.J., Cnudde, N., Enel, P. & Gouvernet, J. (1992) Campagne de détection précoce du mélanome dans la région Provence-Alpes-Côte d'Azur-Corse en 1989. *Annales de Dermatologie et Vénéreologie*, **119**, 105–109.

Creagan, E.T. (1989) Malignant melanoma: cost and reimbursement issues. *Seminars in Oncology*, **16** (S1), 45–50.

Cristofolini, M., Bianchi, R., Boi, S. *et al.* (1993a) Effectiveness of the health campaign for early diagnosis of cutaneous melanoma in Trentino, Italy. *Journal of Dermatology and Surgery in Oncology*, **19**, 117–120.

Cristofolini, M., Bianchi, R., Boi, S. *et al.* (1993b) Analysis of the cost-effectiveness ratio of the health campaign for the early diagnosis of cutaneous melanoma in Trentino, Italy. *Cancer*, **71**, 370–374.

Drummond, M.F., Stoddart, G.L. & Torrance, G.W. (1987) *Methods for the Economic Evaluation of Health Care Programmes*. Oxford University Press, Oxford.

English, D.R. & Armstrong, B.K. (1988) Identifying people at high risk of cutaneous malignant melanoma: results from a case-control study in Western Australia. *British Medical Journal*, **296**, 1285–1288.

Gafni, A. & Torrance, W. (1984) Risk attitudes and time preference in health. *Management Science*, **30**, 440–451.

Grob, J.J., Guglielmina, C., Gouvernet, J., Zarour, H., Noé, C. & Bonerandi, J.J. (1993) Study of sunbathing habits in children and adolescents: application to the prevention of melanoma. *Dermatology*, **186**, 84–98.

Jarrett, P., Sharp, C. & McLelland, J. (1993) Protection of children by their mothers against sunburn. *British Medical Journal*, **306**, 1448.

Hellinger, F.J. (1989) Expected utility theory and risk choices with health outcomes. *Medical Care*, **27**, 273–279.

Keeler, E. & Cretin, S. (1983) Discounting of lifesavings and other non-monetary effects. *Management Science*, **29**, 300–306.

Koh, H.K., Lew, R.A. & Prout, M.N. (1990) Evaluation of melanoma/skin cancer screening in Massachusetts: preliminary results. *Cancer*, **65**, 375–379.

MacKle, R.M. & Hole, D. (1992) Audit of public education campaign to encourage earlier detection of malignant melanoma. *British Medical Journal*, **304**, 1012–1015.

Melia, J., Ellman, R. & Chamberlain, J. (1994) Meeting the Health of the Nation target for skin cancer: problems with tackling prevention and monitoring trends. *Journal of Public Health Medicine*, **16**, 225–232.

Pehamberger, H., Binder, M., Knollmayer, S. & Wolff, K. (1993) Immediate effects of public education campaign on prognostic features of melanoma. *Journal of the American Academy of Dermatology*, **29**, 106–109.

Rhodes, A.R. (1995) Public education and cancer of the skin. *Cancer*, **75** (S2), 613–636.

Slovic, P. (1987) Perception of risk. *Science*, **236**, 280–285.

Slovic, P., Fischoff, B. & Lichtenstein, S. (1978) Accident probabilities and seat belt usage: a psychological perspective. *Accident Analysis and Prevention*, **10**, 281–285.

Smith, T. (1979) The Queensland melanoma project — an exercise in health education. *British Medical Journal*, **i**, 253–254.

Tversky, A. & Kahneman, D. (1974) Judgment under uncertainty: heuristics and biases. *Science*, **185**, 1124–1131.

UK Secretary of State for Health (1992) *The Health of the Nation*. HMSO, London.

Von Neumann, J. & Morgenstern, O. (1947) *Theories of Games and Economic Behavior*. Princeton University Press, Princeton.

Weinstein, M.C. & Fineberg, H.V. (1980) *Clinical Decision Analysis*. W.B. Saunders, Philadelphia.

4

Evaluation of Quality of Life in Dermatology: Application to Psoriasis

A.Y. FINLAY

Introduction

'While psoriasis is not a killer, living with it is murder.' This quote from a psoriasis sufferer encapsulates the myriad effects that this chronic disease has on people. In this chapter the ways in which psoriasis impacts on lives are reviewed, and the reasons for trying to measure this impact are given. The methods available for this measurement are described, along with recent results of their use. Advice is given about which techniques may be of practical help, and there is speculation about the further research work required in this area. Although this chapter focuses on psoriasis, the techniques and concepts described are applicable to a wide range of different skin diseases.

The impact of psoriasis on people's lives

There is nothing new about the realization that psoriasis causes handicap disability. In his Watson Smith lecture, Ingram (1954) commented on 'the cruel fate of leaving a trail of silver scale about the house and bloodstains on the sheets'. In 1970, in an attempt to create a scale to objectively measure severity of psoriasis, the features judged by 56 patients with psoriasis to be the first, third and fifth most important in reflecting psoriasis severity were embarrassment over appearance, scales in bedding and scales on clothing (Baughman & Sobel, 1970). Molin (1973), in his detailed survey of 408 patients, recorded a significant increase in days lost from work in psoriatics compared to controls. Other surveys have highlighted the embarrassment that inhibits daily activities and choice of clothing (Stankler, 1981), the psychological, social and physical discomfort of

psoriasis (Jobling, 1976) and the feelings of stigmatization and despair experienced by sufferers (Ginsburg & Link, 1989). Ramsay and O'Reagan (1988) recorded that 50% of people with psoriasis experienced inhibition of their sexual relationships, and most patients had avoided common social activities such as swimming and sports. Methods of addressing the psychological factors experienced by patients with psoriasis have been described (Dooley & Finlay, 1990; Gupta *et al.*, 1990; Dooley, 1993) and patients' own accounts of their lives affected by psoriasis provide further insights into this area (Weingarten, 1995). An effective way of drawing to the attention of the general public the impact of skin disease on people's lives is for a media personality who coincidentally has psoriasis to publish their experiences (Elton & Finlay, 1995).

Why we need to measure quality of life

Although there are many descriptions of the ways in which psoriasis affects lives, until recently there have been no attempts to measure this consequence of disease. Measurement methods are required for clinical, research, audit and for political purposes.

In everyday clinical practice, all clinicians take into account their view of the extent to which they think their patient's life is being affected when they take clinical decisions about the most appropriate form of management for that person. A typical example in psoriasis is when a decision is being taken about whether to start someone on second-line therapy such as methotrexate. The clinician weighs up the risks and potential benefit to the patient of starting the drug, and clearly if the patient's life is being severely affected by the disease, this will make it more likely that the drug is started. If it were possible to have a very simple, quick and more comprehensive or accurate view of the impact of the disease on the patient, this might be very valuable in aiding this clinical decision.

Clinical research into the effectiveness of new therapies in psoriasis has used several methods of assessing disease activity (Marks *et al.*, 1989), largely based on recording extent of involvement and the presence of various signs. Quality of life measures may add a further dimension to this assessment process, as they provide a 'user'-oriented view, and quality of life information does not necessarily directly parallel other measurement methods. It might be possible, for example, for a treatment to reduce the scores of redness and scaling of a plaque of psoriasis by 50%, but if the plaque was still visible over the dorsum of the hand there might be no improvement in the patient's life. Some licensing authorities may request that this information be presented as part of the application for approval of new therapies.

In many health-care systems, audit of dermatology services is either being encouraged or has become a requirement. A key measure of the quality of a service is the effectiveness of that service in providing management which is successful in improving the quality of life that was adversely affected by the skin disease. Simple quality of life measures may be ideally suited to audit this.

Because skin disease is rarely fatal, resources in many health-care systems are not directed sufficiently to the management of skin disease. Dermatologists, however, well understand the importance of the skin diseases to their patients. The use of quality of life measures may be able to provide politically important information to clearly demonstrate this impact of skin disease, and so add strength to the arguments for more resources for dermatology. These arguments are even stronger if they are also coupled with clear information concerning the economic impact of skin diseases, such as psoriasis, both on the patient and on the health-care system (Finlay, 1995).

During clinical consultations when simple quality of life measures are being used, it is our experience that patients are universally interested in the questions being put to them, recognize the relevance to them of the questions posed and appreciate that these issues are being raised. Generally, the use of the questionnaires adds to the value of the consultation by allowing an opening for issues which are of importance to the patient to be explored.

Methods of measuring quality of life in psoriasis

There are several ways in which quality of life can be measured in psoriasis. These are all questionnaire-based and include psoriasis-specific, dermatology-specific, general health measures and utility methods.

Disease-specific questionnaires

The first disease-specific quality of life questionnaire described for psoriasis was the Psoriasis Disability Index (PDI) (Finlay & Kelly, 1987). To create this, a series of patients with psoriasis were interviewed about the different ways that psoriasis affected them. A series of 28 questions was identified which covered most reported effects. From these, 10 questions were chosen on the basis of examining the correlation between the questions. The PDI was initially used to demonstrate that the total area of involvement of psoriasis is not a reliable guide to disability, and that there was a significant reduction in disability after in-patient treatment for psoriasis.

The 15-question version of the PDI (Finlay & Coles, 1995) has been validated against two general health measures, the UK Sickness Impact Profile (SIP) (Finlay *et al.*, 1990) and the General Health Questionnaire (Root *et al.*, 1994). The substructure and specificity of the PDI to psoriasis have been examined, and a factor analysis indicated that the PDI contained two subscales, one concerning most aspects of everyday activities, the other concerning specific public situations such as the use of communal facilities (Kent, 1993).

The PDI has been used to assess the level of disability experienced by patients who were either about to be admitted to hospital for treatment of their psoriasis, or who were about to be started on systemic therapy (Finlay & Coles, 1995). There was a substantial correlation between the PDI score and the amount that a patient indicated they would pay for a cure, if a cure were possible. In a postal survey of 538 patients with psoriasis in The Netherlands (Haisman *et al.*, 1995), the items that most disturbed this group of patients were identified, and there was an inverse relationship between the PDI score and the level of education of the patient. The PDI has also been used in the assessment of the value of a clinical psychology liaison service for patients with psoriasis (Gledhill *et al.*, 1995). In an audit of UVB phototherapy, the mean PDI fell from 42.6 to 32.2 in 58 patients studied before and after standard UVB treatment (Parry *et al.*, 1995). The PDI was used in a study to assess the effectiveness of cyclosporin: there was a significant reduction in disability at the end of 12 weeks of therapy, as well as an improvement in the clinical sign score (Salek & Finlay, 1993).

Questionnaires other than the PDI have also been used to measure quality of life in psoriasis (McHenry & Doherty, 1992). McKenna and Stern (1995) reported the impact of psoriasis on the quality of life of patients from the 16-centre psoralens and ultraviolet A therapy (PUVA) follow-up cohort in the USA. For this study, physical, psychological, social and total quality of life impact indexes were constructed, and these demonstrated that the most significant impact of psoriasis is upon the psychological dimension of patients' lives. Gupta *et al.* (1989) have described the Psoriasis Life Stress Inventory which codifies major stressful events in the lives of patients with psoriasis.

General health measures

The major advantage of using general health measures in the assessment of the impact of skin diseases is that this provides comparative information between skin diseases and diseases affecting other systems. The UK SIP was used in 32 in-patients and out-patients with psoriasis: this group had a mean score of 9.9 (Finlay *et al.*, 1990). This score compared with a mean SIP score of 7.0 for patients with hypertension, 8.2 for angina and 10.4 for cardiac failure. However, these comparisons must be treated with caution as the criteria for entry of each of these different groups into these separate studies were not necessarily comparable. The SIP has also been used in another study in parallel with the PDI in the assessment of the effects of cyclosporin (Salek & Finlay, 1993), providing

detailed information about which facets of patients' lives were most affected by psoriasis, and which changed following this therapy.

The General Health Questionnaire has also been used in psoriasis (Root *et al.*, 1994), providing the potential for similar comparisons. Another general health measure that is being very widely used in many medical specialities is the SF-36. The PDI and the SF-36 have been used together in a multicentre study in the USA (Nichol *et al.*, 1996) and in a community study in the UK (O'Neil & Kelly, 1996).

One disadvantage of using general health measures in psoriasis is that these questionnaires are usually lengthy, as the questions have to cover all the potential impact of all diseases. This leads to the second major disadvantage: as many of the questions are not directly relevant to psoriasis, their presence blurs and may dilute the measurement of the specific impact of this disease.

Speciality-specific questionnaires

There are many different skin diseases and it would, in theory, be possible to create disease-specific quality of life questionnaires for each one. However, most skin diseases, especially widespread chronic inflammatory conditions such as psoriasis or eczema, affect people's lives in very similar ways, and it would therefore seem more sensible to use a dermatology-specific questionnaire which could be used across all skin diseases. The Dermatology Life Quality Index (DLQI) (Finlay & Khan, 1994) and the children's version, the Children's Dermatology Life Quality Index (CDLQI) (Lewis-Jones & Finlay, 1995), have been described for this use. Both indices consist of 10 questions and are answered with tick boxes: each answer is scored from 0 to 3. These indices have been used in patients with psoriasis, and both in children and in adults, psoriasis is one of the highest scoring skin diseases.

The DLQI has been used to audit the effectiveness of in-patient management of patients with psoriasis and eczema (Kurwa & Finlay, 1995). In both conditions, there was a highly significant improvement in mean scores between the time of admission and 4 weeks after discharge.

Quality of life measures created and validated in one culture are not necessarily valid for use in different cultures. However, both the DLQI and the CDLQI have been translated into several different languages for use in multicentre trials.

Utility measures

Utility measures are used to assess the value that patients put on their disease state. The value may be in terms of hypothetical time or money, or comparisons can be drawn with different diseases. The purpose of this type of assessment is to gain insight into the values or attitudes of patients concerning their disease, and the information gained may be used to guide resource allocation.

The standard utility assessment techniques of vertical rating scale, time trade-off and standard gamble were used in 87 patients with psoriasis, using an interactive, computer-based questionnaire (Zug *et al.*, 1995). These utility measures varied widely for mild, moderate and for severe psoriasis, confirming that the impact of psoriasis on a patient's life is not necessarily related to the extent of the disease (Finlay & Kelly, 1987). The gathering of individual patient's preferences and values using this type of computer software may potentially allow easier and more accurate patient preferences to be incorporated into clinical decision-taking.

In a multicentre study in the UK (Finlay & Coles, 1995), information was gathered from 369 patients with severe psoriasis. Despite having severe psoriasis, the majority felt that it would be worse to have diabetes, asthma or bronchitis than to have psoriasis; 46, 42 and 32% considered it would be either 'better' or 'the same' to have diabetes, asthma or bronchitis, respectively. However, in those patients who also had the comparative disease, 87, 80 and 77% considered it would be 'better' or 'the same' to have the comparative disease. This gives an insight into attitudes of patients with psoriasis who consider that others are worse off than themselves, unless they have the direct experience of those other diseases!

In the same study, 98.9% of patients stated that they would prefer to have a complete cure of their disease rather than be given £1000 (approximately US$1500); 71% of patients said they would be prepared to pay £1000 or more, and 38% said they would pay £10000 for a cure for their psoriasis, if one existed. Time comparisons revealed that 49% of patients with severe psoriasis would be prepared to spend 2 or 3 hours each day on treatment if this might result in normal skin for the rest of the day.

Further developments

Methods to quantify the impact of psoriasis on patients' lives are still at an early stage of development. This review has described the current techniques that have been used over the last 10 years and their, as yet, limited usage. It seems clear, however, that over the coming decade many clinical studies assessing new therapies for psoriasis will use quality of life measures as one means of assessment.

It has been proposed by Katsambas (1990) that the European Academy of Dermatology and Venereology should support these recommendations:

1 Dermatologists should incorporate quality of life measurements to help assess and monitor the progress of their patients.

2 Research is required to develop and refine quality of life measurements.

3 Therapy should clearly demonstrate a positive influence on quality of life.

Although this review focuses on psoriasis, information concerning the measurement of quality of life in acne is given by Motley and Finlay (1992) and by Salek *et al.* (1996), and in eczema is given by Finlay (1996).

By focusing on quality of life as one of the goals to be measured and improved, management methods which address the practical problems of patients with psoriasis and other skin diseases may be encouraged.

References

Baughman, R.D. & Sobel, R. (1970) Psoriasis — a measure of severity. *Archives of Dermatology*, **101**, 390–395.

Dooley, G. (1993) Psychological factors in psoriasis. *Dermatology in Practice*, **1**(7), 14–15.

Dooley, G. & Finlay, A.Y. (1990) Personal construct systems of psoriatic patients. *Clinical and Experimental Dermatology*, **15**, 401–405.

Elton, B. & Finlay, A.Y. (1995) Psoriasis — it's not a laughing matter. *Dermatology in Practice*, **3**(4), 5–8.

Finlay, A.Y. (1995) Quality of life issues and economic burden of psoriasis and atopic dermatitis. *Clinical Drug Investigation*, **10** (Suppl. 1), 1–6.

Finlay, A.Y. (1996) Measurement of disease activity and outcome in atopic dermatitis. *British Journal of Dermatology,* **135**, 509–515.

Finlay, A.Y. & Coles, E.C. (1995) The effect of severe psoriasis on the quality of life of 369 patients. *British Journal of Dermatology,* **132**, 236–244.

Finlay, A.Y. & Kelly, S.E. (1987) Psoriasis — an index of disability. *Clinical and Experimental Dermatology,* **12**, 8–11.

Finlay, A.Y. & Khan, G.K. (1994) Dermatology Life Quality Index (DLQI): a simple practical measure for routine clinical use. *Clinical and Experimental Dermatology,* **19**, 210–216.

Finlay, A.Y., Khan, G.K., Luscombe, D.K. & Salek, M.S. (1990) Validation of Sickness Impact Profile and Psoriasis Disability Index in psoriasis. *British Journal of Dermatology,* **123**, 751–756.

Ginsburg, I.H. & Link, B.G. (1989) Feelings of stigmatization in patients with psoriasis. *Journal of the American Academy of Dermatology,* **20**, 53–63.

Gledhill, K., Keller-Jackson, L. & Cheesebrough, M. (1995) Clinical psychology liaison in a dermatology clinic: a demonstration project. Presented at *6th International Congress on Dermatology and Psychiatry, Amsterdam, The Netherlands, 20–22 April 1995.*

Gupta, M.A., Gupta, A.K., Kirkby, S., Schork, N., Gorr, S., Ellis, C.N. & Voorhees, J.J. (1989) A psychocutaneous profile of psoriasis patients who are stress reactors. *General Hospital Psychiatry,* **11**, 166–173.

Gupta, M.A., Gupta, A.K., Ellis, C.N. & Voorhees, J.J. (1990) Some psychosomatic aspects of psoriasis. *Advances in Dermatology,* **5**, 21–32.

Ingram, J.T. (1954) The significance and management of psoriasis. *British Medical Journal,* **ii**, 823–828.

Jobling, R.G. (1976) Psoriasis — a preliminary questionnaire study of sufferers' subjective experience. *Clinical and Experimental Dermatology,* **1**, 233–236.

Haisma, H.H., Kaptein, A.A., Thio, B. & Vermeer, B.-J. (1995) Social aspects of psoriasis, the Psoriasis Disability Index. Presented at *6th International Congress on Dermatology and Psychiatry, Amsterdam, The Netherlands, 20–22 April 1995.*

Katsambas, A. (1990) Quality of life in dermatology and the EADV. *Journal of the European Academy of Dermatology and Venereology,* **3**, 211–214.

Kent, G. & Al-Abadie, M. (1993) The Psoriasis Disability Index — further analyses. *Clinical and Experimental Dermatology,* **18**, 414–416.

Kurwa, H. & Finlay, A.Y. (1995) Dermatology inpatient admission greatly improves life quality. *British Journal of Dermatology,* **133**, 575–578.

Lewis-Jones, M.S. & Finlay, A.Y. (1995) The Children's Dermatology Life Quality Index (CDLQI): initial validation and practical use. *British Journal of Dermatology,* **132**, 942–949.

Marks, R., Barton, S.P., Shuttleworth, D. & Finlay, A.Y. (1989) Assessment of disease progress in psoriasis. *Archives of Dermatology,* **125**, 235–240.

McHenry, P.M. & Doherty, V.R. (1992) Psoriasis: an audit of patients' views on the disease and its treatment. *British Journal of Dermatology,* **127**, 13–17.

McKenna, K.E. & Stern, R.S. (1995) The impact of psoriasis on the quality of life of patients from the 16-Center PUVA follow-up cohort. *British Journal of Dermatology,* **133** (Suppl. 45), 17.

Molin, L. (1973) Psoriasis. *Acta Dermato-Venereologica,* **53** (Suppl. 72), 87.

Motley, R.J. & Finlay, A.Y. (1992) Practical use of a disability index in the routine management of acne. *Clinical and Experimental Dermatology,* **17**, 1–3.

Nichol, M.B., Margolies, J.E., Lippa, E., Rowe, M. & Quell, J. (1996) The application of multiple quality of life instruments in individuals with mild to moderate psoriasis. *PharmacoEconomics,* **10**, 644–653.

O'Neill, P. & Kelly, P. (1996) Postal questionnaire study of disability in the community associated with psoriasis. *British Medical Journal,* **313**, 919–921.

Parry, E.J., Tillman, D.M., Long, J. & MacKie, R.M. (1995) Audit of UVB phototherapy in the treatment of psoriasis. *British Journal of Dermatology,* **133** (Suppl. 45), 16.

Ramsay, B. & O'Reagan, M. (1988) A survey of the social and psychological effects of psoriasis. *British Journal of Dermatology,* **118**, 195–201.

Root, S., Kent, G. & Al-Abadie, M.S.K. (1994) The relationship between disease severity, disability and psychological distress in patients undergoing PUVA treatment for psoriasis. *Dermatology,* **189**, 234–237.

Salek, M.S. & Finlay, A.Y. (1993) Cyclosporin improves quality of life in psoriasis — does this matter? *British Journal of Dermatology,* **129** (Suppl. 42), 32.

Salek, M.S., Khan, G.K. & Finlay, A.Y. (1996) Questionnaire techniques in assessing acne handicap: reliability and validity study. *Quality of Life Research,* **5**, 131–138.

Stankler, L. (1981) The effect of psoriasis on the sufferer. *Clinical and Experimental Dermatology,* **6**, 303–306.

Weingarten, S. (1995) Psoriasis — how we coped. *British Medical Journal,* **310**, 1076–1077.

Zug, K.A., Littenberg, B., Baughman, R.D. *et al.* (1995) Assessing the preferences of patients with psoriasis. A quantitative, utility approach. *Archives of Dermatology,* **131**, 561–568.

5

Epidemiology and the Study of Genetic Diseases

J.-D. FINE

Many of the most devastating dermatological diseases are rare, inherited ones. Unfortunately, with few recent exceptions, little is known about most of these diseases at the molecular, clinical or even population levels. To some extent, this is due to the inaccessibility of sufficient patients for comprehensive, longitudinal study. In the absence of such data, much of our present knowledge about the genodermatoses is based on findings observed in small series of patients. Unfortunately, such reports may not adequately reflect the true clinical or laboratory spectrum of each disease entity. Similarly, this paucity of data impairs the validation testing of laboratory studies which may be used for the purposes of postnatal and prenatal diagnosis and disease subclassification, as well as the development of specific therapies.

There are now numerous examples of the usefulness of epidemiological principles and techniques for the study of chronic, non-infectious diseases. Indeed, many of our current clinical approaches to the management of hypercholesterolaemia, hypertension, coronary artery disease, stroke and obesity are based on the results of longitudinal epidemiological studies involving at least tens of thousands of patients. More recently, based on the latter successes in other chronic diseases, epidemiological approaches have been applied to the study of rare, genetic diseases. The best example of the impact of epidemiology in dermatological research, as will be illustrated, is in the area of inherited epidermolysis bullosa (EB).

Epidemiological applications to the study of genetic diseases

Study design

Case-control studies and rare diseases

Sound clinical research is dependent on properly designed and executed studies. This demands a thorough understanding of the appropriate choice of study design for a given hypothesis. This also involves knowledge and experience in the estimation of subjects needed to achieve statistical significance, the use of stratification, matching and, where appropriate, different randomization schemes, and the choice and calculation of those statistics most appropriate for the chosen study design.

Determination of the possible association of a rare disease with a preceding exposure is best accomplished by way of a case-control study, once an adequate number of affected individuals can be identified. A critical concern in the design of a case-control study is the proper selection of the control population, since the validity of any associations detected between exposure and disease is very dependent on the correct choice of controls. Traditionally, this involves identification of patients with a rare disease of interest (i.e. adenocarcinoma of the vagina), the selection of two- to threefold that number of control subjects who are otherwise matched (i.e. by age, sex, ethnicity, parity, etc.) to those with the given disease, and then the determination of the presence or absence (by history) of exposure to that agent which is hypothesized to be causally linked to that outcome (i.e. diethylstilbœstrol use by the diseased subjects' mothers).

This scheme can be further modified, when indicated,

in the setting of rare, genetic diseases. First, one or more case-control studies can be nested within a much larger longitudinal cohort study (to include a longitudinal rare disease registry), thus preventing reduplication of efforts, patients and the costs associated with patient surveys and physical examinations. Second, the choice of what constitutes outcome versus exposure can be adjusted to meet the specific needs of the questions being asked. For example, a traditional approach can be taken if one is asking whether exposure to something possibly teratogenic just before or during earliest pregnancy results in a higher frequency of the genetic disease of interest, particularly if the affected patients are believed to represent spontaneous mutations for a dominant disease. That is, if one postulates that mutation for the Koebner subtype of EB simplex is associated with the parents having lived near a source of high electromagnetic radiation, one can assemble an appropriate number of patients and controls and then seek out exposure during that time period hypothesized to be biologically relevant. In this case, the disease of interest is the Koebner subtype of EB simplex and the exposure is high electromagnetic radiation. Alternatively, if one is interested in knowing via case-control design whether patients with the Hallopeau–Siemens subtype of recessive dystrophic EB are at higher risk than patients with other forms of EB for the development of squamous-cell carcinomas, disease and exposure in this particular example become squamous-cell carcinoma and Hallopeau–Siemens disease, respectively, with non-exposure being represented by those subjects having a form of EB other than the Hallopeau–Siemens subtype.

Cohort studies and rare diseases

In general, a cohort study of a population at risk is not optimal for the study of a rare disease, if the identification of new cases of this disease is considered the outcome or endpoint of interest. This study design is a poor choice due to the excessive costs, time and technical labour that would be required to identify sufficient numbers of new cases of a rare disease arising from such a necessarily large study population at risk. These problems are further compounded if the inherited disease of interest (for example, Huntington's chorea) remains clinically dormant for years or even

decades. On the other hand, a longitudinal approach is a reasonable way to assess the magnitude of occurrence of specific outcomes of interest within a rare disease if a substantial number of patients with the disease of interest can be identified, recruited and subsequently systematically followed over time. These efforts can be greatly facilitated by the establishment of a multicentre project involving those investigators most likely to be referred such patients. Alternatively, it is possible to be at least as successful in enrolment if patients are recruited by a national disease registry which is based at a single institution; one advantage of the latter design is the likely marked reduction in interobserver variability, due to the presence of fewer data collectors. In addition, it is preferable that such a rare disease registry be of retrospective longitudinal design so as to include both prevalent and incident cases. The retrospective nature of this study design will further permit the earlier assessment of a population of patients who represent a wide range of ages. Since older individuals will be included, it is likely that some, or many, may have already developed one or more outcomes of interest. As but one example of the utility of such an approach, prior to 1986 only limited numbers of patients with inherited EB were being followed by individual investigators, making any longitudinal data being collected rather uninterpretable, due to a variety of inherent problems in study design, to include selection bias and statistically inadequate numbers of subjects. In contrast, since 1986 virtually all newly identified patients with inherited EB who have resided within the continental United States, as well as many of those previously diagnosed, have been enrolled in the National EB Registry (Fine *et al.*, 1994c). As of 1 December 1995, this amounts to extensive data collection on over 2500 EB patients, making longitudinal surveillance for various outcomes in this disease now very possible.

Clinical trials and genetic diseases

Properly planned and executed clinical trials are invaluable in determining the therapeutic benefit of new treatments, especially in diseases such as the genodermatoses, in which only limited numbers of patients exist or can be recruited for study. When coordinated through a mechanism such as a rare disease registry, multiple interventions may be assessed simultaneously, especially when a crossover design is employed, thereby reducing the total number of study subjects required to be able to detect clinically relevant differences among compared therapies. In addition, pursuit of clinical trials under the auspices of, or with the active assistance of, a disease registry should enhance the likelihood that only well-characterized and otherwise matched subjects are selected for participation. Although a number of different designs for clinical trials exist within the epidemiological literature, the randomized, double-blind approach is generally considered to be most optimal, since it best controls for potential confounders. Not surprisingly, the creation of a clinical trial requires detailed knowledge of a variety of epidemiological and biostatistical principles, including randomization and stratification. They should, therefore, be undertaken only after considerable imput has been provided by epidemiologists and biostatisticians experienced not only in their design and execution but also in all aspects of subsequent data management and analysis.

Estimates of incidence and prevalence

Data are lacking on the incidence and prevalence of most of the genodermatoses. This is particularly problematic in the United States, since the absence of such data prevents any estimates of the financial impact of these diseases on the American health-care system, which in turn potentially jeopardizes future allocation of adequate federal funds for the management of these diseases in the setting of evolving health-care reform. Reasonably accurate estimations of these parameters may be possible in those European countries in which demographic data are maintained on all medical conditions and the provision of health care is highly structured by their governments. In contrast, such estimates are nearly impossible to generate in the United States in the absence of available disease registries having very high rates of patient identification and enrolment. Some affected individuals, for example, may choose not to participate in a project which is focused on data acquisition rather than patient care, and there is no mandatory centralized mechanism in the United States for the reporting of new cases of most non-infectious

diseases. Furthermore, many patients with milder forms of some genetic diseases, who are members of large affected kindreds, may choose not to be seen by another physician since they are already well aware of both their diagnosis and the usual lack of effective treatments.

We have recently attempted to estimate both incidence and prevalence of the major EB subtypes within the United States, using data which have been collected on behalf of the National EB Registry (Fine *et al.*, 1996). After adjustments were made for regional differences in enrolment in the project, we estimated the prevalence of inherited EB to be approximately 2044 in 1990 (i.e. 8.2 EB cases per one million population). We assume that this figure includes most of the severely affected EB patients, since these patients are almost always referred to the National EB Registry early in the course of their disease for the performance of confirmatory diagnostic testing. On the other hand, we are undoubtedly underestimating milder disease, particularly EB simplex. Unfortunately, for the purpose of estimating the overall prevalence of EB, this underreported EB subtype is the most common form of EB in the United States. At present, we have no way of knowing to what extent the latter patients have been underreported to the Registry. Assuming identification and enrolment of only 10 and 5% of all American EB simplex cases, however, we would estimate overall prevalence to be 12 340 and 23 780 patients, respectively. This can be contrasted with Scotland, where the overall prevalence of inherited EB is estimated by Tidman and colleagues to be 45 cases per million (Fine, 1994). Similarly, we estimated that the overall incidence (as new cases per one million live births in the United States) for inherited EB during this same time period was 19.6, and that the incidences for the Weber–Cockayne subtype of EB simplex and the Hallopeau–Siemens variant of recessive dystrophic EB were 6.8 and 0.4 per million, respectively.

Use of epidemiological techniques to determine disease spectrum in genetic diseases

Every well-designed longitudinal epidemiological study is based on the meticulous, systematic collection of data. Often such surveys include a large number of responses encompassing a wide variety of questions, which then can be analysed separately from those addressing the primary hypothesis of the study. An example of such a broadly focused epidemiological study based on a genetic skin disease is the National EB Registry (Fine *et al.*, 1994c). This project's database contains nearly 1000 possible responses to a variety of questions about the subjects' present and past medical histories, family histories, patient demographics, laboratory findings and socio-economic status. Using this database, it has been possible to more precisely determine the range in clinical findings, both cutaneous and extracutaneous, which are present in this group of patients, as stratified by EB type and subtype and, when appropriate, by age (Fine *et al.*, 1994b,d). Many of the resultant findings are in marked disagreement with currently held generalizations about the significance of specific morphological features in given EB subtypes. For example, it is commonly believed that patients with EB simplex, regardless of disease subtype, lack evidence of milia, atrophic scarring or nail dystrophy. Similarly, it has been suggested that the presence of intra-oral disease activity is incompatible with the diagnosis of EB simplex. However, the collective data from the Registry demonstrate that 10–25% of EB simplex patients, particularly those with more generalized distribution of lesions, have one or more of these 'atypical' cutaneous findings (Fine *et al.*, 1994a), and that about 35% of all EB simplex patients have some discernible intra-oral erosions during at least early infancy (Wright *et al.*, 1993). It is similarly believed that exuberant granulation tissue and pseudosyndactyly are features seen exclusively in the Herlitz subtype of junctional EB and the Hallopeau–Siemens subtype of recessive dystrophic EB, respectively. Although these latter two findings are indeed most commonly seen in patients with these specific EB subtypes, they may also be seen infrequently in other forms of inherited EB, suggesting the lack of sensitivity and specificity of these particular findings as surrogate diagnostic markers.

Validation of diagnostic testing in genetic diseases

It is possible to determine the sensitivity (Se) and specificity (Sp) of different diagnostic laboratory techniques if appropriate data are collected as part of a well-planned epidemiological study. Determination of these testing parameters is extremely important, since the use of an insensitive or non-specific diagnostic test will result in patient misclassification, thereby invalidating the results of any further analyses as well as possibly deleteriously influencing the proper choice of therapy in a given patient. These types of analyses have been performed on the following diagnostic laboratory tests using the database of the National EB Registry — transmission electron microscopy, immunofluorescence antigenic mapping, routine histology and several EB-specific monoclonal antibody studies. In general, the findings of electron microscopy and immunofluorescence antigenic mapping were of equally high sensitivity and specificity. In contrast, routine light microscopy proved to be highly unreliable in differentiating among the three major EB types. When two anchoring filament-associated monoclonal antibodies (GB3; 19-DEJ-1) were compared as probes for junctional EB, GB3 was found to be highly specific (Sp = 0.99) but insensitive (Se = 0.67), whereas 19-DEJ-1 was found to have perfect sensitivity (Se = 1.0) but only moderate specificity (Sp = 0.81) (Fine *et al.*, 1993a). Furthermore, neither antibody could be used to reliably differentiate Herlitz from non-Herlitz disease, making the results of these antibody studies useless for the purpose of subclassifying junctional EB patients. Similarly, it was shown that altered staining in skin samples by a monoclonal antibody to type VII collagen was a very specific (Sp = 0.99) but somewhat insensitive (Se = 0.83) marker of recessive dystrophic EB (Fine *et al.*, 1993b).

Outcome analyses and genetic diseases

Many genodermatosis patients develop clinically significant, if not potentially disabling, sequelae over time. In the case of inherited EB, these may include, but are not limited to, progressive involvement of the upper airway, oral cavity, oesophagus, external eyes, hands and feet, and lower gastrointestinal tract. Such disease activity, if persistent or severe, may eventuate in life-threatening stenosis of the upper airway (necessitating tracheostomy), widespread scarring of the soft tissues within the mouth, premature loss of teeth (due to rampant caries or altered soft-tissue anatomy), severe dysphagia, reduction or loss of vision in one or both eyes, disabling acral musculoskeletal deformities, chronic diarrhoea or constipation, or profoundly diminished absorption of nutrients across the mucosa of the small intestine. It is similarly known that patients representing some of the EB subtypes have an increased risk of eventually developing one or more malignancies of the skin. In addition, patients with some types or subtypes of EB are believed to be at increased risk of premature death. With few exceptions, however, data are lacking as to the actual frequency of such occurrences, either over the lifetime of an individual or during specific windows of time.

Data on outcomes such as these are readily forth-coming if traditional epidemiological and biostatistical techniques are applied to the analysis of a well-designed database which contains sufficient amounts of longitudinal data. Overall frequencies for selected outcomes in individual EB subtypes can be easily determined if the dataset is first stratified. While such frequency data may be of some practical use to the clinician in attempting to counsel an individual patient about the course of disease that will likely occur over his or her lifetime, such data provide no insight into when such events are most likely to occur, nor do they provide exact probabilities for the occurrence of each event. The latter, however, can be accurately determined if the dataset is analysed instead by the lifetable technique. With the latter approach, it is possible to determine the cumulative risk of a given event at any age of interest (i.e. by age 37 years), as well as the risk of an outcome occurring during any designated period of time (i.e. between the ages of 2 and 6 years). Such information can be extremely useful in the long-term management of patients, since it alerts both the physician and patient to those specific ages or time periods during which more intensive medical surveillance for particular outcomes will be most appropriate and cost-effective.

Lifetable analysis of the National EB Registry dataset has confirmed that tracheolaryngeal involvement occurs almost exclusively in junctional EB (Fine *et al.*, 1995g). By ages 2, 3 and 5 years, the cumulative prob-abilities of this outcome having occurred in the Herlitz subtype were 9.4%, 20.1% and 20.1%, respectively,

compared to 9.6% at all three ages for patients with the non-Herlitz subtypes of junctional EB. The cumu-lative probability of this particular out-come reached a plateau by the age of 6 years, with 26.7% and 11.0% of patients with Herlitz and non-Herlitz junctional EB, respectively, at risk. There are two important con-clusions that can be made. First, the risk of tra-cheolarygeal involvement in junctional EB is confined to early childhood, suggesting a need for careful surveillance for early disease activity within the upper airway during the first 5 years of life in every child with junctional EB. Second, it is clear that both major junctional EB subtypes are at risk, confirm-ing the need for serial observations in non-Herlitz as well as Herlitz patients.

We have similarly employed lifetable analyses to determine cumulative and interval probabilities for the occurrence of several other outcomes of possible clinical importance within each of the major EB sub-types. These outcomes include pseudosyndactyly formation, oesophageal strictures or stenosis and the development of pigmented and non-pigmented skin cancers (Fine *et al.*, 1995a,c,f). Details of many of these findings may be found elsewhere. With regard to malignancies, our analyses revealed for the first time that patients with the Hallopeau–Siemens subtype of recessive dystrophic EB are at risk of developing malignant melanoma, and that this tumour may arise as early as age 4 years in these patients; on or after the age of 12 years the cumulative risk of developing a malignant melanoma is 3.2% in this specific EB subtype (Fine *et al.*, 1995f). In contrast, squamous-cell carcinomas, another tumour which arises only in those EB patients having recessive dystrophic disease, are first detectable on or after the age of 15 years, with cumulative risks in Hallopeau–Siemens disease of 9.1%, 27.0%, 43.6% and 61.6% at ages 20, 25, 30 and 35 years, respectively. These data not only demon-strate the magnitude of risk for this tumour but also emphasize the lack of need for surveillance for squamous-cell carcinoma until the second decade of life. When similar analyses were performed on the risk of death due to squamous-cell carcinoma, the cumulative risks were virtually identical, although offset by 5 years, consistent with the usual time course for death resulting from eventual distant metastases from squamous-cell carcinomas of skin origin (Fine *et al.*, 1995b,e).

Another area in which a large epidemiological database can be of great importance is in the correlations of genotype with phenotype and genotype with specific outcomes of interest. In EB, for example, dozens of different mutations have now been reported in patients affected with simplex, junctional and dystrophic EB. What is as yet unclear is whether the identification of specific mutations in additional patients can be used as a means of improved patient subclassifications. For example, does the presence of a mutation within a specific portion of the type VII collagen gene result in a clinically unique phenotype, such that its identification in a newborn would allow the physician, in the absence of other affected family members within that kindred, to predict the eventual morphologies, distribution and extent of cutaneous involvement that will occur? Of even greater importance, does the presence of a specific mutation imply that the patient is at significantly higher or lower risk of eventually developing severe acral deformities, malignancy, oesophageal stenosis or any of the other major extracutaneous outcomes of clinical relevance? Neither of these latter questions can be reliably answered at the present time, although they can be in the future, once genotypic characterization is performed on a much greater proportion of the enrollees in the National EB Registry, about whom extensive clinical data already have been collected.

Disease impact and quality of life measurements in genetic diseases

As previously discussed, data are lacking on the financial impact of any of the genodermatoses on affected individuals, their families and the American health-care system. The availability of this information will be critical in the near future if adequate allowances are made for third-party coverage of medical expenses in inherited EB, particularly if potentially highly expensive therapies, such as gene therapy, become available. Recently we have attempted to generate preliminary data on the economic impact of EB on patients and their families (Fine *et al.*, 1995d). In so doing, we assessed the extent of different kinds of third-party coverage which have been available to Registry enrollees for a variety of needed services (i.e. in-patient and out-patient medical expenses; medications; nutritional support; medical and surgical supplies and appliances; other). Analyses were controlled for several variables (to include race, educational background of parents and total family income) which might act as confounders. Details of our initial analyses have been published in abstract form recently. In general, we found that patients with inherited EB, especially those with more severe disease activity, have major limitations in both the availability and extent of health-care coverage, and that this may be further influenced by ethnicity or educational background. Although there are many possible explanations to such data, they may suggest inequality in access to health-care coverage or to referral to tertiary centres such as the National EB Registry. Work is now underway to further explore these possible relationships by way of a more detailed survey of our targeted EB study population.

Similarly, data are lacking on the effect of disease, as stratified by EB subtype, on the quality of life in affected patients and their immediate families. This includes but is not limited to considerations of the psychological impact of EB on patients and their relatives, to include various concerns which collectively contribute to global quality of life assessments. For example, data are lacking on the frequency and severity of depression in patients and their families, and on the risk of divorce in parents of affected children. Anecdotally, some EB patients have committed suicide, although data are lacking to assess the frequency and relative relationship, if any, of this event to EB. It is also presumed that major financial resources are rapidly depleted by families having one or more members affected by severe disease, although there are no data to document the magnitude of this likely problem, nor are there data on how such financial burdens may affect the employment status of one or more parents or the educational opportunities (i.e. college or private education) of unaffected siblings. Each of these issues, however, can be rigorously addressed if proper epidemiological techniques are applied to a database which has been so constructed as to include detailed responses on these and other socio-economic concerns.

Summary

Inherited diseases, especially the genodermatoses, pose many challenges to the research community. Recent experience has demonstrated that laboratory tools and techniques are now available to characterize mutational defects at the molecular level in many of these diseases. Despite these major technological breakthroughs, however, it is remarkable that many basic clinical questions have yet to be similarly addressed. It is quite clear that this type of clinically relevant information will be forthcoming only when large cohorts of patients with these rare genetic diseases are systematically identified within the general population and then are critically studied by way of a variety of well-established epidemiological and biostatistical techniques. Such endeavours will likely be best facilitated by the establishment of either additional rare disease registries or equivalent multi-centre projects which can adequately screen a large target population and actively recruit representative participants.

References

Fine, J.D. (1994) International Symposium on Epidermolysis Bullosa. *Journal of Investigative Dermatology*, **103**, 839–843.

Fine, J.D., Daniels, A. & Zeng, L. (1993a) Comparative analysis of the sensitivity and specificity of 19-DEJ-1 and GB3 monoclonal antibodies for diagnosis and subclassification of junctional epidermolysis bullosa subsets. *Journal of Investigative Dermatology*, **100**, 531.

Fine, J.D., Daniels, A., Zeng, L., Cronce, D. & Briggaman, R.A. (1993b) Comparative analysis of the sensitivity and specificity of anchoring fibrils and type VII collagen for diagnosis and subclassification of dystrophic epidermolysis bullosa subsets. *Journal of Investigative Dermatology*, **100**, 532.

Fine, J.-D., Johnson, L.B., Tien, H. *et al.* (1994a) The diversity of cutaneous and extracutaneous findings in epidermolysis bullosa (EB) simplex is a function of severity of disease subtype. *Journal of Investigative Dermatology*, **103**, 847.

Fine, J.-D., Johnson, L.B., Tien, H. *et al.* (1994b) The protean nature of cutaneous manifestations in inherited epidermolysis bullosa — analysis of the frequency of findings by major subtype of disease in a large, well-defined cohort of patients. *Journal of Investigative Dermatology*, **103**, 847.

Fine, J.D., Johnson, L.B. & Suchindran, C.M. (1994c) The National Epidermolysis Bullosa Registry. *Journal of Investigative Dermatology*, **102**, 54S–56S.

Fine, J.D., Johnson, L.B., Tien, H. *et al.* (1994d) The National Epidermolysis Bullosa (EB) Registry — differences in frequencies of selected gastrointestinal manifestations and cancers across major disease types. *Journal of Investigative Dermatology*, **103**, 846.

Fine, J.-D., Johnson, L.B., Tien, H. *et al.* (1995a) Esophageal stenosis and inherited epidermolysis bullosa (EB): cumulative risk, as assessed by lifetable analysis of the National EB Registry dataset. *Journal of Investigative Dermatology*, **104**, 621.

Fine, J.-D., Johnson, L.B., Tien, H. *et al.* (1995b) Premature death and inherited epidermolysis bullosa (EB): cumulative risk, as assessed by lifetable analysis of the National EB Registry dataset. *Journal of Investigative Dermatology*, **104**, 621.

Fine, J.-D., Johnson, L.B., Tien, H. *et al.* (1995c) Pseudo-syndactyly and inherited epidermolysis bullosa (EB): cumulative risk, as determined by lifetable analysis of the National EB Registry dataset. *Journal of Investigative Dermatology*, **104**, 667.

Fine, J.-D., Johnson, L.B., Tien, H. *et al.* (1995d) Socio-economic considerations of inherited epidermolysis bullosa (EB). *Journal of Investigative Dermatology*, **104**, 621.

Fine, J.-D., Johnson, L.B., Tien, H. *et al.* (1995e) Squamous cell carcinoma (SCC) and recessive dystrophic EB of the Hallopeau–Siemens (RDEB-HS) subtype: analysis of the influence of the extracutaneous disease activity, *in vivo* expression of type VII collagen, and race on both presence and number of tumors, and risk of subsequent death. *Journal of Investigative Dermatology*, **104**, 621.

Fine, J.-D., Johnson, L.B., Tien, H. *et al.* (1995f) Squamous cell carcinomas, basal cell carcinomas, and malignant melanomas in inherited epidermolysis bullosa (EB): cumulative risk, as assessed by lifetable analysis of the National EB Registry dataset. *Journal of Investigative Dermatology*, **104**, 620.

Fine, J.-D., Johnson, L.B., Tien, H. *et al.* (1995g) Tracheolaryngeal stenosis and inherited epidermolysis bullosa (EB): cumulative risk, as assessed by lifetable analysis. *Journal of Investigative Dermatology*, **104**, 621.

Fine, J.D., Johnson, L.B., Tien, H. *et al.* (1996) Estimated incidence and prevalence, and lifetable projection of years of life lost by each major epidermolysis bullosa (EB) subtype. *Journal of Investigative Dermatology*, **106**, 893.

Wright, J.T., Fine, J.-D. & Johnson, L.B. (1993) Hereditary epidermolysis bullosa: oral manifestations and dental management. *Pediatric Dentistry*, **15**, 242–248.

Section 2
Skin Cancers

6

Descriptive Epidemiology of Skin Cancers

B.K. ARMSTRONG

Introduction

Epidemiology is the study of the frequency, distribution and determinants of health-related states or events (primarily diseases) in populations and the application of this study to the improvement of health. *Descriptive epidemiology* deals with the frequency and distribution part of this definition.

The fundamental measure of the frequency of diseases in populations is the *incidence rate*. This rate is usually expressed as the number of new cases of the disease per 100 000 of the population per year or, equivalently, per 100 000 person-years. *Mortality rates* (numbers of deaths per 100 000 person-years) have often been used to describe frequency of disease because of unavailability of data on the numbers of new cases. Melanoma incidence, however, has been measured by cancer registries in many countries for many years. In addition, mortality rates reflect trends in survival as well as trends in incidence and may be more difficult to interpret than incidence rates. In describing the distribution of disease, populations are usually subdivided according to a number of common demographic characteristics: sex, age, place of birth, ethnic origin, area of residence, socio-economic status, occupation, etc. Because the incidence of cancer is usually strongly related to age, differences in the age distribution of populations must be taken into account when comparing incidence rates. This is usually done by calculating *age-standardized rates* which, in essence, treat the populations being compared as if they had the same age distribution. Here, age-standardized rates have been used for all comparisons of incidence rates between populations and population subgroups.

This coverage of the descriptive epidemiology of cutaneous melanoma is based, in part, on earlier reviews, especially Armstrong and Kricker (1995) and Armstrong and English (1996).

World burden of melanoma

An estimated 92 000 new cases of invasive melanoma of the skin (hereafter referred to simply as 'melanoma') occurred worldwide in 1985, which represented 1.2% of all new cancers worldwide or 7% of new cancers in men and 8.5% in women in developed countries (Parkin *et al.*, 1993). The increasing incidence of melanoma in populations of European origin has made it, in the USA, the eighth most common cancer in males and the ninth in females (Parkin *et al.*, 1992). In the country with the highest rates in the world, Australia, it is the fourth most common cancer in males, after non-melanocytic skin cancer and cancers of the lung and prostate, and the fourth most common in females, after non-melanocytic skin cancer, cancer of the colon and cancer of the breast (Jelfs *et al.*, 1996).

Incidence patterns

The incidence of melanoma of the skin varies over 100-fold around the world. Among countries included in *Cancer Incidence in Five Continents, Volume VI*, the lowest rates reported around 1983–87 were 0.5 per 100 000 person-years, or less, in parts of Asia (e.g. China, Japan, Singapore, India, Philippines, Thailand) and in Asian and black people in the USA, while the highest were about 27 per 100 000 person-years in the Australian Capital Territory (Parkin *et al.*, 1992); the most recent estimate for Australia as a whole was 34 per 100 000 (Jelfs *et al.*, 1996).

While melanoma incidence increases with increasing proximity to the Equator in many populations

(Armstrong, 1984), this pattern is by no means consistent. In Europe, for example, it is higher in Norway and Sweden than in France, Italy and Spain (Parkin *et al.*, 1992). This anomaly may be due to the tendency for skin colour to increase in darkness with increasing proximity to the Equator in Europe and the influence of intermittent sun exposure from, for example, summer vacations in southern Europe on melanoma risk in populations resident in northern Europe (Armstrong, 1984).

Incidence trends

A comprehensive analysis of trends in melanoma incidence between the early 1960s and about 1987 in 24 populations of mainly European origin (Armstrong & Kricker, 1994) in North America, Europe and New Zealand showed average increases in incidence of between 3 and 7% a year.

In some populations, notably in Scotland (MacKie *et al.*, 1992), Australia (MacLennan *et al.*, 1992; Burton *et al.*, 1993) and New Zealand (Cooke *et al.*, 1992), quite sharp increases were observed in recorded incidence rates in the 1980s, doubling in as short a period as 2 years in some cases. In other populations, such as Norway (Magnus, 1991), the increases have been reported to have become less steep recently and in the population covered by the USA, SEER registry incidence rates actually fell in women and were relatively stable in men in the early 1980s (Scotto *et al.*, 1991). Very recent evidence indicates that both incidence and mortality rates may have stopped rising in Australia (Jelfs *et al.*, 1996; Giles *et al.*, 1996).

In contrast to populations of mainly European origin, there has been no consistent upward or downward trend over the full period from the early 1960s to the late 1980s in populations of mainly non-European origin (Armstrong & Kricker, 1994).

The recent sharp increases in recorded incidence of melanoma in parts of Australia (and evident also in Scotland and New Zealand at least) have excited some attention (Burton *et al.*, 1993; Burton & Armstrong, 1994). These increases lie outside the long-term trend, have been mainly in thin melanoma and have occurred in association with increased public and professional attention to melanoma and parallel sharp increases in the rates of excision of all kinds of skin

lesions. This suggests that they are due, in part at least, to advancement of the time of diagnosis. The absence of a following fall in incidence in one population (Burton *et al.*, 1993), even after a number of years of observation, may indicate that there has also been increasing ascertainment of a form of melanoma which appears innocuous clinically and is unlikely to cause death if not treated (Burton & Armstrong, 1994).

In spite of this possibly artefactual increase in melanoma incidence in some populations in recent years, there seems little doubt that the major long-term trend in incidence rates in populations of European origin has been real. This is because it has been largely mirrored by increases in mortality. The reasons for this increase are not known with any certainty. While increasing recreational sun exposure, or a change from a predominantly occupational to a predominantly recreational pattern of sun exposure, may be the most likely cause (Armstrong & Kricker, 1994), there are few data on population trends in sun exposure that would allow this hypothesis to be examined directly. Indirectly, it gains some support from the lack of increase in melanoma incidence in most populations of mainly non-European origin (including those, such as Americans of African origin, which are intermingled with populations of European origin), the apparent lack of an increase in melanoma of non-exposed sites (e.g. melanoma of the vulva, vagina, anus and rectum; Ragnarsson-Olding *et al.*, 1993; Weinstock, 1993), the comparatively high rates of increase on the trunk and low rates of increase on the face and the lack of any plausible alternative explanation.

Variation by body site

In people of European origin, melanomas occur most frequently on the trunk in males and the lower limbs in females (Green *et al.*, 1993). Lentigo maligna melanoma differs from the other histological types of melanoma in occurring almost exclusively on the head and neck and other habitually exposed surfaces (English *et al.*, 1987).

It is important to note that when the frequency of melanoma by body site is expressed in terms of density per unit area of skin rather than as a simple percentage distribution, a rather different pattern emerges. In a recent Australian study (Green *et al.*, 1993) its highest density in both sexes was on the usually exposed parts of the head and neck; its lowest density was on the rarely exposed sites (buttocks and abdomen in both sexes and scalp in women); its density was low on the usually exposed forearms and backs of hands and sometimes exposed upper arms and lower limbs; and it was intermediate on the sometimes exposed shoulders and back in both sexes and the chest in males. Thus, while the greatest numbers are found on the intermittently exposed back and legs, the greatest density is on the more continuously exposed head and neck.

The anatomical site distribution of melanoma in black people and people of Asian origin is quite different from that in people of European origin. Most melanomas in black and Asian people occur on the soles of the feet (Higginson & Oettlé, 1960; Mori, 1971). This observation, first made among rural black people in Africa, led to speculation that trauma was a cause of melanoma. However, Stevens *et al.* (1990) used US SEER data to show that the excess on the soles in black people, at least in the USA, was a *relative* excess but not an *absolute* excess, since the incidence rate on the soles in black people was no higher than in white.

Recent increases in incidence of melanoma in populations of European origin have been most pronounced on the trunk, particularly in men, while the incidence of melanoma of the face has remained reasonably stable over time (Armstrong & Kricker, 1994). An interesting trend has been reported from Norway. The incidence of melanoma on the breast has increased in young women since a specific code was allocated to this site in response to the advent of topless sunbathing around the end of the 1960s (Magnus, 1991).

In most populations in which it has been studied, incidence of thin melanoma has increased more than incidence of thick melanoma (Armstrong & Kricker, 1994).

Variation by personal characteristics

Age

Unlike many tumours of adults, melanoma occurs frequently among the young and middle aged. The most recent data on the pattern of incidence by age in Australia are shown in Fig. 6.1. In these data, melanoma was very rare before 15 years of age. Thereafter, it climbed steadily and more or less linearly with age in both sexes to 45–49 years of age, with rates a little higher in women than in men. From 50–55 years of age the curves diverged with rates climbing much more steeply in men than in women

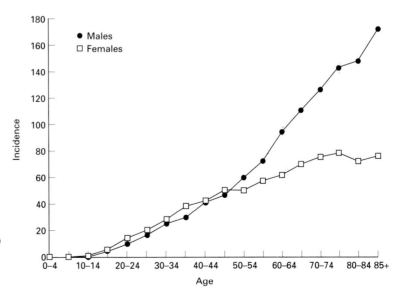

Fig. 6.1 Variation in incidence of melanoma (per 100 000 person-years) with age in males and females in Australia in 1986 to 1990. (After Jelfs *et al.*, 1994a, 1996.)

and more steeply in older men than in younger men. There was a discontinuity in the upward trend between 75–79 and 80–84 years of age in both men and women. There was a similar discontinuity between 45–49 and 50–54 years of age in women only. This pattern is not dissimilar from those in other countries with high rates. For example, the US SEER registries in 1983 to 1987 (Parkin *et al.*, 1992) showed a divergence in rates between men and women from 45 to 49 years of age. However, the rates in US women showed only a 23% increase after 50–54 years of age while those in Australian women increased by 51%.

Patterns of change in incidence with age differ between melanomas on different body sites. On the face, there is a near exponential increase in incidence with increasing age (Magnus, 1981), much as would be expected for a tumour caused by long-term exposure to an environmental agent. On other body sites, the incidence is highest among the middle-aged and falls thereafter (Magnus, 1981). Most, if not all, of the fall in old age may be due to rapid, cohort-based increases in incidence on most of these sites (Magnus, 1981). As noted above, most of the recent increases in incidence have been on sites other than the face.

Sex

The incidence of melanoma tends, generally, to be slightly higher in women than in men. Among 70 registries covering populations of European origin in Europe, North America, Australia and New Zealand (Muir *et al.*, 1987), the average age-standardized incidence rate was 1.0 per 100 000 person-years higher in women (95% confidence interval, assuming normality of rates, 0.60 to 1.37 per 100 000) than in men (Armstrong & English, 1996). As shown in Fig. 6.1, the higher incidence in women occurs mainly during the reproductive period (ages 20–24 to 45–49 years). This difference may be due to a hormone-dependent factor influencing melanoma rates in women of reproductive age (Lee & Storer, 1980). Beyond this period, melanoma rates increase little, if at all, in women while they generally increase throughout life in men. Men generally have thicker melanomas at diagnosis than women (Jelfs *et al.*, 1994b).

Ethnicity

Melanoma is predominantly a disease of populations of European origin. In the USA, for example, melanoma incidence in 1983–87 was some 20-fold higher in white than in black people; the incidence in black people (originally of African origin) was under 1 per 100 000 person-years (Parkin *et al.*, 1992). Rates of melanoma were also very low in populations of Asian origin. For example, in Los Angeles County the incidence rates in people of Japanese, Chinese, Filipino and Korean origin were all near to or below 1 per 100 000 person-years and a tenth or less of those in people of European origin living in the same area.

Among people of European origin there is also evidence of ethnic variation in melanoma incidence. Within Europe, the incidence rates in populations in the south of Italy and Spain in 1983–87 were of the order of 2 per 100 000 person-years (and less than those in more northerly parts of these countries; Parkin *et al.*, 1992) while those in the populations of Denmark, Finland, Norway and Sweden ranged between 6.6 and 13.5 per 100 000. Hispanics (identified as people with Spanish surnames) in Los Angeles had incidence rates between 2 and 3 per 100 000 person-years, while those in other white people were over 11 per 100 000 (Parkin *et al.*, 1992). This is consistent with a general inverse association between skin pigmentations and risk of melanoma.

Country of birth

Migrants who move from areas of low incidence to areas of high incidence with sunny climates, such as Australia, Israel and New Zealand, generally have lower rates of melanoma than the native-born residents of the host countries (see, for example, Khlat *et al.*, 1992). British immigrants to Australia and New Zealand, where the populations are of predominantly British origin, had mortality rates about half those of the native-born residents (Cooke & Fraser, 1985; Khlat *et al.*, 1992); similar differences were observed in incidence rates in Western Australia (Holman *et al.*, 1980). Age at arrival in Australia appeared to be a more powerful predictor of risk than duration of residence (Khlat *et al.*, 1992). Arrival before 10 years of age was associated with no decrease in risk of melanoma relative to that among the Australian-born, but those who arrived after that age had mortality rates of melanoma less than half those in people born in Australia. Similar results were obtained in a study of internal migration within the USA (Mack & Floderus, 1991).

Socio-economic status

Incidence and mortality rates of melanoma are highest among high social classes (Holman *et al.*, 1980; Cooke *et al.*, 1984). Differences in rates among the social classes, imputed from occupation, vary up to twofold. It seems likely that effects of social class are partly (if not wholly) due to differences in behavioural patterns and constitutional risk factors among the various social class groups.

Occupation

An increased incidence of melanoma has been observed in professional or indoor occupations in a number of populations (see, for example, Holman *et al.*, 1980) while both increased and decreased rates of melanoma have been observed in farmers (Fincham *et al.*, 1992). Melanoma on usually exposed body sites such as the head and neck has been reported to be commoner in people who work outdoors (Vågerö *et al.*, 1986) while the opposite was the case for melanoma on occasionally exposed sites.

Previous melanoma

In a population of 14 590 patients with primary melanoma recorded by the New South Wales and Victoria cancer registries in Australia, 496 were recorded with second primary melanomas, 153 diagnosed simultaneously with the first and 343 diagnosed subsequently (Giles *et al.*, 1995). The incidence rate of melanoma in those who had already had one was some 10 times higher than the incidence in those who had never had one. It was estimated that 4.5% of people with a diagnosis of melanoma would develop a second melanoma within 5 years. This probability varied little with age, but was greater in males than females. There was substantial concordance between the site of the first primary and that of the second, especially when on the head and neck or trunk.

Conclusion

Cutaneous melanoma is predominantly a disease of populations of European origin, reaching its highest incidence in Australians, people of mainly European origin who live in a country close to the Equator with high ambient solar radiation. The disease is rare in black people of African origin, other heavily pigmented populations and people of Asian origin. That melanoma incidence is not consistently related to latitude in Europe may be explained by the conflicting trends of increasing ambient solar radiation and increasing skin pigmentation with proximity to the equator.

Melanoma incidence has been increasing in almost all populations of European origin for at least the past 30 years. There is evidence now, however, that this rising trend has come to an end in the USA, Australia and, possibly, some other countries. Recent sharp and substantial increases in melanoma incidence (doubling in some cases) are likely to be due to increasingly early diagnosis of melanoma, or increasing diagnosis of a form of melanoma which appears innocuous clinically and may have been overlooked previously. That melanoma incidence rates have increased little, if at all, in black and Asian populations suggests that the trends in populations of European origins have been largely due to increasing sun exposure.

While melanoma is commonest on the back and legs in populations of European origin, its density of occurrence per unit surface area of skin is greatest on the head and neck. After that, it is most dense on skin which is sometimes exposed to the sun; it is rare on rarely exposed skin. The increasing incidence has mainly affected the trunk. These trends are consistent with an important effect of pattern of sun exposure on incidence of melanoma.

Melanoma incidence begins to increase from about 15 years of age and is generally higher in women before 50 years of age and, thereafter, higher in men. Overall, melanoma incidence is slightly higher in women. Migrants from areas of low to areas of high incidence of melanoma generally have lower rates of melanoma than those born in the country to which they migrate unless they migrate before 10 years of age. Melanoma incidence is higher in people of high socio-economic status than people of low socio-economic status and, generally, higher in people who work indoors than those who work outdoors. Many of these differences may be explicable in terms of differences in sun exposure, particularly pattern of exposure.

People who have had one melanoma have a substantially higher risk of further melanoma than those who have never had a melanoma.

References

Armstrong, B.K. (1984) Melanoma of the skin. *British Medical Bulletin*, **40**, 346–350.

Armstrong, B.K. & English, D.R. (1996) Cutaneous malignant melanoma. In: *Cancer Epidemiology and Prevention* (eds D.R. Schottenfeld and J.F. Fraumeni), pp. 1282–1312, 2nd edn. Oxford University Press, New York.

Armstrong, B.K. & Kricker, A. (1994) Cutaneous melanoma. *Cancer Surveys*, **19**, 219–240.

Armstrong, B.K. & Kricker, A. (1995) Skin cancer. *Dermatologic Clinics*, **13**, 583–594.

Burton, R.C. & Armstrong, B.K. (1994) Recent incidence trends imply a non-metastasizing form of invasive melanoma. *Melanoma Research*, **4**, 107–113.

Burton, R.C., Coates, M.S., Hersey, P. *et al.* (1993) An analysis of a melanoma epidemic. *International Journal of Cancer*, **55**, 765–770.

Cooke, K.R. & Fraser, J. (1985) Migration and death from malignant melanoma. *International Journal of Cancer*, **36**, 175–178.

Cooke, K.R., Skegg, D.C.G. & Fraser, J. (1984) Socio-economic status, indoor and outdoor work, and malignant melanoma. *International Journal of Cancer*, **34**, 57–62.

Cooke, K.R., McNoe, B., Hursthouse, M. & Taylor, R. (1992) Primary malignant melanoma of skin in four regions of New Zealand. *New Zealand Medical Journal*, **105**, 303–306.

English, D.R., Heenan, P.J., Holman, C.D.J. *et al.* (1987) Melanoma in Western Australia in 1981: Incidence and characteristics of histological types. *Pathology*, **19**, 383–392.

Fincham, S.M., Hanson, J. & Berkel, J. (1992) Patterns and risks of cancer in farmers in Alberta. *Cancer*, **69**, 1276–1285.

Giles, G., Staples, M., McCredie, M. & Coates, M. (1995) Multiple primary melanomas: an analysis of cancer registry data from Victoria and New South Wales. *Melanoma Research*, **5**, 433–438.

Giles, G.G., Armstrong, B.K., Burton, R.C., Staples, M.P. &

Thursfield, V.J. (1996) Has melanoma mortality in Australia stopped rising? *British Medical Journal*, **312**, 1122–1125.

Green, A., MacLennan, R., Youl, P. & Martin, N. (1993) Site distribution of cutaneous melanoma in Queensland. *International Journal of Cancer*, **53**, 232–236.

Higginson, J. & Oettle, A.G. (1960) Cancer incidence in the Bantu and 'Cape Colored' races of South Africa: report of a cancer survey in the Transvaal (1953–55). *Journal of the National Cancer Institute*, **24**, 589–671.

Holman, C.D.J., Mulroney, C.D. & Armstrong, B.K. (1980) Epidemiology of pre-invasive and invasive malignant melanoma in Western Australia. *International Journal of Cancer*, **25**, 317–323.

Jelfs, P., Giles, G., Shugg, D. *et al.* (1994a) *Cancer in Australia 1986–1988*. Australian Institute of Health and Welfare, Canberra.

Jelfs, P.L., Giles, G., Shugg, D. *et al.* (1994b) Cutaneous malignant melanoma in Australia, 1989. *Medical Journal of Australia*, **161**, 182–187.

Jelfs, P., Coates, M., Giles, G. *et al.* (1996) *Cancer in Australia 1989–1990 (with projections to 1995)*. Australian Institute of Health and Welfare, Canberra.

Khlat, M., Vail, A., Parkin, M. & Green, A. (1992) Mortality from melanoma in migrants to Australia: Variation by age at arrival and duration of stay. *American Journal of Epidemiology*, **135**, 1103–1113.

Lee, J.A.H. & Storer, B.E. (1980) Excess of malignant melanomas in women in the British Isles. *Lancet*, **ii**, 1337–1339.

Mack, T.M. & Floderus, B. (1991) Malignant melanoma risk by nativity, place of residence at diagnosis, and age at migration. *Cancer Causes and Control*, **2**, 401–411.

MacKie, R., Hunter, J.A.A., Aitchison, T.C. *et al.* (1992) Cutaneous malignant melanoma, Scotland, 1979–89. *Lancet*, **339**, 971–975.

MacLennan, R., Green, A.C., McLeod, G.R.C. & Martin, N.G. (1992) Increasing incidence of cutaneous melanoma in Queensland, Australia. *Journal of the National Cancer Institute*, **84**, 1427–1432.

Magnus, K. (1981) Habits of sun exposure and risk of malignant melanoma: An analysis of incidence rates in Norway 1955–1977 by cohort, sex, age and primary tumor site. *Cancer*, **48**, 2329–2335.

Magnus, K. (1991) The Nordic profile of skin cancer incidence: A comparative epidemiological study of the three main types of skin cancer. *International Journal of Cancer*, **47**, 12–19.

Mori, W. (1971) A geo-pathological study on malignant melanoma in Japan. *Pathology and Microbiology*, **37**, 169–180.

Muir, C.S., Waterhouse, J., Mack, T. *et al.* (1987) *Cancer Incidence in Five Continents, Volume V*. International Agency for Research on Cancer, Lyon.

Parkin, D.M., Muir, C.S., Whelan, S.L. *et al.* (1992) *Cancer*

Incidence in Five Continents, Volume VI. International Agency for Research on Cancer, Lyon.

Parkin, D.M., Pisani, P. & Ferlay, J. (1993) Estimates of the worldwide incidence of eighteen major cancers in 1985. *International Journal of Cancer*, **54**, 594–606.

Ragnarsson-Olding, B., Johansson, H., Rutqvist, L.E. & Ringborg, U. (1993) Malignant melanoma of the vulva and vagina. Trends in incidence, age distribution and long-term survival among 245 consecutive cases in Sweden 1960–1984. *Cancer*, **71**, 1893–1897.

Scotto, J., Pitcher, H. & Lee, J.A.H. (1991) Indications of future decreasing trends in skin melanoma mortality among whites in the United States. *International Journal of Cancer*, **49**, 490–497.

Stevens, N.G., Liff, J.M. & Weiss, N.S. (1990) Plantar melanoma: Is the incidence of melanoma of the sole of the foot really higher in blacks than whites? *International Journal of Cancer*, **45**, 691–693.

Vågerö. D., Ringbäck, G. & Kiviranta, H. (1986) Melanoma and other tumours of the skin among office, other indoor and outdoor workers in Sweden 1961–1979. *British Journal of Cancer*, **53**, 507–512.

Weinstock, M.A. (1993) Epidemiology and prognosis of anorectal melanoma. *Gastroenterology*, **104**, 174–178.

7

Sun Exposure and Skin Cancers

Melanoma and Sun Exposure

J.M. ELWOOD

It is now well established that the predominant cause of cutaneous melanoma is sun exposure, the evidence being best reviewed in the monograph by the International Agency for Research on Cancer which concluded: 'there is sufficient evidence for the carcinogenicity of solar radiation. Solar radiation causes cutaneous malignant melanoma and non melanocytic skin cancer.'

The evidence for this relationship in humans has come from several methods of inquiry. Clinical observation demonstrates that cutaneous melanomas are relatively rare on sun-protected sites on the skin, although they do not show the dominance of incidence on highly exposed sites which is seen for squamous-cell and to a lesser extent basal-cell carcinomas. The body site distribution varies clearly by gender, the differences following differences in exposure related to conventional clothing practices and body hair. Cutaneous melanoma is rare in dark-skinned subjects, and clinical observation, confirmed by later analytical studies, shows that it is most common in subjects with light skin and sensitivity to the acute effects of sun exposure such as sunburn. Geographical epidemiology shows that in relatively homogeneous populations in terms of skin characteristics, melanoma is more frequent at areas closer to the Equator, this being seen, for example, in the approximately fourfold higher rates of melanoma in Australia than in the UK. More careful exploration of melanoma in migrant populations confirms these trends, and shows that the major effect of migration relates to movement around the adolescent years; subjects who moved from the

UK to Australia after adolescence have substantially lower risks of melanoma throughout life, whereas those who moved earlier in childhood adopt rates more similar to the Australian-born population.

These observations led to the hypothesis that melanoma was related to sun exposure, and to the more specific hypothesis of a relationship to intermittent severe exposure on relatively untanned skin, in contrast to the then prevailing opinion on the origins of squamous-cell carcinoma, which was assumed to be closely related to total dose. These hypotheses have been tested in what is now a large number of case-control studies, which have compared melanoma patients and comparison groups in terms of the extent and nature of previous sun exposure. Because of the rarity of the disease, there have been no major cohort or experimental studies of the aetiology of melanoma in humans. The contribution from animal work has been limited because there is no clearly analogous animal model of human melanoma. Melanoma can be induced experimentally in some unusual species, with some very fascinating results, but the direct relevance of these models to humans has to be debated. The assumption that squamous-cell carcinoma has a simple relationship to previous total exposure to sunlight has come under question with more detailed analytical studies and intermittent exposures now appear to have a role for that disease in addition.

We can, therefore, now accept it as established that the cause of most cutaneous melanoma in lightly pigmented human subjects is previous sunlight exposure. Exposure from other sources of ultraviolet radiation is likely to also increase risk.

The details of this relationship, however, are extremely complex. The action spectrum for the production of melanoma in humans in still unknown;

the intensity, duration, frequency and intermittency of the doses received may all affect the outcome. The external dose of ultraviolet radiation is modified by many factors before the biologically effective dose to the target cell is determined. There may be a large number of modifying factors at extracellular, cellular and intracellular levels. There may be a number of different target cells. The effects of ultraviolet radiation may be restricted to those cells directly affected or may also involve systemic effects. Many biological mechanisms may be relevant to the development of melanoma; these may include initiation, promotion and both local and systemic immunosuppressive actions. Ultraviolet radiation is also likely to be involved in the development, progression and transformation of naevi. The time relationships between exposure and biological outcome are likely to be complex and to be different for different biological effects.

In the following three sections, these questions are explored. Elwood and Jopson review the substantial evidence from case-control studies relating cutaneous melanoma, of any body site, to previous sun exposure, concentrating on the differences between the effects of intermittent exposure through leisure and recreational activities, and more regular exposure through occupation. They conclude that in temperate climates, such as Europe and North America, there is good evidence that melanoma risk is increased by intermittent exposure, but risk may be decreased in subjects who have high levels of regular occupational exposure. In areas with much higher levels of solar ultraviolet radiation such as Queensland, these relationships may be different, and the distinction between different exposure patterns is less clear.

Weinstock discusses the issue of local versus systemic effects, which were first hypothesized by Lee and Merrill in a landmark paper which used descriptive and clinical epidemiological observations to suggest that a systemic effect, via an unidentified 'solar circulating factor' could be involved in melanoma production. Weinstock presents data on the occurrence of melanomas at sites which are not directly exposed, such as the soles of the feet, the skin of the vulva, and other internal sites, and demonstrates that the epidemiology of these conditions seems considerably different to that of most cutaneous melanoma, suggesting that the

effects of sun exposure are not, in general, systemic. However, the evidence for purely localized effects is not all that clear, and studies have failed to show a clear relationship between site-specific sunburn and melanoma occurring at that site.

Armstrong reviews the information on the time relationships between sun exposure and melanoma, reviewing the important evidence from the Australian migrant studies, and the growing evidence that naevi are themselves caused by sun exposures and are precursors to at least some melanomas. Recent Australian data show that naevus development relates to sun exposure even in very early childhood. These observations demonstrate the importance of a relatively long time interval between exposure and outcome. However, there is also evidence suggesting short-term effects, with sun exposure relating to the modification of naevi producing junctional activity, and perhaps having a short-term promotional effect on melanoma occurrence.

None of these three reviews presents evidence which leads to a parsimonious single mechanism hypothesis to explain the entire relationship between sun exposure and melanoma occurrence. It seems unlikely that this is possible. It is more likely that there are several important causal chains, each with their own modifying factors and dose and time characteristics. The epidemiological data are particularly weak in giving indications of the action spectrum of ultraviolet radiation in melanoma production. Information on melanoma in relationship to exposure to artificial sources of ultraviolet radiation, which can be more clearly specified in terms of their action spectrum, is helpful in this regard but the evidence is very limited.

Thus we have a complex situation. It is not, however, so complex that conclusions with clinical and public health relevance cannot be made. We can assume with some confidence that most cutaneous melanomas are produced by sun exposure, and that intermittent severe exposure on relatively unacclimatized skin is the most important risk factor, at least in temperate countries. Therefore, reductions in total sun exposure, or in severe intermittent sun exposure, should lead to a reduction in melanoma incidence. There is indeed evidence that the long-term increasing trend of melanoma in some temperate countries is beginning to abate or even reverse in younger adults, which may be due to changes in behaviour over the last 20 or more years as a result of public knowledge and education. In contrast, there is a continuing increasing incidence of melanoma in the highest risk area in Queensland, despite very intensive educational efforts.

The results are sufficiently strong to justify clinical and educational efforts aimed at primary prevention. The limitations to our current understanding, however, show the need for continued research efforts, both to understand the fundamental relationships, and to evaluate critically the results of proposed interventions.

The Role of Different Types of Sun Exposure in the Aetiology of Cutaneous Melanoma

J.M. ELWOOD AND J. JOPSON

Sun exposure and melanoma

The complexity of the dose and time–response relationships between solar exposure and the development of cutaneous melanoma in humans should not be surprising, as sun exposure has a wide range of effects on the skin. Ultraviolet radiation can act as an initiator, a promoter, a co-carcinogen and an immunosuppressive agent. These effects occur after absorption by DNA, or by other chromophores such as melanin or urocanic acid, and may involve the release of free radicals (International Agency for Research on Cancer, 1992). Ultraviolet radiation also stimulates a number of feedback mechanisms which protect the skin against further ultraviolet radiation damage. These include proliferation of melanocytes, increased deposition of melanin in keratinocytes and skin thickening, and may involve both direct effects and effects through the melanocyte stimulating hormone mechanism. Little has been done in animal or experimental systems which helps distinguish the effects of different patterns of sun exposure. Many of the animal models are chosen to exclude some of these processes, such as the use of albino mice, while others have extra mechanisms which humans do not have, such as light activated photorepair systems (International Agency

for Research on Cancer, 1992).

In humans, the risk of cutaneous melanoma has been shown to increase with measures of 'potential' sun exposure, defined as residence in more sunny rather than less sunny places; these results come from case-control studies, geographical studies and, most powerfully, migrant studies. Consistent positive associations have been seen with biological markers which are likely to reflect cumulative sun exposure, such as a history of non-melanocytic skin cancer, actinic tumours or cutaneous microtopographic changes. It should be noted, however, that recent studies of non-melanotic skin cancer cast doubt on the conventional assumption that this disease is simply related to cumulative sun exposure, as associations with intermittent exposure are also important (Kricker *et al.*, 1994, 1995a,b).

Most of the evidence relevant to the effects of different patterns of ultraviolet exposure on the human skin thus comes from epidemiological studies. These are also limited. Epidemiological methods are strongest for comparisons between groups of people who have a major quantitative or qualitative difference in an exposure. The separation of the effects of different types or patterns of exposure to a single (although complex) agent pushes epidemiological methods to their limits. The surprising thing is not that there are still uncertainties about effects of different patterns of sun exposure, but that considerable consistency emerges from the available human evidence.

Studies of melanoma and sun exposure

There have been some 40 published case-control studies of cutaneous melanoma and sun exposure, involving over 11 000 patients with melanoma (Table 7.1). The first was by Lancaster and Nelson in Australia in 1957 (Lancaster & Nelson, 1957). The most important of these were the major studies carried out in the 1970s and 1980s in Canada, Australia (Western Australia and Queensland) and Denmark. These were sufficiently large and sophisticated in data collection and in analysis to have the potential to separate the competing hypotheses of a total dose effect of sun exposure and a specific effect of intermittent exposure, which had been suggested on the basis of descriptive and clinical studies (Elwood & Hislop, 1982; Holman *et al.*, 1983).

Table 7.1 Case-control studies of melanoma assessing sun exposure*.

Reference	Location	Cases (*n*)
Lancaster & Nelson, 1957	Eastern Australia	173
Gellin *et al.*, 1969	New York	79
Beardmore, 1972	Queensland	468
Paffenbarger *et al.*, 1978	Eastern USA	45
Klepp & Magnus, 1979	Norway	78
Adam *et al.*, 1981	England	111
MacKie & Aitchison, 1982	West of Scotland	113
Lew *et al.*, 1983	Boston, USA	111
Rigel *et al.*, 1983	New York, USA	114
Green, 1984; Green *et al.*, 1985	Queensland	183
Elwood *et al.*, 1984, 1985a,b	Western Canada	595
Holman & Armstrong, 1984a,b	Western Australia	511
Brown *et al.*, 1984	New York, USA	74
Graham *et al.*, 1985	Buffalo, USA	404
Sorahan & Grimley, 1985	Birmingham, UK	58
Dubin *et al.*, 1986	New York, USA	1103
Elwood *et al.*, 1986	Nottingham, UK	83
Østerlind *et al.*, 1988a,b; Østerlind, 1990	Eastern Denmark	474
Cristofolini *et al.*, 1987	Trento, Italy	103
Holly *et al.*, 1987	San Francisco, USA	121
Zanetti *et al.*, 1988	Turin, Italy	208
Garbe *et al.*, 1989	Berlin, Germany	200
Weinstock *et al.*, 1989	USA	130
MacKie *et al.*, 1989	Scotland	280
Dubin *et al.*, 1989	New York	289
Beitner *et al.*, 1990	Stockholm, Sweden	523
Elwood *et al.*, 1990	England, Midlands	195
Weiss *et al.*, 1990	Germany	1079
Grob *et al.*, 1990	South-east France	207
Dubin *et al.*, 1990	New York, USA	289
Weinstock *et al.*, 1991	Boston, USA	186
Zanetti *et al.*, 1992	Turin, Italy	260
Zaridze *et al.*, 1992	Moscow, Russia	96
Dunn-Lane *et al.*, 1993	Ireland	100
Herzfeld *et al.*, 1993	New York, USA	324
Autier *et al.*, 1994	Belgium, France and Germany	420
Nelemans *et al.*, 1994	The Netherlands	128
Westerdahl *et al.*, 1994	Sweden	400
White *et al.*, 1994	Washington state	256
Holly *et al.*, 1995	California	452

* Total number of studies = 40. Total number of patients with melanoma = 11 023.

At that time, at least in Canada and Europe, the prevailing medical opinion was against the concept that melanoma could be related to sun exposure, primarily because of the differences in its clinical features, such as site distribution, from non-melanoma skin cancer. Therefore (except possibly in Australia), there was little public knowledge of the issue, and little publicity about the dangers of sun exposure. As a result, these studies were probably less prone to recall bias than subsequent studies. It is now more difficult to be sure that questionnaires on sun exposure result in unbiased answers, because of the high public profile of sun awareness in many countries. It may be that the next set of valuable studies will come from less propagandized areas, such as Eastern Europe, and from countries with different cutaneous characteristics, such as oriental countries.

The available case-control studies vary enormously in their sophistication. Some use questionnaires which would not be sensitive to differences in patterns or timing of sun exposure. There are therefore dangers in oversimplistic reviews which count only the number of positive or negative results, or in meta-analyses based on the least common denominator in terms of questions, which may be so simple as to be uninformative. A more helpful approach is to concentrate on the major studies which have the power to investigate these different effects, as has been done in several major reviews (Elwood, 1992a,b; Elwood & Gallagher, 1993). Studies of sun exposure have also a particular difficulty which is not shared by studies of, for example, smoking or diet, in that the exposure itself is variable. Sun exposure is usually measured in hours of exposure. An hour or exposure at the latitude of, for example, Queensland, Australia, gives about threefold the ultraviolet exposure of an hour of exposure in mid-latitude Europe, and the relative intensities of UVA and of UVB, and the relative importance of average daily compared to peak exposures, differ at different latitudes (Diffey & Elwood, 1993; Elwood & Diffey, 1993).

Case-control studies are efficient in the numbers of subjects required, but have the major disadvantage that the information collected relates to exposure in the past. For melanoma, the pattern of sun exposure several decades before diagnosis is the important factor, yet this will be difficult to ascertain by a retrospective study. Prospective studies, collecting exposure data before disease onset, would be better. The lack of cohort studies is because melanoma, even in high-risk countries, is still in absolute terms a rare disease, and sun exposure is not systematically recorded in any existing database, in the way, for example, that oral contraceptive use can be ascertained from medical records. So it has been impossible, so far, to set up prospective studies. Two of the case-control studies are nested case-control studies within a cohort (Paffenbarger *et al.*, 1978; Weinstock *et al.*, 1991), and have used information collected before disease occurrence, although in one of them, supplementary

information had to be obtained after melanoma occurrence (Weinstock *et al.*, 1991). We should look for opportunities for cohort studies of groups which have characteristics associated with high or low sun exposure. For example, servicemen who served in particularly sunny environments such as the Pacific or the North African desert in the Second World War (a case-control study based on this contrast has been done (Brown *et al.*, 1984)); or, surfers, beach guards or outdoors swimmers in countries like Australia. Groups with less sun exposure include members of religious orders with traditional clothing; this concept has been explored in a descriptive study of different Jewish communities (Gutman *et al.*, 1993). Intervention trials pose even greater logistical problems. Two recent European studies challenge the conventional doctrine that the use of sunscreens should reduce melanoma risk (Autier *et al.*, 1995; Westerdahl *et al.*, 1995). The most satisfactory solution to this would be a randomized trial comparing sunscreens with and without active ingredients, but the logistic and ethical problems of this may be insurmountable. A randomized trial has been used to show that sunscreens reduce the prevalence of solar keratoses in a high-risk population who already have non-melanoma skin cancer (Thompson *et al.*, 1993). Similarly, randomized trials have been mounted to demonstrate the impact of education programmes in reducing sun exposure behaviour (Girgis *et al.*, 1993, 1994) and in children this approach could be combined with a measurement of the frequency of naevi as a biological endpoint, and as an indicator of melanoma risk. Opportunities for ethical trials of sunscreens should be sought; this may be an important method, perhaps the only method in humans, to assess the wavelength dependence or other characteristics of melanoma.

Intermittent exposure

Of the 40 published case-control studies, 20 involving over 7000 patients have published results assessing one or more factors which can be considered to represent intermittent exposure. Of these 20 studies, 14 show substantial and/or significant positive associations with measures of intermittent exposure (Fig. 7.1). The measures used have been recreational or vacation exposure, either in general or related to specific activities such as outdoor sports or sunbathing.

Five of the remaining six studies show no major association, and only one study shows a significant protective effect of intermittent exposure. Thus there is reasonably consistent evidence for a positive association with intermittent sun exposure. Positive results have been reported from several recent detailed studies carried out in Europe. Of particular interest is the strong positive result seen in an Italian study (Zanetti *et al.*, 1992), as some previous work had raised the question of whether Italian residents, who are generally not very sun sensitive, might be protected against intermittent exposure (Cristofolini *et al.*, 1987). However, a recent large study with population-based controls in Sweden did not show any significant positive association with measures such as frequency of sunny holidays (Westerdahl *et al.*, 1994), although other studies in Scandinavian countries have shown increased risks with intermittent exposure.

Another major study not showing an association with intermittent sun exposure was that in Queensland (Green *et al.*, 1986), suggesting that the distinction between different patterns of exposure may not apply at very high sun exposure levels. The very detailed study carried out in Western Australia (Holman *et al.*, 1986) showed positive associations with some, but not all, measures of intermittent exposure, and its results suggest that in that situation with very high overall sun exposure levels, activities such as swimming or sunbathing, which might be expected to be associated

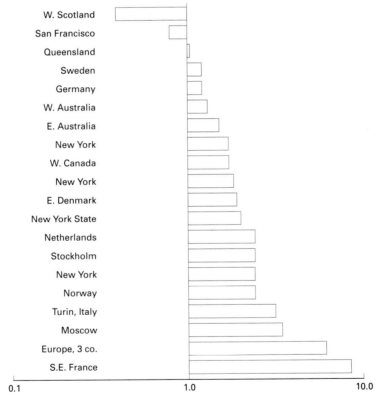

Fig. 7.1 Relative risks (log scale) for intermittent exposure from different studies.
Key to studies: W. Scotland (MacKie & Aitchison, 1982); San Francisco (Holly *et al.*, 1995); Queensland (Beardmore, 1972); Sweden (Westerdahl *et al.*, 1994); Germany (Weiss *et al.*, 1990); W. Australia (Holman *et al.*, 1986); E. Australia (Lancaster & Nelson, 1957); New York (Dubin *et al.*, 1986); W. Canada (Elwood *et al.*, 1985b); New York (Dubin *et al.*, 1990); E. Denmark (Østerlind *et al.*, 1988b); New York State (Herzfeld *et al.*, 1993); Netherlands (Nelemans *et al.*, 1994); Stockholm (Beitner *et al.*, 1990); New York (Rigel *et al.*, 1983); Norway (Klepp & Magnus, 1979); Turin, Italy (Zanetti *et al.*, 1988); Moscow (Zaridze *et al.*, 1992); Europe, 3 co. (Autier *et al.*, 1994); S.E. France (Grob *et al.*, 1990). (From J.M. Elwood (1996) Melanoma and sun exposure. *Seminars in Oncology*.)

with the maximum sun exposure, are not accompanied by an increased risk, while those which may have less severe sun exposure, such as boating or fishing, do show an increase.

Occupational exposure

Assessing the same studies in terms of occupational exposure shows a much more varied pattern (Fig. 7.2). Four of the studies show a significant increase in risk with occupational exposure and a further five show a non-significant increased risk. In contrast, four studies show significant reductions in risk and a further five show non-significant reductions in risk. However, the more detailed studies suggest that there may be a pattern if particularly high levels of exposure can be identified. In the western Canada study, which overall shows a non-significant reduced risk of 0.9, there is a significantly reduced risk for the maximum exposure

category in males, but an increased risk with moderate amounts of sun exposure, which is likely to be related to short-term or seasonal employment (Elwood *et al.*, 1985b). This suggests that short-term or irregular occupational exposure may increase risk, while long-term continued exposure may reduce risk. This mixed overall pattern may explain the inconsistent results from many other studies which do not assess the topic in enough detail. Of other detailed studies, significant protective effects of high levels of occupational exposure are seen in the major Swedish (Westerdahl *et al.*, 1994) and Danish (Østerlind *et al.*, 1988b) studies, and, at least in regard to superficial spreading melanoma, in the Western Australia study (Holman *et al.*, 1986). The most detailed study showing a strong positive association with outdoor occupation is that of Zanetti *et al.* (1988) in Italy.

A recent large study in the USA (White *et al.*, 1994) shows a decreased risk (non-significant) with

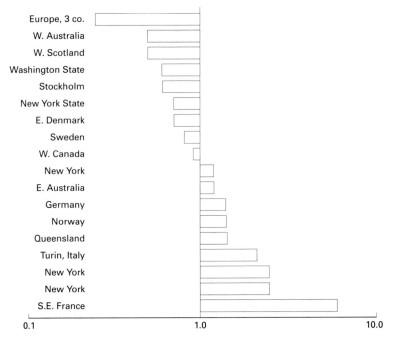

Fig. 7.2 Relative risks (log scale) for occupational exposure from different studies.
Key to studies: Europe 3 co. (Autier *et al.*, 1994); W. Australia (Holman *et al.*, 1986); W. Scotland (MacKie & Aitchison, 1982); Washington State (White *et al.*, 1994); Stockholm (Beitner *et al.*, 1990); New York State (Herzfeld *et al.*, 1993); E. Denmark (Østerlind *et al.*, 1988b); Sweden (Westerdahl *et al.*, 1994); W. Canada (Elwood *et al.*,

1985b); New York (Rigel *et al.*, 1983); E. Australia (Lancaster & Nelson, 1957); Germany (Weiss *et al.*, 1990); Norway (Klepp & Magnus, 1979); Queensland (Beardmore, 1972); Turin, Italy (Zanetti *et al.*, 1988); New York (Dubin *et al.*, 1990); New York (Dubin *et al.*, 1986); S.E. France (Grob *et al.*, 1990). (From J.M. Elwood (1996) Melanoma and sun exposure. *Seminars in Oncology*.)

occupational exposure, but this was assessed as a proportion of total exposure, which raises a difficulty as this proportion could be raised either by increased occupational exposure, or by a relative decrease in other forms of outdoor exposure, making it particularly difficult to interpret. So perhaps the most useful of the new results is that from the large European study (Autier *et al.*, 1994); with a useful definition, having 30 years or more in an outdoor occupation, and in an analysis adjusted for host factors, this showed a significant decrease in melanoma risk, with a relative risk of 0.25.

Contrasts between intermittent and occupational exposure

For each of the 17 studies giving results for both intermittent and occupational exposure, we can assess the ratio of the risk ratios for intermittent

compared to occupational exposure. This is a crude approach because the different measures may not be comparable, and in many studies there are several different measures which could be chosen; but the results are interesting (Fig. 7.3). Some of these studies used hospital-based control groups, which included or totally consisted of patients with skin diseases or other cancers, and these are particularly difficult to interpret. For these studies, the ratios of intermittent to chronic exposure measures are close to 1. In these seven studies, the average relative risk (weighted by the number of subjects in each study), for measures of occupational exposure, was around 1.9, and the average for measures of intermittent exposure was about 1.5. Thus the effects of intermittent and of chronic exposure are not distinct. However, for the studies with a control group drawn from the community, or a hospital control group which excludes patients with skin diseases or other cancers, the ratios

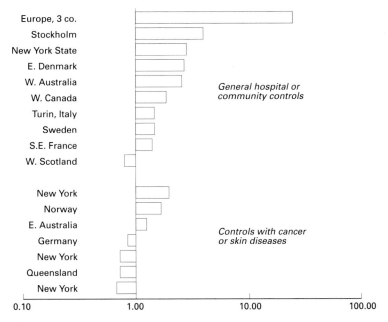

Fig. 7.3 Relative risks (log scale) for ratio of intermittent to occupational exposure from different studies.
Key to studies: Europe, 3 co. (Autier *et al.*, 1994); Stockholm (Beitner *et al.*, 1990); New York State (Herzfeld *et al.*, 1993); E. Denmark (Østerlind *et al.*, 1988b); W. Australia (Holman *et al.*, 1986); W. Canada (Elwood *et al.*, 1985b); Turin, Italy (Zanetti *et al.*, 1988); Sweden (Westerdahl *et al.*, 1994); S.E. France (Grob *et al.*, 1990); W. Scotland (MacKie & Aitchison, 1982); New York (Rigel *et al.*, 1983); Norway (Klepp & Magnus, 1979); E. Australia (Lancaster & Nelson, 1957); Germany (Weiss *et al.*, 1990); New York (Dubin *et al.*, 1990); Queensland (Beardmore, 1972); New York (Dubin *et al.*, 1986). (From J.M. Elwood (1996) Melanoma and sun exposure. *Seminars in Oncology.*)

of intermittent to chronic exposure measures tend to be larger. The weighted average odds ratio for intermittent exposure was 2.7, and for occupational exposure was 1.0, although for each of these there is a considerable range.

The major studies which have appropriate control groups are thus reasonably consistent in showing positive associations with measures of intermittent exposure, but do not show any regular association with occupational exposure. This conclusion is supported by the meta-analysis of published studies conducted by Nelemans *et al.* (1993) which did not include some of the more recent studies mentioned here, and also by the preliminary results of a detailed meta-analysis using the original data which is being carried out on several of the major studies under the auspices of the IMAGE International Epidemiology Group (Coldman & Gallagher, 1993).

The conclusion is that we can support the positive association between melanoma and intermittent exposure, certainly in regard to moderate incidence areas such as Europe and North America. Because the results are more mixed in the Western Australian study and there is no clear distinction between occupational and recreational exposure reported from Queensland, this situation may be different in countries with particularly high levels of sun exposure. On the other hand, overall there is no consistent association with occupational exposure, but several studies show protective effects in those subjects with very high occupational exposure levels.

Total sun exposure

One would predict from this that the association with total sun exposure is likely to be inconsistent. Some studies have reported on total sun exposure without attempting to separate chronic from intermittent exposures, and other studies have reported on the two components, without attempting to look at total exposure. For the set of studies which have reported on total exposure, there is little consistency (Fig. 7.4). The results vary from strong positive effects reported from Queensland and France, to a significant negative effect reported in a recent major case-control study from Washington state. This study is methodologically strong, although it uses a rather complex estimate of sun exposure (White *et al.*, 1994). One analysis is based on having more than 500 hours' yearly exposure in the 10 years before diagnosis, a measure of heavy total exposure, and this shows no significant effect. The other results are based on a 'sun exposure index', which is estimated from the number of days per year spent in the sun, with adjustment for clothing habits, and shows significantly reduced risk of melanoma, for

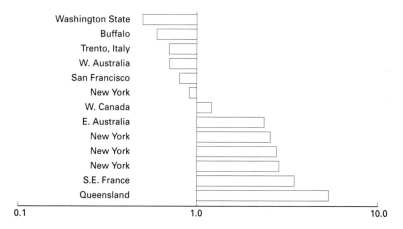

Fig. 7.4 Relative risks (log scale) for total sun exposure from different studies.
Key to studies: Washington State (White *et al.*, 1994); Buffalo (Graham *et al.*, 1985); Trento, Italy (Cristofolini *et al.*, 1987); W. Australia (Holman *et al.*, 1986); San Francisco (Holly *et al.*, 1995); New York (Dubin *et al.*,

1986); W. Canada (Elwood *et al.*, 1985b); E. Australia (Lancaster & Nelson, 1957); New York (Rigel *et al.*, 1983); New York (Dubin *et al.*, 1990); New York (Gellin *et al.*, 1969); S.E. France (Grob *et al.*, 1990); Queensland (Green, 1984). (From J.M. Elwood (1996) Melanoma and sun exposure. *Seminars in Oncology.*)

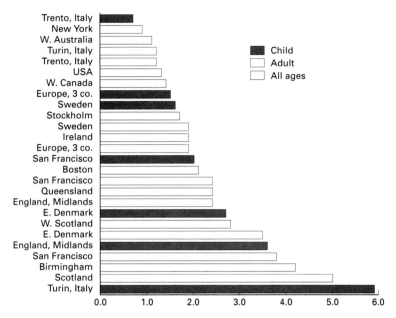

Fig. 7.5 Relative risks (arithmetic scale) for sunburn from different studies.
Key to studies: Trento, Italy (Cristofolini *et al.*, 1987); New York (Dubin *et al.*, 1990); W. Australia (Holman *et al.*, 1986); Turin, Italy (Zanetti *et al.*, 1992); Trento, Italy (Cristofolini *et al.*, 1987); USA (Weinstock *et al.*, 1989); W. Canada (Elwood *et al.*, 1985a); Europe, 3 co. (Autier *et al.*, 1994); Sweden (Westerdahl *et al.*, 1994); Stockholm (Beitner *et al.*, 1990); Sweden (Westerdahl *et al.*, 1994); Ireland (Dunn-Lane *et al.*, 1993); Europe, 3 co. (Autier *et al.*, 1994); San Francisco (Holly *et al.*, 1995); Boston (Lew *et al.*, 1983); San Francisco (Holly *et al.*, 1995); Queensland (Green *et al.*, 1985); England, Midlands (Elwood *et al.*, 1990); E. Denmark (Østerlind *et al.*, 1988b); W. Scotland (MacKie & Aitchison, 1982); E. Denmark (Østerlind *et al.*, 1988b); England, Midlands (Elwood *et al.*, 1990); San Francisco (Holly *et al.*, 1987); Birmingham (Sorahan & Grimley, 1985); Scotland (MacKie *et al.*, 1989); Turin, Italy (Zanetti *et al.*, 1992). (From J.M. Elwood (1996) Melanoma and sun exposure. *Seminars in Oncology.*)

exposure both at ages 2–10 years and at ages 11–20 years. It is debatable whether this should be regarded as a measure of total or of intermittent exposure, and the negative effect seen is a result different from any reported before; no other major studies show a protective effect of high levels of sun exposure in childhood and adolescence. Another recent US study (Holly *et al.*, 1995) also shows a weak negative trend, for a variable of total weekday exposure, which could be interpreted as total or as occupational sun exposure.

Sunburn

The other variable which has been commonly assessed is a history of sunburn. Nearly all studies show positive associations, often strong and significant (Fig. 7.5). In many studies the association with the history of sunburn is stronger than the association with other measures of intermittent sun exposure. But this is difficult to interpret. A stronger association with one factor than with another may mean that one association is the stronger biological relationship, but it also may occur because that factor has been recorded with less random error, which may be because it is easier to recall. Most of the epidemiological studies have used definitions of quite severe sunburn, such as sunburns severe enough to cause blistering, or pain lasting at least 2 days. This would be an easily remembered event, even from many years previously. In contrast, a question on the extent of sunbathing during holidays, or the degree of participation in outdoor sports at various ages, would be open to a considerably larger degree of random error. Sunburn is likely to be simply a good indicator of excessive acute sun exposure, rather than having any specific direct role in melanoma causation. As such, it can legitimately be used as a target for educational activities and an indicator for their evaluation.

Recent studies have assessed sunburn in considerable detail, and the European three countries study and the Italian study both suggest the greatest increased risk with sunburn in childhood or adolescence (Zanetti *et al.*, 1992; Autier *et al.*, 1994), while in the Swedish study (Westerdahl *et al.*, 1994) the strongest association was with sunburn after the age of 19 years; no clear distinction by age was seen in San Francisco (Holly *et al.*, 1995). No association was seen in the two other recent studies, but in these, a rather simple question was used with much less detail. A recent critical review of the literature on sunburn concludes that attempts to assess differences between the effects of sunburn at different ages have been inadequate, and challenges the conclusion that sunburn confers a greater risk when experienced in early life (Whiteman & Green, 1994).

Effects of skin sensitivity

There is a considerable variability in skin response to acute ultraviolet radiation, as measured by tanning response and minimal erythemal dose. Some studies have shown that the increased risks of melanoma associated with sun exposure are higher in those with high sun sensitivity. This is usually assessed by questions on tendency to burn easily, or to tan, on first exposure to strong sunshine in the summer, often referred to, loosely, as 'skin type'. A higher risk in sun-sensitive subjects was reported from studies in New York, which were however very limited in the data collected (Dubin *et al.*, 1989) (Table 7.2). More convincing results came from the Nurses' Health Study in terms of frequency of swimsuit wearing, although this study has quite small numbers (Weinstock *et al.*, 1991). However, in the western Canada study, with a larger number of cases, there was no consistent association between measures of intermittent or chronic exposure and tanning ability except that the presence of an all-year round tan was associated with a sub-

Table 7.2 Relative risk of melanoma with sun exposure for 'sun-sensitive' and 'sun-resistant' subjects.

Reference	Cases (*n*)	Measure of sun exposure	Relative risk compared to low exposure		Ratio sensitive/ resistant	Statistical significance*
			Sun-sensitive	Sun-resistant		
Dubin *et al.*, 1989	272	High occupational exposure	5.52	1.24	4.45	
		High recreational exposure	2.82	1.13	2.50	
		High total exposure	4.41	1.75	2.52	
		Severe sunburn ever	1.87	0.46	4.07	*
Weinstock *et al.*, 1991	122	High recreational exposure	3.50	0.30	11.67	*
Elwood, 1992a	591	High occupational exposure	0.93	1.02	0.91	
		Max. risk occupational exposure	1.43	1.91	0.75	
		High recreational exposure	1.90	1.36	1.40	
		High vacation exposure	1.44	1.67	0.86	
		Childhood sunburn history	0.60	1.22	0.49	
		All-year-round tan	0.95	0.42	2.26	*
White *et al.*, 1994	239	High total exposure, age 2–10 years	0.88	0.30	2.93	*
		High total exposure, age 11–20 years	1.55	0.31	5.00	*
Cress *et al.*, 1995	337	History of sunburns before age 12 years	1.90	2.70	0.70	
		History of sunburns, high-school age	1.30	2.60	0.50	

* Indicates significant difference in risks at $P < 0.05$.

stantially reduced risk in those who tan readily, but no change in risk in those who did not tan readily (Elwood, 1992a). More recently, the large study in Washington state, which used a measure of total sun exposure in childhood and in teenage years, has shown a significantly reduced risk of melanoma with higher total sun exposure in those who tanned readily, but no significant effect in those who tanned poorly (White *et al.*, 1994). In contrast, in the San Francisco study (Cress *et al.*, 1995), the increased risk of superficial spreading melanoma seen with sunburn was more marked in subjects who tanned easily without burning, than in those who tended to burn easily. Thus the empirical evidence does not show a consistent pattern of risks between greater exposure in sun-sensitive subjects.

Dose–response models

The results reviewed above show that the biologically effective dose of ultraviolet radiation received from intermittent exposure is higher than that received from chronic exposure. The explanation presumably relates to the balance between the direct carcinogenic or other detrimental effects of ultraviolet radiation, and the feedback mechanisms by which ultraviolet radiation stimulates pigmentation and epithelial thickening which reduces the epidermal transmissibility of ultraviolet, or confers protection in other ways. Further exploration will have to assess different body sites individually which has not been done to date, primarily because of limitations in numbers and in detail in the studies. Different body sites may be at different points in the spectrum of acute damage versus chronic protection.

The idea of variation in the effect of sun exposure by tanning ability is intuitively attractive, and has been built into hypothetical models of the overall dose–response relationship. An early model assumed an increase in risk with intermittent exposure followed by a decrease with constant exposure, and a greater effect in sun-sensitive individuals (Holman *et al.*, 1986). A later model added a third upward wave, primarily because of the Australian data at very high exposure levels which suggested that there was a further increase in risk. Armstrong has recently presented a further model, which separates the three components of total dose, pattern of dose and skin type, assuming

that risk in those with intermittent exposure rises with total dose, while with regular exposure it may initially fall and then rise (Armstrong, 1994). Empirical results in at least a partially quantitative form come from the western Canada study, which show an increase in risk in association with either intermittent or small amounts of occupational exposure up to a dose range which is approximately equal to the amount of exposure expected from recreational exposure at peak times during a summer 2-week holiday (Elwood, 1992a; Elwood *et al.*, 1985b). Then at higher dosages, there is a split between high risks continuing with higher dosages if these are achieved by intermittent exposure, and risk falling with high dosages if these are achieved by occupational exposure, the risks coming back towards the null value. Males at the maximum occupational dose show a lower melanoma risk compared to the lowest occupational exposure category.

All these models are based on whole-body exposure, whereas it is likely that different body sites have different previous exposure patterns and therefore may be at different points in any model. Differences in body-site exposure may be the explanation for the rather curious result from the western Canada study which demonstrated that the extra risk conferred by intermittent recreational exposure was seen equally strongly in those with very heavy occupational exposure as well as those with no occupational exposure, although it would be expected on all these models that the occupational exposure would protect against risks of recreational exposure (Elwood, 1992a).

Conclusion

Epidemiological studies have taken us a considerable way in understanding the aetiology of cutaneous melanoma in light-skinned people. There is no doubt that exposure to the sun is the predominant cause, although it does not explain all cases of cutaneous melanoma, and clearly does not explain malignant melanoma occurring in other sites. In moderate incidence countries such as most of Europe and North America, with urbanized populations, the major influence tending to increase the risk of cutaneous melanoma is intermittent sun exposure, achieved through recreational and vacation activities. The opportunities for such exposure have increased greatly since the Second World War, with more leisure time and more opportunities for outdoor activities and for travel. There is substantial evidence that long-term regular occupational exposure, characteristic of traditional occupations such as farming, produces a decrease in melanoma risk. This suggests that the various methods the body has to protect itself against increased external ultraviolet radiation are successful when exposed to that radiation on a long-term regular basis, but an intermittent pattern of exposure can deliver a greater carcinogenic dosage because the protective mechanisms are not fully developed and maintained. Sunburn represents the cutaneous reaction to an acute overexposure to ultraviolet radiation, and its strong association with subsequent melanoma risk is probably a reflection of its role as an indicator of severe intermittent exposure, rather than there being any direct aetiological role of sunburn.

These results have considerable implications for public education programmes. They suggest that these programmes will be effective if they produce a reduction in severe intermittent exposures. Programmes which put great emphasis on the use of ultraviolet blocking sun lotions may fail to achieve this if the behavioural change which they produce is increased recreational and vacational sun exposure, made possible by the use of sunscreens to reduce the risk of acute sunburn. A programme which has a broader message to reduce total sun exposure, by changing patterns of outdoor exposure, use of clothing and shade, with use of sunscreens only as part of that overall message, may ultimately be more successful. There needs to be stringent evaluation of programmes, looking at the behavioural changes they produce, ultimately at the changes in melanoma incidence, and also at intermediate biological endpoints such as the frequency of sunburn or the prevalence of naevi.

Acknowledgements

This chapter is based on: J.M. Elwood (1996) Melanoma and sun exposure. In: *Seminars in Oncology: Malignant Melanoma* (ed. E.F. McClay) by permission of Grune and Stratton, Philadelphia.

This work has been supported by the Cancer Research Trust, Private Bag 1965, Dunedin, and by the Cancer Society of New Zealand.

References

Adam, S.A., Sheaves, J.K., Wright, N.H., Mosser, G., Harris, R.W. & Vessey, M.P. (1981) A case-control study of the possible association between oral contraceptives and malignant melanoma. *British Journal of Cancer*, **44**, 45–50.

Armstrong, B.K. (1994) The epidemiology of melanoma: Where do we go from here? In: *Epidemiological Aspects of Cutaneous Malignant Melanoma* (eds R.P. Gallagher & J.M. Elwood), pp. 307–323. Kluwer Academic Publishers, Boston.

Autier, P., Doré, J., Lejeune, F. *et al.* for the EORTC Malignant Melanoma Cooperative Group (1994) Recreational exposure to sunlight and lack of information as risk factors for cutaneous malignant melanoma. Results of a European Organization for Research and Treatment of Cancer (EORTC) case-control study in Belgium, France and Germany. *Melanoma Research*, **4**, 79–85.

Autier, P., Doré, J., Schifflers, E. *et al.* for the EORTC Malignant Melanoma Cooperative Group (1995) Melanoma and use of sunscreens: an EORTC case-control study in Germany, Belgium and France. *International Journal of Cancer*, **61**, 749–755.

Beardmore, G.L. (1972) The epidemiology of malignant melanoma in Australia. In: *Melanoma and Skin cancer* (ed. W.H. McCarthy), pp. 39–63. Government Printer, Sydney.

Beitner, H., Norell, S.E., Ringborg, U., Wennersten, G. & Mattson, B. (1990) Malignant melanoma: aetiological importance of individual pigmentation and sun exposure. *British Journal of Dermatology*, **122**, 43–51.

Brown, J., Kopf, A.W., Rigel, D.S. & Friedman, R.J. (1984) Malignant melanoma in World War II veterans. *International Journal of Dermatology*, **23**, 661–663.

Coldman, A.J. & Gallagher, R.P. (1993) Re-analysis of four epidemiologic studies of malignant melanoma. *Melanoma Research*, **3**, 59.

Cress, R.D., Holly, E.A. & Ahn, D.K. (1995) Cutaneous melanoma in women. V. Characteristics of those who tan and those who burn when exposed to summer sun. *Epidemiology*, **6**, 538–543.

Cristofolini, M., Franceschi, S., Tasin, L. *et al.* (1987) Risk factors for cutaneous malignant melanoma in a northern Italian population. *International Journal of Cancer*, **39**, 150–154.

Diffey, B.L. & Elwood, J.M. (1993) Tables of ambient solar ultraviolet radiation for use in epidemiological studies of malignant melanoma and other diseases. In: *Epidemiological Aspects of Malignant Melanoma* (eds R.P. Gallagher & J.M. Elwood). Kluwer Academic Press, Basle.

Dubin, N., Moseson, M. & Pasternack, B.S. (1986) Epidemiology of malignant melanoma: pigmentary traits, ultraviolet radiation, and the identification of high risk populations. In: *Epidemiology of Malignant Melanoma: Recent Results in Cancer Research* (ed. R.P. Gallagher), pp. 56–75. Springer-Verlag, Berlin.

Dubin, N., Moseson, M. & Pasternack, B.S. (1989) Sun exposure and malignant melanoma among susceptible individuals. *Environmental Health Perspectives*, **81**, 139–151.

Dubin, N., Pasternack, B.S. & Moseson, M. (1990) Simultaneous assessment of risk factors for malignant melanoma and non-melanoma skin lesions, with emphasis on sun exposure and related variables. *International Journal of Epidemiology*, **19**, 811–819.

Dunn-Lane, J., Herity, B., Moriarty, M.J. & Conroy, R. (1993) A case control study of malignant melanoma. *Irish Medical* Journal, **86**, 57–59.

Elwood, J.M. (1992a) Melanoma and sun exposure: contrasts between intermittent and chronic exposure. *World Journal of Surgery*, **16**, 157–166.

Elwood, J.M. (1992b) Melanoma and ultraviolet radiation. *Clinics in Dermatology*, **10**, 41–50.

Elwood, J.M. & Diffey, B.L. (1993) A consideration of ambient solar ultraviolet radiation in the interpretation of studies of the aetiology of melanoma. *Melanoma Research*, **3**, 113–122.

Elwood, J.M. & Gallagher, R.P. (1993) Sun exposure and the epidemiology of malignant melanoma. In: *Epidemiological Aspects of Cutaneous Malignant Melanoma* (eds R.P. Gallagher & J.M. Elwood). Kluwer Academic Press, Basle.

Elwood, J.M. & Hislop, T.G. (1982) Solar radiation in the etiology of cutaneous malignant melanoma in Caucasians. *National Cancer Institute Monographs*, **62**, 167–171.

Elwood, J.M., Gallagher, R.P., Hill, G.B., Spinelli, J.J., Pearson, J.C.G. & Threlfall, W. (1984) Pigmentation and skin reaction to sun as risk factors for cutaneous melanoma: Western Canada Melanoma Study. *British Medical Journal*, **288**, 99–102.

Elwood, J.M., Gallagher, R.P., Davison, J. & Hill, G.B. (1985a) Sunburn, suntan and the risk of cutaneous malignant melanoma: the Western Canada Melanoma Study. *British Journal of Cancer*, **51**, 543–549.

Elwood, J.M., Gallagher, R.P., Hill, G.B. & Pearson, J.C.G. (1985b) Cutaneous melanoma in relation to intermittent and constant sun exposure: The Western Canada Melanoma Study. *International Journal of Cancer*, **35**, 427–443.

Elwood, J.M., Williamson, C. & Stapleton, P.J. (1986) Malignant melanoma in relation to moles, pigmentation, and exposure to fluorescent and other lighting sources. *British Journal of Cancer*, **53**, 65–74.

Elwood, J.M., Whitehead, S.M., Davison, J., Stewart, M. & Galt, M. (1990) Malignant melanoma in England: risks associated with naevi, freckles, social class, hair colour, and sunburn. *International Journal of Epidemiology*, **19**, 801–810.

Garbe, C., Krüger, S., Stadler, R., Guggenmoos-Holzmann, I. & Orfanos, C.E. (1989) Markers and relative risk in a German population for developing malignant melanoma. *International Journal of Dermatology*, **28**, 517–523.

Gellin, G.A., Kopf, A.W. & Garfinkel, L. (1969) Malignant melanoma: a controlled study of possibly associated factors. *Archives of Dermatology*, **99**, 43–48.

Girgis, A., Sanson-Fisher, R.W., Tripodi, D.A. & Golding, T. (1993) Evaluation of interventions to improve solar protection in primary schools. *Health Education Quarterly*, **20**, 275–287.

Girgis, A., Sanson-Fisher, R.W. & Watson, A. (1994) A workplace intervention for increasing outdoor workers' use of solar protection. *American Journal of Public Health*, **84**, 77–81.

Graham, S., Marshall, J., Haughey, B. *et al.* (1985) An inquiry into the epidemiology of melanoma. *American Journal of Epidemiology*, **122**, 606–619.

Green, A. (1984) Sun exposure and the risk of melanoma. *Australasian Journal of Dermatology*, **25**, 99–102.

Green, A., Siskind, V., Bain, C. & Alexander, J. (1985) Sunburn and malignant melanoma. *British Journal of Cancer*, **51**, 393–397.

Green, A., Bain, C., McLennan, R. & Siskind, V. (1986) Risk factors for cutaneous melanoma in Queensland. In: *Epidemiology of Malignant Melanoma: Recent Results in Cancer Research* (ed. R.P. Gallagher), pp. 76–97. Springer-Verlag, Berlin.

Grob, J.J., Gouvernet, J., Aymar, D. *et al.* (1990) Count of benign melanocytic nevi as a major indicator of risk for nonfamilial nodular and superficial spreading melanoma. *Cancer*, **66**, 387–395.

Gutman, M., Inbar, M., Klausner, J.M. & Chaitchik, S. (1993) Malignant melanoma in different ethnic groups in Israel. Incidence and biologic behaviour. *Cancer*, **71**, 2746–2750.

Herzfeld, P.M., Fitzgerald, E.F., Hwang, S. & Stark, A. (1993) A case-control study of malignant melanoma of the trunk among white males in Upstate New York. *Cancer Detection and Prevention*, **17**, 601–608.

Holly, E.A., Kelly, J.W., Shpall, S.N. & Chiu, S. (1987) Number of melanocytic nevi as a major risk factor for malignant melanoma. *Journal of the American Academy of Dermatology*, **17**, 459–468.

Holly, E.A., Aston, D.A., Cress, R.D., Ahn, D.K. & Kristiansen, J.J. (1995) Cutaneous melanoma in women. I. Exposure to sunlight, ability to tan, and other risk factors related to ultraviolet light. *American Journal of Epidemiology*, **141**, 923–933.

Holman, C.D.J. & Armstrong, B.K. (1984a) Cutaneous malignant melanoma and indicators of total accumulated exposure to the sun: An analysis separating histogenetic types. *Journal of the National Cancer Institute*, **73**(1), 75–82.

Holman, C.D.J. & Armstrong, B.K. (1984b) Pigmentary traits, ethnic origin, benign nevi, and family history as risk factors for cutaneous malignant melanoma. *Journal of the National Cancer Institute*, **72**, 257–266.

Holman, C.D.J., Armstrong, B.K. & Heenan, P.J. (1983) A theory of the etiology and pathogenesis of human cutaneous malignant melanoma. *Journal of the National Cancer Institute*, **71**, 651–656.

Holman, C.D.J., Armstrong, B.K. & Heenan, P.J. (1986) Relationship of cutaneous malignant melanoma to individual sunlight-exposure habits. *Journal of the National Cancer Institute*, **76**, 403–414.

International Agency for Research on Cancer (1992) *IARC Monographs on the Evaluation of Carcinogenic Risks to Humans; Ultraviolet Radiation*, Vol. 55. IARC, Lyon.

Klepp, O. & Magnus, K. (1979) Some environmental and bodily characteristics of melanoma patients. A case-control study. *International Journal of Cancer*, **23**, 482–486.

Kricker, A., Armstrong, B.K. & English, D.R. (1994) Sun exposure and non-melanocytic skin cancer. *Cancer Causes and Control*, **5**, 367–392.

Kricker, A., Armstrong, B.K., English, D.R. & Heenan, P.J. (1995a) A dose–response curve for sun exposure and basal cell carcinoma. *International Journal of Cancer*, **60**, 482–488.

Kricker, A., Armstrong, B.K., English, D.R. & Heenan, P.J. (1995b) Does intermittent sun exposure cause basal cell carcinoma? A case-control study in Western Australia. *International Journal of Cancer*, **60**, 489–494.

Lancaster, H.O. & Nelson, J. (1957) Sunlight as a cause of melanoma: a clinical survey. *Medical Journal of Australia*, **i**, 452–456.

Lew, R.A., Sober, A.J., Cook, N., Marvell, R. & Fitzpatrick, T.B. (1983) Sun exposure habits in patients with cutaneous melanoma: a case control study. *Journal of Dermatologic Surgery and Oncology*, **9**, 981–986.

MacKie, R.M. & Aitchison, T. (1982) Severe sunburn and subsequent risk of primary cutaneous malignant melanoma in Scotland. *British Journal of Cancer*, **46**, 955–960.

MacKie, R.M., Freudenberger, T. & Aitchison, T.C. (1989) Personal risk-factor chart for cutaneous melanoma. *Lancet*, **ii**, 487–490.

Nelemans, P. *et al.* (1993) Cutaneous melanoma and sunlight exposure: an attempt to meta-analyse the results of case-control studies. *Melanoma Research*, **3**, 59.

Nelemans, P.J., Rampen, F.H.J., Groenendal, H., Kiemeney, L.A.L.M., Ruiter, D.J. & Verbeek, A.L.M. (1994) Swimming and the risk of cutaneous melanoma. *Melanoma Research*, **4**, 281–286.

Østerlind, A. (1990) Malignant melanoma in Denmark: occurrence and risk factors. *Acta Oncologica*, **29**, 1–22.

Østerlind, A., Hou-Jensen, K. & Jensen, O.M. (1988a) Incidence of cutaneous malignant melanoma in Denmark 1978–1982. Anatomic site distribution, histologic types, and comparison with non-melanoma skin cancer. *British Journal of Cancer*, **58**, 385–391.

Østerlind, A., Tucker, M.A., Stone, B.J. & Jensen, O.M. (1988b) The Danish case-control study of cutaneous malignant melanoma. II. Importance of UV-light exposure. *International Journal of Cancer*, **42**, 319–324.

Paffenbarger, R.S.J., Wing, A.L. & Hyde, R.T. (1978) Characteristics in youth predictive of adult-onset malignant lymphomas, melanomas, and leukemias: brief communication. *Journal of the National Cancer Institute*, **60**, 89–92.

Rigel, D.S., Friedman, R.J., Levenstein, M.J. & Greenwald, D.I. (1983) Relationship of fluorescent lights to malignant melanoma: another view. *Journal of Dermatologic Surgery and Oncology*, **9**, 836–838.

Sorahan, T. & Grimley, R.P. (1985) The aetiological significance of sunlight and fluorescent lighting in malignant melanoma: a case-control study. *British Journal of Cancer*, **52**, 765–769.

Thompson, S.C., Jolley, D. & Marks, R. (1993) Reduction of solar keratoses by regular sunscreen use. *New England Journal of Medicine*, **329**, 1147–1151.

Weinstock, M.A., Colditz, G.A., Willett, W.C. *et al.* (1989) Nonfamilial cutaneous melanoma incidence in women associated with sun exposure before 20 years of age. *Pediatrics*, **84**, 199–204.

Weinstock, M.A., Colditz, G.A., Willett, W.C. *et al.* (1991) Melanoma and the sun: the effect of swimsuits and a 'healthy' tan on the risk of nonfamilial malignant melanoma in women. *American Journal of Epidemiology*, **134**, 462–470.

Weiss, J., Garbe, C., Bertz, J. *et al.* (1990) Risikofaktoren für die Entwicklung maligner Melanome in der Bundesrepublik Deutschland. *Hautarzt*, **41**, 309–313.

Westerdahl, J., Olsson, H. & Ingvar, C. (1994) At what age do sunburn episodes play a crucial role for the development of malignant melanoma? *European Journal of Cancer*, **30A**, 1647–1654.

Westerdahl, J., Olsson, H., Måsbäck, A., Ingvar, C. & Jonsson, N. (1995) Is the use of sunscreens a risk factor for malignant melanoma? *Melanoma Research*, **5**, 59–65.

White, E., Kirkpatrick, C.S. & Lee, J.A.H. (1994) Case-control study of malignant melanoma in Washington state. 1. Constitutional factors and sun exposure. *American Journal of Epidemiology*, **139**, 857–868.

Whiteman, D. & Green, A. (1994) Melanoma and sunburn. *Cancer Causes and Control*, **5**, 564–572.

Zanetti, R., Rosso, S., Faggiano, F., Roffino, R., Colonna, S. & Martina, G. (1988) Étude cas–témoins sur le mélanome de la peau dans la province de Torino, Italie. *Revue d'Epidemiologie et de Sante Publique*, **36**, 309–317.

Zanetti, R., Franceschi, S., Rosso, S., Colonna, S. & Bidoli, E. (1992) Cutaneous melanoma and sunburns in childhood in a southern European population. *European Journal of Cancer*, **28A**, 1172–1176.

Zaridze, D., Mukeria, A. & Duffy, S.W. (1992) Risk factors for skin melanoma in Moscow. (Letter) *International Journal of Cancer*, **52**, 159–161.

Melanoma: Childhood or Lifelong Sun Exposure

B.K. ARMSTRONG

Introduction

The time in life that sun exposure is important in causing melanoma has both biological and preventive implications. From the biological point of view, knowing when sun exposure occurs in relation to when the melanoma that causes occurs can tell us whether it has an *early* or *late stage* effect (Vainio *et al.*, 1992) and, thus, whether its effects may be by way of initiating mutations in melanocytes or by promoting the progression of mutated melanocytes towards melanoma, or both. From the preventive point of view, if it could be shown that the risk of melanoma associated with a particular amount of sun exposure were greater in one period of life than another, this would assist greatly in targeting prevention programs.

Present evidence suggests that sun exposure in childhood is particularly important in causing melanoma and there is also some, generally indirect, evidence that sun exposure near to time of diagnosis of melanoma may also increase its risk. There are few data that suggest a special relationship between melanoma and sun exposure in any other period of life.

Sun exposure in childhood is particularly important in causing melanoma

Evidence from studies of migrants

People who migrate from the UK, an area of low sun exposure, to Australia, an area of high sun exposure, before about 15 years of age have a similar lifetime risk of melanoma as people (mainly of British origin) born in Australia (Table 7.3). People who migrate to Australia from the UK after 15 years of age have about a one-third of the lifetime risk of melanoma experienced by those born in Australia. Stated simply, living in Australia during the first 15 years contributes about two-thirds to the lifetime risk of melanoma of a lifelong resident of Australia. Similar results were obtained in a study of migration to Southern California

from less sunny parts of the United States (Mack & Floderus, 1991). Thus childhood exposure to the sun appears to be particularly important in causing melanoma.

Two other explanations should be considered for these observations. First, it may be that there is an environmental factor other than sun exposure that explains the large difference in incidence of melanoma (approximately sixfold) between Australia and the UK. However, no such environmental factor is currently known. Second, it may be that those who migrate to Australia in childhood have a lifetime pattern of sun exposure which is similar to that in those born in Australia, while those who migrate in late teenage or adulthood expose themselves, on average, much less than do their Australian-born peers. There are currently no data by which this possibility could be evaluated. It seems unlikely, however, that the level of exposure could be sufficiently less to produce one-third the incidence of melanoma.

Assuming that sun exposure in childhood is really of special importance in contributing to lifetime risk of melanoma there are several ways that this effect might be realized. First, incidence of melanoma may bear a power relationship to time since first exposure to the sun. Because exposure to the sun begins at birth and continues throughout life the form of its relationship to melanoma may be similar to that between amphibole asbestos exposure and mesothelioma. This kind of asbestos, once inhaled, remains in the body for the rest of life (i.e. there is lifelong exposure from the time of first exposure). Peto *et al.* (1982) showed that lifetime risk of mesothelioma was related to time since first exposure raised to the power 3.2. In practice this meant that a person exposed first at 20 years of age had about a 17% lifetime risk, at 30 years an 8% risk and at 40 years a 3% risk. Thus, a 20-year delay in beginning exposure to asbestos reduced the risk of mesothelioma to under one-fifth of what it would otherwise have been.

Second, there may be some special susceptibility to carcinogenic effects of sun exposure in childhood. While there is no need to argue that this is so, the relationship of prevalence of naevi to age and the role of naevi as precursors to melanoma provide the basis for such an effect.

Table 7.3 Relative risks of melanoma in Australia according to age at arrival of immigrants as estimated by analyses based on incident cases in Western Australia (Holman & Armstrong, 1984) and national mortality data (Khlat *et al.*, 1992).

Authors	Country of origin of migrants	Age at arrival in Australia (years) (relative risks and 95% CI)			
		Birth	<15	15–29	>30
Holman & Armstrong, 1984	All countries	1.00	0.89 (0.44–1.80)	0.34 (0.16–0.72)	0.30 (0.08–1.13)
Khlat *et al.*, 1992	England	1.00	0.86 (0.73–1.00)	0.42 (0.34–0.52)	0.32 (0.28–0.34)
	Rest of UK and Ireland	1.00	0.74 (0.57–0.97)	0.48 (0.36–0.64)	0.36 (0.24–0.39)

Evidence from studies of naevi

The number of melanocytic naevi a person has is the strongest measurable predictor, after age and ethnic origin, of their risk of melanoma. It is likely, also, that some if not most melanomas have their origin in melanocytic naevi (Elder *et al.*, 1981).

The prevalence of one or more naevi on the skin increases from about 1% at birth to near 100% by the teenage years in populations of European origin. A person's complement of naevi is probably achieved by about 15 years of age and the density per unit surface area of the skin reaches a plateau after about 9 years of age (Nicholls 1973; English & Armstrong, 1994). Thus, while questions remain about the turnover of naevi in adult life, particularly in people with dysplastic naevi (Halpern *et al.*, 1993), it seems reasonable to conclude that childhood is the most important time of life for the development of new naevi. It follows then, given the importance of naevi as determinants of risk of melanoma, that childhood events that determine number of naevi are very important in determining lifetime risk of melanoma.

What are these events? Present evidence points to sun exposure as the main environmental determinant of number of naevi (see Chapter 10). Thus, an effect of sun exposure in childhood on risk of subsequent melanoma may be mediated, at least in part, by its effect in increasing the number of precursor naevi.

Evidence from case-control studies of sun exposure

Risk of melanoma is consistently and quite strongly related to a past history of one or more sunburns (Armstrong & English, 1996). It is often stated, also, that sunburn in childhood is especially important in increasing risk of melanoma. To evaluate the evidence for this statement, all case-control studies of melanoma published up to the end of 1992 in which sunburn was recorded were reviewed and measures of sunburn classified according to whether they related to early life (generally under 20 years of age), adult life (generally over 20 years of age) or the whole of life (Table 7.4). Altogether, 27 measures of history of sunburn were reported in 18 studies. Most of those relating to early life (80%) and the whole of life (91%) were significantly associated ($P < 0.05$) with melanoma; only one of six (17%) associations with measures in adult life were so associated. When a similar review of measures of recreational exposure to the sun was carried out, there was little difference between the proportions positive in adult life and early life (Table 7.4), but few studies had measures specific to these periods of life.

Thus, sunburn in early life may be a more potent cause of melanoma than sunburn in adult life. This would, in any case, be expected from the data in migrants and need have nothing special to say about sunburn *per se*.

Table 7.4 Observations in case-control studies of associations between measures of sunburn and recreational sun exposure at different times of life and risk of melanoma.

Type and time reference of exposure	Associations reported (*n*)	Percentage significantly positive
Sunburn		
All measures	27	67
Whole of life	11	91
Early life	10	80*
Adult life	6	17
Recreational sun exposure		
All measures	30	63
Whole of life	23	65
Adult life	3	67
Early life	4	50

* $P = 0.05$ for difference from proportion positive in adult life.

Sun exposure near to the time of diagnosis may also influence risk of melanoma

Evidence from fluctuations in ambient solar irradiance

Two studies show descriptive evidence of a peak in melanoma incidence following periods of probable increased UV irradiance at the surface of the earth.

Houghton *et al.* (1978) reported that incidence of melanoma in Connecticut and New York state varied cyclically in phase with, but peaking 2 years after, variation in sunspot activity. A similar pattern was observed in data from Finland, without the 2-year lag, but not in Norway. Sunspots are associated with increases in cosmic radiation entering the stratosphere. Cosmic radiation depletes stratospheric ozone and thus may increase ambient UV radiation at the surface of the earth.

Using a different model, Swerdlow (1979) found that year-by-year variations in melanoma incidence in males and females in England and Wales were significantly correlated one with the other, and that incidence in females was significantly correlated with the average daily hours of bright sunshine 2 years before. Incidence in males was positively correlated with hours of sunshine in this period, but not significantly so.

Evidence from seasonal variation in melanoma and naevi

The diagnosis of melanoma peaks in spring and summer and reaches a trough in winter (Schwartz *et al.*, 1987). While this pattern could indicate a very short latency effect of sun exposure on melanoma occurrence, it is more plausibly explained by behavioural factors — melanomas being more likely to be seen, and therefore presented for diagnosis, in warmer weather.

This explanation would probably stand except for some additional observations. First, seasonal variation is not confined to melanoma on sites usually clothed in the winter, it is seen also in melanomas on the head and neck (Schwartz *et al.*, 1987). Second, seasonal variation also occurs in excision of naevi, and naevi excised during spring and summer are more likely to show inflammation and regression than naevi excised during less sunny periods (Armstrong *et al.*, 1984). This may suggest that sun exposure is increasing the probability of malignant change in naevi (and may have a similar effect on more advanced lesions). Finally, melanomas diagnosed on exposed body sites in summer were found to have a higher mean proliferation fraction (2.60 with standard error of the mean (S.E.) 0.48) than those on non-exposed sites (1.29, S.E. 0.57) and those diagnosed in winter (1.80, S.E. 0.39, on exposed sites and 1.49, S.E. 0.52, on non-exposed sites; Fleming *et al.*, 1991).

Mixed evidence from case-control studies

There is an almost complete lack of any evidence from case-control studies that usual total sun exposure near to the time of diagnosis of melanoma has materially increased its risk (Armstrong & English, 1996). However, Klepp and Magnus (1979) in Norway found a moderate association with sunbathing holidays in southern Europe in the preceding 5 years (relative risk 2.4, 95% confidence interval 1.0–5.8) and Grob *et al.* (1990) found a strong association with outdoor leisure exposure in the past 2 years (relative risk 8.4, 95% confidence interval 3.6–19.7).

Conclusion

The epidemiological evidence is consistent with the view that sun exposure beginning in childhood gives rise to the first mutational step in the development of melanoma. This step may be visibly represented by a melanocytic naevus. Because of the need for further, probably also mutational steps, the earlier in life the initial mutation occurs, the higher the probability that a melanoma will result from it.

Sun exposure at any age stimulates proliferation of melanocytes, most likely as a response to DNA damage (Morpugo *et al.*, 1980). This proliferative stimulus in already mutated melanocytes, lacking the capacity to protect themselves against further mutation, may promote the late stages in development of melanoma. The epidemiological evidence for such an effect, however, is both indirect and weak.

References

Armstrong, B.K. & English, D.R (1996) Cutaneous malignant melanoma. In: *Cancer Epidemiology and Prevention* (eds D.R. Schottenfeld and J.F. Fraumeni), pp. 1282–1312, 2nd edn. Oxford University Press, New York.

Armstrong, B.K., Heenan, P.J., Caruso, V., Glancy, R.J. & Holman, C.D.J. (1984) Seasonal variation in the junctional component of pigmented naevi. *International Journal of Cancer*, **34**, 441–442.

Elder, D., Greene, M.H., Bondi, E.E. *et al.* (1981) Acquired melanocytic nevi and melanoma. The dysplastic nevus syndrome. In: *Pathology of Malignant Melanoma* (ed. A.B. Ackerman), pp. 185–215. Masson, New York.

English, D.R. & Armstrong, B.K. (1994) Melanocytic nevi in children. I. Anatomic sites and demographic and host factors. *American Journal of Epidemiology*, **139**, 390–401.

Fleming, M.G., Swan, L.S. & Heenan, P.J. (1991) Seasonal variation in the proliferation fraction of Australian common nevi. *American Journal of Dermatopathology*, **13**, 463–466.

Grob, J.J., Gouvernet, J., Aymar, D. *et al.* (1990) Count of benign melanocytic nevi as a major indicator of risk for nonfamilial nodular and superficial spreading melanoma. *Cancer*, **66**, 387–395.

Halpern, A.C., Guerry, Du P. IV, Elder D.E. *et al.* (1993) Natural history of dysplastic nevi. *Journal of the American Academy of Dermatology*, **29**, 51–57.

Holman, C.D.J. & Armstrong, B.K. (1984) Pigmentary traits, ethnic origin, benign naevi and family history as risk factors for cutaneous malignant melanoma. *Journal of the National Cancer Institute*, **72**, 257–266.

Houghton, A., Munster, E.W. & Viola, M.V. (1978) Increased incidence of malignant melanoma after peaks of sunspot activity. *Lancet*, **i**, 759–760.

Khlat, M., Vail, A., Parkin, M. & Green, A. (1992) Mortality from melanoma in migrants to Australia: Variation by age at arrival and duration of stay. *American Journal of Epidemiology*, **135**, 1103–1113.

Klepp, O. & Magnus, K. (1979) Some environmental and bodily characteristics of melanoma patients. A case-control study. *International Journal of Cancer*, **23**, 482–486.

Mack, T.M. & Floderus, B. (1991) Malignant melanoma risk by nativity, place of residence at diagnosis, and age at migration. *Cancer Causes and Control*, **2**, 401–411.

Morpugo, G., Porro, M.N., Passi, S. & Fanelli, C. (1980) The role of UV light in the control of melanogenesis. *Journal of Theoretical Biology*, **83**, 247–254.

Nicholls, E.M. (1973) Development and elimination of pigmented moles, and the anatomical distribution of primary malignant melanoma. *Cancer*, **32**, 191–195.

Peto, J., Seidman, H. & Selikoff, J.J. (1982) Mesothelioma mortality in asbestos workers: implications for models of carcinogenesis and risk assessment. *British Journal of Cancer*, **45**, 125–135.

Schwartz, S.M., Armstrong, B.K. & Weiss, N.S. (1987) Seasonal variation in the incidence of cutaneous malignant melanoma — An analysis by body site and histologic type. *American Journal of Epidemiology*, **126**, 104–111.

Swerdlow, A.J. (1979) Incidence of malignant melanoma of the skin in England and Wales and its relationship to sunshine. *British Medical Journal*, **ii**, 1324–1327.

Vainio, H., Magee, P.N., McGregor, D.B. & McMichael, A.J. (eds) (1992) *Mechanisms of Carcinogenesis in Risk Identification.* International Agency for Research on Cancer, Lyon.

Melanoma: Site-Specific or Systemic Effect of Sun Exposure?

M.A. WEINSTOCK

Humans frequently wear clothing while outdoors. On these occasions, some areas of the skin are largely shielded from solar radiation while others are directly exposed. This chapter discusses whether the melanomas that arise due to sun exposure indeed arise as a result of direct exposure of the primary site to the sun, or whether a systemic (generalized whole-body) effect of sun exposure plays an important role.

Systemic effects of sun exposure are biologically

plausible. In response to local ultraviolet irradiation, both local and systemic immune suppression has been experimentally observed (Kripke, 1984). Other evidence in humans has linked immunosuppression to melanoma risk, although based on the scarce available data, the magnitude of this association appears quite modest (Bouwes Bavinck *et al.*, 1996). However, alternative mechanisms may explain a systemic effect, including a potential systemic melanocytic activation induced by ultraviolet rays (Stierner *et al.*, 1989).

Analytical epidemiology

Analytical studies have not focused on linking the site of sun exposure to the site of melanoma, perhaps because the former is rather difficult to measure, and the validity of such measures can be called into question. This is particularly true for case-control studies, where the relevant exposures may have occurred decades earlier. Two types of approach have been tried. One sought to compare the site of the melanoma to the sites which had been sunburned. It is known that susceptibility to sunburn varies by anatomical site, hence interpretation of associations may be difficult (Olson *et al.*, 1966). Nevertheless, no site-specific association was noted with this approach (Green *et al.*, 1986).* The second approach compares the site of the melanoma to the sites protected from intense sun exposure. This approach has taken advantage of the fact that swimsuits are worn during particularly intense sun exposures, and that among women, swimsuits of different styles vary substantially in the areas of skin they protect from the sun. Furthermore, the style of swimsuit worn may be more accurately recalled than other measures of site-specific sun exposure. Inquiries regarding style of swimsuit worn at ages 15–24 years were included in the now classic study of Holman and colleagues in Western Australia (Holman *et al.*, 1986). They observed that women who reported wearing bikinis during that period were at a 13-fold higher risk of melanoma of the trunk than those who reported wearing one-piece swimsuits with

---

*After this chapter was accepted for publication, a case-control study was published which suggested an association between site of sunburn and site of subsequent melanoma (Chen *et al.*, 1996)

a high backline, i.e. on or above the shoulder blades. This magnitude of relative risk was several times greater than other observed relative risks for sun-related factors, and had a broad confidence interval (from 2 to 84). A second study of this association was based upon inquiries into swimsuit styles of nurses in the United States when they were 15–20 years of age (Weinstock *et al.*, 1991). This study noted a relative risk of 0.8 for women who wore bikinis compared to those who wore one-piece swimsuits with high backlines. The 95% confidence interval, however, was also broad (0.3–2.6), and did have a small interval of overlap with the confidence interval of the prior study. The estimated relative risk for melanoma at any site among women who wore bikinis was 1.8 (95% confidence interval 0.9–3.5) in the later study.

Descriptive epidemiology

The descriptive epidemiology of melanoma provides more insights into this issue than the limited data from case-control studies. Basal and squamous-cell carcinoma of the skin are widely accepted as largely due to the direct effects of sun exposure on the skin at the site of exposure. In light-skinned populations, the vast majority of both of these tumour types occur on the face (Scotts *et al.*, 1983), yet the same is not true of melanoma. Indeed, melanoma is most common on the trunk, and among women, on the legs, both sites which are less frequently exposed to the sun than the face (Østerlind *et al.*, 1988).

This observation regarding the site distribution of melanoma was used more than 25 years ago to support the hypothesis that there exists a 'solar circulating factor', inducible by sunlight in exposed skin, that travels throughout the body to increase melanoma risk in both exposed and unexposed areas (Lee & Merrill, 1970). However, other explanations may be entertained. Specifically, a large body of evidence has accumulated to suggest that, at least in temperate climates, intense intermittent exposure is particularly effective in the induction of melanoma when compared to more frequent, less intense exposures (Elwood, 1992) (see Chapter 7, pp. 50–62). When outdoors, the face is generally exposed, whereas the trunk is more typically exposed only when the sun is relatively intense, e.g. in summer at the beach. Hence, although the face may have greater cumulative exposure, the trunk would have more intense exposures on non-acclimated (perhaps untanned; Weinstock *et al.*, 1991) skin, hence relatively high incidence of melanoma.

Numerous studies of secular and cohort trends in melanoma incidence by site have now been published. The general observation over the past several decades is that melanomas on the face have changed relatively little in frequency, but that there has been an explosive increase of melanomas on the trunk and, among women, on the extremities, particularly the lower extremity (Houghton *et al.*, 1980; Magnus, 1981; Thörn *et al.*, 1990; Dennis *et al.*, 1993; Armstrong & Kricker, 1994). If the overall increase in melanoma incidence is due to a systemic effect of sun exposure, the substantial differences among anatomical sites would not be expected. Alternatively, the increasing recreational sun exposures over this time period may be expected to have led to more intermittent intense exposure to the trunk, and therefore to the observed pattern. A notable exception to the above pattern involves Queensland, an area relatively close to the Equator that has extremely high melanoma incidence. Incidence increased substantially there during the 1980s (MacLennan *et al.*, 1992), yet the proportional increase did not differ substantially by site (Green *et al.*, 1993).

Among the various reports of melanoma frequency by body site are several that express frequency in proportion to the skin surface area at that site (Elwood & Lee, 1975; Magnus, 1981; Elwood & Gallagher, 1983; Pearl & Scott, 1986; Østerlind *et al.*, 1988; Green *et al.*, 1993). Two of these are particularly notable for describing recent population-based incidence data that more precisely identify anatomical site of melanoma. The report from the very high incidence area of Queensland demonstrates clear evidence of high incidence in sites receiving intense (although not necessarily intermittent) sun exposure, and low incidence in areas not frequently exposed (see Fig. 7.6). These data are also notable for revealing striking gender differences. Sun protection by gender-specific patterns of hair styles is indicated by the fourfold higher incidence of ear and neck melanomas among men and the even greater disparity of scalp melanoma, despite relatively similar incidence of facial melanoma. Sun protection by gender-specific patterns of clothing

are suggested by the approximately twofold increased risk among men of melanoma on the chest, abdomen and back, in contrast to the opposite trend on the lower extremities and upper arms (but not forearms) (see Fig. 7.6) (Green *et al.*, 1993). The second report derives from Denmark, a relatively low incidence area, but describes generally similar patterns (see Fig. 7.7) (Østerlind *et al.*, 1988).

Melanoma at anatomical sites rarely or never sun exposed

Further insight may be gleaned from examination of the incidence of melanoma at anatomical sites which are consistently sun protected. If the effect of sun exposure is systemic, trends at these sites should parallel those observed for exposed sites. However, there should be no relation of incidence at these sites to general sun exposure if the effect of exposure is completely site-specific. Some data are available regarding incidence trends at two rarely or never exposed cutaneous sites: the sole of the foot and the vulvar skin. Overall, melanoma incidence is quite low among non-Caucasian groups, whether of Asian or African origin (Parkin *et al.*, 1992). Among these groups, the sole of the foot is typically the most common site of melanoma. Other melanomas in these groups tend to occur on the palms, nailbeds and mucous membranes (Giraud *et al.*, 1975; Suseelan & Gupta, 1977; Seiji *et al.*, 1983; Collins, 1984; Crowley *et al.*, 1991; Hudson & Krige, 1995). This difference among races is due to the almost total lack of melanomas on sun-exposed skin of dark-skinned individuals; there appears to be no substantial variation in incidence of plantar melanoma among the races (Stevens *et al.*, 1990). Furthermore, while melanoma has been increasing substantially among whites in recent decades, there has been no substantial increase among blacks, again consistent with the hypothesis that incidence is rising only for melanomas on sun-exposed areas (Ries *et al.*, 1994).

Direct estimates of sun exposure in vulvar melanoma patients compared to controls are not available. However, an analysis of vulvar melanoma incidence in Sweden over a 25-year period revealed a steady decline in incidence rate, despite large increases in incidence of sun-related cutaneous melanoma overall (Thörn *et al.*, 1990; Ragnarsson-Olding *et al.*, 1993).

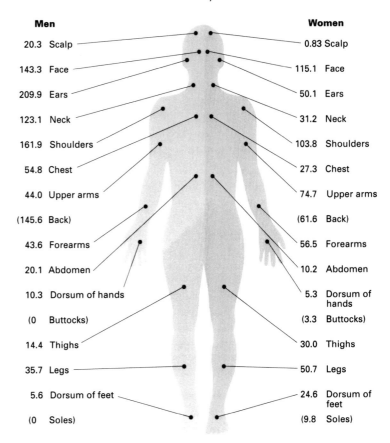

Men		Women
20.3	Scalp	0.83 Scalp
143.3	Face	115.1 Face
209.9	Ears	50.1 Ears
123.1	Neck	31.2 Neck
161.9	Shoulders	103.8 Shoulders
54.8	Chest	27.3 Chest
44.0	Upper arms	74.7 Upper arms
(145.6	Back)	(61.6 Back)
43.6	Forearms	56.5 Forearms
20.1	Abdomen	10.2 Abdomen
10.3	Dorsum of hands	5.3 Dorsum of hands
(0	Buttocks)	(3.3 Buttocks)
14.4	Thighs	30.0 Thighs
35.7	Legs	50.7 Legs
5.6	Dorsum of feet	24.6 Dorsum of feet
(0	Soles)	(9.8 Soles)

Fig. 7.6 Age and surface area-adjusted incidence of invasive malignant melanoma by anatomical site in Queensland, Australia, 1987 (Green *et al.*, 1993).

In the United States, no change in incidence was noted over a 15-year period despite substantial increases in overall melanoma incidence (Ries *et al.*, 1994; Weinstock, 1994). The American study did note that vulvar melanoma was more common among the white than the black people, but the observed relative risk (2.6; 95% confidence interval 1.2–6.0) was substantially less than the observed relative risk for melanoma overall. Furthermore, the vulvar melanomas were more common in the northern United States than in the south, the opposite of expectation if melanoma incidence were substantially related to a systemic effect of sun exposure (Weinstock, 1994).

Limited incidence data are available for melanomas arising on certain mucosal sites, including the anorectal, vaginal, oral and nasal mucosa. These data are derived from population-based cancer registration in approximately 10% of the US population. No significant racial gradient was observed for any of these sites, although modest racial differences could not be excluded due to small numbers of cases of these rare tumours among minority races. There was an increase over 19 years in the incidence of nasal melanoma, but no secular trend was observed for anorectal, vaginal or oral melanoma. Nasal and anorectal melanomas were more common in northern latitudes, however. Oral melanoma was more common in the south, and no significant latitude gradient could be documented for vaginal melanoma (Weinstock, 1993, 1994; Chiu & Weinstock, 1996).

Conclusion

Early observations regarding the differences in anatomical distribution of melanomas compared to sun-induced basal and squamous-cell carcinomas of the skin resulted in speculation regarding possible increased systemic susceptibility to melanoma in-

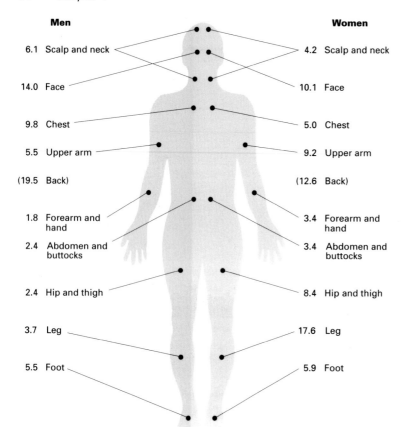

Men

6.1 Scalp and neck

14.0 Face

9.8 Chest

5.5 Upper arm

(19.5 Back)

1.8 Forearm and
     hand

2.4 Abdomen and
     buttocks

2.4 Hip and thigh

3.7 Leg

5.5 Foot

Women

4.2 Scalp and neck

10.1 Face

5.0 Chest

9.2 Upper arm

(12.6 Back)

3.4 Forearm and
     hand

3.4 Abdomen and
     buttocks

8.4 Hip and thigh

17.6 Leg

5.9 Foot

Fig. 7.7 Age and surface area-adjusted incidence of invasive malignant melanoma by anatomical site in Denmark, 1978–82 (Østerlind *et al.*, 1988).

duced by sun exposure on limited areas of the skin. Laboratory investigations confirmed the existence of systemic effects of localized ultraviolet radiation exposures. Case-control studies of location of sunburns received and style of swimsuits worn have not provided adequate evidence to distinguish site-specific from systemic effects of sun exposure on melanoma risk. However, analysis of the detailed site distribution of melanoma in sun-exposed skin, including relatively gender-specific patterns suggestive of skin shading by hair and clothing, support the site-specific hypothesis.

Finally, trends with person, place and time in incidence of melanoma arising at sun-exposed sites have been observed to differ sharply from trends of melanoma arising at rarely or never sun-exposed cutaneous sites (the plantar foot and vulva) and of melanoma arising at absolutely sun-unexposed mucosal sites. This contrast suggests distinct aetiologies for melanomas on sun-protected sites and the absence of a substantial systemic effect of sun exposure on melanoma risk.

Acknowledgements

The author is supported by grants AR43051, CA49531 and CA50087 from the National Institutes of Health and by the Department of Veterans Affairs Cooperative Studies Program.

References

Armstrong, B.K. & Kricker, A. (1994) Cutaneous melanoma. *Cancer Surveys,* **19**, 219–240.

Bouwes Bavinck, J.N., Hardie, D.R., Green, A. *et al.* (1996) The risk of skin cancer in renal transplant recipients in Queensland, Australia: a follow-up study. *Transplantation,* **61**, 715–721.

Chiu, N.T. & Weinstock, M.A. (1996) Melanoma of oronasal

mucosa: population-based analysis of occurrence and mortality. *Archives of Otolaryngology, Head and Neck Surgery,* **122**, 985–988.

Collins, R.J. (1984) Melanoma in the Chinese of Hong Kong: emphasis on volar and subungual sites. *Cancer,* **54**, 1482–1488.

Crowley, N.J., Dodge, R., Vollmer, R.T. & Seigler, H.F. (1991) Malignant melanoma in black Americans: a trend toward improved survival. *Archives of Surgery,* **126**, 1359–1365.

Dennis, L.K., White, E. & Lee, J.A.H. (1993) Recent cohort trends in malignant melanoma by anatomic site in the United States. *Cancer Causes and Contributions,* **4**, 93–100.

Elwood, J.M. (1992) Melanoma and sun exposure: contrasts between intermittent and chronic exposure. *World Journal of Surgery,* **16**, 157–166.

Elwood, J.M. & Gallagher, R.P. (1983) Site distribution of malignant melanoma. *Canadian Medical Association Journal,* **128**, 1400–1404.

Elwood, J.M. & Lee, J.A.H. (1975) Recent data on the epidemiology of malignant melanoma. *Seminars in Oncology,* **2**, 149–154.

Giraud, R.M.A., Rippey, E. & Rippey, J.J. (1975) Malignant melanoma of the skin in black Africans. *South African Medical Journal,* **49**, 665–668.

Green, A., Bain, C., McLennan, R. & Siskind, V. (1986) Risk factors for cutaneous melanoma in Queensland. *Recent Results in Cancer Research,* **102**, 76–97.

Green, A., MacLennan, R., Youl, P. & Martin, N. (1993) Site distribution of cutaneous melanoma in Queensland. *International Journal of Cancer,* **53**, 232–236.

Holman, C.D.J., Armstrong, B.K. & Heenan, P.J. (1986) Relationship of cutaneous malignant melanoma to individual sunlight-exposure habits. *Journal of the National Cancer Institute,* **76**, 403–414.

Houghton, A., Flannery, J. & Viola, M.V. (1980) Malignant melanoma in Connecticut and Denmark. *International Journal of Cancer,* **25**, 95–104.

Hudson, D.A. & Krige, J.E.J. (1995) Melanoma in black South Africans. *Journal of the American College of Surgeons,* **180**, 65–71.

Kripke, M.L. (1984) Immunologic unresponsiveness induced by ultraviolet radiation. *Immunological Review,* **80**, 87–102.

Lee, J.A.H. & Merrill, J.M. (1970) Sunlight and the aetiology of malignant melanoma: a synthesis. *Medical Journal of Australia,* **ii**, 846–851.

MacLennan, R., Green, A.C., McLeod, G.R.C. & Martin, N.G. (1992) Increasing incidence of cutaneous melanoma in Queensland, Australia. *Journal of the National Cancer Institute,* **84**, 1427–1432.

Mangus, K. (1981) Habits of sun exposure and risk of malignant melanoma: an analysis of incidence rates in Norway 1955–77 by cohort, sex, age, and primary tumor site. *Cancer,* **48**, 2329–2335.

Olson, R.L., Sayre, R.M. & Everett, M.A. (1966) Effect of anatomic location and time on ultraviolet erythema. *Archives of Dermatology,* **93**, 211–215.

Østerlind, A., Hou-Jensen, K. & Jensen, O.M. (1988) Incidence of cutaneous malignant melanoma in Denmark 1978–1982. Anatomic site distribution, histologic types, and comparison with non-melanoma skin cancer. *British Journal of Cancer,* **58**, 385–391.

Parkin, D.M., Muir, C.S., Whelan, S.L., Gao, Y.T., Ferlay, J. & Powell, J. (eds) (1992) *Cancer Incidence in Five Continents.* Vol. VI. International Agency for Research on Cancer, Lyon.

Pearl, D.K. & Scott, E.L. (1986) The anatomic distribution of skin cancers. *International Journal of Epidemiology,* **15**, 502–506.

Ragnarsson-Olding, B., Johansson, H., Rutqvist, L-E. & Ringborg, U. (1993) Malignant melanoma of the vulva and vagina: trends in incidence, age distribution, and long-term survival among 245 consecutive cases in Sweden 1960–1984. *Cancer,* **71**, 1893–1897.

Ries, L.A.G., Miller, B.A., Hankey, B.F., Kosary, C.L., Harras, A. & Edwards, B.K. (eds) (1994) *SEER Cancer Statistics Review, 1973–1991* (NIH Publication No. 94-2789). National Cancer Institute, Bethesda, Maryland

Scotto, J., Fears, T.R. & Fraumeni, J.F. (1983) *Incidence of Nonmelanoma Skin Cancer in the United States* (NIH Publication No. 83-2433). Public Health Service, Washington, DC.

Seiji, M., Takematsu, H., Hosokawa, M. *et al.* (1983) Acral melanoma in Japan. *Journal of Investigative Dermatology,* **80**, 56s–60s.

Stevens, N.G., Liff, J.M. & Weiss, N.S. (1990) Plantar melanoma: is the incidence of melanoma of the sole of the foot really higher in blacks than whites? *International Journal of Cancer,* **45**, 691–693.

Stierner, U., Rosdahl, I., Augustsson, A. & Kagedal, B. (1989) UVB irradiation induces melanocyte increase in both exposed and shielded human skin. *Journal of Investigative Dermatology,* **92**, 561–564.

Suseelan, A.V. & Gupta, I.M. (1977) Malignant melanoma in Nigeria — pathological studies. *African Journal of Medical Science,* **6**, 209–213.

Thörn M., Bergström, R., Adami, H.-O. & Ringborg, U. (1990) Trends in the incidence of malignant melanoma in Sweden, by anatomic site, 1960–1984. *American Journal of Epidemiology,* **132**, 1066–1077.

Weinstock, M.A. (1993) Epidemiology and prognosis of anorectal melanoma. *Gastroenterology,* **104**, 174–178.

Weinstock, M.A. (1994) Malignant melanoma of the vulva and vagina in the United States: patterns of incidence and population-based estimates of survival. *American Journal of Obstetrics and Gynecology,* **171**, 1225–1230.

Weinstock, M.A., Colditz, G.A., Willet, W.C. *et al.* (1991) Melanoma and the sun: the effect of swimsuits and a 'healthy' tan on the risk of nonfamilial malignant melanoma in women. *American Journal of Epidemiology*, **134**, 462–470.

Sun Exposure and Non-Melanocytic Skin Cancer

R.P. GALLAGHER

Introduction

Non-melanocytic skin cancer, comprised of basal-cell and squamous-cell carcinoma, is the most common tumour among white-skinned populations around the world (Giles *et al.*, 1988; Levi *et al.*, 1988; Gallagher *et al.*, 1990; Roberts, 1990; Miller & Weinstock, 1994). These cancers are almost uniformly non-fatal (Weinstock, 1993) and perhaps because of this, the true importance of non-melanocytic skin cancer has been underestimated. However, if diagnosis is overly delayed, they can cause substantial morbidity and their treatment can result in disfigurement. Their care also consumes a substantial proportion of health budgets in Western countries, particularly in areas of maximal incidence such as Australia.

The single most important environmental risk factor for both basal and squamous-cell skin cancers is sunshine or, more properly, solar ultraviolet radiation (International Agency for Research on Cancer, 1992); however the effect of sunlight is modified substantially by host and pigmentary factors of populations at risk. The important host factors which modify risk are briefly discussed here with a review of what has been learned about the relationship between these common skin cancers and sun exposure.

Host factors

As has been noted in international comparative data, skin cancers are substantially less common in Asian and other non-white populations (Muir *et al.*, 1987). Even accounting for possible ascertainment problems, heavily pigmented ethnic groups have rates of basal and squamous-cell carcinoma which are one to two orders of magnitude lower than whites. Case-control studies have shown that ethnic origin is also important

among white populations; individuals of southern European origin (Kricker *et al.*, 1991; Gallagher *et al.*, 1995a,b) have lower risks of non-melanocytic skin cancer than those of Scandinavian and Celtic origin, who are generally accepted to be at the highest risk (Giles *et al.*, 1988; Kricker *et al.*, 1991; Gallagher *et al.*, 1995b).

Light skin colour is known to increase risk of basal (Green *et al.*, 1988; Kricker *et al.*, 1991; Gallagher, *et al.*, 1995a) or squamous-cell carcinoma (Aubrey & MacGibbon, 1985; Green *et al.*, 1988; Gallagher *et al.*, 1995b) and is sometimes an independent prognostic risk factor even after control for ethnic origin (Gallagher *et al.*, 1995a). Similarly, light and particularly red hair colour (Hogan *et al.*, 1989; Hunter *et al.*, 1990; Vitasa *et al.*, 1990; Gallagher *et al.*, 1995a,b) and sometimes light eye colour (Aubrey & MacGibbon, 1985; Vitasa *et al.*, 1990) also appear to place subjects at elevated risk of non-melanocytic skin cancer although hair and eye colour seldom persist as independent risk indicators after adjustment for ethnic status and other host characteristics (Kricker *et al.*, 1991; Gallagher *et al.*, 1995a).

Propensity to burn rather than tan upon exposure to the sun has been found to be a consistent indicator of elevated risk for both basal (Hunter *et al.*, 1990; Vitasa *et al.*, 1990; Kricker *et al.*, 1991; Gallagher *et al.*, 1995b) and squamous-cell carcinoma (Kricker *et al.*, 1991; Gallagher *et al.*, 1995b; Grodstein *et al.*, 1995) although this sometimes disappears as a predictive factor after control for other phenotype variables (Gallagher *et al.*, 1995a,b; Grodskin *et al.*, 1995).

Factors combining host characteristics and sunlight exposure

A number of factors which combine host characteristics and sunlight exposure, namely freckling, sunburns, presence of acquired melanocytic naevi and indicators of chronic sun damage, have also been investigated in relation to non-melanocytic skin cancer. Kricker *et al.* (1991) found that adult or childhood freckling on the arm increased risk of both basal-(BCC) and squamous-cell carcinoma (SCC) and similar findings were seen in a Canadian study (Gallagher *et al.*, 1995a,b). In both studies, however, freckling was an independent predictor of risk only for BCC, not for

SCC. The study of Maryland watermen, traditional American East-coast fishermen, showed childhood freckling to be a risk factor for both tumour types (Vitasa *et al.*, 1990).

History of sunburn has been associated with elevated risk of both BCC (Hogan *et al.*, 1989; Hunter *et al.*, 1990; Gallagher *et al.*, 1995a) and SCC (Gallagher *et al.*, 1995b; Grodstein *et al.*, 1995). In some (Gallagher *et al.*, 1995a,b) but not all of these studies, childhood burns seemed to be more important than those suffered as an adult.

Naevus prevalence as a risk factor for non-melanocytic skin cancer has been investigated in the Australian study of Kricker *et al.* (1991), and presence of four or more naevi $\geqslant 5$ mm on the back was an independent risk factor for BCC after control for other host and pigmentary factors. This is a potentially important finding, as presence of acquired melanocytic naevi has also been shown to be a strong predictor of cutaneous melanoma risk (Holman & Armstrong, 1984b; Holly *et al.*, 1987), and thus may indicate similarities in the aetiology of melanoma and BCC.

A number of indicators of solar-induced skin damage have been assessed as potential risk indicators for BCC and SCC. Presence of solar elastosis on the neck was found to be a risk factor for both BCC and SCC (Kricker *et al.*, 1991) and, in addition, telangiectasia of the face has been related to SCC risk (Green *et al.*, 1988; Kricker *et al.*, 1991) but not to BCC risk (Kricker *et al.*, 1991). Presence of solar keratoses is also important in predicting risk of SCC (Kricker *et al.*, 1991). Finally, loss of fine textured skin markings on the hand as assessed by a technique known as cutaneous microtopography has been shown to be predictive of elevated risk of both BCC (Kricker *et al.*, 1991) and cutaneous melanoma (Holman & Armstrong, 1984a).

Sunlight exposure

Latitude as an indicator of exposure

A number of studies have addressed the issue of the relationship between solar exposure and non-melanocytic skin cancer by examining cancer incidence data for gradients of risk by latitude within homogeneous populations. An inverse association between latitude and non-melanocytic skin cancer incidence has been noted in the United States (Scotto *et al.*, 1983). This study showed a strong relationship between ground level UVB irradiation as measured by Robertson–Berger meters at different latitudes within the country and incidence of both BCC and SCC. A similar latitude gradient was seen for both types of non-melanocytic skin cancer in Norway (Magnus, 1991). In the Southern hemisphere, an analogous effect is seen in Australia, where incidence rates for non-melanocytic skin cancer rise from south to north toward the Equator (Giles *et al.*, 1988).

Residence as an indicator of exposure

More detailed data on the relationship of sun exposure and non-melanocytic skin cancer have recently become available from a series of analytical studies (Table 7.5). Residence in high versus low sun areas has been used as a surrogate for sun exposure in several of these studies. Hunter *et al.* (1990), in a cohort study of nurses, showed an elevated risk for BCC among women residing in California or in Florida, by comparison with cohort members resident in other parts of the USA. Similar results were seen for SCC (Grodstein *et al.*, 1995). Results for both BCC and SCC persisted after control for host and pigmentation factors, suggesting that residence in sunny places and, by extension, increased sun exposure elevates risk. Kricker *et al.* (1991) demonstrated a substantially reduced risk of both BCC and SCC in Australian residents who were born in other countries and migrated to Australia — a generally higher sunlight area than their place of birth — later in life. For BCC, the strongest protection was afforded to those who migrated to Australia from lower sunlight areas after their first decade of life.

Indicators of recreational or intermittent sun exposure

There is strong evidence that intermittent sun exposure, particularly on unacclimatized skin, is important in accounting for risk of cutaneous malignant melanoma (Elwood *et al.*, 1985; Østerlind *et al.*, 1988). Recently, epidemiological studies have begun to evaluate the effect of intermittent versus constant and cumulative exposure on risk of non-melanocytic skin cancer. A Canadian case-control study of BCC reported a positive gradient of risk with childhood and adolescent recreational sun exposure (Gallagher *et al.*, 1995a). The effect was most pronounced in subjects who were unable to tan.

Kricker *et al.* (1995b) showed a positive relationship between risk of BCC and sun exposure on non-working weekend days, especially exposure in teenage years. Risk of BCC increased substantially with proportion of sun exposure achieved in an intermittent fashion in subjects who tanned poorly, but not at all in subjects who tanned easily. Again this was most pronounced at age 15–19 years. Other potential measures of intermittent strong sun exposure showed no association, however, including lifetime frequency of sunbathing and participation in most outdoor sports.

Green and Battistutta found no difference in risk of BCC between subjects who spent their recreational time outdoors compared with those who spent most of it indoors (Green & Battistutta, 1990). No data were presented on exposure in childhood or in the teenage years.

Studies of recreational or intermittent sun exposure and risk of SCC have shown different results from those seen for BCC. No association with lifetime recreational sun exposure or with childhood exposure was seen in the Canadian study (Gallagher *et al.*, 1995), while in the investigation of Grodstein *et al.* (1995) no measures of such exposure were available. A non-significant elevated risk of SCC was detected by Green and Battistutta (1990) in subjects whose leisure time was spent mainly or partly outdoors.

Sunburn as an indicator of intermittent exposure

Sunburn is a measure of intermittent heavy sun exposure on susceptible skin. A number of studies have found frequent painful or blistering sunburns to be associated with elevated risk of BCC (Hogan *et al.*, 1989; Hunter *et al.*, 1990; Gallagher *et al.*, 1995a; Kricker *et al.*, 1995b) although some have not (Green *et al.*, 1990). In the study of Gallagher *et al.* (1995a),

Table 7.5 Recent analytical studies: non-melanocytic skin cancer and sun exposure.

Place	Type of study	Cases (*n*)	Comparison subjects (*n*)	Control source	Reference
Western Australia	Case control	226 BCC 45 SCC	1015	Population	Kricker *et al.* (1991a, 1995a,b)
Queensland	Cross-sectional	42 BCC *or* SCC	2095 total subjects	Population	Green *et al.* (1988)
Queensland	Cross-sectional	66 BCC 21 SCC	1770 total subjects	Population	Green & Battistutta (1990)
Canada	Case control	225 BCC 180 SCC	406	Population	Gallagher *et al.* (1995a,b)
Canada	Case control	92 SCC	174	Hospital skin patients	Aubrey & McGibbon (1985)
Canada	Case control	538 BCC	738	Population	Hogan *et al.* (1989)
USA	Cross-sectional	33 BCC 35 SCC	808 total subjects	Population of fishermen	Vitasa *et al.* (1990) Strickland *et al.* (1989)
USA	Cohort	771 BCC	Cohort of 73 366	Nurses	Hunter *et al.* (1990)
USA	Cohort	197 SCC	Cohort of 107 900	Nurses	Grodstein *et al.* (1995)
Sicily	Case control	108 BCC 25 SCC	266	Hospital	Gafa *et al.* (1991)
Egypt	Case control	99 BCC 37 SCC	145	Hospital	Khwsky *et al.* (1994)

* BCC = basal-cell carcinoma; SCC = squamous-cell carcinoma.

from Canada, the effect was seen largely for severe burns in childhood and adolescence. Studies of SCC have also shown an association between sunburn history and risk (Green & Battistutta, 1990; Gallagher *et al.*, 1995b; Grodstein *et al.*, 1995). In the only study which addressed the issue of timing of sunburns, both childhood and recent adult (in the 10 years prior to diagnosis) burns were important in SCC (Gallagher *et al.*, 1995b).

Chronic occupational and cumulative sun exposure

Only one study of BCC has reported a positive relationship between risk of this tumour and either chronic occupational sunlight or cumulative sunlight exposure (Hogan *et al.*, 1989) and this investigation reported the association to be with winter rather than summer exposure. Most other studies have found no association (Strickland *et al.*, 1989; Green & Battistutta, 1990; Hunter *et al.*, 1990; Vitasa *et al.*, 1990; Gallagher *et al.*, 1995a).

Kricker *et al.* (1995a), after analysis of Australian data, proposed that risk of BCC initially increases with total solar ultraviolet exposure, but reaches a plateau and may actually decline in those with the highest exposure. If other studies confirm this exposure pattern then BCC incidence will have demonstrated a relationship with solar ultraviolet radiation similar to that thought to govern cutaneous malignant melanoma (Armstrong, 1988).

Studies of SCC and chronic occupational or cumulative sun exposure have been more fruitful than investigations of BCC, and positive associations have been seen with several measures of chronic occupational sun exposure (Green & Battistutta, 1990; Gallagher *et al.*, 1995b) or total exposure (Strickland *et al.*, 1989). These findings indicate that SCC incidence may be more closely related to the total lifetime solar UV dose than BCC.

Other results

Findings from several other case-control studies are somewhat ambiguous, as the authors have combined BCCs and SCCs in the analysis. An investigation carried out among subjects from Egypt (Khwsky *et al.*, 1994)

demonstrated an elevated risk of non-melanocytic skin cancer in subjects reporting an outdoor job, and also a gradient of risk with degree of sun exposure. A study of skin cancer in Sicily showed a slightly elevated risk for non-melanocytic skin cancer in agricultural workers, presumably due to chronic sun exposure, and in addition a higher risk for subjects reporting ≥ 6 hours of sun exposure per day (Gafa *et al.*, 1991). On multivariate analysis, only the latter finding persisted.

Summary

Sunlight is the single most important environmental cause of both major forms of non-melanocytic skin cancer (International Agency for Research on Cancer, 1992) and there is strong evidence that incidence of both BCC and SCC is increasing rapidly. Findings emerging from recent studies have demonstrated clear differences in the relationship of each type of skin cancer to solar ultraviolet radiation. Basal-cell carcinoma demonstrates a surprising similarity to cutaneous malignant melanoma, in that intermittent patterns of sun exposure (Kricker *et al.*, 1995b) and perhaps childhood and early life exposure (Kricker *et al.*, 1991; Gallagher *et al.*, 1995a) may play a critical role in development of these cancers. Squamous-cell carcinoma, on the other hand, seems to more closely fulfil the traditional association which classically was thought to exist between chronic or cumulative sunlight and non-melanocytic skin cancers.

All three types of skin cancer, melanoma, BCC and SCC, share roughly the same relationship with phenotypic characteristics, however, and this is of value in the design of both primary and secondary skin cancer prevention programmes.

References

Armstrong, B.K. (1988) Epidemiology of malignant melanoma: intermittent or total accumulated exposure to the sun? *Journal of Dermatology, Surgery and Oncology*, **18**, 835–849.

Aubrey, F. & MacGibbon, B. (1985) Risk factors for squamous cell carcinoma of the skin. *Cancer*, **55**, 907–911.

Elwood, J.M., Gallagher, R.P., Hill, G.B. & Pearson, J.B. (1985) Cutaneous melanoma in relation to intermittent and constant sun exposure: The Western Canada Melanoma Study. *International Journal of Cancer*, **35**, 427–433.

Gafa, L., Filippazzo, M., Tumino, R., Dardanoni, G., Lanzarone, F. & Dardanoni, L. (1991) Risk factors for non-melanoma skin cancer in Ragusa, Sicily: a case-control study. *Cancer Causes and Control*, **2**, 395–399.

Gallagher, R.P., Ma, B., McLean, D.I., Yang, C.P., Ho, V., Carruthers, J.A. & Warshawski, L.M. (1987) Trends in basal cell carcinoma, squamous cell carcinoma and melanoma of the skin from 1973 through 1987. *Journal of the American Academy of Dermatology*, **23**, 413–421.

Gallagher, R.P., Hill, G.B., Bajdik, C.D. *et al.* (1995a) Sunlight exposure, pigmentation factors and risk of non-melanocytic skin cancer. I. Basal cell carcinoma. *Archives of Dermatology*, **131**, 157–163.

Gallagher, R.P., Hill, G.B., Bajdik, C.D. *et al.* (1995b) Sunlight exposure, pigmentation factors and risk of non-melanocytic skin cancer. II. Squamous cell carcinoma. *Archives of Dermatology*, **131**, 164–169.

Giles, G.C., Marks, R. & Foley, P. (1988) Incidence of non-melanocytic skin cancer treated in Australia. *British Medical Journal*, **296**, 13–17.

Green, A. & Battistutta, D. (1990) Incidence and determinants of skin cancer in a high risk Australian population. *International Journal of Cancer*, **46**, 356–361.

Green, A., Beardmore, G., Hart, V., Leslie, D., Marks, R. & Staines, D. (1988) Skin cancer in a Queensland population. *Journal of the American Academy of Dermatology*, **19**, 1045–1052.

Grodstein, F., Speizer, F. & Hunter, D. (1995) A prospective study of incident squamous cell carcinoma of the skin in the Nurses' Health Study. *Journal of the National Cancer Institute*, **87**, 1061–1066.

Hogan, D.J., To, T., Gran, L., Wong, D. & Lane, P. (1989) Risk factors for basal cell carcinoma. *International Journal of Dermatology*, **28**, 591–594.

Holly, E.A., Kelly, J.W., Shpall, S.N. & Chiu, S.-H. (1987) Number of melanocytic nevi as a major risk factor for malignant melanoma. *Journal of the American Academy of Dermatology*, **17**, 459–468.

Holman, C.D.J. & Armstrong, B.K. (1984a) Cutaneous malignant melanoma and indicators of total accumulated exposure to the sun: an analysis separating histologic type. *Journal of the National Cancer Institute*, **73**, 75–82.

Holman, C.D.J. & Armstrong, B.K. (1984b) Pigmentary traits, ethnic origin, benign nevi and family history as risk factors for cutaneous malignant melanoma. *Journal of the National Cancer Institute*, **72**, 257–266.

Hunter, D.J., Colditz, G., Stamfer, M., Rosner, B., Willett, W. & Speizer, F. (1990) Risk factors for basal cell carcinoma in a prospective cohort of women. *Annals of Epidemiology*, **1**, 13–23.

International Agency for Research on Cancer (1992) *IARC Monographs on Evaluation of Carcinogenic Risk to Humans*. Vol. 55. *Solar and Ultraviolet Radiation*, IARC, Lyon.

Khwsky, F.E., Bedwani, R., d'Avanzo, B. *et al.* (1994) Risk factors for non-melanocytic skin cancer in Alexandria, Egypt. *International Journal of Cancer*, **56**, 375–378.

Kricker, A., Armstrong, B., English, D. & Heenan, P. (1991) Pigmentary and cutaneous risk factors for non-melanocytic skin cancer — a case-control study. *International Journal of Cancer*, **48**, 650–662.

Kricker, A., Armstrong, B.K., English, D.R. & Heenan, P.J. (1995a) A dose–response curve for sun exposure and basal cell carcinoma. *International Journal of Cancer*, **60**, 482–488.

Kricker, A., Armstrong, B.K., English, D.R. & Heenan, P.J. (1995b) Does intermittent sun exposure cause basal cell carcinoma? A case-control study in Western Australia. *International Journal of Cancer*, **60**, 489–494.

Levi, F., La Vecchia, C., Te, V.-C. *et al.* (1988) Descriptive epidemiology of skin cancer in the Swiss Canton of Vaud. *International Journal of Cancer*, **42**, 811–816.

Magnus, K. (1991) The nordic profile of skin cancer incidence. A comparative epidemiological study of the three main types of skin cancer. *International Journal of Cancer*, **47**, 12–19.

Miller, D.L. & Weinstock, M.A. (1994) Non-melanoma skin cancer in the United States: incidence. *Journal of the American Academy of Dermatology*, **30**, 774–778.

Muir, C., Waterhouse, J., Mack, T., Powell, J. & Whelan, S. (1987) *Cancer Incidence in Five Continents, Vol. V.* IARC Scientific Publication No. 88, pp. 880–881. IARC, Lyon.

Østerlind, A., Tucker, M.A., Stone, B.J. & Jensen, O.M. (1988) The Danish case-control study of cutaneous malignant melanoma. II. Importance of UV light exposure. *International Journal of Cancer*, **42**, 319–324.

Roberts, D.L. (1990) Incidence of non-melanoma skin cancer in West Glamorgan, South Wales. *British Journal of Dermatology*, **122**, 399–403.

Scotto, J., Fears, T.R. & Fraumeni, J.F. (1983) *Incidence of Non-melanoma Skin Cancer in the United States*, US DHSS, Public Health Service (Publication No. (NIH) 83-2433), April 1983. DHHS, Washington DC.

Strickland, P.T., Vitasa, B., West, S., Rosenthal, F., Emmett, E. & Taylor, H. (1989) Quantitative carcinogenesis in man: solar ultraviolet B dose dependence of skin cancer in Maryland watermen. *Journal of the National Cancer Institute*, **81**, 1910–1913.

Vitasa, B.C., Taylor, H.R., Strickland, P.T. *et al.* (1990) Association of non-melanoma skin cancer and actinic keratosis with cumulative solar ultraviolet exposure in Maryland watermen. *Cancer*, **65**, 2811–2817.

Weinstock, M.A. (1993) Non-melanoma skin cancer mortality in the United States, 1969 through 1988. *Archives of Dermatology*, **129**, 1286–1290.

Ozone Depletion and Skin Cancers

B.L. DIFFEY

Introduction

In 1974, Molina and Rowland, who along with Paul Crutzen were awarded the 1995 Nobel Prize for Chemistry, predicted that man-made chlorine compounds released at ground level would diffuse into the upper atmosphere and destroy the ozone resident there (Molina & Rowland, 1974). It was not for another 10 years that scientists from the British Antarctic Survey (Farman *et al.*, 1985) showed that each year since the mid-1970s there had been an unexpected decrease in the abundance of springtime ozone over the Antarctic — the so-called *ozone hole*. For the past decade there has been increasing public concern about just what is going on in the skies above us, fuelled by media speculation of skin cancer epidemics. Yet the media coverage of this topic often contains significant misreporting (Bell, 1994) and has been unnecessarily alarmist.

Skin cancers are the most common human cancer and their incidence is increasing in many countries. It is well recognized that chronic exposure to sunlight is a causal factor in the development of human skin cancer, particularly non-melanoma skin cancers (NMSC). Concern has been expressed widely that depletion of stratospheric ozone by chemical reactions involving the degradation products of chlorofluorocarbons will lead to a rise in the incidence of skin cancers as a consequence of increased levels of solar ultraviolet radiation (UVR) at the Earth's surface (Russell Jones, 1987; MacKie & Rycroft, 1988; UNEP, 1989, 1991).

Trends in atmospheric ozone and ambient ultraviolet radiation

Significant global scale decreases in total ozone have been occurring since the late 1970s, and the loss of ozone in the northern hemisphere is now proceeding with a rate of loss over mid-latitudes (30–50°N) seen in winter and early spring in the range 6–7% per decade. The loss in summer months, when ultraviolet (UV) levels are much higher and people are exposed more frequently to the sun, is less at about 2–3% per decade (Frederick, 1993).

Calculations for the northern hemisphere based on the measured ozone trends for the period 1979–89 indicate that, all other factors being constant, the terrestrial erythemally-effective ultraviolet radiation (which lies mainly within the UVB waveband) should have increased by less than 1% at 15°N to between 4.0 and 4.7% at 35°N and poleward during this decade (Frederick, 1993). Paradoxically these predictions have not generally been borne out by ground-based UV monitoring programmes (Diffey, 1996). Reasons offered to account for this apparent discrepancy include the limited period of most UV monitoring networks, accuracy of instrument calibration and long-term stability of monitoring equipment, year-to-year fluctuations in cloud cover (Frederick & Erlick, 1995) and an increase in ozone and aerosols present in the lower atmosphere due to pollution (Bruhl & Crutzen, 1989). Despite the record low in total ozone which occurred in the northern winters of 1992 and 1993 (Bojkov *et al.*, 1993), measurements in the Austrian Alps showed no significant increase of cumulative erythermal exposure compared with a reference series of measurements obtained between 1981 and 1988 (Blumthaler & Ambach, 1994).

In the southern hemisphere, the influence of Antarctic ozone depletion on ambient UVB in Melbourne (latitude 38°S) has been reported by Roy and Gies (1992). Continuous monitoring of ambient UVB showed that the levels recorded in February 1991 were 37% and 27% higher than for the same month in 1990 and 1989, respectively. February 1991 had the lowest ozone values recorded for this period, but also very low cloud cover compared with recent years. These two important factors reinforce each other and illustrate the difficulty of separating the effects of ozone depletion from climate on ambient UVB. So whilst there is unequivocal evidence concerning stratospheric ozone depletion, we cannot be sure, as yet, whether this depletion is accompanied by increases in terrestrial UVR. This does not mean that no systematic trend exists, simply that the 95% confidence interval on estimated trends is likely to encompass zero.

Risk analysis of human skin cancer

Estimates of the risk of inducing skin cancer from exposure to ultraviolet radiation demand knowledge of dose–response relationships and the relative effectiveness of different wavelengths in the spectral power distribution of the source in causing skin cancer. These data remain unknown for malignant melanoma and so it is unwise to make predictions about the consequences ozone depletion may have on the incidence of melanoma. However, data on dose–response relationships and action spectra are available to some extent to allow quantitative estimates to be made of the risk of inducing NMSC from solar UVR exposure.

Dose–response relationships

Application of multivariate analysis to population-based epidemiology of NMSC skin cancer has shown that, for a group of subjects with a given genetic susceptibility, age and environmental ultraviolet exposure are the two most important factors in determining the relative risk. Other epidemiological studies have confirmed these findings, and this has led to a simple power law relationship which expresses the risk in terms of these factors (Slaper & van der Leun, 1987):

$$risk \propto (annual\ UV\ dose)^\beta\ (age)^\alpha.$$

The symbols α and β are numerical constants associated with the age dependence of the incidence and the biological amplification factor, respectively, and are normally derived from surveys of skin cancer incidence and ultraviolet climatology. This equation is applicable to situations where the annual exposure received by an individual remains unaltered throughout life. In most instances changes in lifestyle with age mean that the annual UV exposure does not remain constant.

The situation of changes in annual exposure was examined in a series of experiments with mice (de Gruijl, 1982), and led Slaper and van der Leun (1987) to modify the above equation to estimate the risk of NMSC at age, T, as:

$$risk \propto (cumulative\ UV\ dose\ at\ age\ T)$$

$$^{\beta-1} \sum_{t=0}^{T} (annual\ dose\ at\ age\ [T-t]) \cdot t^{\alpha-\beta}$$

Age exponent α

The value of the parameter α can be estimated from

| | Exponent ± standard error | | |
Country	Males	Females	Reference
BCC			
USA	3.54 ± 0.24	2.89 ± 0.22	Scotto *et al.*, 1983
USA	–	2.82 ± 0.37	Hunter *et al.*, 1990
USA	3.49 ± 0.11	2.93 ± 0.13	Chuang *et al.*, 1990
Switzerland	4.03 ± 0.33	3.16 ± 0.17	Levi *et al.*, 1988
Netherlands	4.21 ± 0.15	3.70 ± 0.13	Coebergh *et al.*, 1991
Wales	3.38 ± 0.47	3.44 ± 0.54	Roberts, 1990
Australia	2.63 ± 0.29	1.96 ± 0.32	Marks *et al.*, 1993
SCC			
USA	4.44 ± 0.25	4.19 ± 0.08	Scotto *et al.*, 1983
USA	5.56 ± 0.27	5.44 ± 0.27	Glass & Hoover, 1989
Switzerland	6.47 ± 0.22	4.91 ± 0.40	Levi *et al.*, 1988
Netherlands	6.32 ± 0.55	5.26 ± 0.60	Coebergh *et al.*, 1991
England	5.64 ± 0.53	4.47 ± 0.38	Whitaker *et al.*, 1979
Australia	4.71 ± 0.79	3.30 ± 1.12	Marks *et al.*, 1993

Table 7.6 Estimates of the age exponent α obtained using a power function model of BCC and SCC incidence.

published incidence data on basal-cell cancer (BCC) and squamous-cell cancer (SCC) from the slope of the logarithm of incidence plotted against the logarithm of age. Estimates of the exponent α for BCC and SCC are given in Table 7.6. The value is greater for SCC than for BCC, and for men than for women.

Biological amplification factor β

Estimates of the biological amplification factor (β) from epidemiological studies carried out in the United States and Norway are summarized in Table 7.7. The estimates of β from the United States were based on the 1977–78 survey of NMSC incidence in eight regions of the USA with corresponding measurements of ambient erythemal UVR obtained from Robertson–Berger meters (Scotto *et al.*, 1983). The difference in the ranges of values shown for Scotto *et al.* (1983) and Rundel (1983) arises because the former used an eponential model of age-standardized incidence, whereas Rundel fitted a log-normal distribution to the age-incidence data in each geographical area and estimated the mean onset time for both BCC and SCC. The reciprocal mean onset times were then modelled as a linear function of erythemal UVR dose across the different geographical areas.

The estimates of β from Norway were derived from incidence data on BCC and SCC collected by the Norwegian Cancer Registry (Moan *et al.*, 1989) and estimates of erythemal UVR obtained by modelling solar spectral irradiance and combining with the CIE reference action spectrum for ultraviolet erythema in human skin (McKinlay & Diffey, 1987).

Mean values of α and β (pooled for males and females) from the data given in Tables 7.6 and 7.7 are summarized in Table 7.8. Both the age exponents α and the biological amplification factors β are higher for SCC than for BCC.

Action spectrum for photocarcinogenesis

Clearly an action spectrum for skin cancer can only be obtained from animal experiments. The most extensive investigations to date are those from groups at Utrecht and Philadelphia. These workers exposed a total of about 1100 albino hairless mice to 14 different broad-band ultraviolet sources and by a mathematical optimization process derived an action spectrum referred to as the *Skin Cancer Utrecht–Philadelphia (SCUP)* action spectrum (de Gruijl *et al.*, 1993). The SCUP action spectrum is that for skin tumour induction in hairless mice, a species which has a thinner epidermis than humans.

By taking into account differences in the optics of human epidermis and hairless albino mouse epidermis, the experimentally determined action spectrum for tumour induction in mouse skin can be modified to arrive at a postulated action spectrum for human skin cancer (de Gruijl & van der Leun, 1994). The resulting action spectrum resembles the action spectrum for erythema (McKinlay & Diffey, 1987) (Fig. 7.8) suggesting that this action spectrum may be used as a surrogate for human skin cancer. For this reason erythemal doses expressed in units of *minimal erythema dose (MED)* can be used to express carcinogenic-effective exposure. It is important to appreciate, however, that the MED is used as an exemplary measure of *exposure* rather than as the dose necessary to cause a biological outcome in any given individual. Here 1 MED is defined as equivalent to an erythemally-weighted radiant exposure of $200 \, J/m^2$ which has been shown to approximate the exposure dose necessary to result in a barely perceptible erythema in unacclimatized white skin.

Table 7.7 Estimates of the biological amplification factors β for BCC and SCC.

| Country | Biological amplification factors | | Reference |
	Males	Females	
BCC			
USA	1.3–2.6	1.1–2.1	Scotto *et al.*, 1983
USA	1.8–2.2	1.1–1.5	Rundel, 1983
Norway	1.5–2.0	1.6–2.1	Moan *et al.*, 1989
SCC			
USA	2.1–4.1	2.2–4.3	Scotto *et al.*, 1983
USA	2.4–2.8	1.6–2.1	Rundel, 1983
Norway	1.2–1.5	1.6–1.8	Moan *et al.*, 1989

Table 7.8 Summary of age exponents and biological amplification factors for BCC and SCC (mean ± standard deviation).

Parameter	BCC	SCC
Age exponent	3.2 ± 0.6	5.1 ± 0.9
Biological amplification factor	1.7 ± 0.3	2.3 ± 0.5

Human exposure to solar UVR

The solar UVR exposure received by an individual depends on three factors:
• Ambient solar ultraviolet radiation.
• The fraction of ambient exposure received on appropriate anatomical sites.
• Behaviour outdoors.

Estimates of personal exposure can be obtained in two ways: by direct measurement using UV-sensitive film badges normally worn on the lapel site or by modelling the variables above (Diffey, 1992). The results obtained from both methods indicate that indoor workers in the UK receive around 100 MED per year mainly from weekend and vacational exposure, and principally to the hands, forearms and face. This value is approximately 6% of the total ambient available. Children have a greater opportunity for outdoor exposure and receive an annual dose of around 150 MED. For indoor workers, the annual exposure associated with occupation (travelling to and from work, going outside at lunchtime) is about 20 MED, about 40 MED is contributed by weekend exposure, and the remaining 30 MED from vacational exposure. In the case of children, 'occupational' exposure (playtime and lunchtime exposure) may be about 30 MED, recreational about 90 MED (because children are at school for only about 190 days per year) and vacation with parents giving about 30 MED. It must be stressed, however, that there will be large variations in the annual exposure doses received by individuals within a given population group depending upon propensity for outdoor activities and to what extent these are influenced by shade. This has been demonstrated in a recent large-scale study of the outdoor ultraviolet exposure of 180 children and adolescents in three geographically distinct regions of England over a period of 3 months (Diffey *et al.*, 1996).

Stratospheric ozone depletion and the risk of non-melanoma skin cancer

A 1% decrease in ozone will lead to a 1.2–1.4% increase in carcinogenic-effective UVB radiation (Health Council of The Netherlands, 1994). For every 1% increase in carcinogenic-effective UVB radiation, it is estimated (Health Council of The Netherlands, 1994) that there will be an approximate 2.5% increase of SCC incidence, with a corresponding figure of approximately 1.5% for BCC. Combining these we arrive at overall amplification factors, which can be summarized as:

$$1\% \downarrow \text{ in } O_3 \rightarrow 1.4 \times 2.5 = 3.5\% \uparrow \text{SCC}$$
$$\rightarrow 1.4 \times 1.5 = 2.1\% \uparrow \text{BBC}.$$

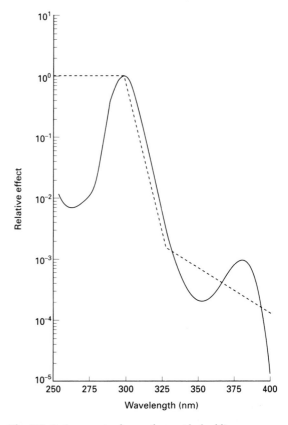

Fig. 7.8 Action spectra for erythema (dashed line; McKinlay & Diffey, 1987) and for non-melanoma skin cancer (solid line; de Gruijl & van der Leun, 1994) in human skin.

We can use this approach to estimate the consequence of a sustained 10% stratospheric ozone depletion in the UK. The most recent figures for skin cancer incidence in the UK are based on 1989 data and are obtained from the Office of Population Census and Surveys for England and Wales, Information and Statistics Division of the National Health Service (NHS) Directorate of Information Services for Scotland, and the Northern Ireland Cancer Registry. These sources yield a combined figure of just over 40 000 cases of skin cancer annually in the UK. Of these, about 30 000 are BCC, about 6000 are SCC and the remaining 4000 are malignant melanoma. However, because of underrecording of non-melanoma skin cancers (BCC and SCC) in the UK and the rising incidence, the number of these cancers occurring each year is probably closer to double these figures. So, for a sustained 10% ozone depletion, we might expect an increase of 21% and 35% in the incidence of BCC and SCC, respectively, giving an additional 12 000 cases of BCC and 4000 cases of SCC each year in the UK.

Whilst this approach may be applicable to future generations, it is not appropriate to British people alive today. By combining ultraviolet climatological data for the UK with models of human behaviour (Diffey, 1992) it is possible to estimate the monthly exposure to the face (the most common site for NMSC) in subjects taken to be representative of different population groups. These exemplary exposures are given for a child aged 10 years and an adult indoor worker in Table 7.9.

In the absence of ozone depletion, the adult indoor worker continues to receive an annual facial exposure dose of 100 MED. The child receives 150 MED per year until the age of 18 years and thereafter 100 MED each year (assuming he/she becomes an indoor worker). However if ozone depletion continues indefinitely at the rates shown in Table 7.9, it is possible to calculate the expected lifetime exposure, and hence the increased risk of developing skin cancer, for each subject compared with that expected if ozone levels remained at present values (Table 7.10). Implicit in these estimates is that behaviour, time spent outdoors and climate remain unchanged, and that terrestrial UVB will increase even though there are no conclusive measurement data to confirm this at present.

The above calculations of the lifetime risk of skin cancer assume that ozone depletion continues indefinitely at present rates. However, if there is global adherence to international undertakings for the phasing out of ozone depleting chemicals, as agreed in the Montreal Protocol (UNEP, 1987), ozone levels should begin to recover slowly in the next century.

Models of atmospheric chemistry and transport are not capable of predicting reliably the details of any future ozone depletion resulting from the increasing concentrations of chlorine compounds which are largely responsible (SORG, 1990, 1991). There will also be a time lag of several years before stratospheric chlorine concentrations respond to a decrease in chlorine loading. The implication is that stratospheric ozone destruction may continue to increase for several years after the chlorine loading of the troposphere has passed its peak value (SORG, 1993).

Given these uncertainties the approach used here is to assume that ozone depletion continues at present rates for a period T_c years from now and thereafter the ambient ultraviolet levels at that time return exponentially to present levels with a half recovery time of τ years. The child's risk of BCC and

Table 7.9 Estimated monthly solar UVR exposure dose to the face of a child and adult indoor worker, and total ozone trends for UK latitudes and longitudes (from Niu *et al.*, 1992).

Month	Exposure dose to face (MED)		Ozone decrease per year (%)
	Child	Adult	
January	0.3	0.2	0.6
February	1	0.5	0.3
March	3	1	0.8
April	14	6.4	0.6
May	20	13	0.8
June	25	16	0.3
July	32	22	0.3
August	40	33	0.1
September	10	6	0.3
October	3.5	1.6	0.6
November	1	0.2	0.5
December	0.2	0.1	0.4
Annual	150	100	0.4

Table 7.10 Cumulative solar ultraviolet exposure dose to face, and the risk of skin cancer assuming ozone depletion continues indefinitely at current rates relative to an intact ozone layer, calculated for a child aged 10 years and an adult indoor worker aged 35 years.

| Age (years) | Cumulative dose to face (MED) | | | Risk of skin cancer | | | |
| | No ozone depletion | Ozone depletion at current rates | | BCC | | SCC | |
		Child	Adult	Child	Adult	Child	Adult
50	5900	6265	5954	1.07	1.01	1.10	1.01
60	6900	7454	7044	1.09	1.02	1.13	1.03
70	7900	8678	8175	1.11	1.03	1.16	1.05

SCC at age 70 years for a range of T_c and τ have been calculated and the results are shown in Table 7.11, where it can be seen that if ozone depletion continues at present rates for another 20 years, say, and then recovers with a half recovery time of 20 years, the risk of SCC by age 70 years will be 1.07 compared with 1.16 if ozone depletion continues indefinitely at present rates.

Conclusion

For British adults alive today, ozone depletion continuing indefinitely at current rates is predicted to result in a relatively small additional lifetime risk (<5%; Table 7.10) of non-melanoma skin cancer, assuming no changes in climate, time spent outdoors, behaviour or clothing habits. The lifetime risk incurred by today's children, however, is predicted to be 10–16% greater than expected in the absence of ozone depletion. However, if the production and use of substances which deplete ozone are reduced as expected under the current provisions of the Montreal Protocol, the increased lifetime risk of skin cancer is likely to be less than these estimates (Table 7.11). It is to be hoped that public awareness about the adverse health effects of sun exposure will achieve these changes, which could lead to a reduction — rather than the anticipated increase — in skin cancer incidence. If there is no change in sun exposure habits and the rate of ozone depletion the calculations suggest that 50 years from now the number of skin cancers occurring each year in the UK will increase from

the present number of about 80 000 to around 88 000. This is a much smaller relative increase than has occurred over the previous 50 years and illustrates that changes in leisure time, fashion and activities in the sun — factors which are commonly believed to be important in the rising incidence of skin cancers — have had a much greater effect on skin cancer rates

Table 7.11 The risk of skin cancer in a child presently aged 10 years when aged 70 years relative to that under an intact ozone layer. Data are given assuming that ozone depletion continues at present rates until a period T_c years from now and thereafter the ambient ultraviolet levels at that time return exponentially to present levels with a half recovery time of τ years.

| T_c (years) | τ years | | | | | |
	5	10	15	20	25	30
Basal-cell carcinoma						
10	1.02	1.02	1.03	1.03	1.03	1.03
20	1.04	1.05	1.05	1.05	1.06	1.06
30	1.06	1.07	1.07	1.08	1.08	1.08
40	1.08	1.09	1.09	1.10	1.10	1.10
50	1.10	1.11	1.11	1.11	1.11	1.11
60	1.11	1.11	1.11	1.11	1.11	1.11
Squamous-cell carcinoma						
10	1.02	1.03	1.03	1.04	1.04	1.04
20	1.05	1.06	1.06	1.07	1.07	1.08
30	1.07	1.09	1.10	1.10	1.10	1.11
40	1.11	1.12	1.12	1.13	1.13	1.13
50	1.14	1.14	1.15	1.15	1.15	1.15
60	1.16	1.16	1.16	1.16	1.16	1.16

than expected as a consequence of ozone depletion. Clearly it will prove difficult to identify the real effect of ozone depletion on skin cancer incidence over the next few decades. So whilst we are right to be alarmed at continuing damage to the atmosphere, predictions of skin cancer epidemics as a result are probably alarmist.

References

Bell, A. (1994) Media (mis)communication on the science of climate change. *Public Understanding of Science*, **3**, 259–275.

Blumthaler, M. & Ambach, W. (1994) Health and climate change. *Lancet*, **343**, 303.

Bojkov, R.D., Zerefos, C.S., Balis, D.S., Ziomas, I.C. & Bais, A.F. (1993) Record low total ozone during northern winters of 1992 and 1993. *Geophysics Research Letters*, **13**, 1351–1354.

Bruhl, C. & Crutzen, P.J. (1989) On the disproportionate role of tropospheric ozone as a filter against solar UVB radiation. *Geophysics Research Letters*, **16**, 703–706.

Chuang, T-Y., Propesca, A., Su, W.P.D. & Chute, C.G. (1990) Basal cell carcinoma: a population-based incidence study in Rochester, Minnesota. *Journal of the American Academy of Dermatology*, **22**, 413–417.

Coebergh, J.W.W., Neumann, H.A.M., Vrints, L.W., van der Heijden, L., Meijer, W.J. & Verhagen-Teulings, M.T. (1991) Trends in the incidence of non-melanoma skin cancer in the SE Netherlands 1975–1988: a registry-based study. *British Journal of Dermatology*, **125**, 353–359.

de Gruijl, F.R. (1982) *The dose–response relationship for UV tumorigenesis*. PhD thesis, University of Utrecht.

de Gruijl, F.R. & van der Leun, J.C. (1994) Estimate of the wavelength dependency of ultraviolet carcinogenesis in humans and its relevance to the risk assessment of a stratospheric ozone depletion. *Health Physics*, **67**, 319–325.

de Gruijl, F.R., Sterenborg, H.J.C.M., Forbes, P.D. *et al.* (1993) Wavelength dependence of skin cancer induction by ultraviolet irradiation of albino hairless mice. *Cancer Research*, **53**, 53–60.

Diffey, B.L. (1992) Stratospheric ozone depletion and the risk of non-melanoma skin cancer in a British population. *Physical Medicine and Biology*, **37**, 2267–2279.

Diffey, B.L. (ed.) (1996) *Measurement and Trends of Terrestrial UVB Radiation in Europe*. Organizzazione Editoriale Medico Farmaceutica, Milan.

Diffey, B.L., Gibson, C.J., Haylock, R. & McKinlay, A.F. (1996) Outdoor ultraviolet exposure of children and ado-lescents. *British Journal of Dermatology*, **134**, 1030–1034.

Farman, J.C., Gardiner, B.G. & Shanklin, J.D. (1985) Large losses of total ozone in Antarctica reveal season $ClO_x NO_x$ interaction. *Nature*, **315**, 207–210.

Frederick, J.E. (1993) Ultraviolet sunlight reaching the Earth's surface: a review of recent research. *Photochemistry and Photobiology*, **57**, 175–178.

Frederick, J.E. & Erlick, C. (1995) Trends and interannual variations in erythema sunlight, 1978–1993. *Photochemistry and Photobiology*, **62**, 476–484.

Glass, A.G. & Hoover, R.N. (1989) The emerging epidemic of melanoma and squamous cell skin cancer. *Journal of the American Medical Association*, **262**, 2097–2100.

Health Council of The Netherlands (1994) *Risks of UV Radiation Committee. UV Radiation from Sunlight* (publication no. 1994/05E). Health Council of The Netherlands, The Hague.

Hunter, D.J., Colditz, G.A., Stampfer, M.J., Rosner, B., Willet, W.C. & Speizer, F.E. (1990) Risk factors for basal cell carcinoma in a prospective cohort of women. *Annals of Epidemiology*, **1**, 13–23.

Levi, F., LaVecchia, C., Te, V-C. & Mezzanotte, G. (1988) Descriptive epidemiology of skin cancer in the Swiss Canton of Vaud. *International Journal of Cancer*, **42**, 811–816.

MacKie, R.M. & Rycroft, M.J. (1988) Health and the ozone layer: skin cancers may increase dramatically. *British Medical Journal*, **297**, 369–370.

Marks, R., Staples, M. & Giles, G.G. (1993) Trends in non-melanocytic skin cancer treated in Australia: the second national survey. *International Journal of Cancer*, **53**, 585–590.

McKinlay, A.F. & Diffey, B.L. (1987) A reference action spectrum for ultraviolet induced erythema in human skin. *CIE Journal*, **6**, 17–22.

Moan, J., Dahlback, A., Henriksen, T. & Magnus, K. (1989) Biological amplification factor for sunlight-induced non-melanoma skin cancer at high latitudes. *Cancer Research*, **49**, 5207–5212.

Molina, M. & Rowland, F.S. (1974) Stratospheric sink for chlorofluoromethanes chlorine atom catalyzed destruction of ozone. *Nature*, **249**, 810–812.

Niu, X., Frederick, J.E., Stein, M.L. & Tiao, G.C. (1992) Trends in column ozone based on TOMS data: dependence on month, latitude and longitude. *Journal of Geophysics Research*, **97**, 14661–14669.

Roberts, D.L. (1990) Incidence of non-melanoma skin cancer in West Glamorgan, South Wales. *British Journal of Dermatology*, **122**, 399–403.

Roy, C.R. & Gies, H.P. (1992) Results from an Australian solar UVR measurement network and implications for radiation protection policy. In: *Proceedings of the 8th International Congress of the International Radiation Protection Association, 17–22 May, 1992, Montreal*, Vol. 1, pp. 759–762.

Rundel, R.D. (1983) Promotional effects of ultraviolet radiation on human basal and squamous cell carcinoma. *Photochemistry and Photobiology*, **38**, 569–575.

Russell Jones, R. (1987) Ozone depletion and cancer risk. *Lancet*, **ii**, 443–446.

Scotto, J., Fears, T.R. & Fraumeni, J.F. (1983) *Incidence of Non-melanoma Skin Cancer in the United States* (NIH publication no. 83-2433). US Department of Health and Human Sciences, Bethesda.

Slaper, H. & van der Leun, J.C. (1987) Human exposure to ultraviolet radiation: quantitative modelling of skin cancer incidence. In: *Human Exposure to Ultraviolet Radiation: Risks and Regulations* (eds W.F. Passchier & B.F.M. Bosnjakovic), pp. 155–171. Elsevier, Amsterdam.

Stratospheric Ozone 1990. United Kingdom Stratospheric Ozone Review Group. Third Report. HMSO, London.

Stratospheric Ozone 1991. United Kingdom Stratospheric Ozone Review Group. Fourth Report. HMSO, London.

Stratospheric Ozone 1993. United Kingdom Stratospheric Ozone Review Group. Fifth Report. HMSO, London.

United Nations Environment Programme (1987) *Montreal Protocol on Substances that Deplete the Ozone Layer*. UNEP Conference Service Number 87-6106.

United Nations Environment Programme (1989) *Environmental Effects Panel Report*. UNEP, Nairobi.

United Nations Environment Programme (1991) *Environmental Effects of Ozone Depletion: 1991 Update*. UNEP, Nairobi.

Whitaker, C.J., Lee, W.R. & Downes, J.E. (1979) Squamous cell skin cancer in the north-west of England, 1967–69, and its relation to occupation. *British Journal of Industrial Medicine*, **36**, 43–51.

8
Other Environmental Risk Factors for Skin Cancers

PUVA and Non-Melanoma Skin Cancer

R.S. STERN

Introduction

In 1974, oral methoxsalen and ultraviolet A (PUVA) therapy was shown to be highly effective in the treatment of severe psoriasis (Parrish *et al.*, 1974). Within a year, PUVA became widely used for the treatment of psoriasis and other skin diseases including atopic eczema and cutaneous T-cell lymphoma. Since 1974, hundreds of thousands of persons have been treated with PUVA for skin and other diseases.

Even before its effectiveness for the treatment of skin disease was demonstrated, the carcinogenic risk of PUVA in animals was known (Urbach, 1959). Additional recent work demonstrates that PUVA is an efficient cause of skin cancer in animals. In fact, exposure to PUVA is often used as a positive control in animal studies designed to assess the photocarcinogenic potential of other compounds (Dunnick *et al.*, 1991).

Despite the clear evidence in animals that exposure to PUVA greatly increases the risk of skin cancer, there has been substantial debate in the medical literature whether, as used in humans, PUVA increases the risk of non-melanoma skin cancer, particularly squamous-cell carcinoma of the skin. Here, evidence from studies of the carcinogenic risk of PUVA in humans is reviewed. Differences in study design, population treated and method of analysis that might explain the differences in the conclusions of these studies are discussed. Potential biases that may explain differences between studies as well as power of alternative studies to detect

the carcinogenic effects of high levels of exposure to PUVA are noted. In addition, the evidence that relates risk to dose of PUVA and potential interactions between PUVA and other psoriasis therapies as risk factors for the development of non-melanoma skin cancer are assessed. The natural history of these tumours, especially their metastatic risk and the relative susceptibility of different anatomical sites to PUVA-induced non-melanoma skin cancer, is reviewed. The relative advantages and disadvantages of different methods of study to assess the relationship between the incidence of squamous-cell carcinoma and exposure to PUVA are also discussed.

PUVA and squamous-cell carcinoma

Cohort studies

One method for evaluating the long-term risk of a therapy is the prospective cohort study. Such studies identify a group of exposed patients and follow them to document their exposure to the treatment of interest (i.e. PUVA) as well as alternative possible causes of the toxicity (i.e. UVB, methotrexate and ionizing radiation). Well-done prospective cohort studies are more likely to have accurate and complete ascertainment of cases (i.e. skin cancers) than are retrospective studies. For a cohort study to be efficient, it must have sufficient power to detect what would be a clinically important increase in risk. For example, if one expected 1 out of every 500 persons in a year in the population not exposed to PUVA to develop a skin tumour during follow-up, following a population of 1000 individuals exposed to PUVA for 5 years would have a power of <80% of detecting a doubling of incidence due to PUVA if it existed (i.e. would have less than a 4/5 chance of demonstrating such an increase with statistical significance). The power of a study is even more limited if only a portion of the treated group (i.e. the cohort) had received high enough doses to be at increased risk. For example, if only 10% of 1000 patients had received such doses, the chances of a study of 1000 patients for 5 years demonstrating a significant increase in risk that was, in fact, truly a twofold increase, but was limited to the high-dose group, would be less than 1 in 10. The chances of detecting even a fivefold increase in relative risk in this small high-dose group compared to the larger low-dose patients would be <70%.

The PUVA Follow-up Study

A few months after the effectiveness of PUVA in the treatment of psoriasis was documented, 16 centres organized a study to determine the safety of this treatment. With sponsorship from the National Institutes of Health (NIH), the study enrolled 1380 patients first treated in 1975 and 1976 at these 16 centres (Stern *et al.*, 1979). Known as the PUVA Follow-up Study, this study has followed these patients with periodic dermatological examinations and patient interviews for nearly 20 years. Reported tumours are confirmed from pathology reports, and patient exposures to both PUVA therapy and other potential carcinogens such as UVB, tar and methotrexate are prospectively documented. For each cycle of examinations, follow-up has usually exceeded 90% of eligible patients.

In 1979, an increase in the incidence of cutaneous carcinoma was detected among members of this cohort. Most notable was the higher incidence of squamous- than basal-cell carcinoma (rate ratio 3:2 compared to a usual ratio of $\geq$1:6 in the general population) (Stern *et al.*, 1979). The anatomical distribution of squamous-cell carcinomas was also different than that observed in the general population. More than 80% of these tumours were on the trunk, lower extremities and genitals. Prior exposure to ionizing radiation for the treatment of psoriasis, having had a prior skin cancer and being skin type I or II were all identified as risk factors for the development of skin cancer for squamous-cell but not basal-cell carcinomas. There was also a significant relation between number of

PUVA treatments and the risk of squamous-cell cancer. Taken together, these data suggested that 2 years of intense exposure to PUVA increased the risk of squamous-cell carcinoma among individuals with substantial past exposure to other cutaneous carcinogens or who were fair skinned and who easily sunburn. These data suggested that PUVA therapy promoted the development of squamous-cell cancer. These early findings did not address the issue of whether PUVA is a complete carcinogen, as had been demonstrated in animals (Urbach, 1959).

In 1984, additional data from the PUVA Follow-up Study demonstrated a significant dose-dependent relation between exposure to PUVA and the risk of squamous-cell carcinoma (Stern *et al.*, 1984). Overall, the risk of squamous-cell carcinoma was 16-fold higher among PUVA-treated patients compared to that expected from general population rates. Some of these observed increases are undoubtedly due to these patients' other exposures to other carcinogens such as UVB, tar and ionizing radiation. However, when low- and high-dose patients exposed to PUVA are compared and Poisson logistic regression is utilized to estimate the relative risk attributable to tar, ionizing radiation and level of exposure to PUVA simultaneously, high-dose PUVA patients had an adjusted relative standard morbidity ratio 12.8-fold that of patients exposed to low doses of PUVA.

After an average of 6 years of follow-up, a total of 54 of the original 1380 patients had developed 169 squamous-cell carcinomas (Stern *et al.*, 1984). After an additional nearly 8 years of follow-up, the number of patients with these tumours had increased by 166% (from 54 to 144) and the number of squamous-cell carcinomas had increased by 265% (from 169 to 618 squamous-cell cancers) (Stern *et al.*, 1984; Stern & Laird, 1994). After nearly 14 years of follow-up, similar relations in this cohort between PUVA dose level and risk of squamous-cell carcinoma were noted. After adjusting for exposure to other carcinogens, the relative risk of squamous-cell carcinoma was 5.9-fold higher for patients exposed to high doses of PUVA compared to those exposed to low doses (Stern & Laird, 1994).

Additional observations that link exposure to PUVA to an increased risk of squamous-cell carcinoma include the association between the occurrence of tumours at unusual anatomical sites and the level exposure to PUVA. Among those who develop squamous-cell carcinomas after low exposures to PUVA (i.e. < 160 treatments 11 years after beginning treatment), 29% were on the lower extremities. Among those who developed squamous-cell carcinomas after high-dose exposure only 8% were on the head and neck, and 60% were on the lower extremities. After 14 years, > 25% of surviving patients exposed to more than 300 treatments with PUVA had developed one or more squamous-cell carcinomas (Stern & Laird, 1994).

Other cohort studies

A number of other cohort studies provide varying assessments of the association between exposure to PUVA and the risk of squamous-cell carcinoma. With one exception, these studies include substantially fewer patients than the PUVA Follow-up Study. Uniformly in these studies, rates of follow-up and duration of follow-up are substantially lower than those for the United States PUVA Follow-up Study funded by the NIH.

Forman and colleagues studied 551 patients in seven medical centres for up to 10 years (Forman *et al.*, 1989). By the criteria of the United States PUVA Follow-up Study, most of these patients had low-dose exposure. Still, these authors noted a trend toward increasing numbers of squamous-cell carcinoma in patients with higher exposure to PUVA. In the majority of cases, squamous-cell carcinomas occurred on sites that were not sun-exposed.

A European group followed 1643 of 3175 patients for an average of 8 years. They detected nearly twice as many squamous and basal carcinomas, but denied a 'clinically relevant increase in the risk of tumors induced by PUVA' (Henseler *et al.*, 1987). A closer analysis of these data demonstrates the clear increased risk of squamous-cell carcinoma but not basal-cell carcinoma in patients exposed to 'high doses of PUVA'. High dose was defined as $3000 \, J/cm^2$, a dose approximately equivalent to the 300 treatment high-dose criteria used in the United States PUVA Follow-up Study. The authors report about 10% of their patients had these doses. In contrast, 56% of patients

with squamous-cell carcinoma, but no patients with basal-cell carcinoma, were high-dose patients. Further, high-dose patients with squamous-cell carcinoma were an average of 15 years younger than low-dose patients with squamous-cell carcinoma. In fact, a recalculation of their data yields a crude estimate of 12-fold higher risk of squamous-cell carcinoma in high-dose European patients compared to low-dose patients reported in this study.

A Dutch group using the same treatment protocol took issue with the assertion by some members of the European PUVA study that the protocol utilized in Europe reduced the risk of squamous-cell cancer associated with PUVA (Bruynzeel *et al.*, 1991). After 13 years of follow-up, the Dutch group demonstrated a dose-dependent increase in the incidence of squamous-cell cancer among their patients. A group of English physicians examined their patients who had received PUVA and noted of those who had > 2000 J/cm^2 (a dose lower than the criteria used to define high dose for either the PUVA Follow-up Study or the European PUVA Study), 19% had developed squamous-cell carcinomas and 46% had histologically atypical squamous keratoses.

Torinuki studied a small group of Japanese who had received PUVA (108 patients). Only one patient developed a squamous-cell carcinoma and this was attributed to prior ionizing radiation. Given the low incidence of squamous-cell carcinoma in the Japanese population, the small number of patients followed and the small number of patients with substantial exposure to PUVA, the power of this study is low and this negative result is not surprising (Torinuki & Tagami, 1988).

Chuang and colleagues did a retrospective study of patients treated with PUVA. The definition of high-dose PUVA used was a fraction of the dose that defined high dose in both the European and the United States PUVA Follow-up Study. Even with this less stringent criteria for high-dose exposure, this study also noted an increase in the risk of squamous-cell carcinoma among patients who received 'high doses of PUVA' (Chuang *et al.*, 1992). It would be expected, given the much lower number of exposures used as the criteria to define high dose, that the magnitude of this increased risk was much lower than that observed in the PUVA Follow-up Study.

Record linkage study

Prospective cohort studies have many advantages for studying the association of skin cancer and treatment with PUVA. Cohort studies are, however, expensive, time-consuming and difficult. Using the unique resources of the Swedish Cancer Registry which enables linking of patients identified by their having had PUVA with the cancer reports collected in this registry, Lindelof and colleagues studied 4799 Swedish patients who had ever received PUVA therapy (Lindelöf *et al.*, 1991). Duration of follow-up averaged 7 years. These authors noted a dose-dependent increase in the risk of squamous-cell carcinoma, as well as a 30-fold increase in incidence of squamous-cell carcinoma among patients with >200 treatments compared to that expected from rates for the general Swedish population. Within and between dose groups, their findings closely parallel those observed in the United States study at the end of a similar period of follow-up (Lindelöf *et al.*, 1991).

These authors also noted fewer squamous-cell carcinomas in patients receiving bath rather than oral PUVA. The number of exposures in the bath PUVA group was, however, lower (Lindelöf *et al.*, 1991, 1992). Therefore, whether bath PUVA treatment is, in fact, safer than oral PUVA is not yet established.

Other risk factors

Methotrexate

Early results from the United States PUVA Follow-up Study indicated that ionizing radiation and high levels of exposure to tar or UVB were independent risk factors for the development of squamous-cell carcinoma in the study population (Stern *et al.*, 1979). Less clear is the evidence concerning either the independent or synergistic carcinogenic potential of methotrexate at doses used to treat psoriasis. Based on observations in a small group of patients, a synergistic carcinogenic potential for methotrexate when used in combination with PUVA has been suggested (Fitzsimons *et al.*, 1983). A nested case-control study by Lindelöf suggested that prior therapy with methotrexate might be a risk factor for skin cancer in PUVA-treated patients (Lindelöf & Sigurgeirsson, 1993). Using Poisson regression, the data from the United States PUVA Follow-up Study assessed methotrexate as an independent risk factor for squamous-cell carcinoma as well as possible interaction between methotrexate use and level of exposure to PUVA as risk factors for these tumours. At high levels of exposure (more than 3 years of use), methotrexate is a significant independent risk factor for the development of squamous-cell carcinoma (relative risk equals 2.1) (Stern & Laird, 1994). No synergy between high levels of exposure to methotrexate and the carcinogenic effects of increasing doses of PUVA was noted.

Morbidity of PUVA tumours

Until recently, it was thought that PUVA-associated squamous-cell carcinomas had limited associated morbidity and did not cause deaths. In the PUVA study, however, recently the proportion of patients with squamous-cell carcinoma who developed metastases has increased to 4% (Stern, 1994). Metastases from presumed PUVA-associated skin tumours have been reported by others (Lewis *et al.*, 1994). Clearly, these findings increase concern about the clinical importance of these tumours.

Susceptibility

Susceptible sites

The lower extremities appear to be especially susceptible to the carcinogenic effect of PUVA (Stern *et al.*, 1984; Stern & Laird, 1994). Probably, even more susceptible to the carcinogenic effects of PUVA are the male genitalia. After 12 years, the PUVA Follow-up Study demonstrated a nearly 100-fold increase in the risk of male genital neoplasms for PUVA-treated patients. Among males exposed to high levels of PUVA, the incidence of invasive tumours was nearly 300-fold higher than that observed in the general population and there was a strong and significant relation between level of exposure to PUVA and risk of genital neoplasms (Stern, 1990). Others have since confirmed these observations (de la Brassinne & Richert, 1992). As a result, genital protection is now a standard part of therapy.

Susceptibility factors

Certain phenotypic characteristics are associated with increased risks of skin cancer independent of PUVA. For example, easy sunburning and poor ability to tan with sun exposure are associated with two- to threefold increases in the risk of non-melanoma skin cancer compared to that for other individuals of European ancestry in the general population (Vitaliano & Urbach, 1980). These phenotypic features are associated with similar increases in the risk of PUVA-exposed patients. PUVA patients who are skin type I and II have a two- to threefold higher risk of non-melanoma cancer than skin type III and IV patients also exposed to PUVA (Stern & Momtaz, 1984).

Conclusion

The studies of the carcinogenic risks of PUVA illustrate how a variety of epidemiological approaches can be used to assess the safety of a new treatment and how findings from epidemiological studies help to refine estimates of the risks and benefits of a treatment. Continued studies of PUVA-treated patients, especially the original cohort of patients who have been studied for nearly 20 years as part of the United States PUVA Follow-up Study, will help determine the ultimate risk and morbidity of this very effective treatment for psoriasis.

References

Bruynzeel, I., Bergman, W., Hartevelt, H.M. *et al.* (1991) 'High single-dose' European PUVA regimen also causes an excess of non-melanoma skin cancer. *British Journal of Dermatology*, **124**, 49–55.

Chuang, T.Y., Heinrich, L.A., Schultz, M.D., Reizner, C.T., Kumm, R.C. & Cripps, D.J. (1992) PUVA and skin cancer. A historical cohort study on 492 patients. *Journal of the American Academy of Dermatology*, **26**, 173–177.

de la Brassinne, M. & Richert, B. (1992) Genital squamous-cell carcinoma after PUVA therapy. *Dermatology*, **185**, 316–318.

Dunnick, J.K., Forbes, P.D., Eustis, S.L., Hardisty, J.F. & Goodman, D.G. (1991). Tumors of the skin in the HRA/Skh mouse after treatment with 8-methoxypsoralen and UVA radiation. *Fundamentals of Applied Toxicology*, **16**, 92–102.

Fitzsimons, C.P., Long, J. & MacKie, R.M. (1983) Synergistic carcinogenic potential of methotrexate and PUVA in psoriasis. *Lancet*, **i**, 235–236.

Forman, A.B., Roenigk, H.H., Caro, W.A. & Magid, M.L. (1989) Long-term follow-up of skin cancer in the PUVA-48 cooperative study. *Archives of Dermatology*, **125**, 515–519.

Henseler, T., Christophers, E., Honigsmann, H. & Wolff, K. (1987) Skin tumors in the European PUVA Study. Eight-year follow-up of 1643 patients treated with PUVA for psoriasis. *Journal of the American Academy of Dermatology*, **16**, 108–116.

Lewis, F.M., Shah, M., Messenger, A.G. & Thomas, W.E. (1994) Metastatic squamous-cell carcinoma in patient receiving PUVA. *Lancet*, **344**, 1157.

Lindelöf, B. & Sigurgeirsson, B. (1993) PUVA and cancer: a case-control study. *British Journal of Dermatology*, **129**, 39–41.

Lindelöf, B., Sigurgeirsson, B. Tegner, E. *et al.* (1991). PUVA and cancer; a large-scale epidemiological study. *Lancet*, **338**, 91–93.

Lindelöf, B., Sigurgeirsson, B., Tegner, E., Larko, O. & Berne, B. (1992) Comparison of the carcinogenic potential of trioxsalen bath PUVA and oral methoxsalen PUVA. A preliminary report. *Archives of Dermatology*, **128**, 1341–1344.

Parrish, J.A., Fitzpatrick, T.B., Tanenbaum, L. *et al.* (1974) Photochemotherapy of psoriasis with oral methoxsalen and longwave ultraviolet light. *New England Journal of Medicine*, **291**, 1207–1211.

Stern, R.S. (1990) Genital tumors among men with psoriasis exposed to psoralens and ultraviolet A radiation (PUVA) and ultraviolet B radiation. The Photochemotherapy Follow-up Study. *New England Journal of Medicine*, **322**, 1093–1097.

Stern, R. (1994) Metastatic squamous-cell cancer after psoralen photochemotherapy. *Lancet*, **344**, 1644–1645.

Stern, R.S. & Laird, N. (1994) The carcinogenic risk of treatments for severe psoriasis. *Cancer*, **73**, 2759–2764.

Stern, R.S. & Momtaz, K. (1984) Skin typing for assessment of skin cancer risk and acute response to UVB and oral methoxsalen photochemotherapy. *Archives of Dermatology*, **120**, 869–873.

Stern, R.S., Thibodeau, L.A., Kleinerman, R.A. *et al.* (1979) Risk of cutaneous carcinoma in patients treated with oral methoxsalen photochemotherapy for psoriasis. *New England Journal of Medicine*, **300**, 809–813.

Stern, R.S., Laird, N., Melski, J., Parrish, J.A., Fitzpatrick, T.B. & Bleich, H.L. (1984) Cutaneous squamous-cell carcinoma in patients treated with PUVA. *New England Journal of Medicine*, **310**, 1156–1161.

Torinuki, W. & Tagami, H. (1988) Incidence of skin cancer in Japanese psoriatic patients treated with either methoxsalen phototherapy, Goeckerman regimen, or both therapies. A

10-year follow-up study. *Journal of the American Academy of Dermatology*, **18**, 1278–1281.

Urbach, F. (1959) Modification of ultraviolet carcinogenesis by photoactive agents: preliminary report. *Journal of Investigative Dermatology*, **32**, 373–378.

Vitaliano, P.P. & Urbach, F. (1980) The relative importance of risk factors in nonmelanoma carcinoma. *Archives of Dermatology*, **116**, 454–456.

Fluorescent and Halogen Sources, Suntanning Lamps and Skin Cancers

J.-P. CESARINI

Exposure to ultraviolet (UV) radiation occurs from both natural and artificial sources. The sun is the principal source of exposure for most people. With the depletion of stratospheric ozone, people and the environment will be exposed to higher intensities of UV. At the World Environment Conference (Rio de Janeiro, 1992), it was specifically recommended to 'undertake, as a matter of urgency, research on the effect on human health of the increasing ultraviolet radiation reaching the earth surface'. There is also, as a consequence, a necessity to undertake measurements and scientific approaches on artificial sources of UV expressing a potential hazard in addition to the natural solar UV source. Various lamps are used in medicine, industry, commerce, research and at home. Acute effects of UV radiation on the skin consist of: (i) solar erythema, 'sunburn', which may result, when severe, in blistering and destruction of the surface of the skin (similar to those effects resulting from first- or second-degree heat burns); (ii) chronic skin changes, consisting of benign abnormalities of keratinocytes and/or melanocytes; and (iii) skin cancer (melanoma and non-melanocytic). In these conditions, UV-specific mutations of the tumour-suppressor gene *P53* have been observed in two studies (Volkenandt *et al.*, 1991; Florenes *et al.*, 1994). In solar elastosis, 'photoageing', and all skin cancer conditions the p53 protein is overexpressed, as evaluated in numerous immuno-histochemical studies (Asklen & Morkve, 1992).

UV exposure conditions

In outdoor conditions, the UVA and UVB content of solar exposure can be predicted from the thickness of the ozone layer, season, hour of the day, altitude, cloudiness, nebulization and pollution (dust). The total yearly dose received at a given location by a given population can be roughly estimated and averaged on the number of years spent in the location. Of course, human behaviour is widely different according to the attitude towards solar exposure, but, at the individual level, a more or less precise count can be achieved. In outdoor conditions, humans can be exposed to both natural and artificial sources, the dose being much more difficult to evaluate. Solar radiations are filtered by window glass, windshield and car windows, eye-glasses and plastic covers; enormous variations in filtered UVA and UVB, according to the glass composition or the plastic nature, are experienced. In domestic and commercial conditions, artificial sources are fluorescent tubes for lighting, desk-top and general halogens, and UV sources for cosmetic tanning. All these sources are based on one principle: electrical discharge of ionizing gas in a quartz envelope. The composition of the gas and the chemical nature of the envelope determine the spectrum of emitted radiations. Workers are exposed to artificial sources: welding or foundry work, film projection, high-intensity discharge lamps in crack detection, printing and dyeline copying, insecticidal UV sources in catering and restaurants. UVA, UVB and UVC radiations are emitted by the sources to which workers are exposed. Duration of irradiation, intensity and composition of the spectrum of the sources differ widely.

Potential detrimental effects from artificial light sources

Numerous questions have been raised after the analysis of epidemiological studies or from reports of accidents. International organizations in charge of the security of users have brought some responses to the questions (IRPA, 1991). There are several bodies which, independently, are in charge of surveillance for the safety of users of artificial sources: Commission Internationale de l'Eclairage (CIE) and its Technical

Committees, the International Electrotechnical Commission (IEC), the International Commission for Non-Ionizing Radiation Protection (ICNIRP), the International Labour Organization (ILO) and the World Health Organization (WHO). The documents issued by these commissions provide the industrial community with some guidelines, such as normalization by the European Economic Community (EEC) and compliances to the limits of exposure (ACGIH, 1992). International conferences are regularly organized by health authorities, and documents are issued, keeping the organizations in charge of the population security informed of the progress in the knowledge of the ultraviolet impact on human health (WHO, 1994) and making the industry aware of the potential risks in their practice from lighting devices developed from new technologies. Figure 8.1 (Muel, 1987) illustrates the power spectrum distribution of several UV-emitting artificial sources and the solar spectrum as a reference.

The action spectrum for erythema produced by the CIE Technical Committee has been adopted by the international community as a reference spectrum (McKinlay & Diffey, 1987) and is considered as representative for every UV hazard until the adoption of specific action spectra for specific detrimental effects. It does not differ much from the American Conference Governmental Industrial Hygienists (ACGIH)-recommended occupational maximum permissible exposure levels (Fig. 8.2).

Fluorescent tubes for lighting

Several epidemiological studies on malignant melanoma have suggested a link between skin cancers and occupational or domestic exposure to fluorescent lighting (Beral *et al.*, 1982; Pasternack *et al.*, 1983). They show a trend in a positive association. More than 10 other studies excluded a link between fluorescent exposure and malignant melanoma (Sorahan & Grimley, 1985; Swerdlow *et al.*, 1988).

A fluorescent lighting tube is a source of radiation created by a gas discharge in a glass tube, internally

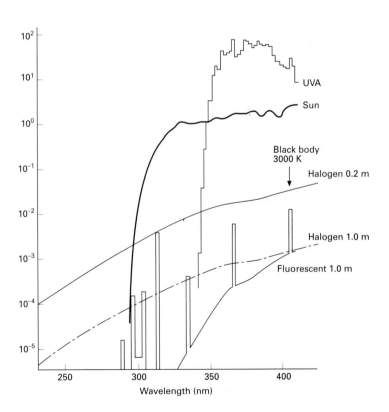

Fig. 8.1 Spectral power distribution of fluorescent tube for lighting, halogen, UVA suntanning lamp and sunlight. (From Muel, 1987.)

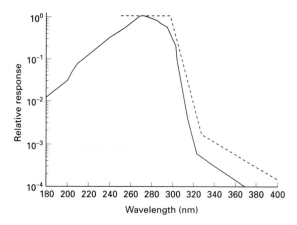

Fig. 8.2 UV-induced erythemal action spectrum [CIE (dashed line); McKinlay & Diffey, 1987] and IRPA/ICNIRP (1991) (solid line) relative spectral effectiveness. (From WHO, 1994.)

coated with photoluminescent substances (powder). The nature of the powder is responsible for the spectrum of the emission (Fig. 8.3). For example, a cool white fluorescent lamp (illuminance of 500 lux) has an average total UV irradiance of 0.3 W/m². Weighted by the reference erythema action spectrum of ACGIH limit values, no erythemal risk below general level of 1 minimal erythema dose (MED) has been detected. If one estimates the average MED per year from environmental exposure to 150 MED and the average MED per year from fluorescent light environment at 50 MED, the calculated risk for additional skin cancers is not negligible. However, Lytle *et al.* (1993) found a relative risk for office workers to be 4.3 for exposure longer than 20 years and 4.5 for >7 hours exposure per day.

A survey of more than 10 fluorescent tubes manufactured and traded worldwide has shown that some tubes were above the maximal threshold limits and should be withdrawn from the market. It has been shown that a simple change in the glass envelope composition, resulting from a change in the source of the sand, dramatically changed the emission spectrum of the tube. Periodic checking of the spectrum of such light sources in order to avoid unintentional overexposure of the users is strongly recommended.

From a CIE Research Note (Technical Committee TC6-09) (Muel *et al.*, 1988), it can be said that:

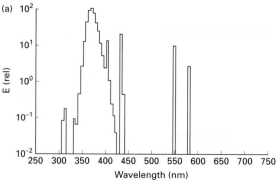

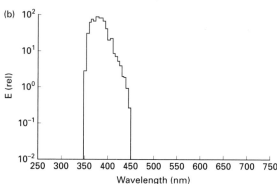

Fig. 8.3 Spectral power distribution of (a) UVA fluorescent tube (low pressure) and (b) UVA metal halide source (high pressure). The two sources are typical of suntanning sources. (From Mutzhas, 1986.)

the available evidences do not support the existence of any substantial association between melanoma risk and exposure to fluorescent lighting. The Committee has evaluated the UV radiations, weighted by the CIE erythema action spectrum, received from fluorescent lighting, and found that the doses are normally not above a few percent of the doses received from the sun. The evidence for risk of melanoma is too uncertain to merit any regulatory control. There is a recommendation for using diffusers in styrene or any other devices to quench the potential UV radiations emitted by the sources able to reach the user's tegument and eyes.

Nevertheless, the lifetime exposure of indoor workers to unfiltered fluorescent lighting may add 3.9% to the risk from solar UV. There is a small increased risk of squamous-cell carcinoma from exposure to UV-emitting fluorescent lamps. However, significant differences in the spectrum distribution between manufacturers still exist and might be of importance. As an example, in a recent study (Cebula *et al.*, 1995), the illumination of *Salmonella* by GE F15T8, GE F15T12 and Sylvania F15T8 15 W cool white (fluorescent lamp with 6% of irradiance in UV spectrum) induces lethality and mutagenicity, while, under the same conditions, Philips 15 W cool white fluorescent lamp (1% of irradiance in UV spectrum) has no detectable effects. This work pointed out the necessity of increasing attention at home and in the workplace and the necessity of regular checks in industrial production.

Desk-top and general lighting halogens

Erythema and skin hardening on the hands of office workers have been described (Césarini & Muel, 1989). Melanoma has been reported in the personnel of retail shops lit with quartz halogen spotlamps. The spectral distribution of different halogen sources has revealed emission of UVC, UVB and UVA (Fig. 8.3). We succeeded (Césarini & Muel, 1992) in inducing actinic erythema on the backs of volunteers in 30 min at a 30-cm distance from a halogen source, and pigmentation on their hands after 5 days of consecutive 2-hour exposure at a distance of 50 cm. We have calculated the erythemal irradiance of two different sources and found a source emitting $0.09 \, W/m^2$ and a source emitting $0.4 \, W/m^2$. As a comparison, the solar erythemal irradiance at $40°$ zenith angle is $0.25 \, W/m^2$ (Fig. 8.1).

A CIE Research Note (TC6-18) has concluded that different irradiances given by desk-lamps and halogen lamps accidentally directed on any part of the body may be potentially dangerous. It is recommended avoiding unnecessary irradiation on the hands and possibly on the eyes and filtering of the emitted radiation (McKinlay *et al.*, 1989). Specific notes have

subsequently been written on the labels of naked bulbs used in indirect lighting and in slide projectors. For the home use of direct light devices, halogen sources must be covered with built-in plastic covers.

Suntanning lamps

Several investigations on epidemiology of skin malignant melanoma established a relation between the use of sunbeds or sunlamps and malignant melanoma (Diffey, 1987; Swerdlow *et al.*, 1988; Walter *et al.*, 1990; Westerdahl *et al.*, 1994). More recently, it has been clearly demonstrated that more than 10 exposures per year to tanning devices induces a significant risk for the development of squamous-cell carcinoma, basal-cell carcinoma and melanoma (Autier *et al.*, 1994). Autier *et al.* have calculated risk factors (Table 8.1). Several reports on artificial tanning in European countries pointed out the need for regulation and estimated the risks for the general public use of UV sources (Césarini *et al.*, 1987).

The motives for exposure to UV are numerous, mostly due to an association of a tan with good health. The publicity surrounding tanning saloons is largely oriented around the absolute safety of the use of UVA-emitting lamps. In fact, a survey of the public sources sold by catalogue or used in beauty saloons and fitness centres revealed that the sources emitted UVA and UVB in different ratios (Fig. 8.3a & 8.3b). Low-pressure UVA fluorescent tubes (Fig. 8.3a) are more or less contaminated with UVB (0.5–4% of the UV power output) which may represent more than one-half of the erythemal weighted irradiance. The high-pressure filtered UVA discharge lamp (Fig. 8.3b) emits pure UVA but 10 times the irradiance of natural solar UVA irradiance.

The emission spectrum weighted by the erythema CIE action spectrum demonstrated that, in general, the erythemal effective radiant exposure per session

Table 8.1 Conditions of exposure and risks of melanoma.		
	Exposure for tanning before 1980	OR = 2.71 ($P \leqslant 0.05$)
	Exposure for tanning after 1980	OR = 1.11 (Not significant)
	Exposure for tanning, no skinburn	OR = 0.92 (Not significant)
	Exposure for tanning + skinburn	OR = 8.97 ($P < 0.001$)

OR, Odds ratio.

(20–30 min) can be estimated at 150 J/m² (equivalent to 0.8 MED for averagely sensitive skin). The total annual exposure is estimated at 25 MED (30 sessions) with extension up to 100 MED for some addicted users. It should be realized that under the same conditions, some equipment may emit 400 J/m² (2 MED per session). This level has to be compared with the 150–200 MED received yearly during everyday life in temperate countries. The population of Australia, receiving 300–400 MED, has a skin cancer incidence eightfold the cancer incidence of northern Europe. So the cumulative dose received by regular users of tanning saloons approaches the level of populations living in subtropical areas (van Weelden *et al.*, 1988). Beside the long-term risks (Roza *et al.*, 1989), reports of severe sunburns, phototoxicity and idiopathic photodermatosis have drawn the attention of the regulatory authorities (IRPA/INIRC, 1991). In some countries, like France, where psoralen pills can be easily obtained, or where psoralen-containing suntan preparations were, up till recently, advertised and freely available on the market (Autier *et al.*, 1995), a significant number of people had to be admitted to intensive care units for severe burns. Careful questioning of tanning saloon users revealed that the incidence of itching, nausea, skin rashes and pigmented dermatitis was not insignificant (>20% of users) (Mawn & Fleischer, 1993).

UVA artificial tanning should no longer be considered as the safest way to get a tan (de Gruijl *et al.*, 1993; de Gruijl, 1993) if the importance of radiation in the UVA range, according to the carcinogenic action spectrum, is considered (Fig. 8.4).

Conclusion

Several direct artificial sources of UV are present in the human environment. The risks from radiation of these sources have been evaluated through hundreds of epidemiological studies, spectral power distribution of source analysis and, when available, weighted by biological action spectra. The risk of developing non-melanocytic skin cancers and malignant melanoma from fluorescent light is estimated to be very low. The risk from halogen light sources, especially when used at a short distance (<1 m) is not negligible and requires filtering measures (styrene or glass). The risk from

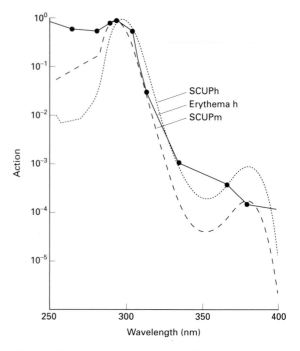

Fig. 8.4 Carcinogenic action spectrum for mouse (SCUPm), and proposed human carcinogenic action spectrum (SCUPh), compared with human erythemal action spectrum. The human epidermis is much thicker than murine epidermis. A correction for a correspondence in UV transmission should be made. (From de Gruijl *et al.*, 1993.)

tanning equipment appears much higher. Some data indicate that 10 exposures per year have significant adverse effects, i.e. the possibility of malignant melanoma. The risks from artificial tanning sources have been found as high as eightfold for populations with very sensitive skin and under 30 years of age. This is independent of constitutional and sun-exposure factors. The possible causal relation between malignant melanoma and tanning devices should be a warning to public health authorities in terms of the possible detrimental health consequences of irresponsible exposure to tanning equipment.

References

ACGIH (1992) *Threshold Limit Values and Biological Exposure Indices*, pp. 124–127. ACGIH, Cincinnati.

Asklen, L.A. & Morkve, O. (1992) Expression of p53 protein in cutaneous melanoma. *International Journal of Cancer*, **52**, 13–16.

Autier, P., Dore, J.F., Lejeune, F. *et al.* (1994) Cutaneous malignant melanoma and exposure to sunlamps or sunbeds: An EORTC multicenter case-control study in Belgium, France and Germany. *International Journal of Cancer*, **58**, 809–813.

Autier, P., Dore, J.F., Schifflers, E. *et al.* (1995) Melanoma and use of sunscreens: an EORTC case-control study in Germany, Belgium and France. *International Journal of Cancer*, **61**, 749–755.

Beral, V., Evans, S., Shaw, H. & Milton, G. (1982) Malignant melanoma and exposure to fluorescent lighting at work. *Lancet*, **ii**, 290–293.

Cebula, T.A., Henrikson, E.N., Hartman, P.E. & Biggley, W.H. (1995) Reversion profiles of coolwhite fluorescent light compared with far ultraviolet light: homologies and differences. *Photochemistry and Photobiology*, **61**, 353–359.

Césarini, J.P. & Muel, B. (1989) Erythema induced by quartz-halogen sources. *Photodermatology*, **6**, 222–227.

Césarini, J.P. & Muel, B. (1992) Risques dermatologiques des sources quartz-halogène. *Annales de Dermatologie et de Vénéréologie*, **119**, 349–353.

Césarini, J.P., Muel, B. & Bastie, J. (1987) The French project for sunlamp regulations. In: *Human Exposure to Ultraviolet Radiation: Risks and Regulations* (eds W.F. Passchier & B.F.M. Bosnjakovic), pp. 497–501. Excerpta Medica, Amsterdam.

de Gruijl, F.R. (1993) UV-induced skin cancer: man and mouse. In: *Symposium on The Dark Side of Sunlight*, pp. 111–124. Utrecht University, The Netherlands.

de Gruijl, F.R., Sterenborg, H.J.C.M., Forbes, P.D. *et al.* (1993) Wavelength dependence of skin cancer induction by ultraviolet irradiation of albino hairless mice. *Cancer Research*, **53**, 53–60.

Diffey, B.L. (1987) Analysis of the risk of skin cancer from sunlight and solaria in subjects living in northern Europe. *Photodermatology*, **4**, 118–126.

Florenes, V.A., Oyjord, T., Holm, R. *et al.* (1994) *TP53* allele loss, mutations and expression in malignant melanoma. *British Journal of Cancer*, **69**, 253–259.

IRPA (1991) *Guidelines on Protection against Non-Ionizing Radiation* (eds A.S. Duchêne, J.R.A. Lakey & M.H. Repacholi). Pergamon Press, New York.

IRPA/INIRC (1991) Health issues of ultraviolet 'A' sunbeds used for cosmetic purposes. *Health Physics*, **61**, 285–288.

Lytle, C.D., Cyr, W.H., Beer, J.Z. *et al.* (1993) An estimation of squamous cell carcinoma risk from ultraviolet radiation emitted by fluorescent lamps. *Photodermatology Photoimmunology and Photomedicine*, **9**, 268–274.

Mawn, V.B. & Fleischer, A.B. Jr. (1993) A survey of attitudes, beliefs, behavior regarding tanning bed use, sunbathing,

and sunscreen use. *Journal of the American Academy of Dermatology*, **29**, 959–962.

McKinlay, A.F. & Diffey, B.L. (1987) A reference action spectrum for ultraviolet induced erythema in human skin. *CIE Journal*, **6**, 17–22.

McKinlay, A.F., Whillock, M.J. & Meulemans, C.C.E. (1989) Ultraviolet radiation and blue-light emissions from spotlights incorporating tungsten halogen lamps. *Report of the National Radiological Protection Board* (NRPBR228). NRPB, Chilton.

Muel, B. (1987) Spectral measurements of irradiances at skin level from sunlamps and other sources. In: *Human Exposure to Ultraviolet Radiation: Risks and Regulations* (eds W.F. Passchier & B.F.M. Bosnjakovic), pp. 259–264. Excerpta Medica, Amsterdam.

Muel, B., Césarini, J.P. & Elwood, J.M. (1988) Malignant melanoma and fluorescent lighting. *CIE Journal*, **7**, 29–33.

Mutzhas, M.F. (1986) UVA-emitting light sources. In: *The Biological Effects of UVA Radiation* (eds F. Urbach & R.W. Gange), pp. 10–29. Praeger, New York.

Pasternack, B.S., Dubin, N. & Moseson, M. (1983) Malignant melanoma and exposure to fluorescent lighting. (Letter.) *Lancet*, **i**, 704.

Roza, L., Baan, R.A., van der Leun, J.C., Kligman, L. & Young, A.R. (1989) UVA hazards in skin associated with the use of tanning equipment. *Journal of Photochemistry and Photobiology, B: Biology*, **3**, 281–287.

Sorahan, T. & Grimley, R.P. (1985) The aetiological significance of sunlight and fluorescent lighting in malignant melanoma: a case control study. *British Journal of Cancer*, **52**, 765–769.

Swerdlow, A.J., English, J.S.C., Mackie, R.M. *et al.* (1988) Fluorescent lights, ultraviolet lamps, and risk of cutaneous melanoma. *British Medical Journal*, **297**, 647–650.

van Weelden, H., de Gruijl, F.R., van der Putte, S.C.J., Toonstra, J. & van der Leun, J.C. (1988) The carcinogenic risks of modern tanning equipment: is UV-A safer than UV-B? *Archives of Dermatological Research*, **280**, 300–307.

Volkenandt M., Schelgel, U., Nanus D.M. *et al.* (1991) Mutational analysis of the human *p53* gene in malignant melanoma. *Pigment Cell Research*, **4**, 35–40.

Walter, S.D., Marrett, L.D., From, L. *et al.* (1990) The association of cutaneous malignant melanoma with the use of sunbeds and sunlamps. *American Journal of Epidemiology*, **131**, 232–243.

Westerdahl, J., Olsson, H., Måsbäck, A. *et al.* (1994) Use of sunbeds or sunlamps and malignant melanoma in southern Sweden. *American Journal of Epidemiology*, **140**, 691–699.

WHO (1994) *Environmental Health Criteria 160*, p. 61. WHO, Geneva.

Melanoma: Risk Factors Other Than Sun Exposure

F.H.J. RAMPEN

The incidence of cutaneous melanoma has been rising for many decades in nearly all affluent countries with a predominantly fair-skinned population. Epidemiological evidence suggests that sun exposure or ultraviolet radiation is a strong and consistent environmental risk factor for melanoma. However, sun exposure cannot explain every case of the disease (Williams, 1995). Non-solar factors are probably also involved. Up till now, the causal inference of factors other than ultraviolet exposure has been poorly studied and understood. Here, challenges are made to the ultraviolet theory and non-solar factors in the risk of melanoma are reviewed.

Sun exposure

The role of cumulative sunlight exposure in the aetiology of non-melanoma skin cancer is now evident. These tumours predominantly appear on sun-exposed areas and occur more frequently among outdoor workers. In contrast, the incidence of melanoma is higher among indoor than outdoor workers (Lee & Strickland, 1980). Melanoma does not predominantly occur on body sites that are most exposed to the sun (Crombie, 1981).

To explain these inconsistencies, the 'intermittent' sunlight theory was launched (Fears *et al.*, 1977): short bursts of intense ultraviolet exposure during recreational activities should increase the risk for melanoma; more regular, chronic exposure has a neutral or even protective effect. No valid explanation has ever been given why little (intermittent) exposure to the sun causes many melanomas, and much (chronic) exposure causes only a few. In the northern hemisphere, the intermittent exposure hypo thesis is supported by much evidence in the literature, but in Australian studies the distinction between intermittent and chronic exposure is far from clear (Elwood, 1992). Complex and speculative exposure–response models have been proposed to explain all discrepancies: risk rises initially with moderate levels of intermittent exposure, then falls at the levels of regular occu-

pational exposure, but then rises again with more intense intermittent exposure (Armstrong, 1988).

Our meta-analysis of population-based studies disclosed odds ratios of only 1.57 (95% confidence interval 1.29–1.91) for intermittent sunlight exposure and 0.75 (confidence interval 0.60–0.89) for chronic exposure (Nelemans *et al.*, 1995). In epidemiological terms, relative risks or odds ratios < 2.0 are regarded as weak evidence. It is also worthy of note that studies which excluded lentigo maligna melanoma and/or applied some blinding strategy to reduce recall bias yielded lower odds ratios than other studies. The lack of standardization of measures for sun exposure and outcome measures warrants cautious interpretation of published results.

The intermittent sun exposure theory was designed to explain the predominance of melanomas on body sites that are usually covered by clothing (intermittently sun-exposed sites). However, intermittent sun exposure showed a stronger association with melanomas on chronically sun-exposed sites than on intermittently sun-exposed sites (Nelemans *et al.*, 1993a). This association is unexpected.

The spectacular increase of incidence of cutaneous melanoma over the past decades can best be explained by a single aetiological factor. It is highly unlikely that two or more causal factors are responsible for the observed trends. Most investigators agree that the sunlight saga is too simplistic and that other factors must be involved (Armstrong & Kricker, 1995). This creates serious doubt on the sunlight hypothesis. The cause of melanoma remains an enigma and most probably ultraviolet radiation has little, if anything, to do with it (Rampen & Fleuren, 1987). Provocative as this statement may seem, there are indications that a hitherto unknown environmental factor, associated with sunworshipping, is involved (see below).

Interestingly, human melanoma models provide patchy and controversial information. If ultraviolet radiation is an important cause of melanoma, one would expect incidence rates to increase in persons who are disproportionally exposed to ultraviolet rays (e.g. photochemotherapy) or have a genetic or acquired susceptibility to ultraviolet-induced cancers (e.g. xeroderma pigmentosum, albinism, organ-transplant recipients, acquired immunodeficiency syndrome). The data currently available are insufficient to incriminate ultraviolet radiation as of particular relevance (Weinstock, 1992). Potential human models are consistently related to extraordinarily high rates of non-melanoma skin cancer, but there is a scarcity of reports of melanomas in these groups. For instance, in a Swedish study describing the long-term follow-up of 4799 PUVA-treated patients, 28 squamous-cell carcinomas were reported (4.5 expected) against five melanomas (5.1 expected) (Lindelöf *et al.*, 1991). The incidence of melanoma in albino patients is not increased by several orders of magnitude, as is observed with non-melanoma skin cancer (Weinstock, 1992). Only for xeroderma pigmentosum does there appear to be a strikingly high melanoma incidence (Kraemer *et al.*, 1987). The main problem with the published data on this issue is the fact that specific histogenetic melanoma types are rarely reported. The melanomas in xeroderma pigmentosum patients might be predominantly of the lentigo maligna line-age, rather than of the superficial spreading/nodular lineage. This association would be of no relevance to the current increase in melanoma incidence which concerns primarily superficial spreading and nodular melanomas.

Occupation

In reviewing published associations between melanoma and occupational exposures, three major methodological shortcomings are encountered: (i) incompleteness of exposure information; (ii) lack of control for other risk factors; and (iii) limited comparability of the occupational and reference populations (Nelemans *et al.*, 1992). In very few studies was adjustment made for skin complexion characteristics, mole counts, socioeconomic class and sun exposure habits.

Exposure to occupational hazards may play a part in the aetiology of cutaneous melanoma. Exposure to chemicals at the workplace, however, cannot account for a substantial proportion of melanoma cases. In Europe, female melanoma patients outnumber males considerably. Conceivably, occupational exposure to specific compounds is much more frequent and intense in males than in females. The low melanoma risk of blue-collar factory workers relative to white-collar workers with cleaner jobs is notable (Lee & Strickland, 1980; Beral & Robinson, 1981; Pion *et al.*, 1995).

Literature data, however, indicate an increased risk for melanoma in certain chemical and technically advanced industries (Austin & Reynolds, 1986; Nelemans *et al.*, 1992). Increased risks have been reported for workers in the petrochemical, chemical, electronics, printing, textile, rubber, vinyl chloride and synthetic fibres industries (for a review, see Nelemans *et al.*, 1992). This myriad of associations precludes meaningful identification of incriminated chemicals or groups of chemicals.

We found an increased risk for melanoma for subjects who had at some time worked in the electronics, metal or transport and communication industries (Nelemans *et al.*, 1993b). The results were adjusted for age and sex, education level, skin complexion characteristics and sunlight exposure. No increased risks were encountered for working in the chemical and textile industries. Stratification by duration of industrial exposure did not result in increases in relative risks with longer exposures. Analyses according to contact with specific groups of chemicals did not yield consistent results.

The study of Pion *et al.* (1995) deserves closer consideration. These authors explored the relation between occupation and melanoma risk through a large case-control study in the United States. A total of 2780 melanoma patients were included. Occupations were classified by pay scale, 'collar' criteria and location of workplace. Men with higher incomes and those holding white-collar jobs were more prone to developing melanoma. No risk differences were noted between men with indoor versus outdoor jobs. No significant differences could be demonstrated for women in any of the occupation groups. This may be explained by the fact that most women in this study were married to higher-paid husbands. It is likely that women are exposed to the same lifestyle risk factors as are their partners. Table 8.2 lists the five occupations with the highest and lowest odds ratios for men only. The high melanoma risks of firemen and dentists are noteworthy.

Pion *et al.* (1995) also examined several specific chemical exposures as well as exposure to X-rays. The following associations were found: X-rays, odds ratio = 1.37 (95% confidence interval 1.12–1.67; P = 0.002); pesticides, odds ratio = 1.19 (confidence interval 0.99–1.43; P = 0.07); and substances added to

Table 8.2 Occupations with the five highest and five lowest odds ratios for cutaneous melanoma for men (after Pion *et al.*, 1995).

Occupation	Number of exposed subjects	Odds ratio (95% confidence interval)
Firemen	16	2.29 (0.85–6.16)
Dentists	37	2.01 (1.04–3.88)
Social workers	10	1.96 (0.55–6.96)
Architects	10	1.96 (0.55–6.96)
Executives	171	1.67 (1.22–2.30)
Painters	21	0.49 (0.14–1.67)
Auto workers	121	0.45 (0.26–0.76)
Technicians	46	0.44 (0.19–1.04)
Factory workers	26	0.38 (0.12–1.28)
Plumbers	15	0.21 (0.03–1.60)

drinking water, odds ratio = 1.14 (confidence interval 0.98–1.33; $P = 0.08$). All other exposures, including asbestos, formaldehyde, tar products, solvents, dyes, diesel and gasoline exhausts, textile fibres and well water, had no influence on melanoma risk.

Other risk indicators

The most important environmental and other risk factors for melanoma, other than sunlight exposure and occupation, will be discussed here briefly (for a review, see Nelemans *et al.*, 1992).

The relationship of coffee, tea, artificial sweeteners, dietary fat and alcohol to cutaneous melanoma has remained relatively unexplored. Consistent associations with melanoma risk have never been reported. The role of retinoids, dietary antioxidants and dietary fat has been concisely reviewed by le Marchand (1992). Dietary antioxidants may reduce and polyunsaturated fat may increase the risk for melanoma through interaction with the carcinogenic effect of ultraviolet radiation. Retinoids may inhibit the growth of melanoma. Alcohol intake may have a causal or growth-promoting effect on melanoma (Williams & Horm, 1977; Stryker *et al.*, 1990). It has been suggested that alcohol stimulates the anterior pituitary secretion of melanocyte-stimulating hormone (Williams, 1976). With all these dietary factors, it is not clear whether there is an independent association and, if so, whether this relates to aetiological influences or to growth-modifying effects.

Smoking habits have never been reported to be associated with melanoma risk. The same applies to the use of soaps, shampoos, hair dyes and other cosmetics. Sunscreen preparations, on the other hand, have been associated with significantly elevated relative risks (Graham *et al.*, 1985). The most plausible explanation for this finding is that the use of sunscreens can be regarded as an indicator of fair-skin complexion. Thus, sunscreen use is an indirect measure of melanoma proneness.

There is a possible relation between (prior) skin disease and melanoma. Psoriasis and acne patients are treated with a variety of topical and systemic agents, among which is phototherapy. An increased incidence of melanoma has been described among psoriasis patients (Beral *et al.*, 1983). However, PUVA-treated patients are not at particular risk for developing melanoma (Gupta *et al.*, 1988; Lindelöf *et al.*, 1991). Results from studies on the effect of a history of acne on melanoma risk are not consistent. Acne may have a protective effect (Beral *et al.*, 1983). *Propionibacterium acnes* shares immunogenic properties with *Corynebacterium parvum*. Hence, *P. acnes* may confer some protection against melanoma. However, the role of *P. acnes* on susceptibility to cancer is not fully understood (Rampen & Mohan, 1985; Sheenan-Dare *et al.*, 1988).

Oncogenic viruses have been implicated. Virus-like particles have been detected in melanoma biopsies (Parsons *et al.*, 1976). A relation with cervical intra-epithelial neoplasia (human papillomavirus) has also been reported (Hartveit & Maehle, 1988; Hartveit *et al.*, 1988). Whether these findings reflect merely a coincidental phenomenon in lifestyle remains to be elucidated.

Levodopa therapy is suspected by many authors to enhance melanoma growth. However, the case reports of melanoma in patients with Parkinson's disease are very few and probably meaningless in the light of the large numbers of patients under long-term levodopa therapy (Rampen, 1985). Chemotherapy for childhood cancer may be more important. Increased naevus counts have been documented in children after prolonged treatment with cytostatics (Hughes *et al.*, 1989; de Wit *et al.*, 1990). Induction or activation of naevocellular naevi by cytostatic drugs may herald an increase in the occurrence of melanomas in this susceptible population.

As already mentioned, a positive association with exposure to X-rays has been reported by Pion *et al.* (1995). These authors found an excess of melanoma cases among dentists and hypothesized that exposure to X-rays may be responsible. On the other hand, dentists might have a high relative risk for melanoma because of their high incomes and attendant lifestyle. The relation between ionizing radiation exposure and melanoma risk among employees of nuclear plants is not constant (Austin *et al.*, 1981; Acquavella *et al.*, 1982; Austin & Reynolds, 1986). An interesting theory is the suggested radon-associated cancer/melanoma risk (Henshaw *et al.*, 1990; Bridges *et al.*, 1991). There is a remarkable association between mutation frequencies and indoor radon concentrations.

Water pollution

Among the various alternative hypotheses, the water pollution theory is probably the most promising (Rampen *et al.*, 1992). This theory may also explain the current intermittent sunlight concept, since sun exposure habits and aquatic sports are highly correlated.

In a recent study, we found that melanoma patients reported regular swimming in swimming pools and/or open waters more often than control patients with other types of cancer (Nelemans *et al.*, 1994). The adjusted odds ratios for regular swimming in any type of polluted water before the age of 15 years was 2.36 (95% confidence interval 1.31–4.26). Exposure after the age of 25 years was not associated with increased risk. These findings are in accord with the current opinion that cutaneous melanoma is induced especially during childhood. In our study, adjustment was made for age and sex, socio-economic status, skin complexion characteristics and sun-exposure variables.

We also found that the age at which swimming was learned was an important risk indicator (Nelemans *et al.*, 1994). Those who learned to swim before the age of 9 years had the highest risk. There was also a positive association between the number of swimming certificates and melanoma risk. Interestingly, persons swimming exclusively in relatively unpolluted waters such as fens and (Alpine) lakes showed no increased risk.

Two other reports have addressed the relation between swimming and melanoma risk (Holman *et al.*, 1986; Østerlind *et al.*, 1988). Although the odds ratios for swimming were slightly elevated, the results remain inconclusive since swimming was considered as a measure of acute, intermittent ultraviolet exposure; various types of swimming water were not specified.

In an investigation from Norway it was demonstrated that melanoma risk increased with increasing chlorine levels of tapwater (Flaten, 1992). It should be noted that often the same chlorinated tapwater is used to fill swimming pools. Also, people take their daily bath or shower with the same tapwater.

Environmental compounds from waste discharges have been found to induce chromatophoromas in fish (Kinae *et al.*, 1990). The authors held halogenated contaminants from pulp-mill wastewater responsible for the high occurrence of this type of pigment-cell neoplasms. In adjacent unpolluted bay water, no fish melanomas were discovered.

Malignant melanoma clustering in a Florida county appeared to be associated with high levels of trihalomethane in water (Aldrich & Peoples, 1982). Trihalomethanes are chlorination byproducts with very potent carcinogenic properties.

Increased risks for melanoma have been reported for firemen (Howe & Burch, 1990; Sama *et al.*, 1990). In the study by Pion *et al.* (1995) on occupation and melanoma risk, firemen topped the list for occupations among men. It is tempting to speculate that firemen regularly have close and prolonged contact with chlorine compounds in water. Surprisingly, Pion *et al.* (1995) found that occupational exposure to substances added to drinking water was a risk factor for melanoma at a near-significant level ($P = 0.08$). On the other hand, exposure to unpolluted well water was not associated with a higher risk.

Conclusion

Several case-control studies have evaluated the sunlight–melanoma relationship. Generally, only weak associations have been reported. Weak associations are often due to undetected biases. Information and recall biases as well as misclassification of sunlight-exposure variables could be responsible for the alleged relationship. Patients with melanoma tend to have enhanced recall of past ultraviolet exposure because they know that sunlight is the suspected risk denominator (Rampen & Fleuren, 1987).

Too much emphasis is laid on the so-called 'intermittent' sunlight exposure postulate. This theory was designed to explain the differences in risk for melanoma, on the one hand, and non-melanoma skin cancer on the other, among indoor versus outdoor occupation groups and according to body site. However, the intermittent sunlight hypothesis has everything of a *deus ex machina*.

Occupational exposure to specific chemical compounds cannot account for the majority of melanoma cases. The possible direct and indirect interrelationships between occupation and melanoma risk are best explained by socio-economic status and attendant lifestyle characteristics.

An attractive alternative to the puzzling aetiology of cutaneous melanoma is the water-pollution concept (Rampen *et al.*, 1992). Swimming pools are usually decontaminated by chlorination with sodium hypochlorite. Open waters nowadays are heavily polluted with chlorine compounds from industrial and domestic sources. Many chlorination byproducts are mutagenic. It is hypothesized that chlorine substances in swimming pools and open waters are the main risk factor for cutaneous melanoma, and that ultraviolet exposure is a confounding factor. Several reports point to carcinogenic substances in water, possibly chlorination byproducts, as serious candidates in the aetiology of melanoma. Although it is extremely difficult to unravel the genuine influences of exposure to chlorinated water and exposure to sunlight, increased risk from contact with polluted water can be explained epidemiologically and biologically.

References

Acquavella, J.F., Wilkinson, G.S., Tietjen, G.L. *et al.* (1982) Malignant melanoma incidence at the Los Alamos National Laboratory. *Lancet*, **ii**, 883–884.

Aldrich, T.E. & Peoples, A.J. (1982) Malignant melanoma and drinking water contamination. *Bulletin of Environmental Contamination and Toxicology*, **28**, 519.

Armstrong, B.K. (1988) Epidemiology of malignant melanoma: Intermittent or total accumulated exposure to the sun? *Journal of Dermatologic Surgery and Oncology*, **14**, 835–849.

Armstrong, B.K. & Kricker, A. (1995) Skin cancer. *Dermatology Clinics*, **13**, 583–594.

Austin, D.F. & Reynolds, P.J. (1986) Occupation and malignant melanoma of the skin. In: *Epidemiology of Malignant Melanoma: Recent Results in Cancer Research* (ed. R.P. Gallagher), Vol. 102, pp. 98–107. Springer-Verlag, Berlin.

Austin, D.F., Snyder, M.A., Reynolds, P.J. *et al.* (1981) Malignant melanoma among employees of Lawrence Livermore National Laboratory. *Lancet*, **ii**, 712–716.

Beral, V. & Robinson, N. (1981) The relationship of malignant melanoma, basal and squamous skin cancers to indoor and outdoor work. *British Journal of Cancer*, **44**, 886–891.

Beral, V., Evans, S., Shaw, H. & Milton, G. (1983) Cutaneous factors related to the risk of malignant melanoma. *British Journal of Dermatology*, **109**, 165–172.

Bridges, B.A., Cole, J., Arlett, C.F. *et al.* (1991) Possible association between mutant frequency in peripheral lymphocytes and domestic radon concentrations. *Lancet*, **337**, 1187–1189.

Crombie, I.K. (1981) Distribution of malignant melanoma on the body surface. *British Journal of Cancer*, **43**, 842–849.

Elwood, J.M. (1992) Melanoma and ultraviolet radiation. *Clinics in Dermatology*, **10**, 41–50.

Fears, T.R., Scotto, J. & Schneidermann, M.A. (1977) Mathematical models of age and ultraviolet effects on the incidence of skin cancer among whites in the United States. *American Journal of Epidemiology*, **105**, 420–427.

Flaten, T.P. (1992) Chlorination of drinking water and cancer incidence in Norway. *International Journal of Epidemiology*, **21**, 6–15.

Graham, S., Marchall, J. & Haughey, B. (1985) An inquiry into the epidemiology of melanoma. *American Journal of Epidemiology*, **122**, 606–619.

Gupta, A.K., Stern, R.S., Swanson, N.A. *et al.* (1988) Cutaneous melanomas in patients treated with psoralens plus ultraviolet A: A case report and the experience of the PUVA Follow-up Study. *Journal of the American Academy of Dermatology*, **19**, 67–76.

Hartveit, F. & Maehle, B.O. (1988) A link between malignant melanoma and cervical intra-epithelial neoplasia? *Acta Dermato-Venereologica (Stockholm)*, **68**, 140–143.

Hartveit, F., Maehle, B.O., Skaarland, E. *et al.* (1988) Cervical lesions in patients with malignant melanoma. *Acta Dermato-Venereologica (Stockholm)*, **68**, 144–148.

Henshaw, D., Eatough, J.P. & Richardson, R.B. (1990) Radon: A causative factor in the introduction of myeloid leukaemia and other cancers in adults and children? *Lancet*, **335**, 1008–1012.

Holman, C.D.J., Armstrong, B.K. & Heenan, P.J. (1986) Relationship of cutaneous malignant melanoma to individual sunlight-exposure habits. *Journal of the National Cancer Institute*, **76**, 403–414.

Howe, G.R. & Burch, J.D. (1990) Fire fighters and risk of cancer: An assessment and overview of the epidemiologic evidence. *American Journal of Epidemiology*, **132**, 1039–1050.

Hughes, B.R., Cunliffe, W.J. & Bailey, C.C. (1989) Excess benign melanocytic naevi after chemotherapy for malignancy in childhood. *British Medical Journal*, **299**, 88–91.

Kinae, N., Yamashita, M., Tomita, I. *et al.* (1990) A possible correlation between environmental chemicals and pigment cell neoplasia in fish. *Science of the Total Environment*, **94**, 143–153.

Kraemer, K.H., Lee, M.M. & Scotto, J. (1987) Xeroderma pigmentosum: Cutaneous, ocular, and neurologic abnormalities in 830 published cases. *Archives of Dermatology*, **123**, 241–250.

Lee, J.A.H. & Strickland, D. (1980) Malignant melanoma: Social status and outdoor work. *British Journal of Cancer*, **41**, 757–763.

le Marchand, L. (1992) Dietary factors in the etiology of melanoma. *Clinics in Dermatology*, **10**, 79–82.

Lindelöf, B., Sigurgeirsson, B., Tegner, E. *et al.* (1991) PUVA and cancer: A large scale epidemiological study. *Lancet*, **338**, 91–93.

Nelemans, P.J., Verbeek, A.L.M. & Rampen, F.H.J. (1992) Nonsolar factors in melanoma risk. *Clinics in Dermatology*, **10**, 51–63.

Nelemans, P.J., Groenendal, H., Kiemeney, L.A.L.M., Rampen, F.H.J., Ruiter, D.J. & Verbeek, A.L.M. (1993a) The association between melanoma and sunlight exposure: An age- and site-specific analysis. In: *Environmental Risk Indicators for Cutaneous Melanoma* (ed. P.J. Nelemans), pp. 111–128. Quickprint, Nijmegen.

Nelemans, P.J., Scholte, R., Groenendal, H. *et al.* (1993b) Melanoma and occupation: Results of a case-control study in The Netherlands. *British Journal of Industrial Medicine*, **50**, 642–646.

Nelemans, P.J., Rampen, F.H.J., Groenendal, H., Kiemeney, L.A.L.M., Ruiter, D.J. & Verbeek, A.L.M. (1994) Swimming and the risk of cutaneous melanoma. *Melanoma Research*, **4**, 281–286.

Nelemans, P.J., Rampen, F.H.J., Ruiter, D.J. & Verbeek, A.L.M. (1995) An addition to the controversy of sunlight exposure and melanoma risk: A meta-analytical approach. *Journal of Clinical Epidemiology*, **48**, 1331–1342.

Østerlind, A., Tucker, M.A., Stone, B.J. & Jensen, O.M. (1988) The Danish case-control study of cutaneous malignant melanoma. II. Importance of UV-light exposure. *International Journal of Cancer*, **42**, 319–324.

Parsons, P.G., Klucis, E., Goss, P.D. *et al.* (1976) Oncornavirus-like particles in malignant melanoma and control biopsies. *International Journal of Cancer*, **18**, 757–763.

Pion, I.A., Rigel, D.S., Garfinkel, L., Silverman, M.K. & Kopf, A.W. (1995) Occupation and the risk of malignant melanoma. *Cancer*, **75**, 637–644.

Rampen, F.H.J. (1985) Levodopa and melanoma: Three cases and review of literature. *Journal of Neurology, Neurosurgery and Psychology*, **48**, 585–588.

Rampen, F.H.J. & Fleuren, B.A.M. (1987) Melanoma of the skin is not caused by ultraviolet radiation but by a chemical xenobiotic. *Medical Hypotheses*, **22**, 341–346.

Rampen, F.H.J. & Mohan, G. (1985) Role of *Propionibacterium acnes* in cancer risk. *IRCS Medical Science*, **13**, 972.

Rampen, F.H.J., Nelemans, P.J. & Verbeek, A.L.M. (1992) Is water pollution a cause of cutaneous melanoma? *Epidemiology*, **3**, 263–265.

Sama, S.R., Martin, T.R., Davis, L.K. & Kriebel, D. (1990) Cancer incidence among Massachusetts firefighters, 1982–1986. *American Journal of Industrial Medicine*, **18**, 47–54.

Sheenan-Dare, R.A., Cunliffe, W.J., Simmons, A.V. *et al.* (1988) Acne vulgaris and malignancy. *British Journal of Dermatology*, **119**, 669–673.

Stryker, W.S., Stampfer, M.J., Stein, E.A. *et al.* (1990) Diet plasma levels of beta-carotene and alpha-tocopherol, and risk of malignant melanoma. *American Journal of Epidemiology*, **131**, 597–611.

Weinstock, M.A. (1992) Human models of melanoma. *Clinics in Dermatology*, **10**, 83–89.

Williams, H.C. (1995) Melanoma with no sun exposure. *Lancet*, **346**, 581.

Williams, R.R. (1976) Breast and thyroid cancer and malignant melanoma promoted by alcohol-induced pituitary secretion of prolactin, TSH and MSH. *Lancet*, **i**, 996–999.

Williams, R.R. & Horm, J.W. (1977) Association of cancer sites with tobacco and alcohol consumption and socioeconomic status of patients: Interview study from the Third National Cancer Survey. *Journal of the National Cancer Institute*, **58**, 525–547.

de Wit, P.E.J., de Vaan, G.A.M., de Boo, T.M., Lemmens, W.A.J.G. & Rampen, F.H.J. (1990) Prevalence of naevocytic naevi after chemotherapy for childhood cancer. *Medical and Pediatric Oncology*, **18**, 336–338.

9

Cutaneous Melanoma and Oral Contraceptives: Case-Control and Cohort Studies, 1975–1995

E.A. HOLLY

Several lines of evidence have supported a possible association between cutaneous malignant melanoma and characteristics of female endocrine status promoting considerable interest among those who studied melanoma in the 1980s and the 1990s. Several reports on this association were published from case-control and cohort studies with most studies finding little evidence to support an association. In general, the larger case-control studies conducted later found no association between the use of oral contraceptives (OC) and melanoma, while the smaller studies conducted earlier had reported some positive associations among various subgroups that were investigated.

Biological evidence for an association between malignant melanoma and exogenous or endogenous hormonal factors exists but is somewhat inconsistent. Despite numerous investigations of this topic, controversy persists concerning the presence of oestrogen-receptor proteins in malignant melanoma in humans (Flowers *et al.*, 1987). Oestrogen receptors have been found in human malignant melanoma cells, although the percentage that are oestrogen positive varies greatly by study (Fisher *et al.*, 1976; Creagan *et al.*, 1980). Reports from others have indicated that the apparent oestrogen-binding capacity of human melanoma tissues is the result of interactions other than with oestrogen receptors (Flowers *et al.*, 1987). Following this report, other investigators evaluated melanomas, benign naevi and dysplastic naevi for the presence of sex hormone binding and oestrogen-receptor protein and were unable to demonstrate true oestrogen receptors (Lecavalier *et al.*, 1990). However, oestrogens, whether taken for contraception, administered topically (Jadassohn, 1958) or used to relieve menopausal symptoms (Hamilton, 1939), can produce hyperpigmentation with the degree of darkening increasing

with duration of use (Carruthers, 1966). Further, melanocyte-stimulating hormone rises progressively throughout pregnancy (Ances & Pomerantz, 1974). Age-specific incidence rates also provide support for a hormonal association with melanoma. Rates among women increase sharply with age from puberty until menopause when the rate of increase begins to diminish. However, rates among men have a fairly consistent increase beginning at puberty and continuing into the elderly population. This review updates a report published in 1993 on cutaneous malignant melanoma and OC use in case-control and cohort studies and adds studies published in English through 1995 (Holly, 1994).

Exposure to ultraviolet light also causes the skin pigment to darken and most likely plays some role in the aetiology of melanoma (Holman *et al.*, 1984). Therefore, sunlight exposure history needs to be determined in all studies of hormones and cutaneous melanoma to control, in the analysis, for its possible confounding effect with melanoma. Many of the early studies did not have these data or other risk correlates available for analysis. In spite of this concern, little confounding effect of sunlight has been shown between OC and melanoma in the studies that have had data available to control for sunlight (Adam *et al.*, 1981; Ramcharan *et al.*, 1981; Gallagher *et al.*, 1985; Green & Bain, 1985; Østerlind *et al.*, 1988; Le *et al.*, 1992; Holly *et al.*, 1995c).

The tables and text are presented separately, and in the order published, for the case-control and cohort studies reviewed here. Risk estimates are presented separately for ever-use versus never-use of OCs and for long-term versus short-term or no use when the data are available. Risk assessments by histological type of melanoma also are presented for the studies that had adequate data to analyse their results separately. When available in the original papers, confidence intervals (95%) and/or *P* values are presented in the text. The data presented in the tables will not be discussed in the text unless the association is noteworthy. The footnotes for Table 9.1 (see p. 106) provide the definitions for long-term use and latency periods when this clarification is required.

Table 9.1 Case-control studies of melanoma and oral contraceptives published up to 1996 (adapted, with permission, from Kluwer Publications; Holly, 1994).

Year published. First author. Study population. Location	*n* cases *n* controls	Odds ratios for oral contraceptive use		Other hormone-related factors of interest	Comments
		Ever use vs. never use	Long-term use** vs. short-term use or no use		
1977. Beral. Kaiser Health Plan. Record review; controls randomly chosen from same plan. California, USA	37 74	1.8	No data	Association between melanoma and use of hormones for menopause	Information on sunlight exposure, complexion, etc. not available; small numbers prevented subgroup analysis
1981. Adam. Population-based record review and postal survey. Oxford, UK	158 503	1.1* 1.3	1.6 ⩾ 5 years	–	OC use not related to any risk factors for melanoma; postal survey obtained data on sun exposure, hair, eye and skin colour
1982. Bain. Postal survey, registered nurses. 11 states in USA	141 2820	0.93** 1.4 <40 years	2.3 3.0†	–	Married women; adjusted for geographical area, parity, age first birth; control for sun exposure, complexion and histological type not possible
1983. Holly. Population-based cases and controls. Seattle, USA	87 863	1.2	2.4† SSM 3.6† 4.4† 5.1†	Association between melanoma and age at birth of first child at ⩾31 years†	Information on sun exposure, complexion, etc. not available; risk by time interval was assessed
1984. Helmrich. Hospital-based cases and controls. Boston, USA	160 640	0.8	1.0 1.2 1.1 0.7	–	Hospitalized cases were a subgroup of all melanoma patients; hospitalized controls may have used OCs at higher rate than general population; histology, sun exposure, complexion, hair colour, etc. not available

Continued on p. 104.

Table 9.1 *Continued.*

Year published. First author. Study population. Location	*n* cases *n* controls	Odds ratios for oral contraceptive use		Other hormone-related factors of interest	Comments
		Ever use vs. never use	Long-term use** vs. short-term use or no use		
1984. Beral, Melanoma Clinic. Population controls = 74%, hospital controls = 26%. Sydney, Australia	287 574	1.0	1.5†	Association between melanoma and use of hormones for menopause, to suppress lactation and to regulate periods	Controlled for sun exposure, hair and skin colour, number of naevi and other variables; risk by time interval was assessed
1984. Holman. Population-based cases, controls from registered voters and public schools. Western Australia	276 276	1.0 1.1 SSM	1.1 1.5 SSM 4.7 0.33	Borderline association between melanoma and menopausal oestrogen use	Controlled for sun exposure, hair and skin colour, height and weight; risk by time interval was assessed
1985. Gallagher. Population-based cases and controls. Western Canada	361 361	1.0	0.9 SSM ≥ 5 years	Association between lowered incidence of melanoma and more live births† and bilateral oophorectomy†	Controlled for sun exposure, hair and skin colour, freckling, education, weight, height and other variables; risk by time interval was assessed
1985. Green. Population-based cases and controls. Queensland, Australia	91 91	0.7	1.0 1.6 0.5 0.4	Elevated risk with over six live births, older age at first birth, increasing years of ovulatory life,† late age at menarche	Insufficient data to analyse by hormones other than OC; controlled for sun exposure, hair and skin colour and number of naevi; risk by time interval was assessed
1988. Østerlind. Population-based cases and controls. Denmark	280 536	0.8 0.9 SSM	0.8 0.8 0.8 1.0 1.3 SSM	Age at menopause; suggestion of increased risk with menopausal replacement oestrogen	Adjusted for age, number of naevi and sun exposure; data on hair, skin and eye colour and freckles also collected
1990. Zanetti. Population-based cases and controls. Turin, Italy	110 123	1.1 1.3 SSM	0.94 0.98	Decreased risk for parity three or more†	Controlled for age, education, sun exposure and holiday at beach; data on hair, skin and eye colour also collected; low number of OC users (21%) in sample

Continued.

Table 9.1 *Continued.*

Year published. First author. Study population. Location	*n* cases *n* controls	Odds ratios for oral contraceptive use		Other hormone-related factors of interest	Comments
		Ever use vs. never use	Long-term use** vs. short-term use or no use		
1992. Le. Cases and controls were patients in five medical centres. France	91 149	No data	0.9 2.0 2.7 2.3 4.4†	Increased risk for young age at menarche†	Controlled for sun exposure and age at menarche; data on hair, skin and eye colour, age at menarche and other reproductive factors also were collected
1992. Palmer. Cases and controls were patients in hospitals and at patient clinics. New York and Philadelphia, USA	615 2107	'Non-severe' 1.5† 'Severe' 1.1	'Non-severe' 1.4 1.6† 1.5 2.0 'Severe' 2.4† SSM 2.0† SSM 1.3 SSM 2.0 NM 1.0 NM 1.0 NM	–	Controlled for age, geographical region, year of interview, years of education, religion, body mass index, menopausal status and skin type; also collected data on cigarette smoking, lifetime sun exposure, conjugated oestrogen use, parity, age at first birth and age at menarche; no ORs given by histological type for 'non-severe' cases
1994. Holly.*** Polulation-based cases and controls. San Francisco Bay Area, USA	452 930	–	–	Increased risk of SSM associated with exogenous hormone† and conjugated oestrogen use after hysterectomy; increased risk for SSM associated with use of vaginal creams with oestrogen†	Controlled for age and education; also collected data on sun exposure, hair, skin and eye colour, number of large naevi, demographic and lifestyle factors
1995. Holly.*** Polulation-based cases and controls. San Francisco Bay Area, USA	452 930	0.74 SSM 0.60 NM	0.61† SSM 0.93 SSM 1.0 SSM 2.0† SSM 0.60 NM 0.73 NM 0.37 NM 1.4 NM	Pregnancy-related factors; hormone-related cutaneous variables	Controlled for age; decreased risk associated with use of acne medication;† information about sun exposure, phenotypic characteristics, number of large naevi, demographic and lifestyle factors also were collected

Continued on p. 106.

Case-control studies

Two studies of melanoma, one a case-control study and one a cohort study, were conducted in the Kaiser-Permanente Health Plan in Walnut Creek, California, with the preliminary results from the cohort study reported in the same publication as the case-control study (Beral *et al.*, 1977). The cohort study results are provided as the first entry in Table 9.2 and below in the cohort studies section. The case-control study data from that publication included 37 cases and 74 age-matched controls who were 20–59 years of age (Beral *et al.*, 1977). The odds ratios (OR) for melanoma among ever-users of OCs was 1.8-fold that of women who had never used these agents. The increased risk for use of OCs was noted in age groups 20–34 and 35–59 years when each was analysed separately. The ever-users of OCs or oestrogens had an excess of lesions of the lower limbs. However, the number of cases was small and the associations were not statistically significant. Neither sunlight exposure nor indicators of outdoor activity were available and histological type also was not reported.

An OR of 1.3 (confidence interval, CI = 0.92–2.0) was reported in a medical record review of English women (158 cases and 503 controls) aged 15–49 years for ever-use versus never-use of OCs (Adam *et al.*, 1981). A postal survey of a subset (111 cases, 342 controls) of these women provided a somewhat lower OR of 1.1 (CI = 0.73–1.8) for ever-use versus never-use of these agents. In the postal survey, an OR of 1.6 (CI = 0.83–3.0) was reported for melanoma among women who had used OCs for 5 years or more compared with those who had never used them. The postal survey included questions on exposure to sunlight, outdoor leisure activities, hair, eye and skin colour and occupation. No analyses by histological subcategories of melanoma were presented.

No overall relationship between melanoma and ever-use of OCs in 141 women with melanoma was found from results of a postal survey among married registered nurses in 11 states in the United States. These women were aged 30–55 years and were compared with 2820 age-matched women who were the control subjects for this study (Bain *et al.*, 1982). A crude OR of 0.93 (CI = 0.64–1.36) for ever-use of OCs was observed. Women who were aged < 40 years at diagnosis had elevated odds ratios for use of these agents. The unadjusted OR for this group of women was 1.8 (CI = 1.1–2.9) and this risk diminished to

---

Table 9.1 *Continued from p. 105.*

* 1.1 from postal survey, 1.3 from medical record review.

** Long-term use definitions:

Bain, 1982: ≥ 2 years OC use beginning ≥ 10 years before diagnosis (dx) in women age < 40 years, multivariate analysis then univariate presented.

Holly, 1983: superficial spreading melanoma (SSM) only; 5–9 years, ≥ 10 years, ≥ 5 years use first beginning ≥ 12 years before dx; ≥ 5 years use with at least 5 years since last use, respectively.

Helmrich, 1984: ≥ 5 years use beginning 10 years or more before diagnosis for all cases; ≥ 5 years Clark levels I and II, III, and IV and V, respectively.

Beral, 1984: ≥ 5 years use beginning 10 years or more before diagnosis.

Holman, 1984: all melanomas ≥ 5 years use, SSM ≥ 5 years, Hutchinson melanotic freckle ≥ 2 years use, nodular melanoma (nM) ≥ 2 years use, respectively.

Green, 1985: < 1 year use, 1 to < 2 years, 2 to ≤ 4 years, > 4 years use, respectively.

Østerlind, 1988: < 2 years use, 2–4 years, 5–9 years, ≥ 10 years use, respectively.

Zanetti, 1990: < 3 years use, ≥ 3 years use.

Le, 1992: duration (*D*) < 10 years with latency (*L*) < 15 years, *D* < 10 years with *L* ≥ 15 years, *D* ≥ 10 years with *L* ≥ 15 years and among 30–40 years old: 1–9 years use and ≥ 10 years use, respectively.

Palmer, 1992: < 1 year use, 1–4 years use, ≥ 5 years use, respectively for both SSM and NM in severe disease cases: < 1 year use, 1–4 years use, 5–9 years use, ≥ 10 years use in non-severe cases.

Holly, 1995: < 5 years use, 5–9 years use, ≥ 10 years use, ≥ 5 years use and < 15 years since first use, respectively for both SSM and NM.

*** Same study population.

†*P* < 0.05.

Table 9.2 Cohort studies of melanoma and oral contraceptives published up to 1996 (adapted, with permission, from Kluwer Publications; Holly, 1994).

Year published, First author. Study population. Location.	*n* cases *n* women	Relative risk estimates for oral contraceptive use		Other hormone-related factors of interest	Comments
		Ever use vs. never use	Long-term use vs. short-term or no use		
1977, Beral.* Kaiser Health Plan. California, USA	22 17 942	1.4	1.4 < 4 years 1.7 ⩾ 4 years	Association between melanoma and ever use of oestrogens other than OCs	Information on sunlight exposure, complexion, histology, etc. not available; small number of cases prevented subgroup analysis
1981. Ramcharan. Kaiser Health Plan. California, USA	20 14 104	3.5***	No data	–	Melanoma–OC use association persisted after consideration of other factors; OC use not associated with exposure to sunlight
1981. Kay. Oxford/Family Planning Association. UK	40 306 286**	1.5	No data	–	Brief Letter to the Editor, no mention of exposure to sunlight, complexion or risk by time interval
1991. Hannaford. Oxford/Family Planning Association, 17 family planning clinics. England and Scotland	32 17 032	0.82	1.02 5–10 years 0.98 ⩾ 10 years	Reduced risk of melanoma with an increase in parity***	Adjusted for age, parity at diagnosis, social class and smoking at recruitment; some subgroups of women not followed past age 45 years
1991. Hannaford. Royal College of General Practitioners, physician-based sample. UK	58 46 000	0.92	0.69 5–10 years 1.8 ⩾ 10 years	Reduced risk of melanoma with an increase in parity***	Married women or living as married; controlled for age, parity, social class and smoking

* Includes some patients presented in Ramcharan's 1981 publication.
** Woman-years of observation.
*** Significantly different from 1 ($P < 0.05$).

1.4 (CI = 0.83–2.5) after adjustment for geography, parity, age at first pregnancy, height and prior hair-dye use. The unadjusted odds ratios were 1.4 for women who had used OCs for 1–24 months (CI = 0.71–2.6) and 2.3 (CI = 1.3–4.0) for those who had used them for ⩾ 25 months. With adjustment for the above-mentioned factors, the magnitude of these associations diminished to 1.2 (CI = 0.59–2.5) and 1.7 (CI = 0.88–3.4), respectively, and the risk estimate for longer use was no longer statistically significant. Women who were < 40 years of age and used OCs for at least 2 years beginning 10 years or more before diagnosis had a crude OR of 3.0 (CI = 1.2–7.5). The adjusted analysis reduced this estimate to 2.3 (CI = 0.77–6.9). There was no association with use of OCs in the much smaller group of women who were aged > 40 years.

Inadequate information was available for analysis by histological type or for control of the effects of hair, complexion and eye colour or exposure to sunlight.

A population-based study of 87 white women with melanoma and 863 randomly chosen white control subjects aged 37–74 years was conducted in Seattle and environs in the state of Washington (Holly *et al.*, 1983). Only women who were in an age group that could have used OCs (37–59 years) were considered for the OC analyses. For superficial spreading melanoma (SSM), odds ratios for users of OCs for 5–9 and 10 years or more were 2.4 and 3.6, respectively (for trend, $P = 0.004$). There was no association with risk for use of OCs for 4 years or less. Women at greatest risk of SSM were those who began taking OCs 12 years or more before diagnosis and who took them for at least 5 years (OR = 4.4; CI = 2.0–9.7), and those who took them for at least 5 years ending 5 years or more before diagnosis (OR = 5.1; CI = 2.0–13). The elevated ORs may reflect the effects of the stronger dose pill used in the 1960s, a longer latent period, or both. No elevated risk for OC use and all histological types of melanoma was found. Having a first child after the age of 30 years also was associated with an elevated risk of SSM. Number of live births, hysterectomy status, age at menopause and menopausal oestrogen use were not found to be risk factors for specific histological types of melanoma in this study. The results from the Seattle group provided initial support for analysis by histological type in studies of melanoma.

Study results from 160 hospitalized melanoma patients and 640 hospitalized control subjects aged 20–59 years showed no statistically significant association between ever-use of OCs and melanoma in a study conducted at Boston University (Helmrich *et al.*, 1984). No effect of duration for OC use was noted between hospitalized melanoma patients and years of use or for years since first and last use. Inadequate information was available for analysis by histological subtype. Clark's level of tumour thickness was available on pathology reports for some melanoma patients. Clark levels IV and V are more likely to include more nodular melanomas (NM) because NMs are, in general, thicker tumours, while Clark levels I and II are more likely to include a greater proportion of SSM tumours. While not significant, the reduced odds ratio for Clark

levels IV and V and the slightly elevated odds ratio for Clark levels I and II support the need for subgroup analysis by histological type in studies of melanoma and OC use. Use of Breslow thickness measurements are more precise measures of the tumour type if histological category is unavailable.

Sydney, Australia, was the site for study of women aged 18–54 years that included 287 women with melanoma and 574 mostly population-based controls (26% were hospital-based) (Beral *et al.*, 1984). An elevated risk of 1.5 (CI = 1.03–2.1) was observed for malignant melanoma among women who had taken OCs for at least 5 years beginning 10 years or more prior to diagnosis. Odds ratios for melanoma for women who had taken OCs remained essentially the same after adjustment for reported hair and skin colour, frequency of naevi on the body, place of birth and exposure to sunlight. More melanoma patients than control subjects had begun taking OCs at least 10 years before diagnosis (47% compared to 39%, $P = 0.05$). There was no increased risk for melanoma for ever-use versus never-use of OCs. ORs also were elevated for use of hormones to regulate periods (OR = 1.9), hormone-replacement therapy (OR = 1.4) and use of hormonal injections to sup-press lactation (OR = 1.4), although these results could have been due to chance. There were no statistically significant differences noted by histological subtype for OC use.

No statistically significant relationship was found between any histological subtype of melanoma and OC use among 276 cases and 276 control subjects in a study conducted in Western Australia among girls and women aged 10–79 years (seven cases were <18 years of age) (Holman *et al.*, 1984). With adjustment for phenotypic risk factors, the odds ratios for SSM were 0.78 (CI = 0.32–1.9) for women using OCs for less than 2 years, 2.2 (CI = 0.73–6.8) for 2–4 years of use, and 1.6 (CI = 0.53–4.9) for a history of 5 years or more of use. Sun exposure, skin reaction to sunlight, hair colour and number of raised naevi on the arms were considered in analyses as potential confounding factors. Time periods were considered to assess latency for OC use and histological types of melanoma. Odds ratios were 1.3 for SSM and 2.5 for Hutchinson's melanotic freckle for ever-use of OCs 10 years or more before diagnosis. Numbers in these subgroups were necessarily small and confidence intervals overlapped unity. There was borderline evidence of an association between SSM and duration of use of unopposed oestrogens in this study. Odds ratios for 1–12 months of use and ≥ 13 months were 1.7 and 2.3, respectively (for trend, $P = 0.08$).

No increased risk by histological subtype of melanoma was revealed for ever-use of OCs in a study conducted in western Canada (Gallagher *et al.*, 1985). The group studied included 361 cases and 361 controls aged 20–79 years. When women in age groups 20–39 and 40–69 years were analysed separately, no increased risk for use of OCs was noted in either group. Women who had five or more live births were at a decreased risk of SSM (OR = 0.4; for trend, $P = 0.02$) with a decreased risk associated with increased number of live births. Women with bilateral oophorectomy also were at a decreased risk of SSM (OR = 0.3; $P = 0.001$). Sunlight exposure was not related to OC use when considered in the analyses. Risk estimates for nodular melanoma often were in the opposite direction from those of SSM for some of the hormonally-related factors.

Queensland, Australia, study results showed no increased risk of cutaneous melanoma in relation to OC use (Green & Bain, 1985). This study of 91 cases (excluding lentigo maligna melanoma) and 91 control subjects aged 51–81 years considered sun-related factors in the analysis. When age groups were analysed separately (women < 35 years of age and those 35–49 years), no increased risk for use of OCs was noted in either of the two groups. Other reproductive factors also were not shown to be related consistently to melanoma, with the possible exception of an increased risk with increasing age at menarche and increase in length of ovulatory life. For age of menarche at 12–13, 14–15 and 16–17 years, odds ratios were 1.2, 1.9 and 2.6, respectively (for trend, $P = 0.04$). Odds ratios were 12 for 21–30 years of ovulatory life (CI = 1.4–101) and 21 for ≥ 31 years of ovulatory life (CI = 1.7–252). Risk estimates were elevated for an increase in age at birth of first child and number of live births. However, the trends were inconsistent, confidence limits overlapped 1.0 and numbers were small in each of these groups. Most risk estimates were not altered substantially when adjustment was made for sunlight exposure and phenotypic factors. It was not possible

to compute risk estimates separately for nodular melanoma due to the small number of cases.

A Danish study of melanoma in women reported no elevated risks associated with OC use or with any other hormonal and reproductive factors (Østerlind *et al.*, 1988). These women were 17–92 years of age and the study included 280 cases and 536 control subjects and did not consider lentigo maligna melanoma. Women aged 20–59 years were analysed separately and no increased risk for use of OCs was noted for this group who would have been most likely to have used these agents. Histological type examination revealed a risk of 1.3 for SSM for OC use of 10 years or more (CI = 0.7–2.2; for trend, $P = 0.91$). Age at menarche, menopausal status, age at natural menopause, number of reproductive years, number of pregnancies, number of miscarriages and number of live births were among the reproductive factors that were examined. Other factors that were considered were duration of OC use, type of pill and potency, and menopausal replacement therapy, type and potency. Adjustment was made for age and host factors such as presence of naevi, freckles, hair colour and sunbathing. There was no confounding by endogenous or exogenous hormonal factors, by host factors such as naevi, freckles and light hair colour, nor by sun exposure as measured by sunbathing — little difference was noted between the crude and adjusted values. No other reproductive factors were found to be associated with melanoma risk, except a possible association with age at menopause.

In north-western Italy a study was conducted among a low-OC use population and included 110 cases and 123 control subjects (Zanetti *et al.*, 1990). The women were aged 17–92 years and results showed no significantly elevated risk estimates between cutaneous melanoma and OC use. Analyses were conducted separately by histological type, and also included results by duration of use. The OC analyses considered only women under the age of 60 years, who would have been in the age group most likely to have used OCs. The odds ratio for SSM for ever-use versus never-use was 1.3 (CI = 0.36–4.5). No data were presented on duration of use or dose for SSM. A very small percentage of women had ever used OCs in the overall group of women. A protective effect for having had three or more children was noted in this study with an OR of 0.33 (CL = 0.16–0.70; for trend, $P = 0.02$). The effect was diminished and was no longer significant (OR = 0.62, CL = 0.29–1.3) after adjustment for other factors related to cutaneous melanoma. No association was noted for age at birth of first child.

Five French medical facilities were the site of a study that reported an elevated risk estimate for cutaneous melanoma and OC use among women who had used these agents for 10 years or more (OR = 2.1; CI = 0.7–5.9) (Le *et al.*, 1992). The risk estimate increased somewhat after control for phenotypic and sun-exposure factors (OR = 2.4; CI = 0.4–14.0). Subjects in this study were white hospitalized women with melanoma who were matched to white control subjects who also were hospitalized. Out-patient melanoma subjects also were included and were matched to out-patient control women. OC use of 1–9 years and 10 or more years had risk estimates of 1.1 and 2.1, respectively. After control for phenotypic and sun-exposure factors, the corresponding risk estimates were 1.0 and 2.4 and the elevated risk estimates could have been due to chance. Duration of use and latency risk estimates are presented in Table 9.1 and show increased risk with increased duration of use and increased latency since last use. Since earlier work from these authors had indicated an increased risk among OC users aged 30–40 years and that a latency period of 15 years was required for an increased risk of melanoma, data from women in this age group were analysed separately. Results presented in the long-term use column of the table showed an increasing risk with longer duration of OC use (for trend, $P = 0.03$). With control for phenotypic factors and sun exposure, young age at menarche was reported as a risk factor for malignant melanoma. The sample was too small to demonstrate a difference by histological type and therefore no values were reported.

A large hospital- and clinic-based study that divided cases into 'severe' and 'non-severe' based on tumour thickness and presence of metastases was conducted in Brookline, Massachusetts (Palmer *et al.*, 1992). Cases included 357 women aged 18–64 years with severe disease and 192 women with non-severe disease. There was no association between OC use and melanoma among the severe cases, although there was a modest adjusted overall risk for ever-use of OCs among the non-severe cases (OR = 1.5; CI = 1.1–2.2). There was a duration-of-use association with adjusted risks rising from 1.4 among women who had used these agents for less than 1 year to 2.0 for women who had used them for 10 years or longer. Information on histological type was available for about half of the cases and risks for SSM ($n = 238$) associated with OC use were elevated, but not consistently by length of use (adjusted OR = 2.4; CI = 1.2–4.6 for less than 1 year of OC use; OR = 2.0; CI = 1.1–3.6 for 1–4 years of use; and OR = 1.3; CI = 0.6–2.6 for at least 5 years of use).

In the San Francisco Bay Area, a large population-based study was conducted among 452 women with melanoma and 930 control subjects (Holly *et al.*, 1995c). The women were 25–59 years of age and showed no consistent association or elevated risk for SSM or NM with use of OCs when examined by histological type for duration of use, latency, age at diagnosis, age at first use and time period of first use. All pathological materials were reviewed by two dermatopathologists to determine histological classification. There was an elevated risk for melanoma only among the subgroup who had used OCs for 5 years or more and who had used them fewer than 15 years prior to diagnosis, with an increased risk reported for all cutaneous melanoma combined (OR = 1.7; CI = 1.1–2.7), for SSM (OR = 2.0; CI = 1.2–3.3) and for nodular melanoma (OR = 1.4; CI = 0.50–4.1).

Other factors that were related to hormones also were reported from this study. An increase in pigmentation on the face while pregnant (OR = 0.54; CI = 0.36–0.83) and an increase in pigmentation of other body sites showed a protective association with SSM (OR = 0.71; CI = 0.48–1.0), while an increase in pigmentation of the face while using OCs (OR = 0.70; CI = 0.43–1.1) and of other body sites while using OCs provided mixed results that could have been due to chance. Use of acne medication was associated with a decreased risk of SSM (OR = 0.55; CI = 0.35–0.84) but not NM. Elevated risks were reported for having had a bilateral oophorectomy 9 years or fewer prior to the melanoma diagnosis for SSM (OR = 2.2; CI = 1.1–4.5) and NM (OR = 2.6; CI = 0.59–10.6) when compared with premenopausal women (Holly *et al.*, 1994). Several other factors related to reproductive life were examined, including age at birth of first child and number of live births, and were found to have no consistent associations with any histological type of melanoma. Hormone-replacement therapy also was considered in this same study population (Holly *et al.*, 1994). There was no overall risk for the majority of women who had used postmenopausal hormones after natural menopause. However, risks for melanoma were somewhat elevated for some subgroups of women who had used these agents, particularly among women with SSM who had used them for more than 2 years after a hysterectomy in which one or no ovaries were removed (OR = 5.4; CI = 1.5–19.3). There was some indication of a dose–response effect for SSM when 0.625 mg and 1.25 mg doses were considered (OR = 2.3; CI = 0.93–5.7 for 0.625 mg and OR = 2.8; CI = 1.2–6.4 for 1.25 mg; for trend, *P* = 0.02). The number of women in the subgroups were small and the attributable risk for SSM likewise is modest.

Cohort studies

A prospective study was conducted to evaluate the non-contraceptive effects of OCs among the members of Kaiser-Permanente Health Plan in northern California (Beral *et al.*, 1977). Preliminary results were published from this study of 17 942 women aged 17–59 years. Of this group, 22 women were diagnosed as having melanoma with pathological confirmation during the follow-up period of approximately 90 000 person-years of observation. Relative risks of 1.4 were observed for melanoma among users of OCs for fewer than 4 years use and 1.7 for use for 4 years or more when compared with women who had never used these agents. Increased risk associated with ever-use of non-contraceptive oestrogens was reported with a relative risk of 1.8, although all of these associations could have been due to chance. Small numbers precluded analysis by histological type.

Results from the same cohort study conducted in the Kaiser-Permanente Health Plan population in northern California were reported later for women aged 18–64 years (Ramcharan *et al.*, 1981). Overlap exists between the subjects in the earlier report (Beral *et al.*, 1977) and these data (Ramcharan *et al.*, 1981), but the groups cannot be clearly distinguished using the available data. The study population for this report (Ramcharan *et al.*, 1981) included 20 melanoma cases

in a population of 14 104 women who responded to the 1977 interim questionnaire. For ever-use of OCs the risk for melanoma was 3.5 over all age groups combined (CI = 1.4–9.0). Hours of exposure to sunlight by current, past or never-use of OCs were not a confounder as the percentage distribution of this exposure was nearly identical in each of the three OC use groups. Histological type was not considered in the analysis due to sample-size limitations.

The Oxford/Family Planning Association follow-up study on OC use and health published a brief Letter to the Editor in which they reported preliminary results for 40 women who were diagnosed with melanoma through 1979 (Kay, 1981). Based on a total of 306 286 woman-years of observation in the UK, the adjusted relative risk for ever-use versus never-use of OCs was 1.5 (CI = 0.73–2.9). This brief Letter presented no data on subjects' ages, histological diagnosis or risk by time interval. Results with more information from this follow-up study were reported in 1991 (Hannaford *et al.*, 1991).

Later results from the Oxford/Family Planning Association study and the Royal College of General Practitioners study, both prospective studies conducted in the UK, were published together in one report (Hannaford *et al.*, 1991). No excess risk of melanoma was reported in women who had ever used OCs and who were in the Oxford/Family Planning Association study that included 32 cases of melanoma among 17 032 women. No elevated risk estimates were reported for OC use by duration of use, and time since last OC use was not linearly related to melanoma incidence, although the standardized rate of melanoma more than doubled among women who had used OCs from 4 to 6 years prior to diagnosis of their melanoma. This result was similar in both the Oxford/Family Planning Association study women and the Royal College of General Practitioners study population. However, the rates dropped among the women for whom it had been more than 6 years since last use. Neither parity nor social class were related to melanoma risk in the Oxford/Family Planning Association study group that included only women who were married or living as married. No data were available for analyses by histological type.

A total of 58 of 46 000 women were diagnosed with melanoma among those who were followed in the

Royal College of General Practitioners prospective study (Hannaford *et al.*, 1991). One-half of these women were using OCs at the time the study began and all of the study population were married or living as married. Although results could have been due to chance, an elevated risk of 1.8 was reported for 10 years or more of use. No excess risk of melanoma was noted for ever-use of OCs. Oestrogen and progestogen contents of the OCs were analysed and no evidence of increased risk was found by pill dose. With an increase in parity, the authors reported a decline in incidence rates of melanoma, although this could have been a chance finding. Histological type was not reported. The authors noted that the Royal College of General Practitioners study has had a substantial loss to follow-up of 31 000 women. Both studies should provide more meaningful data in another decade or two if study retention is adequate.

Discussion

When *ever-use* of OCs for all age, histological types and length of use groups are considered together, there appears to be only a modest effect of OCs on melanoma. Only the follow-up study from the Kaiser-Permanente Health Plan in California showed strong evidence of an association between *ever-use* of OCs and risk for all histological types of melanoma (Ramcharan *et al.*, 1981). An 1984 weighted average of estimates of risk from seven of the studies reviewed above suggested that if *ever-use* of OCs is a risk factor for melanoma, the overall increased risk due to these substances is not more than one-third above that of women who have never used these agents (Holman *et al.*, 1984). Several additional studies of this topic have been completed with few new positive results to change the above conclusions for ever-use of these agents. When subgroup analyses are considered, the concern about an effect of use of OCs becomes more complex because many dissimilar subgroups and time periods were analysed in the numerous studies reviewed here. Different long-term use definitions were used, making it difficult to compare results directly. Nevertheless, results from the more recent studies and time periods in which low-dose OCs were used are reassuring.

If more research is to be conducted on the effects of endogenous and exogenous oestrogens on melanoma, several factors should be considered to obtain a better understanding of the complex interrelationships among the variables of interest. Examples of the factors of interest are: case and control group selection; the possible different effects OCs may have on histological types of melanoma; age groups of subjects; stronger dose of OCs used in the 1960s; latency and duration of use by time period; other potential confounders, such as sunlight; and other reproductive factors. Large samples are required and subgroup analyses must be carefully planned. Some of these factors and others are briefly discussed below.

Selection of case and control groups

Use of population-based case and control groups in the study of melanoma will help to circumvent selective subject ascertainment and other problems inherent in use of hospital or neighbourhood subjects in epidemiological studies. Hospitalized cases do not necessarily present a problem for the study of many cancers. However, because the vast majority of melanoma patients, particularly those with SSM, are diagnosed and managed as out-patients for their primary tumour, a study using only hospitalized patients is likely to have a highly select case population and perhaps a larger proportion of patients with NM than would be found in a population-based study. Therefore, it is most appropriate to include population-based subject recruitment in a study of malignant melanoma and OC use.

Control group selection has the potential to be a significant factor in the study of melanoma and OC use. Hospitalized control groups may underestimate the strength of an association between melanoma and OC use. A $\geq 20\%$ increase in hospitalized rates among OC users in the Boston area, when compared with non-users, was reported in a study of 66 000 women conducted by a group from the Department of Epidemiology at Harvard University (Hoover *et al.*, 1978). An increase in hospitalization rates was reported even for conditions such as trauma and appendectomy that are unlikely to be related biologically to OC use (Hoover *et al.*, 1978). These two subsets of patients made up nearly 50% of the Boston University control group population (Helmrich *et al.*, 1984).

Neighbourhood controls used in studies of associations between melanoma and OC use may overmatch case and control populations on some factors of interest. Because OC use varies with social and reproductive factors (Hoover *et al.*, 1978) and persons of like socio-economic status tend to have similar health habits and live in similar neighbourhoods, use of neighbourhood controls may overmatch on OC use and other factors of interest.

Histological type

In the studies reviewed above, risk of melanoma associated with OC use, if present, was minimal when all age groups, histological types and OC ever-use groups were considered together. Random fluctuation and small numbers are likely to account for some of the associations found by histological type in the above studies. However, SSM and NM appeared to present enough variation by histological subtype to warrant separate analysis. The studies reviewed here and other evidence (Holman & Armstrong, 1984) indicate the importance of conducting analyses by histological type, although there is some controversy about the relevance of type-specific analyses. In western Canada, melanoma data that included both men and women showed SSM and NM to have similar risk ratios for some factors. However, SSM was more common among women, while NM was equally distributed by gender (Elwood *et al.*, 1987). For the studies reviewed, most provided few patients with NM and rarely provided data by histological type. For this reason, few data were presented for NM in this review. Although few NM patients were available in studies that presented data for this subtype, odds ratios for NM in relation to OC use often were in the opposite direction of those for SSM, particularly when long-term use was considered (Helmrich *et al.*, 1984; Gallagher *et al.*, 1985) (Clark levels IV and V were used as rough indicators for NM) (Holly *et al.*, 1983, 1994, 1995c; Holman *et al.*, 1984; Palmer *et al.*, 1992).

To better understand whether there are differences between SSM and NM, aetiological clues should be sought in a large population-based study or from a pooled analysis of available population-based data. In our work, the SSM cases were slightly younger at 41 years compared to 44 years for the NM subjects (Holly *et al.*, 1995b), and number of years living in a sunny climate had ORs for SSM that were elevated and ORs for NM that were below unity (Holly *et al.*, 1995a). Ever having been overweight by 9 kg provided ORs of 0.89 for SSM and 2.1 for NM in our population-based study of women (Holly *et al.*, 1995b). The age differences found in our study would be consistent with SSM being diagnosed earlier than NM, whereas the suggested protective association with number of years living in a sunny climate has no immediate biological relevance. If significant opposite effects for NM and SSM are found in relation to OC use in a pooled analysis of the existing studies, thought must be given to a biological rationale for this possible difference in association. Further, personal and sociological characteristics could be explored that might explain these differences.

Factors related to time and formulation of oral contraceptives

Many characteristics of subjects and other variables in a melanoma–OC study are integrally associated with time and aetiology and need to be considered in analyses — age of the subjects may affect duration of use and the latency period, and the OC oestrogen content has been drastically reduced over the years. Young women who currently are using OCs have not been exposed to the higher oestrogen content OCs available in the 1960s. Data analysis should be stratified to consider younger women separately from older women who may have taken OCs with different formulations available decades ago and who would have had an opportunity for longer latency subsequent to the high-dose formulation. In contrast, women currently >70 years at diagnosis would have been in an age group less likely to have used OCs and so should not be routinely included in OC-use analyses. The same policy should apply for menopausal oestrogens: only women who were in an age group eligible to use postmenopausal oestrogens should be included in the analyses of an association between melanoma and use of these preparations.

Age groups in each of the studies reviewed were analysed differently and many reported all age groups together. In some reports data were age-adjusted, while in others age-specific subgroup analyses were done, with the latter occasionally providing associations with OC use.

To determine whether there is an effect of the stronger formulation pill, dose of OCs also should be considered within the appropriate age groups. Precise dosage is often difficult to determine because women tend to recall the number of years they took OCs, but they are less likely to remember when they took a specific brand, especially if they used several brands and they were used decades ago. Providing colour photographs of OC packages is helpful to assist in subject recall. Both current formulations and those from the 1960s should be provided for study subject review. While photo books and reproductive calendars used to assist in recall are beneficial, it is difficult to assess dosage accurately for each individual because of the difficulty in recall of precise timing of OC use. Consideration of the time period when the women used OCs provides an estimate of the dosage effect since the preparations available in the 1960s were considerably stronger than those most commonly used in the 1980s. Dose, duration of use by time period and latency may be estimated simultaneously by considering, for example, only women who had taken OCs for at least 5 years and who began to take them at least 10 or 15 years ago.

If there is an adequate number of women with melanoma in a study and a large control group, other combinations of the data that take into account age, dose, duration by time period and latency may be considered. Detailed subgroup analyses require sample sizes found only in very large studies. Sample size may be a problem inherent in the study of melanoma and use of OCs particularly when histological type is considered. Even the largest population-based studies conducted to date have been too small to permit adequate subgroup analyses by histological type and other factors of interest for all but SSM.

Sunlight

Exposure and skin sensitivity to sunlight were not measured in most of the earlier studies reviewed here, but were considered in many of the more recent larger studies. Sunlight is unlikely to have been a confounding factor in these earlier reports as it was unrelated to OC use in most of the studies of mela-

noma conducted to date in several regions of the world: California (Ramcharan *et al.*, 1981; Holly *et al.*, 1995a), England (Adam *et al.*, 1981), western Canada (Gallagher *et al.*, 1985), Australia (Green & Bain, 1985), Denmark (Østerlind *et al.*, 1988) and in France (Le *et al.*, 1992). Effects of OCs and other reproductive factors might possibly be modified in geographical areas with intense sunlight and high incidence rates of melanoma, although this was not the case in Australia. It is unknown whether variation in ex-posure to sunlight may partially explain differences between results in studies from areas of low and high exposure such as Seattle, Canada and Australia.

Other reproductive factors

Several studies reported positive associations with use of replacement oestrogen therapy, although some of these results could have been due to chance (Beral *et al.*, 1977, 1984; Holman *et al.*, 1984; Østerlind *et al.*, 1988; Holly *et al.*, 1994). Single reports noted statistically significant associations between melanoma and diverse reproductive factors — age at birth of first child at ⩾ 31 years was reported as a risk factor in one study (Holly *et al.*, 1983). Younger age at menarche conveyed an increased risk in one report after adjustment for other factors (Zanetti *et al.*, 1990). A decrease in melanoma risk was noted for women who had had bilateral oophorectomies (Gallagher *et al.*, 1985), and a decrease in risk was noted for women with greater numbers of live births (Gallagher *et al.*, 1985; Zanetti *et al.*, 1990), although this risk was somewhat diminished in the latter report after control for other factors (Zanetti *et al.*, 1990). Two other studies also reported decreased risks with more children, although these results could have been due to chance (Holly *et al.*, 1983; Holman *et al.*, 1984), and a larger study by one of the same research groups did not confirm their earlier results in a separate larger study (Holly *et al.*, 1995c). Older age at natural menopause was shown to be related to SSM in one of the larger more recent studies (Holly *et al.*, 1995c), and history of hot flashes among premenopausal women was of borderline significance in the same study population. Women who used hormones to regulate their periods or to stop lactation were at an increased risk of melanoma, although this result could have been due to chance (Beral *et al.*, 1984).

Many of the factors related to more detailed measures of hormonal life among women have been considered in few of the separate studies. It would be useful to include each of them in any future research on melanoma in women.

Future directions

A possible association between either endogenous or exogenous oestrogens and melanoma is a complex topic. Since most women use OCs for a relatively brief period, studies that investigate the risk for ever-use include a large proportion of subjects who had only short-term exposure to these agents. Unless the study is large, it is difficult to find an association between long-term use and increased risk, particularly among women who used the higher oestrogen content OCs for sale decades ago. The results become even more complicated and require even more subjects to properly assess interrelationships when long-term use of OCs is considered by amount of oestrogen in these agents, histology, latency and the specific time period that the OCs were used. Some associations discussed in this presentation were not statistically significantly related to melanoma but are presented here as clues to the primary areas that should be considered in future studies of melanoma and endogenous and exogenous hormones. Several large, well-conducted studies of melanoma and hormonal factors have been completed in the last several years that provided support for the lack of an association with *ever-use* of these agents. More time to assess latency and large numbers of subjects will be required to answer some of the questions that have arisen in the studies reviewed above. There currently is a need for a careful, pooled analysis of the large population-based studies to address the unresolved concerns outlined above. A grant was funded in 1995 in the United States to address these questions. Dr Margaret Karagus at Dartmouth University in New Hampshire is the principal investigator who currently is undertaking a pooled analysis of several large studies of melanoma in women that meet specific criteria. This pooled analysis will address questions of long-term use of OCs, hormonal replacement therapy and other reproductive, endogenous and exogenous hormonal events that have been shown to be related to cutaneous melanoma.

The study will include > 2500 subjects with melanoma and 3500 control subjects who are 20–79 years of age. The original studies were conducted in Australia, Canada, Denmark, Italy, Scotland and the United States. A uniform coding scheme will be used for all relevant variables and investigators from each study will help to plan analyses and interpret results. The study goal will be to resolve some of the still outstanding questions regarding the possible association between OC use, reproductive factors and melanoma by histological type. Data from the large studies on melanoma and OC use are reassuring in that the risk of melanoma with short-term use of the more recent formulations appears to be negligible.

References

Adam, S.A., Sheaves, J.K., Wright, N.H., Mosser, G., Harris, R.W. & Vessey, M.P. (1981) A case-control study of the possible association between oral contraceptives and malignant melanoma. *British Journal of Cancer*, **44**, 45–50.

Ances, I.G. & Pomerantz, S.H. (1974) Serum concentrations of β-melanocyte-stimulating hormone in human pregnancy. *American Journal of Obstetrics and Gynecology*, **119**(8), 1062–1068.

Bain, C., Hennekens, C.H., Speizer, F.E., Rosner, B., Willett, W. & Belanger, C. (1982) Oral contraceptive use and malignant melanoma. *Journal of the National Cancer Institute*, **68**(4), 537–539.

Beral, V., Ramcharan, S. & Faris, R. (1977) Malignant melanoma and oral contraceptive use among women in California. *British Journal of Cancer*, **36**, 804–809.

Beral, V., Evans, S., Shaw, H. & Milton, G. (1984) Oral contraceptive use and malignant melanoma in Australia. *British Journal of Cancer*, **50**, 681–685.

Carruthers, R. (1966) Chloasma and oral contraceptives. *Medical Journal of Australia*, **ii**, 17–20.

Creagan, E.T., Ingle, J.N., Woods, J.E., Pritchard, D.J. & Jiang, N.S. (1980) Estrogen receptors in patients with malignant melanoma. *Cancer*, **46**, 1785–1786.

Elwood, J.M., Gallagher, R.P., Worth, J.A., Wood, W.S. & Pearson, J.C.G. (1987) Etiological differences between subtypes of cutaneous malignant melanoma: Western Canada Melanoma Study. *Journal of the National Cancer Institute*, **78**(1), 37–44.

Fisher, R.I., Neifeld, J.P. & Lippman, M.E. (1976) Oestrogen receptors in human malignant melanoma. *Lancet*, **ii**, 337–338.

Flowers, J.L., Seigler, H.F., McCarty, Sr, K.S., Konrath, J. & McCarty, Jr, K.S. (1987) Absence of estrogen receptor in human melanoma as evaluated by a monoclonal antiestrogen receptor antibody. *Archives of Dermatology*, **123**, 764–765.

Gallagher, R.P., Elwood, J.M., Hill, G.B., Coldman, A.J. Threlfall, W.J. & Spinelli, J.J. (1985) Reproductive factors, oral contraceptives and risk of malignant melanoma: Western Canada Melanoma Study. *British Journal of Cancer*, **52**, 901–907.

Green, A. & Bain, C. (1985) Hormonal factors and melanoma in women. *Medical Journal of Australia*, **142**, 446–448.

Hamilton, J.B. (1939) Significance of sex hormones in tanning of the skin in women. *Proceedings of the Society for Experimental Biology and Medicine*, **40**, 502–503.

Hannaford, P.C., Villard-Mackintosh, L., Vessey, M.P. & Kay, C.R. (1991) Oral contraceptives and malignant melanoma. *British Journal of Cancer*, **63**, 430–433.

Helmrich, S.P., Rosenberg, L., Kaufman, D.W. *et al.* (1984) Lack of an elevated risk of malignant melanoma in relation to oral contraceptive use. *Journal of the National Cancer Institute*, **72**(3), 617–620.

Holly, E.A. (1994) *Cutaneous Melanoma and Oral Contraceptives*. Kluwer Academic Publishers, Dordrecht.

Holly, E.A., Weiss, N.S. & Liff, J.M. (1983) Cutaneous melanoma in relation to exogenous hormones and reproductive factors. *Journal of the National Cancer Institute*, **70**(5), 827–831.

Holly, E.A., Cress, R.D. & Ahn, D.K. (1994) Cutaneous melanoma in women: Ovulatory life, menopause, and use of exogenous estrogens. *Cancer Epidemiology, Biomarkers and Prevention*, **3**, 661–668.

Holly, E.A., Aston, D.A., Ahn, D.K. & Kristiansen, J.J. (1995a) Cutaneous melanoma in women. I. Exposure to sunlight, ability to tan, and other UV related risk factors. *American Journal of Epidemiology*, **141**, 923–933.

Holly, E.A., Aston, D.A., Ahn, D.K. & Kristiansen, J.J. (1995b) Cutaneous melanoma in women. II. Phenotypic characteristics and other host-related factors. *American Journal of Epidemiology*, **141**, 934–942.

Holly, E.A., Cress, R.D. & Ahn, D.K. (1995c) Cutaneous melanoma in women. III. Reproductive factors and oral contraceptive use. *American Journal of Epidemiology*, **141**(10), 943–950.

Holman, C.D.J. & Armstrong, B.K. (1984) Cutaneous malignant melanoma and indicators of total accumulated exposure to the sun: An analysis separating histogenetic types. *Journal of the National Cancer Institute*, **73**, 75–82.

Holman, C.D.J., Armstrong, B.K. & Heenan, P.J. (1984) Cutaneous malignant melanoma in women: Exogenous sex hormones and reproductive factors. *British Journal of Cancer*, **50**, 673–680.

Hoover, R., Bain, C., Cole, P. & MacMahon, B. (1978) Oral contraceptive use: Association with frequency of hospitalization and chronic disease risk indicators. *American Journal of Public Health*, **68**, 335–341.

Jadassohn, W. (1958) Art for art's sake in medicine. *Archives of Dermatology*, **78**, 427–437.

Kay, C.R. (1981) Malignant melanoma and oral contraceptives. *British Journal of Cancer*, **44**, 479.

Le, M.G., Cabanes, P.A., Desvignes, V., Chanteau, M.F., Mlika, N. & Avril, M.F. (1992) Oral contraceptive use and risk of cutaneous malignant melanoma in a case-control study of French women. *Cancer Causes and Control*, **3**, 199–205.

Lecavalier, M.A., From, L. & Gaid, N. (1990) Absence of estrogen receptors in dysplastic nevi and malignant melanoma. *Journal of the American Academy of Dermatology*, **23**, 242–246.

Østerlind, A., Tucker, M.A., Stone, B.J. & Jensen, O.M. (1988) The Danish case-control study of cutaneous malignant melanoma. III. Hormonal and reproductive factors in women. *International Journal of Cancer*, **42**, 821–824.

Palmer, J.R., Rosenberg, L., Strom, B.L. *et al.* (1992) Oral contraceptive use and risk of cutaneous malignant melanoma. *Cancer Causes and Control*, **3**, 547–554.

Ramcharan, S., Pellegrin, F.A., Ray, R. & Hsu, J.P. (1981) *The Walnut Creek Contraceptive Drug Study. A Prospective Study of the Side Effects of Oral Contraceptives*. Vol. 3. US Government Printing Office, Washington, DC.

Zanetti, R., Franceschi, S., Rosso, S., Bidoli, E. & Colonna, S. (1990) Cutaneous malignant melanoma in females: The role of hormonal and reproductive factors. *International Journal of Epidemiology*, **19**(3), 522–526.

10

Epidemiology of Melanocytic Naevi

Naevi: Appearance, Prevalence and Involution

R.P. GALLAGHER

Introduction

It has been known for some time that there is an association between acquired melanocytic naevi and risk of cutaneous malignant melanoma, but it was not until relatively recently that the strength of that relationship was demonstrated in a series of well-conducted population-based epidemiological studies (Holman & Armstrong, 1984; Green *et al.*, 1986). The relationship between naevi and melanoma persists after control of other host factors known to be associated with melanoma risk such as skin colour, hair colour and sun sensitivity. Furthermore, the relationship remains strong whether counts on the arms only (Holman & Armstrong, 1984; Green *et al.*, 1986) are employed or whether whole-body counts are used (Holly *et al.*, 1987; Garbe *et al.*, 1989). Recently, Holly *et al.* (1994) demonstrated a high degree of correlation between total body naevus counts and counts on individual anatomical subsites, including constantly, intermittently and non-sun exposed sites, and this may suggest a generalized susceptibility of the melanocyte layer to solar ultraviolet radiation in individuals who develop many naevi.

This review will concentrate on the evidence concerning the appearance and involution of naevi, with emphasis on their relationship to age, gender and anatomical distribution. Risk factors for the evolution of naevi such as host pigmentation factors, sunburn history and solar exposure are described elsewhere in this volume.

Appearance of naevi

In order to examine the process of appearance of acquired melanocytic naevi, it is necessary to seek data on children, as it has been demonstrated that most naevus formation takes place early in life. It is generally agreed that only about 1–2% of white children are born with one or more congenital naevi (Kroom *et al.*, 1987; Rivers *et al.*, 1990). Early in life, acquired naevi begin to develop, although there is, as yet, limited information as to exactly how the process begins. Australian investigators (Harrison *et al.*, 1994) examined a sample of children aged one to six years and demonstrated the appearance of acquired naevi in children by age one year, with a steady rise in total body naevus counts through to age six. The increase in naevi was not due simply to the rapid increase in body size which takes place in the early years, as there was a similar increase in naevus density expressed as the number of naevi per square metre of body surface area.

Increases of naevi with age

Most of the information on increases in naevi with age comes from recent studies conducted on school-age children; that is, on subjects aged 6–18 years. Such studies have been conducted in Australia, a high sunlight area, and also lower sunlight areas such as Canada and Europe. It should be noted that direct comparisons of results obtained in naevus studies conducted in different parts of the world are difficult due to the slightly different protocols used for counting by each investigation. Nonetheless, comparisons can be very useful in suggesting mechanisms by which naevi might be generated. Figure 10.1 shows a

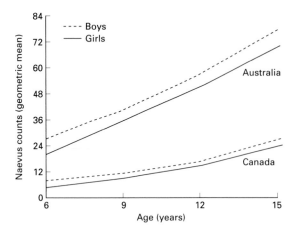

Fig. 10.1 Naevus counts in Australian and Canadian children; naevi ≥ 2 mm. (After Gallagher *et al.*, 1990; Kelly *et al.*, 1994.)

comparison of naevus counts from boys and girls resident in three Australian cities (Melbourne, Sydney and Townsville) (Kelly *et al.*, 1994), relatively high sunlight areas, with counts made in Vancouver Canada (Gallagher *et al.*, 1990b), a low sunlight area. The graphs show that absolute numbers of prevalent naevi increase in a linear fashion from 6 to 15 years in Australia, as well as in Canada. However, when naevus density (Fig. 10.2) is examined (that is, the number of naevi per square metre of body surface area), the

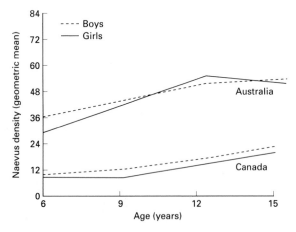

Fig. 10.2 Naevus density in Australian and Canadian children; naevi ≥ 2 mm/m² BSA. (After Gallagher *et al.*, 1990; Kelly *et al.*, 1994.)

increase in density appears to peak in the Australian children at about the age of 12 years, while in Canada the increase continues until at least the age of 15 years. Further data (not shown) are available from the study of English and Armstrong (1994) showing that the increase in naevus density in Western Australia may stop as early as age 9 years. These data suggest that, except in the case of a few children who develop large numbers of naevi due to inherited factors, all the melanocytes prone to proliferation and naevus formation are activated early in life by the high degree of sun exposure in Australia, while in Canada, a low sunlight area, such activation is not completed until later in adolescence, due to the more gradual accumulation of sun exposure. Furthermore, although caution is required because counting techniques are not identical in these studies, it appears that the ultimate naevus density in Australian children at the age of 15 years is higher than that in Canadian children. Thus, early intense sun exposure may be strongly related to naevus density. This may suggest that lowering early age solar exposure could reduce naevus counts in adolescents and young adults, and perhaps by extension their adult risk of melanoma.

Gender and anatomical site distribution

In most studies conducted to date in children, males appear to have both higher naevus counts than females and higher naevus density (Green *et al.*, 1989; Sigg & Pelloni, 1989; Gallagher *et al.*, 1990b; Coombs *et al.*, 1992; English & Armstrong, 1994; Kelly *et al.*, 1994). Furthermore, the rate of increase in naevi by age and anatomical site appears to differ in males and females. In Canadian boys, there is a consistent excess of naevi by comparison with girls at all ages on both the head and neck and the trunk (Gallagher *et al.*, 1990b). For the upper limb, young females (age 6–12 years) have similar naevus prevalence figures to boys; however, in adolescence (aged 13–18 years) girls develop a substantially higher naevus prevalence rate at this site than boys. In the Canadian study, the upper limbs had the highest naevus density of any anatomical site among adolescent females. Naevus density on the lower limbs is similar in young boys and girls, but by adolescence, density is higher among females. Similar distribution patterns by gender are seen in the Australian study of Nicholls (1973) although the more recent study of English and Armstrong (1994) does not show pronounced differences between boys and girls on upper and lower limbs at any age. The differences between males and females in naevus density may be due to clothing preferences and patterns of sunlight exposure in childhood and adolescence. It may be that boys get more exposure playing outside while young (up to age 12 years), and girls, as they approach adolescence, selectively get more sun exposure or sunburns to specific body sites such as the upper and lower limbs. One of the more interesting findings in both the Australian and Canadian studies is the very low naevus density on the lower limbs in female children. In the lower limbs of women there is a high incidence of malignant melanomas, suggesting that a correspondingly high naevus density should have been seen.

In the data collected in Canada (Gallagher *et al.*, 1990b), in which only naevi ⩾ 2 mm in diameter were counted, the highest naevus density was seen on intermittently sun-exposed body sites such as the back and shoulders. In the Australian data collected in Perth (English & Armstrong, 1994), naevi of all sizes were counted as well as those ⩾ 2 mm. For naevi of all sizes, the highest density was seen on a constantly sun-exposed site — the face. However, analysis of data on naevi ⩾ 2 mm shows that the highest density of these larger naevi are on the back.

Data from these studies, taken together, suggest that constant exposure to sunlight, as would occur on anatomical sites such as the face, may be responsible for generating small naevi, while intermittent solar exposure, perhaps in conjunction with sunburn, may be responsible for generation of larger (⩾ 2 mm diameter) naevi, seen to predominate on the back both in Vancouver and in Perth. Perhaps unacclimatized (untanned) skin on the back and other intermittently exposed sites also may allow a greater UV dose to penetrate to the melanocyte layer than might be the case in sites such as the face which would benefit from the protection afforded by tanning and thickening of the epidermis brought about by constant sun exposure.

Finally, low naevus prevalence rates are seen on the hands of children in both Australia and Canada,

and this corresponds to the low incidence rates of malignant melanoma on the hands in males and females in adulthood. This may be partially due to tanning and thickening of the epidermis with consequent solar protection; however, the face has similar constant exposure, and has both considerably higher naevus density and melanoma incidence rates per unit of surface area than the hands (Elwood & Gallagher, 1983).

Further research is needed, focusing specifically on pattern of solar exposure among children at various ages to see whether naevus prevalence and melanoma incidence by gender correspond with either sun exposure or sunburn history. There would be substantial value in carrying out such research in both high and low sunlight areas.

Naevi and puberty

It has been hypothesized that naevus density increases markedly at puberty, suggesting an effect of hormones on the appearance of new naevi (Pack *et al.*, 1952; MacKie *et al.*, 1985). Several recent studies make it possible to address this hypothesis with a greater degree of precision as data are now available on large numbers of children in the relevant age groups. The data from the Canadian study (Gallagher *et al.*, 1990b) indicate an increase in naevus density between age 10 and 13 years in girls, but a much smaller increase in boys. Furthermore, the majority of any increase in boys is seen only on the head and neck and back, and in females predominantly on the head and neck and upper limbs. If the increase was hormonally mediated at puberty, it might be expected that the increase would be seen equally on all sites.

The data of English and Armstrong (1994) indicate that virtually all the increase in naevus density in Western Australian children occurs before the age of puberty and the numbers of prevalent naevi increase evenly over the entire age range 5–14 years. Similarly, the data from Melbourne, Sydney and Townsville (Kelly *et al.*, 1994) show relatively uniform increases in density between the ages of 6, 9 and 12 years, and relatively little if any further increase after the age of 12 years. The British investigation of Pope *et al.* (1992) assesses children from the age of 4 to 11 years and unfortunately does not extend through the ages of puberty; however, the increase in naevus prevalence through ages 4–11 appears quite regular.

It would seem, then, that there is little support from analytical studies for a substantial effect of puberty, independent of age, on the genesis of new naevi. It should be noted, however, that all the recent studies which have evaluated naevus density in children have been cross-sectional rather than longitudinal in nature. It is, therefore, possible — although unlikely — that differing naevus prevalence rates in the cohorts making up the cross-section of children studied may be partially responsible for a failure to detect major changes in naevus density associated with puberty.

Involution and disappearance of naevi

What is known about the factors influencing the involution or disappearance of acquired melanocytic naevi? Examination of the literature suggests that little is known with any certainty, partly due to the fact that, until recently, the importance of naevi had not been recognized. Observational cohorts which might help answer questions about disappearance of naevi have not yet been assembled. Since acquired naevi develop in children, the few cohorts currently under observation do not include subjects who are old enough to have entered the age groups where involution appears to take place.

In New Zealand in 1985, Cooke *et al.* (1985) surveyed 872 adults, counting naevi on all body sites except the scalp, buttocks, genitals and in addition, in women, the breasts. The peak naevus prevalence is seen among subjects aged 20–29 years with numbers declining for older 10-year age groups. The data can be taken to suggest that:

• The number of naevi in successively younger 10-year cohorts of New Zealand whites is increasing, perhaps due to some environmental exposure.
• Naevi increase in prevalence in individuals through childhood and early adulthood but then tend to regress or disappear with age.

A further investigation conducted in Scotland by MacKie *et al.* (1985) examined a total of 432 white subjects of all ages, counting all naevi ⩾ 3 mm in diameter with the exception of those in the genital areas. Counts were higher in females than in males at all

ages in this population. This finding stands in contrast to most other naevus studies which show either higher counts in males or equivalent counts in males and females both in children and adults. The highest counts were seen in subjects aged 20–29 years. In subjects aged 50–59, 60–69 and ⩾ 70 years, naevus counts declined markedly, in a fashion similar to that seen in New Zealand (Cooke *et al.*, 1985). The earlier Australian study of Nicholls shows a similar pattern overall with maximal counts of naevi ⩾ 2 mm in males in their teens, and females in their teens and twenties (Nicholls, 1973). These mean counts progressively declined in each 10-year age group thereafter until counts reached their minimum values in both sexes among subjects aged 60–69 years. Armstrong *et al.* examined the aetiology of melanocytic naevi among 511 normal residents of Western Australia, who had been recruited as control subjects in a case-control investigation of malignant melanoma (Armstrong *et al.*, 1986). Naevi counted in the study consisted only of palpable lesions on the arms below the axillae. Macular naevi were not considered in this study. Naevi were somewhat more common on females than on males, although this may not be surprising, as several other studies also show higher counts on the arms of females than males even though males have higher total body counts (Cooke *et al.*, 1985; Gallagher *et al.*, 1990b). The data suggested that in adults, the maximal naevus prevalence was seen on adults with inter-mediate skin reflectance, intermediate numbers of recent sunburns and intermediate levels of recent sun exposure. Similar findings for childhood sunburns and sun exposure were also detected. Armstrong *et al.* suggested that the findings might be explained by proposing an effect for sunlight exposure in both the appearance and involution of naevi. Sunlight exposure in childhood serves to generate naevi in susceptible children by causing initial mutations in the melanocyte layer which allow some of these cells to escape their usual growth constraints and multiply, forming visible naevi. Further cumulative sunlight exposure accruing with age, however, provokes further mutations along with consequent immune reaction leading to the destruction and disappearance of the naevus.

There is independent evidence for such a mechanism from histological investigations of melanocytic lesions.

Halo naevi are more likely to be excised in the summer months, suggesting an increased immunological reaction against atypical naevi during periods of high sun exposure. In addition, the proportion of excised naevi demonstrating junctional activity is higher in the summer than during the winter (Holman *et al.*, 1983), indicating that in existing naevi, continued sun exposure stimulates potentially mutational changes at the cellular level.

Is naevus density increasing over time?

A significant question in terms of melanoma risk is whether naevus density is increasing in each succeeding cohort among white populations in Western countries. The major difficulty in addressing this question is that none of the investigations conducted from the 1950s to the 1970s which might have facilitated such evaluation used standardized clinical definitions of a naevus. Furthermore, the protocols and techniques used to count naevi were not uniform. Pack *et al.* (1952) in New York counted naevi on 1000 subjects in the early 1950s and found a mean count of 14.6 per subject. Unfortunately, the clinical definition of a naevus or mole as used in this study is not given, and no information on how naevi were distinguished from freckles is present. The age structure of the cohort of subjects was also not well described and hence it is difficult to know how comparable this group is to that of later studies. In 1960 Stegmaier and Becker counted and excised all pigmented lesions thought clinically to be melanocytic naevi on 20 volunteer subjects aged 20–25 years. A total of 1090 melanocytic lesions were removed, of which 815 proved histologically to be melanocytic naevi. Clinically then, each subject had about 54 naevi, although histologically the figure was closer to 41. Again, no definition was given of how naevi were defined clinically, although the authors make it clear that lesions of all sizes were excised and many were pin-head size. Although the counts made by Stegmaier and Becker were considerably higher than those of Pack *et al.* 10 years earlier, it seems likely that the two studies were not counting comparable lesions. In addition, the Stegmaier and Becker study concentrated strictly on subjects who were in the age group now known to exhibit the maximal numbers

of naevi, whereas Pack *et al.* included subjects representing a broad age range.

Nicholls (1973) in a cross-sectional study involving 1518 subjects of all ages residing in the Sydney area found a mean count of naevi $\geq 2\,mm$ in 15-year-old subjects of 43 for males and 20 for females. The study of Kelly *et al.* (1994) which was carried out in the early 1990s also included 15-year-olds from Sydney, and the mean count for males was 98 and for females 80. This study also assessed only naevi $\geq 2\,mm$ in diameter, and the results suggest that naevus density increased substantially over the 20-year period intervening between the two studies. Caution is required in interpreting such a comparison, however, as aspects of the earlier study were not well defined and there are certain to be differences in the counting protocols used in the two studies.

Future comparisons of naevus density should be somewhat easier than today, as workers at the International Agency for Research on Cancer have assembled a standardized protocol for identifying and counting naevi which is well adapted to field studies on large non-hospitalized populations (International Agency for Research on Cancer, 1990). If future investigators undertake to follow the methods outlined in the IARC report, it should be possible to look at differences between populations, and within populations, over time.

Summary

At the present time, with melanoma incidence still rising, there are a number of important questions to be resolved concerning the appearance and disappearance of acquired melanocytic naevi. First of all, why is the anatomical site distribution of naevi not concordant with that of cutaneous melanoma? Perhaps the lack of concordance is due to one being primarily related to sun exposure, while the other is related to sunburn history. Green has suggested that the degree of susceptibility of melanocytes to malignant transformation may vary by anatomical site (Green, 1992).

Data from studies on children suggest that boys tend to develop naevi more quickly or at an earlier age than girls. In addition, the anatomical distribution is different in the two sexes, and females tend to develop more naevi on the upper limbs than males (Holman *et al.*, 1983; Gallagher *et al.*, 1990b), although their melanoma rate at this site is not markedly different from that of males (Gallagher *et al.*, 1990a). Perhaps the differences in naevus prevalence between males and females are due to differences in their patterns of early life sun exposure or of sunburn.

The hand appears to develop relatively few naevi and few melanomas, even though it is constantly exposed to sunlight. Perhaps the constant low-grade trauma from the activities of daily life thicken the epidermis, providing protection for the melanocyte layer. Alternatively, constant sun exposure causing tanning might afford protection for the melanocyte layer, although the face is also sun exposed and has a high prevalence of both naevi and melanoma.

Why is melanoma incidence on the legs of females so high when naevus prevalence is relatively low? Finally, is the prevalence of naevi increasing over time, and can this be directly related to increases in childhood sunlight exposure, sunburn or both?

References

Armstrong, B.K., de Klerk, N. & Holman, C.D.J. (1986) Etiology of common acquired melanocytic nevi: constitutional variables, sun exposure and diet. *Journal of the National Cancer Institute*, **77**, 329–335.

Cooke, K.R., Spears, G.F. & Skegg, D.C. (1985) Frequency of moles in a defined population. *Journal of Epidemiology and Community Health*, **39**, 48–52.

Coombs, B., Sharples, K. & Cooke, K. (1992) Variation and covariates of the number of benign nevi in adolescents. *American Journal of Epidemiology*, **136**, 344–355.

Elwood, J.M. & Gallagher, R.P. (1983) Site distribution of malignant melanoma. *Canadian Medical Association Journal*, **128**, 1400–1404.

English, D.R. & Armstrong, B.K. (1994) Melanocytic nevi in children. I. Anatomic sites and demographic and host factors. *American Journal of Epidemiology*, **139**, 390–401.

Gallagher, R.P., Ma, B., McLean, D.I. *et al.* (1990a) Trends in basal cell carcinoma, squamous cell carcinoma and melanoma of the skin from 1973 through 1987. *Journal of the American Academy of Dermatology*, **23**, 413–421.

Gallagher, R.P., McLean, D.I. & Yang, C.P. *et al.* (1990b) Anatomic distribution of acquired melanocytic nevi in white children. *Archives of Dermatology*, **126**, 466–471.

Garbe, C., Kruger, S., Stadler, R., Guggenmoss-Holzmann, I.

& Orfanos, C.E. (1989) Markers and relative risk in a German population for developing malignant melanoma. *International Journal of Dermatology*, **28**, 517–523.

Green, A. (1992) A theory of site distribution of melanomas: Queensland, Australia. *Cancer Causes and Control*, **3**, 513–516.

Green, A., Bain, C., MacLennan, R. & Siskind, V. (1986) Risk factors for cutaneous melanoma in Queensland. *Recent Results in Cancer Research*, **102**, 76–97.

Green, A., Siskind, V., Hansen, M.E. *et al.* (1989) Melanocytic nevi in school children in Queensland. *Journal of the American Academy of Dermatology*, **20**, 1054–1060.

Harrison, S.L., MacLennan, R., Speare, R. & Wronski, I. (1994) Sun exposure and melanocytic naevi in young Australian children. *Lancet*, **344**, 1529–1532.

Holly, E.A., Kelly, J.W., Shpall, S.N. & Chiu, S.-H. (1987) Number of melanocytic nevi as a major risk factor for malignant melanoma. *Journal of the American Academy of Dermatology*, **17**, 459–468.

Holly, E.A., Kelly, J.W., Ahn, D.K., Shpall, S.N. & Rosen, J.I. (1994) Risk of cutaneous melanoma by number of melanocytic nevi and correlation of nevi by anatomic site. In: *Epidemiological Aspects of Cutaneous Malignant Melanoma* (eds R.P. Gallagher & J.M. Elwood), pp. 159–172. Kluwer Academic Publishers, Boston.

Holman, C.D.J. & Armstrong, B.K. (1984) Pigmentary traits ethnic origin, benign nevi and family history as risk factors for cutaneous malignant melanoma. *Journal of the National Cancer Institute*, **72**, 257–266.

Holman, C.D.J., Heenan, P.J., Caruso, V. & Glancy, R.J. (1983) Seasonal variation in the junctional component of pigmented naevi. *International Journal of Cancer*, **31**, 213–215.

International Agency for Research on Cancer (1990) *Epidemiological Studies on Melanocytic Naevi: Protocol for Identifying and Recording Naevi*. IARC Internal Report No. 90/002. IARC, Lyon.

Kelly, J.W., Rivers, J.K., MacLennan, R., Harrison, S., Lewis, A.E. & Tate, B.J. (1994) Sunlight: a major risk factor associated with development of melanocytic naevi in Australian school children. *Journal of the American Academy of Dermatology*, **30**, 40–48.

Kroon, S., Clemmensen, O.J. & Hastrup, N. (1987) Incidence of congenital melanocytic nevi in newborn babies in Denmark. *Journal of the American Academy of Dermatology*, **17**, 422–426.

MacKie, R.M., English, J., Aitcheson, T.C. *et al.* (1985) The number and distribution of benign pigmented moles in a healthy British population. *British Journal of Dermatology*, **113**, 167–174.

Nicholls, E.M. (1973) Development and elimination of pigmented moles and the anatomical distribution of primary malignant melanoma. *Cancer*, **32**, 191–195.

Pack, G., Lenson, N. & Gerber, D. (1952) Regional distribution of moles and melanomas. *Archives of Surgery,* **65**, 862–870.

Pope, D., Sorahan, T., Marsden, J. *et al.* (1992) Benign pigmented nevi in children. *Archives of Dermatology,* **128**, 1202–1206.

Rivers, J.K., Frederiksen, P.C. & Dibdin, C. (1990) A prevalence survey of dermatoses in the Australian neonate. *Journal of the American Academy of Dermatology,* **23**, 77–81.

Sigg, C. & Pelloni, F. (1989) Frequency of acquired melanocytic nevi and their relationship to skin complexion in 939 school children. *Dermatologica,* **179**, 123–128.

Stegmaier, O. & Becker, S.W. (1960) Incidence of melanocytic nevi in young adults. *Journal of Investigative Dermatology,* **34**, 125-129.

Sun Exposure, Phenotype and Naevus

J.J. GROB AND J.J. BONERANDI

Pigmented naevi are clearly implicated in the epidemiology of melanoma but their exact role remains unclear. They may simply be an indicator of the state of activation of the melanocytic system or more ominously constitute a reservoir of cells ready to degenerate. In other words, they may be risk markers or precursors of melanoma. Since it has been established that sun plays a determinant role in the natural history of melanoma, many epidemiological studies have been undertaken in the last 10 years to assess the role of sun exposure in the development of naevi.

Problems in assessing the relationship between sun exposure and naevi

A number of problems have led to seemingly different and/or contradictory findings and impede comparison of the results of epidemiological studies.

Differences in study design and methodology

A wide range of study designs and methodology have been proposed to study the relationship between naevi, sun exposure and phenotype. These methods can be divided into three main categories. The first consists of evaluating the correlation between number of naevi and phenotype as a marker of sun sensitivity. The second is to assess the relationship between number of naevi and sun-exposure history. The third involves evaluation of density of naevi on different anatomical areas as a function of regional sun exposure.

Even in studies using the same approach, different methodology has been used. Studies assessing the correlation between number of naevi and phenotype have been based on different characteristics such as skin colour, hair colour, eye colour, freckling, propensity to sunburn and ability to tan. Each of these features has different implications (see below). Similarly, studies assessing sun-exposure history and naevi have rarely used the same criteria for evaluation of sun exposure: cumulative amount of sun exposure, specific types of sun exposure (seaside, etc.), frequency of sunburn during childhood and frequency of sunburns. In studies assessing the density of naevi as a function of the regional sun exposure, anatomical areas have rarely been defined the same way. Studies also differ with regard to the type of naevi counted and to the sites on which naevi were counted.

Another source of discrepancy involves demographic factors. Some authors studied only adults (Armstrong *et al.,* 1986; English *et al.,* 1987; Brogelli *et al.,* 1991; Augustsson *et al.,* 1992; Richard *et al.,* 1993) whereas others studied different groups of young people, i.e. children only (Green *et al.,* 1989; Pope *et al.,* 1992; English & Armstrong, 1994a; Harrisson *et al.,* 1994), teenagers (Coombs *et al.,* 1992) and children and teenagers (Sigg & Pelloni, 1989; Gallagher *et al.,* 1990a,b, 1991). Since naevi appear during childhood and adolescence, results of these studies are obviously not comparable. Studies have been performed in a wide range of countries including Australia (Armstrong *et al.,* 1986; Grob *et al.,* 1990; English & Armstrong, 1994a; Fritschi *et al.,* 1987; Harrisson *et al.,* 1992; Kelly *et al.,* 1994), Canada (Gallagher *et al.,* 1990b, 1991), France (Richard *et al.,* 1993; Roudil *et al.,* 1995), Germany (Garbe *et al.,* 1994), Israel (Harth *et al.,* 1992), Italy (Brogelli *et al.,* 1991), The Netherlands (Rampen *et al.,* 1986, 1987), New Zealand (Coombs *et al.,* 1992), Sweden (Augustsson *et al.,* 1990, 1992), Switzerland (Siggs & Pelloni, 1989), the UK (English *et al.,* 1987; Pope *et al.,* 1992; Fritschi *et al.,* 1994) and the USA

(Kopf *et al.*, 1978, 1985, 1986). There are major differences between these countries with regard to the ethnicity, behaviour toward sun and climatic conditions. What is true in a Celtic population in Scotland is not necessarily true in a mixed population in the South of France or even another Celtic population in Australia.

Ambiguities

An unspoken ambiguity of all studies is that a relationship between light phenotype and high number of naevi may be interpreted in two ways. It is usually accepted as evidence of an effect of sun exposure on the development of naevi since light phenotype is considered as a marker of high sun sensitivity. However, it could also be the result of an association between the genes controlling the number of naevi and those controlling characteristics such as hair colour and skin complexion. Criteria used to define phenotype are also a source of ambiguity. Skin colour, hair colour, eye colour, complexion, degree of freckling, propensity to sunburn and tanning ability are very different. Skin, hair and eye colour are strictly descriptive. Freckling is descriptive but also evaluates sun exposure, since freckles depend on UV exposure. Propensity to sunburn and tanning ability assess both the adaptive properties of the skin and sun behaviour. Individuals with a very sensitive skin type who do not expose themselves might say that they are not subject to sunburns, whereas less-sensitive individuals who expose themselves in the middle of the day at sea without protection might say that they burn easily. Furthermore unlike skin, hair and eye colour which can be objectively measured by examiners, freckling, propensity to sunburns and tanning ability are subjective self-reported data.

Another ambiguity in epidemiological studies concerns the interpretation of the relations between number of naevi and skin type. A higher number of naevi in a light-skinned person is considered as an indirect proof that sun exposure promotes naevi, but, to a certain extent, it could be the opposite. Since the same amount of UV exposure is more aggressive in a light-skinned than dark-skinned individual, it is generally reasoned that individuals with lighter skin experience more deleterious effects of UV. However,

this hypothesis assumes that phenotype itself has no influence on sun behaviour. In reality, an individual who easily sunburns may limit his/her exposure more than an individual who tans easily, so that in the end it could be difficult to know who has the higher biological effect of UV.

A last example of the ambiguity of results concerns sunburns. What is the meaning of excess sunburns associated with excess naevi? Does it mean that simply excessive sun exposure, indirectly measured by sunburns, induces naevi or does it mean that severe trauma of the skin induces naevi?

Confounding factors

There are several potential confounding factors which can have an impact on the results of epidemiological studies about sun exposure, phenotype and naevi. Phenotype can be a biasing factor in naevus counting. Freckles can be miscounted as naevi and vice versa. In red-haired people, naevi are less pigmented and thus more difficult to detect and count. Classification of phenotype can also induce a bias. The results of a study can change greatly depending on whether or not red-haired people are included with blond or on how many freckling classes are used. The method of determining skin colour (visual assessment versus measurement of reflectance) can affect results. Age-related changes in the number of naevi are also a major bias in studies using populations with wide-ranging ages. Several approaches have been proposed in recent studies to limit the impact of these biases: studying people of the same age (Coombs *et al.*, 1992; Garbe *et al.*, 1994), or people with the same age, sex and phenotype (Richard *et al.*, 1993) or simply studying very large populations (Pope *et al.*, 1992; English & Armstrong, 1994a; Kelly *et al.*, 1994).

The way of counting naevi is another potential source of bias that must be controlled (Aitken *et al.*, 1994; English & Armstrong, 1994b). Depending on who (dermatologist, other physician or nurse) counts what (palpable naevi, all naevi, naevi >2mm) and where (total body, limited areas), results in the same population sample can be different. Lastly, studies dealing with past sun exposure are also subject to recall bias since the memory of sun exposure more than 20 years before is questionable (Barwick & Ya-Ting, 1995).

Summary of findings from major epidemiological studies

Number of naevi and phenotype

Number of naevi is related to 'descriptive' phenotype defined by characteristics including race and colour of the skin, hair and eyes. It has been established that the number of naevi is higher in Caucasians than in Orientals and that black people have the lowest number of naevi (Pack *et al.*, 1963; Coleman *et al.*, 1980; Gallagher *et al.*, 1991). In Caucasians, most studies have shown that the number of naevi increases as skin colour gets lighter (Armstrong *et al.*, 1986; Green & Swerdlow, 1989; Gallagher *et al.*, 1990a; Pope *et al.*, 1992; Fritschi *et al.*, 1994; Harrisson *et al.*, 1994; Kelly *et al.*, 1994) with the possible exception of very light-skinned people (Armstrong *et al.*, 1994). Results regarding hair colour are somewhat contradictory. A study has suggested that the lighter the hair (Green *et al.*, 1989), the more naevi there are, while others have shown a range of conflicting results, i.e. an association between dark hair and high number of naevi (English *et al.*, 1987; Kelly *et al.*, 1994), a specifically lower number of naevi in red-haired people (Pope *et al.*, 1992; English & Armstrong 1994b; Fritschi *et al.*, 1994; Kelly *et al.*, 1994) or no correlation (Armstrong *et al.*, 1986; Green *et al.*, 1989; Gallagher *et al.*, 1990b; Coombs *et al.*, 1992). Results regarding eye colour are also unclear. Some studies indicate that people with lighter eyes have more naevi (English *et al.*, 1987; Kelly *et al.*, 1994) while others find no correlation (Armstrong *et al.*, 1986; Coombs *et al.*, 1992; Harrisson *et al.*, 1994).

Number of naevi is also related to 'adaptative' phenotype defined as the way the skin adapts to sun exposure: tanning ability, freckling tendency and propensity to sunburns. Two studies demonstrated that ability to get a deeper tan is associated with fewer naevi (Gallagher *et al.*, 1990a; Harrisson *et al.*, 1994) while one showed the opposite (English *et al.*, 1987). Most studies agree that the higher the degree of freckling, the higher the number of naevi (Sigg & Pelloni, 1989; Gallagher *et al.*, 1990a; Coombs *et al.*, 1992; Pope *et al.*, 1992; Fritschi *et al.*, 1994; Harrisson *et al.*, 1994). However in two studies maximal number of naevi was described in people with intermediate freckling (Nicholls, 1968; English & Armstrong, 1994b). All studies have shown that individuals with a greater propensity to sunburns have a higher number of naevi (Green *et al.*, 1989; Gallagher *et al.*, 1990a; Harrisson *et al.*, 1994).

Finally, even when phenotype is defined according to a combination of 'descriptive' and 'adaptive' criteria, it is also correlated with number of naevi. Lighter phenotype and less-adaptative properties are associated with a higher number of naevi (Sigg & Pelloni, 1989; Rampen *et al.*, 1986; Coombs *et al.*, 1992; Richard *et al.*, 1993).

Number of naevi and sun exposure

The density of naevi is different on differently sun-exposed sites. The first study to compare the number of naevi on differently exposed areas of the body showed a higher number of elevated naevi on the lateral than medial aspect of the arms (Kopf *et al.*, 1978). This finding was confirmed by a series of works showing a higher density of naevi on sun-exposed than sun-protected areas (Augustsson *et al.*, 1990, 1992; Gallagher *et al.*, 1990b; Richard *et al.*, 1993; English & Armstrong, 1994a). Further study demonstrated that the density of naevi was higher on intermittently exposed areas than constantly exposed areas (Gallagher *et al.*, 1990b; Richard *et al.*, 1993; English & Armstrong, 1994b).

Number of naevi is correlated with sun-exposure history. A history of many sunburns has generally been associated with a higher number of naevi (Gallagher *et al.*, 1990a; Pope *et al.*, 1992; Richard *et al.*, 1993; Garbe *et al.*, 1994; Harrisson *et al.*, 1994). However, two studies did not confirm this finding with one showing that people with intermediate sunburn history had the highest number of naevi (Armstrong *et al.*, 1986) and the other showing no correlation (Coombs *et al.*, 1992). A clear correlation between sunbathing and a higher number of naevi has been demonstrated (Pope *et al.*, 1992; Richard *et al.*, 1993; Harrisson *et al.*, 1994) although one study did not find such a relation (Rampen & Fleuren, 1987). Ambient solar radiation also influences the number of naevi. This number tends to increase with decreasing latitude of residence in white people (Kelly *et al.*, 1994). Comparison of naevi in Australian and Scottish populations (Fritschi *et al.*, 1994), which are both of Celtic origin and thus of similar phenotype, show that Australians have more naevi.

Type or size of naevi and sun exposure

'Dysplastic naevi', which are in fact 'clinically atypical naevi' in most studies, were reported to be more numerous on sun-exposed areas (Kopf *et al.*, 1985, 1986). We recently found a higher number on intermittently exposed areas suggesting that aggressive sun exposure, i.e. excess sun exposure on unprepared skin, promotes the development of atypical naevi (Richard *et al.*, 1993). This hypothesis is supported by a case-control study showing that, although subjects with atypical mole syndrome were more likely to have naevi on the buttocks, the features of these naevi were not atypical (Abadir *et al.*, 1995). However, distribution of 'dysplastic naevi' was reported to be independent of sun exposure (Rampen & Fleuren, 1987; Augustsson *et al.*, 1992).

Sun exposure may also have an influence on the size of naevi. The number of large naevi is maximum on intermittently-exposed areas (Richard *et al.*, 1993) whereas the number of small naevi is maximum on regularly-exposed areas. The mean number of large naevi is related to beach recreation and history of sunburns only in the red-haired. The ratio of the density of naevi on intermittently exposed area in red-haired people to the density of naevi on intermittently exposed area in dark-haired people is higher for large naevi than for small (Richard *et al.*, 1993). Taken together, these data together suggest that number of large naevi may be related to aggressive sun exposure, which tends to occur more often in most sensitive skin types (Richard *et al.*, 1993).

Age-dependence of the impact of sun exposure on naevi

There is evidence that sun exposure during childhood promotes the development of naevi (Gallagher *et al.*, 1990a; Pope *et al.*, 1992; Richard *et al.*, 1993; Harrisson *et al.*, 1994). In Australia, there are more palpable naevi in people who migrated before the age of 10 years (Holman & Armstrong, 1984). However, sun exposure between 15 and 30 years still promotes naevi. In a study involving monozygotic twins, we showed that the twin who received the more sun exposure between 15 and 30 years of age had a twofold higher risk to present more naevi (Roudil *et al.*, 1995). Paradoxically, chronic exposure in older people appears to contribute to regression of naevi since skin markers for cumulative exposure are associated with a lower number of naevi (Harth *et al.*, 1992).

General mechanisms of naevus development

As stated above, it is difficult to compare previous epidemiological studies and there are many apparent contradictions. However, several points appear to be certain. Sun exposure plays an important role in the development of naevi, which occurs mainly during the first two or three decades of life. Both ambient and occasional sun exposure seem to stimulate appearance of naevi. Sun-sensitive people, by whatever definition, tend to have more naevi. However, no one phenotype criterion is perfectly correlated with the number of naevi.

A number of other points are starting to take shape:
• First, the 'red-phenotype', including not only people with red hair but also people with blond Venetian or auburn hair with freckles, constitute a special subgroup characterized by high sun sensitivity, naevi difficult to count because they are easily confused with freckles and perhaps low genetic tendency to naevogenesis.
• Second, 'traumatizing sun exposure' seems to be the most potent stimulator of naevi and to be responsible for development of large naevi, 'traumatizing sun exposure' being defined not just as sunburn but as any excessive sun exposure on unprepared skin causing important acute biological effects. It is more likely in sun-sensitive phenotypes but can occur in any phenotypes.
• Third, the period for development of naevi is not limited to the first 20 years.
• Fourth, chronic sun exposure is associated with long-term regression of naevi (dermatoheliosis).

Based on these points, it can be hypothesized that the number of naevi ('moliness') depends on three major factors: (i) amount and type of sun exposure mainly but not exclusively during the first 30 years of life; (ii) genetically-determined ability to 'block' UV; and (iii) genetically-determined 'propensity to naevogenesis'. With regard to the last factor, it should be said that the underlying mechanism is unclear. However, there is evidence from studies of so-called 'melanoma/dysplastic naevus syndrome' that the number and type of naevi may be genetically transmitted. Twin studies also suggest that propensity to naevogenesis could be partly genetically determined (Duffie *et al.*, 1992). According to this 'three-factor hypothesis', the number of naevi should be highest in people with 'lighter' phenotype (except red-haired people who may have a low propensity to naevogenesis), with a familial tendency to moliness and who have been highly sun exposed. In this subgroup, the largest and most atypical naevi should be more frequent in people who have experienced more 'traumatizing sun exposure'.

It must be underlined that risk factors for naevi are the same as those classically proposed for melanoma (sun exposure in childhood, light phenotype and low tanning ability). 'Traumatizing sun exposure' is a major risk factor for both large naevi and melanoma. It can thus be understood why the number of large naevi is one of the most important risk markers of melanoma (Grob *et al.*, 1990). In fact, the number and type of naevi in a young adult provides the clinician with an indication of both the genetics and exposure to environmental factors predisposing to melanoma.

We still have much to learn concerning the natural history of naevi and the role of genetic transmission. However, current knowledge provides a basis for evaluating the efficacy of prevention. Any measure that limits development of naevi in infants should reduce the risk of melanoma in adults.

References

Abadir, M.C., Marghoob, A.A., Slade, J., Salopeck, T.G., Yadav, S. & Kopf, A.W. (1995) Case-control study of melanocytic nevi on the buttocks in atypical mole syndrome: role of solar radiation in the pathogenesis of atypical moles. *Journal of the American Academy of Dermatology*, **1**, 31–36.

Aitken, J.F., Green, A., Eldridge, A. *et al.* (1994) Comparability of naevus counts between and within examiners, and comparison with computer image analysis. *British Journal of Cancer*, **69**, 487–491.

Armstrong, B.K., De Klerk, N.H. & Holman, C.J. (1986) Etiology of common acquired melanocytic nevi: constitutional variables, sun exposure and diet. *Journal of the Natural Cancer Institute*, **77**, 329–335.

Augustsson, A., Stierner, U., Rosdahl, I. & Suurkula, M. (1990) Regional distribution of melanocytic naevi in relation to sun exposure, and site-specific counts predicting total number of naevi. *Acta Dermato-Venereologica*, **72**, 123–127.

Augustsson, A., Stierner, U., Rosdahl, I. & Suurkula, M. (1992) Melanocytic naevi in sun-exposed and protected skin in melanoma patients and controls. *Acta Dermato-Venereologica*, **71**, 512–517.

Berwick, M. & Ya-Ting, C. (1995) Reliability of reported sunburn history in a case-control study of cutaneous malignant melanoma. *American Journal of Epidemiology*, **11**, 1033–1037.

Brogelli, L., De Giorgi, V., Bini, F. & Giannotti, B. (1991) Melanocytic naevi: clinical features and correlation with the phenotype in healthy young males in Italy. *British Journal of Dermatology*, **125**, 349–352.

Coleman, W.P., Gately, L.E., Krementz, A.B., Reed, R.J. & Krementz, E.T. (1980) Nevi, lentigines, and melanomas in Blacks. *Archives of Dermatology*, **116**, 548–551.

Coombs, B.D., Sharples, K.J., Cooke, K.R., Skegg, C.G. & Elwood, J.M. (1992) Variation and covariates of the number of benign naevi in adolescents. *American Journal of Epidemiology*, **136**, 344–355.

Duffie, D.L., MacDonald, A.M., Easton, D.F., Ponder, B.A.J. & Martin, N.G. (1992) Is the genetic moliness simply the genetics of sun exposure? An analysis of nevus counts and risk factors in British twins. *Cytogenetics and Cell Genetics*, **59**, 194–196.

English, D.R. & Armstrong, B.K. (1994a) Melanocytic nevi in children. Anatomic sites and demographic and host factors. *American Journal of Epidemiology*, **139**, 390–401.

English, D.R. & Armstrong, B.K. (1994b) Melanocytic nevi in children. Observer variation in counting nevi. *American Journal of Epidemiology*, **139**, 402–407.

English, S.C., Swerdlow, A.J., MacKie, R.M. *et al.* (1987) Relation between phenotype and banal melanocytic nevi. *British Medical Journal*, **294**, 152–154.

Fritschi, L., McHenry, P., Green, A., MacKie, R., Green, L. & Siskind, V. (1994) Naevi in schoolchildren in Scotland and Australia. *British Journal of Dermatology*, **130**, 599–603.

Gallagher, R.P., McLean, D.I., Yang, C.P. *et al.* (1990a) Suntan, sunburn, and pigmentation factors and the frequency of acquired melanocytic nevi in children. *Archives of Dermatology*, **126**, 770–776.

Gallagher, R.P., McLean, D.I., Yang. C.P. *et al.* (1990b) Anatomic distribution of acquired melanocytic nevi in white children. A comparison with melanoma: the

Vancouver Mole Study. *Archives of Dermatology*, **126**, 466–471.

Gallagher, R.P., Rivers, J.K., Yang, P.C., McLean, D.I., Coldman, A.J. & Silver, H.K.B. (1991) Melanocytic nevus density in Asian, Indo-Pakistani, and white children: the Vancouver Mole Study. *Journal of the American Academy of Dermatology*, **25**, 507–512.

Garbe, C., Buttner, P., Weib, J., Soyer, H.P., Stocker, U., Krüger, S. *et al.* (1994) Associated factors in the prevalence of more than 50 common melanocytic nevi, atypical melanocytic nevi, and actinic lentigines: multicenter case-control study of the central malignant melanoma registry of the German dermatological society. *Journal of Investigative Dermatology*, **102**, 700–705.

Green, A. & Swerdlow, V. (1989) Epidemiology of melanocytic nevi. *Epidemiologic Reviews*, **11**, 204–221.

Green, A., Siskind, U., Hansen, M.E., Hansen, L. & Leech, P. (1989) Melanocytic nevi in school children in Queensland. *Journal of the American Academy of Dermatology*, **20**, 1054–1060.

Grob, J.J., Gouvernet, J., Aymar, D. *et al.* (1990) Count of benign melanocytic nevi as a major indicator of risk for non-familial nodular and superficial spreading and nodular melanoma. *Cancer*, **66**, 387–395.

Harrisson, S.L., McLennan, R., Speare, R. & Wronski, I. (1994) Sun exposure and melanocytic naevi in young Australian children. *Lancet*, **344**, 1529–1532.

Harth, Y., Friedman-Birnbaum, R. & Linn, S. (1992) Influence of cumulative sun exposure on the prevalence of common acquired nevi. *Journal of the American Academy of Dermatology*, **27**, 21–24.

Holman, C.D. & Armstrong, B.K. (1984) Pigmentary traits, ethnic origin, benign nevi, and family history as risk factors for cutaneous malignant melanoma. *Journal of the National Cancer Institute*, **72**, 257–266.

Kelly, J.W., Rivers, J.K., MacLennan, R., Harrison, S., Lewis, A.E. & Tate, B.J. (1994) Sunlight: a major factor associated with the development of melanocytic nevi in Australian schoolchildren. *Journal of the American Academy of Dermatology*, **30**, 40–48.

Kopf, A.W., Lazar, M., Bart, R.S., Dubin, N. & Bromberg, J. (1978) Prevalence of nevocytic nevi on lateral and medial aspects of arms. *Journal of Dermatology, Surgery and Oncology*, **4**, 153–158,

Kopf, A.W., Linsday, A.C., Rogers, G.S., Friedman, R.J., Rigel, D.S. & Levenstein, M. (1985) Relationship of nevocytic nevi to sun exposure in dysplastic nevus syndrome. *Journal of the American Academy of Dermatology*, **12**, 656–662.

Kopf, A.W., Gold, R.S. & Rogers, G.S. (1986) Relationship of lumbosacral naevocytic naevi to sun exposure in dysplastic naevus syndrome. *Journal of Dermatology*, **122**, 1003–1006.

Nicholls, E.M. (1968) Susceptibility and somatic mutation in the production of freckles, birthmarks and moles. *Lancet*, **i**, 71–73.

Pack, G.T., Davis, J. & Oppenheim, A. (1963) The relation of race and complexion to the incidence of moles and melanoma. *Annals of the New York Academy of Science*, **100**, 719–742.

Pope, D.J., Sorahan, T., Marsden, J.R., Ball, P.M., Grimley, R.P. & Peck, I.M. (1992) Benign pigmented nevi in children. *Archives of Dermatology*, **128**, 1201–1206.

Rampen, F.H.J. & Fleuren, B.A.M. (1987) Relation between phenotype and banal melanocytic nevi. *British Medical Journal*, **294**, 773.

Rampen, F.H.J., Van der Meer, H.L.M. & Boezeman, J.B.M. (1986) Frequency of moles as a key to melanoma incidence. *Journal of the American Academy of Dermatology*, **13**, 1200–1203.

Roudil, F., Grob, J.J., Gouvernet, J., Richard, M.A., Basseres, N. & Bonerandi, J.J. (1995) Influence on sun exposure after childhood on the development of nevi. *European Journal of Dermatology*, **5**, 477–480.

Richard, M.A., Grob, J.J., Gouvernet, J. *et al.* (1993) Role of sun exposure on nevus. First study in age–sex–phenotype controlled populations. *Archives of Dermatology*, **129**, 1280–1285.

Sigg, C. & Pelloni, F. (1989) Frequency of acquired melanonevocytic nevi and their relationship to skin complexion in 939 schoolchildren. *Dermatologica*, **179**, 123–128.

The Atypical Naevus Syndrome: Towards a Better Definition of the Melanoma-Associated Phenotype

M. PIEPKORN

Introduction

The clinical assessment of risk for melanoma could potentially be founded on genotypic or phenotypic markers, or a combination thereof. Whereas the development of reliable genotypic markers is certainly the ultimate objective because of their theoretical precision, the clinical assessment of melanoma risk is presently limited to phenotypic markers, supplemented by information from the patients' families and personal medical histories. Currently available phenotypic indicators include Fitzpatrick's cutaneous phototype, the global characteristics of the melanocytic naevus (mole) trait as assessed by clinical criteria, and the putative melanoma precursor lesion, the dysplastic naevus (now more commonly referred to as 'naevus with architectural disorder and melanocytic atypia'). The latter is a candidate risk marker that is primarily defined by histological criteria. Among the clinical indicators, the naevus phenotype has been most closely linked to melanoma susceptibility by empirical data ranging from clinical observations to epidemiological evidence. The naevus phenotype is represented by the total number of naevi, number of large (>5 mm) naevi and the extent to which the lesions display atypical features of shape and colour heterogeneity.

Reports documenting the association between the occurrence of melanoma and an atypical naevus trait date back to the early nineteenth century (Norris, 1820). In more recent times, periodic references to the phenomenon have appeared in the literature (Cawley, 1952; Lynch & Krush, 1968; Anderson, 1971). It remained until the latter part of the 1970s, however, before significant interest came to be focused on that association (Frichot *et al.*, 1977; Lynch *et al.*, 1978), much of the credit for which can be given to W.H. Clark and co-workers (Clark *et al.*, 1978, 1984; Reimer *et al.*, 1978; Elder *et al.*, 1980; Greene *et al.*, 1985). The correlation between an atypical naevus trait (increased number and/or sizes of naevi, at least some of which have irregularity of shape and colour) and increased risk for melanoma is one component of the evidence that has been advanced to support the notion that melanocytic naevi are a stage in the development of melanoma (Clark *et al.*, 1984). It is clear from clinical observations, however, that the strength of the correlation varies substantially between melanoma-prone kindreds. This variability of association suggests that melanoma susceptibility and the atypical mole phenotype reflect underlying genetic heterogeneity, i.e. they are the con-sequences of multiple interacting genes. The relevant epidemiological evidence linking the naevus phenotype to melanoma risk is reviewed here with a description of the quantitative characteristics of the association, addressing the limitations in its use for melanoma risk assessment. The importance of developing genetic markers for predisposition to melanoma will accordingly be evident.

Epidemiology of the atypical naevus trait

Pedigrees of melanoma-prone kindreds often exhibit strong concordance between an atypical naevus trait and personal history of melanoma (Greene *et al.*, 1985; Bale *et al.*, 1989). Repeated descriptions of naevus characteristics in such kindreds have suggested autosomal dominant Mendelian inheritance with incomplete penetrance, as inferred from observations of vertical and male-to-male transmission and from an estimated transmission probability of *c.* 50% in the pedigrees (Clark *et al.*, 1978; Lynch *et al.*, 1978; Reimer *et al.*, 1978; Greene *et al.*, 1985; Bale *et al.*, 1989). Major gene effects have also been evident in segregation and pedigree analyses of quantitative naevus traits, such as total naevus number and total density of naevi (Goldgar *et al.*, 1991, 1992; Meyer *et al.*, 1992), and by the observation of strong concordance for total number of naevi between monozygotic, but not dizygotic, twins (Easton *et al.*, 1991).

Outside the setting of familial melanoma, the correlations in instances of sporadic melanoma have been quantified in a number of investigations employing case-control study design (Table 10.1) (Swerdlow *et al.*, 1984, 1986; Nordlund *et al.*, 1985; Holly *et al.*, 1987; Grob *et al.*, 1988, 1990; Roush *et al.*, 1988; Titus-Ernstoff *et al.*, 1988; Augustsson *et al.*, 1990; Halpern *et al.*, 1991; Kruger *et al.*, 1992; Garbe *et al.*, 1994; Rieger *et al.*, 1995). These studies generally confirm the intuitive notion that large numbers of naevi correlate with melanoma risk and specifically establish in a quantitative manner that there is a positive linear relationship between quantitative aspects of the phenotype and relative risk for the cancer (Table 10.1; Fig. 10.3). While each referenced study illustrates the correlation, appreciable differences are nonetheless apparent between them with respect to the risk magnitude at varying quantitative levels of expression of the multiple naevus trait. These differences could reflect variations in study design, but most probably signify effects of heterogeneity in the gene pools and from covariate environmental factors in the respective underlying patient populations. Despite this variability, the basic positive correlation has remained consistent across all studies.

The continuous or quantitative nature of the naevus phenotype is reflected in the case-control literature (Table 10.1; Fig. 10.3,) outlined above. This characteristic obviously limits its utility as a melanoma risk indicator in medical practice because of constraints introduced at several levels in any clinical algorithm derived from the relationship. Among these are setting of a minimum diagnostic threshold and assignment of risk in a dichotomous or stratified fashion. Moreover, only about one-third (34%) of unselected patients with a history of melanoma have an atypical phenotype, defined at a minimal threshold as the presence of one or more atypical naevi > 5 mm in diameter; the frequency for comparison in control subjects is *c.* 12% (Fig. 10.4) (Nordlund *et al.*, 1985; Swerdlow *et al.*, 1986; Holly *et al.*, 1987; Grob *et al.*, 1988; Roush *et al.*, 1988; Augustsson *et al.*, 1990; Garbe *et al.*, 1994). Therefore, the sensitivity and specificity of the phenotype as a melanoma risk indicator are substantially restricted. Due in part to these constraints, as well as to the efforts of Clark and associates, attention came to be focused on the dysplastic naevus.

The dysplastic naevus

The concept of the dysplastic naevus was a central tenet in studies of familial melanoma during the 1980s, but by the end of that decade it had generated

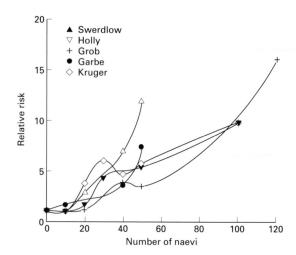

Fig. 10.3 The correlation between naevus phenotype and relative risk for melanoma. This chart, assembled from the indicated sources, illustrates the positive relationship between relative risk for melanoma and numbers of naevi, which is one component of the atypical naevus phenotype.

substantial controversy (National Institutes of Health, 1992). The specific hypotheses developed by Clark from studies of melanocytic naevi were twofold, namely that the dysplastic naevus is both an indicator of risk for melanoma and a formal precursor lesion to that malignancy (Clark *et al.*, 1984). Clinical and investigative attention directed at the dysplastic naevus had the effect of shifting emphasis away from quantitative attributes of the clinical naevus phenotype and toward a constellation of histological criteria that were proposed to indicate genetically increased risk for melanoma (Clark *et al.*, 1984).

The controversy surrounding the dysplastic naevus derives, in part, from the circular nature of the process by which the lesion was described and from insufficient histological controls in the studies that originally described the lesion. In those reports, biopsy specimens were in most instances obtained from large, clinically atypical naevi in subjects with an abnormal naevus phenotype and not from clinically banal naevi or from persons without atypical appearing naevi (Elder *et al.*, 1980; Clark *et al.*, 1984; Greene *et al.*, 1985). This histological examination often disclosed dysplasia, which thus came to be linked with the clinical trait of large, atypical naevi (Elder *et al.*, 1980; Clark *et al.*,

Table 10.1 Case-control studies. Relative risk rates for melanoma according to numbers of naevi*.

| | Naevi (*n*) | | | |
Reference	10–25	25–50	>50	>100
Holly *et al.* (1987)	1.6	4.4	5.4	9.8
Swerdlow *et al.* (1986)	6.7	11	54	
Grob *et al.* (1990)	1.2	3.8		16
Garbe *et al.* (1994)	1.7	3.7	3.7	7.6
Kruger *et al.* (1992)	3.8	6.1		
Average	3	5.8	4.5	11

* The relative risk rates for melanoma are listed for numbers of naevi, according to the indicated pooled intervals, as taken from each of these representative case-control studies and as group averages.

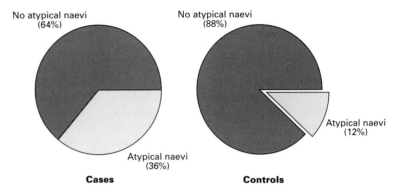

Fig. 10.4 Fraction of melanoma cases and controls with atypical naevi. For this illustration, the definition of affected phenotype is based on the presence of one or more naevi that are ≥5 mm in diameter and that exhibit qualitatively atypical characteristics (see text).

1984; Greene *et al.*, 1985). Essentially, the diagnostic process evolved in a circular fashion, without relevant control biopsy evaluations of clinically banal naevi and of naevi from the general population (Elder *et al.*, 1980). In order to establish that the dysplastic naevus is reasonably predictive of an abnormal genotype, specificity for large atypical naevi and low population prevalence are necessary. The studies of dysplasia did not control for its population prevalence (Elder *et al.*, 1980; Clark *et al.*, 1984; Greene *et al.*, 1985), which is pertinent because subsequent studies by independent groups have indicated histological dysplasia to be common in clinically banal naevi (Grob *et al.*, 1988; Meyer *et al.*, 1988; Curley *et al.*, 1989; Piepkorn *et al.*, 1989, 1990; Cook & Fallowfield, 1990; Klein & Barr, 1990). The dysplastic naevus would lack specificity as an indicator of the melanoma-prone person if it is common in clinically banal naevi and prevalent in the general population. Similar limitations would follow from marginal interobserver variability in applying the histological criteria.

Interobserver concordance rates in the diagnosis of histological dysplasia have been purported to be reasonable (Rhodes *et al.*, 1989). In an attempt to corroborate this assertion, studies from the University of Utah evaluated the population prevalence of dysplasia and the inter-observer reliability in its diagnosis. A panel of five independent experts skilled in the diagnosis of pigmented lesions was assembled to review a set of histological slides from the Utah population-based data set (Piepkorn *et al.*, 1994). In contrast to the design of other studies (Rhodes *et al.*, 1989), there was no advance agreement on criteria. Whereas intra-observer concordance was reasonable, reproduci-

bility between observers averaged only 56% in this multiobserver study (Piepkorn *et al.*, 1994), indicating significant imprecision in applying the diagnostic criteria.

The pathologist panel evaluated one naevus per subject from a set of population controls, where the choice of naevi for microscopic examination was assigned by computer randomization (Piepkorn *et al.*, 1994). The prevalence estimate for the dysplastic naevus ranged from 7 to 32% between the observers. Regardless of the stringency of criteria, the frequency of dysplasia would thus have been quite high in this population-based sample if all naevi from each subject had been examined microscopically. This result corroborates earlier findings from the Utah data set (Meyer *et al.*, 1988; Piepkorn *et al.*, 1989; Piepkorn, 1990) and the studies of others (Grob *et al.*, 1988; Curley *et al.*, 1989; Cooke & Fallowfield, 1990; Klein & Barr, 1990). The predictive value of histological criteria would therefore be low in the clinical assessment of melanoma risk if, as indicated in these studies, dysplasia is common in banal naevi from the general population. Attention should thus be directed once again to the global clinical phenotype.

Quantitative characteristics of the naevus phenotype

Algorithms have been devised by investigators in order to clinically stratify melanoma risk along the multiple naevus phenotype continuum. For example, Newton *et al.* (1993) defined the AMS (atypical mole syndrome) scoring system. In this model, weighted scores were applied for several different attributes, including two or more naevi > 5 mm in diameter, over one hundred naevi 2 mm in diameter, naevi in the anterior scalp and pigmented lesions of the iris. These categorical values were then summed to give a global numerical rating for expression of the trait. By this measure, > 50% of familial melanoma cases had the AMS phenotype according to the threshold that was chosen, followed in decreasing frequency by first-degree relatives in melanoma kindreds, sporadic cases of melanoma and population controls. Because of the continuous (quantitative) nature of the trait, however, the setting of any diagnostic threshold at the lower end of the spectrum will limit specificity of the criteria, and sensitivity will be constrained by the setting of more stringent criteria at the opposite end.

The melanoma-associated trait was quantified in the population-based data set at the University of Utah (Goldgar *et al.*, 1991, 1992; Meyer *et al.*, 1992). The study population comprised 533 subjects, including controls (*n* = 204), probands ascertained on the basis of familial (*n* = 23) and sporadic melanoma (*n* = 33), and family members of the probands. The analyses focused on two quantitative parameters related to the naevus phenotype. These were total number of naevi and a derived parameter, total naevus density, which was calculated as the total area of naevi $\times 10^4$ divided by the total body surface area; the latter measure thus incorporates the effects of both number and size of naevi. Melanoma cases manifested increased mean values for both measures, compared with spouse and random digit dial controls from the population. The effect was strongest in individuals who were members of melanoma-prone families. Mean total number of naevi ± S.D. was 86 ± 44 for familial cases, 42 ± 34 for sporadic cases and 26 ± 23 for controls ($P < 0.0001$ and $P = 0.028$ for the comparison of the former two values, respectively, with controls). Mean total naevus densities for the three groups were, respectively, 192 ± 148, 116 ± 114 and 56 ± 55 ($P < 0.0001$ and $P = 0.011$). The frequency distributions of total naevus densities for the three groups were skewed and broadly overlapped. Relatives of the probands from the multiple melanoma kindreds exhibited a statistically significant increase in both quantitative traits, which increased with increasing degree of kinship to the probands. Pedigree analyses were consistent with the effects of a segregating major gene on the naevus pheno-type (Goldgar *et al.*, 1991, 1992; Meyer *et al.*, 1992).

A locus for melanoma susceptibility on chromosome 9p

The dysplastic naevus assumed a major role in the initial search for melanoma susceptibility loci in the human genome (Greene *et al.*, 1985; Bale *et al.*, 1989). In studies using genetic linkage analysis, the diagnosis of dysplastic naevi on research subjects was taken as sufficient evidence for an abnormal genotype, i.e. for the existence of an inherited mutation at a critical genetic locus that confers susceptibility to melanoma. Because the presence of one or more dysplastic naevi, identified by either clinical or histological criteria, was used to assign gene carrier status for melanoma, the dysplastic naevus thus came to be exploited experimentally as a major phenotypic indicator of an abnormal genotype (Bale *et al.*, 1989). By these means, the study of Bale *et al.* (1989) linked the affected naevus phenotype to the effects of a major locus, which they assigned to the short arm of chromosome 1 by co-segregation with polymorphic genetic probes. This result was notable because it was the first indication of the genomic location of a melanoma susceptibility locus. Unfortunately, multiple attempts by independent investigators to confirm assignment of a melanoma locus to that position in melanoma-prone kindreds have been unsuccessful (reviewed by Piepkorn, 1994).

Subsequently, genomic mapping strategies were exploited by other investigators in order to determine the regions of DNA most commonly deleted in melanoma cell lines (Fountain *et al.*, 1992), under the premise that a tumour suppressor locus important to the development of that cancer should be frequently and non-randomly deleted in the tumour-cell clones. This experimental approach determined that markers for a region on the short arm of chromosome 9 were more commonly deleted than were the other markers that were analysed, strongly pointing to the presence of a major melanoma susceptibility locus mapping to that region (Fountain *et al.*, 1992). The significance of a chromosomal 9p locus in melanoma development was further established by genetic linkage analyses conducted at the University of Utah (Cannon-Albright *et al.*, 1992). Multipoint linkage placed the locus, which has been designated MLM, near the tested 9p markers at band 21–22,with strong statistical significance. Independent corroboration of linkage was first reported in Australian melanoma kindreds, and others have followed (reviewed by Piepkorn, 1994). Collectively, the assignment to chromosome 9p of a major locus for melanoma susceptibility is firmly supported.

The mapping of the chromosome 9p gene provided opportunities to assess the phenotypic effects of the melanoma susceptibility gene (Cannon-Albright *et al.*, 1994). The penetrance of the disease-conferring allele and its effects on the naevus phenotype were evaluated by measuring the quantitative traits described above in subjects from three Utah melanoma kindreds in which mutations at the candidate chromosome 9p melanoma susceptibility locus were known to be segregating (Cannon-Albright *et al.*, 1994). For this analysis, affected individuals were identified by a common haplotype of contiguous restriction fragment-length polymorphisms closely linked to the susceptibility locus. In some of those families, an effect of the disease allele on naevus phenotype was evident. The mean number of naevi in affected individuals from such families was 53, compared with 32 in non-carrier control subjects. Moreover, naevus densities were nearly twice as high in gene carriers compared with the controls. The 9p familial melanoma susceptibility locus, therefore, is partly responsible in some families for quantitative aspects of the naevus phenotype, but a polygenic basis for the trait is suggested by the absence of overt effects of the 9p disease allele in other melanoma kindreds. The penetrance of the locus for melanoma development in those persons carrying a mutant allele is estimated to increase 1% per year over the age of 20 years, such that there is a 30% risk of melanoma by the age of 30 years and a *c.* 60% risk by the age of 80 years. These observations suggest that mutations at the chromosome 9p locus are associated with increased numbers of naevi and that interactions with other loci or with environmental factors are necessary for acquisition of the malignant phenotype, which ultimately occurs in most of those who inherit an abnormal allele.

Prospects for molecular diagnosis

The cloning and nucleotide sequencing of the region on chromosome 9p that is most frequently deleted in melanoma cells eventually led to the identification of the gene for p16, which is a 16 kDa protein that negatively regulates (controls) cell-cycle progression; subsequent mutational analyses have now established the gene to be a strong candidate for the principal familial melanoma susceptibility locus (reviewed by Piepkorn, 1994). These recent advances may eventually lead to effective screening tests for identifying persons at increased melanoma risk. The use of genetic markers, however, is restricted to those with germline mutations in all somatic cells, including the peripheral blood mononuclear cells that would be tested. Moreover, it is likely that there is genetic heterogeneity for melanoma susceptibility, despite the apparently prominent role of the chromosome 9p locus, in that other loci may contribute to the predisposition in some families. The testing of all relevant loci would be required in the design of a comprehensive screening strategy with genetic markers; any such loci not yet discovered will contribute to the risk of false negativity in the testing process. Allelic heterogeneity, defined as the existence of multiple versions of the mutant allele, further complicates screening because effective probes should recognize each mutant version of the disease-associated gene. For these reasons, the prospects for reliable genetic screening are not imminent, but nevertheless hold promise.

Thoughts on the nature of melanocytic naevi

Melanocytic naevi are customarily considered to be precursor lesions in the progression of melanocytes to melanoma cells (Clark *et al.*, 1984). The intuitive appeal of this long-held view follows partly from the correlations between the naevus phenotype and melanoma susceptibility discussed above and from the observation that histological sections of melanomas often contain remnants of naevus tissue. Other empirical observations, however, are not clearly consistent with that model. These include the findings that naevus-cell populations exhibit a low fraction of cycling cells, are quite difficult to cultivate *in vitro*, have normal karyotypes (Cowan *et al.*, 1988) and have not been observed to undergo transformation to melanoma in experimental model systems, for example, in human naevus xenografts on athymic mice or by stimulation with ultraviolet radiation (Meyer *et al.*, 1995). Alternative hypotheses regarding the nature of naevi are necessary. The lesions may not in fact be proximal lesional stages in melanoma development, but rather may reflect an alternative pathway of cellular development. Much of the empirical database can be accommodated by postulating that naevi and melanoma are pleiotropic effects of a common stimulus or origin. One plausible hypothesis is that melanocytic naevi are populations of apoptocytes, acting to divert an altered melanocytic clone down a pathway of terminal differentiation and away from the malignant phenotype. According to this model, evolutionary processes have selected for naevi as a host defence mechanism against transformation into a specific form of cancer.

Conclusions and prospects

Present and past observations, in summary, have established qualitative and quantitative correlations between the naevus phenotype and susceptibility to melanoma. The relationship is continuously variable by its nature, such that life-long relative risk for melanoma is substantial in those with extreme expression of the atypical naevus trait. Such individuals, however, are uncommon among unselected, incident cases of melanoma, of whom less than one-half will be clinically distinguishable by an atypical naevus phenotype. The low sensitivity of the naevus phenotype as a diagnostic marker of those with a predisposition for melanoma underscores the importance of developing molecular probes for melanoma susceptibility genes. Genetic markers will, it is hoped, ultimately permit risk assignment in a more precise fashion, enabling physicians to identify persons in melanoma kindreds who are most at risk for melanoma and who thus would be most likely to benefit from careful prospective surveillance.

References

Anderson, D.E. (1971) Clinical characteristics of the genetic variety of cutaneous melanoma in man. *Cancer*, **28**, 721–725.

Augustsson, A., Stierner, U., Rosdahl, I. & Suurkula, M. (1990) Melanocytic naevi in sun-exposed and protected skin in melanoma patients and controls. *Acta Dermato-Venereologica*, **71**, 512–517.

Bale, S.J., Dracopoli, N.C., Tucker, M.A. *et al.* (1989) Mapping the gene for hereditary cutaneous malignant melanoma–dysplastic nevus to chromosome 1p. *New England Journal of Medicine*, **320**, 1367–1372.

Cannon-Albright, L.A., Goldgar, D.E., Meyer, L.J. *et al.* (1992) Assignment of a locus for familial melanoma, MLM, to chromosome 9p13–p22. *Science*, **258**, 1148–1151.

Cannon-Albright, L.A., Meyer, L.J., Lewis, C.M. *et al.* (1994) Penetrance and expressivity of the chromosome 9p melanoma susceptibility locus. *Cancer Research*, **54**, 6041–6044.

Cawley, E.P. (1952) Genetic aspects of malignant melanoma. *Archives of Dermatology and Syphilis*, **65**, 440–450.

Clark, W.H. Jr, Reimer, R.R., Greene, M. *et al.* (1978) Origin of familial malignant melanoma from heritable melanocytic lesions: 'The B-K mole syndrome'. *Archives of Dermatology*, **114**, 732–738.

Clark, W.J. Jr, Elder, D.E., Guerry, D. IV *et al.* (1984) A study of tumor progression: the precursor lesions of superficial spreading and nodular melanoma. *Human Pathology*, **15**, 1147–1165.

Cook, M.G. & Fallowfield, M.E. (1990) Dysplastic naevi—an alternative view. *Histopathology*, **16**, 29–35.

Cowan, J.M., Halaban, R. & Francke, U. (1988) Cytogenetic analysis of melanocytes from premalignant naevi and melanomas. *Journal of the National Cancer Institute*, **80**, 1159–1164.

Curley, R.K., Cook, M.G., Fallowfield, M.E. & Marsden, R.A. (1989) Accuracy in clinically evaluating pigmented lesions. *British Medical Journal*, **299**, 16–18.

Easton, D.F., Cox, G.M., Macdonald, A.M. & Ponder, B.A.J. (1991) Genetic susceptibility to naevi: A twin study. *British Journal of Cancer*, **64**, 1164–1167.

Elder, D.E., Goldman, L.I., Goldman, S.C. *et al.* (1980) Dysplastic nevus syndrome: A phenotypic association of sporadic cutaneous melanoma. *Cancer*, **46**, 1787–1794.

Fountain, J.W., Karayiorgou, M., Ernstoff, M.S. *et al.* (1992) Homozygous deletions within human chromosome band 9p21 in melanoma. *Proceedings of the National Academy of Science USA*, **89**, 10557–10561.

Frichot, B.C. III, Lynch, H.T., Guirgis, H.A. *et al.* (1977) New cutaneous phenotype in familial malignant melanoma. *Lancet*, **i**, 864–865.

Garbe, C., Buttner, P., Weiss, J. *et al.* (1994) Risk factors for developing cutaneous melanoma and criteria for identifying persons at risk: multicenter case-control study of the central malignant melanoma registry of the German Dermatological Society. *Journal of Investigative Dermatology*,

102, 695–699.

Goldgar, D.E., Cannon-Albright, L.A., Meyer, L.J. *et al.* (1991) Inheritance of naevus number and size in melanoma and dysplastic nevus syndrome kindreds. *Journal of the National Cancer Institute*, **83**, 1726–1733.

Goldgar, D.E., Cannon-Albright, L.A., Meyer, L.J. *et al.* (1992) Inheritance of nevus number and size in melanoma DNS kindreds. *Cytogenetics and Cell Genetics*, **59**, 200–202.

Greene, M.H., Clark, W.H. Jr, Tucker, M.A. *et al.* (1985) High risk of malignant melanoma in melanoma-prone families with dysplastic nevi. *Annals of Internal Medicine*, **102**, 458–465.

Grob, J.J., Andrac, L., Romano, M.H. *et al.* (1988) Dysplastic nevus in non-familial melanoma: a clinico-pathologic study of 101 cases. *British Journal of Dermatology*, **118**, 745–752.

Grob, J.J., Gouvernet, J., Aymar, D. *et al.* (1990) Count of benign melanocytic nevi as a major indicator of risk for nonfamilial nodular and superficial spreading melanoma. *Cancer*, **66**, 387–395.

Halpern, A.C., Guerry, D. IV, Elder, D.E. *et al.* (1991) Dysplastic nevi as risk markers of sporadic (non-familial) melanoma: a case-control study. *Archives of Dermatology*, **127**, 995–999.

Holly, E.A., Kelly, J.W., Shpall, S.N. & Chiu, S.-H. (1987) Number of melanocytic nevi as a major risk factor for malignant melanoma. *Journal of the American Academy of Dermatology*, **17**, 459–468.

Klein, L.J. & Barr, R.J. (1990) Histological atypia in clinically benign nevi: A prospective study. *Journal of the American Academy of Dermatology*, **22**, 275–282.

Kruger, S., Garbe, C., Buttner, P. *et al.* (1992) Epidemiologic evidence for the role of melanocytic nevi as risk markers and direct precursors of cutaneous malignant melanoma. *Journal of the American Academy of Dermatology*, **26**, 920–926.

Lynch, H.T. & Krush, A.J. (1968) Heredity and malignant melanoma: implications for early cancer detection. *Canadian Medical Association Journal*, **99**, 17–21.

Lynch, H.T., Frichot, B.C. & Lynch, J.F. (1978) Familial atypical multiple mole–melanoma syndrome. *Journal of Medical Genetics*, **15**, 352–356.

Meyer, L.J., Piepkorn, M.W., Seuchter, S.A. *et al.* (1988) Genetic and epidemiological evaluation of dysplastic nevi. *Pigment Cell Research*, **1**(Suppl.), 144–151.

Meyer, L.J., Goldgar, D.E., Cannon-Albright, L.A. *et al.* (1992) Number, size, and histopathology of nevi in Utah kindreds. *Cytogenetics and Cell Genetics*, **59**, 167–169.

Meyer, L.J., Schmidt, L.A., Goldgar, D.E. & Piepkorn, M.W. (1995) Survival and histopathologic characteristics of human melanocytic nevi transplanted to athymic (nude) mice. *American Journal of Dermatopathology*, **17**, 368–373.

National Institutes of Health Consensus Conference: Diagnosis and Treatment of Early Melanoma (1992) *Journal of the American Medical Association*, **268**, 1314–1319.

Newton, J.A., Bataille, V., Griffiths, K. *et al.* (1993) How common is the atypical mole syndrome phenotype in apparently sporadic melanoma? *Journal of the American Academy of Dermatology*, **29**, 989–996.

Nordlund, J.J., Kirkwood, J., Forget, B.M. *et al.* (1985) Demographic study of clinically atypical (dysplastic) nevi in patients with melanoma and comparison subjects. *Cancer Research*, **45**, 1855–1861.

Norris, W. (1820) Case of fungoid disease. *Edinburgh Medical and Surgical Journal*, **16**, 562–565.

Piepkorn, M. (1990) A hypothesis incorporating the histologic characteristics of dysplastic nevi into the normal biological development of melanocytic nevi. *Archives of Dermatology*, **126**, 514–518.

Piepkorn, M.W. (1994) Genetic basis of susceptibility to melanoma. *Journal of the American Academy of Dermatology*, **31**, 1022–1039.

Piepkorn, M., Meyer, L.J., Goldgar, D. *et al.* (1989) The dysplastic melanocytic nevus: A prevalent lesion that correlates poorly with clinical phenotype. *Journal of the American Academy of Dermatology*, **20**, 407–415.

Piepkorn, M.W., Barnhill, R.L., Cannon-Albright, L.A. *et al.* (1994) A multi-observer, population-based analysis of histologic dysplasia in melanocytic nevi. *Journal of the American Academy of Dermatology*, **30**, 707–714.

Rieger, E., Soyer, H.P., Garbe, C. *et al.* (1995) Overall and site-specific risk of malignant melanoma associated with nevus counts at different body sites: a multicenter case-control study of the German Central Malignant-Melanoma Registry. *International Journal of Cancer*, **62**, 393–397.

Reimer, R.R., Clark, W.H. Jr, Greene, M.H. *et al.* (1978) Precursor lesions in familial melanoma. A new genetic preneoplastic syndrome. *Journal of the American Medical Association*, **239**, 744–746.

Rhodes, A.R., Mihm, M.C. Jr & Weinstock, M.A. (1989) Dysplastic melanocytic nevi: A reproducible histologic definition emphasizing cellular morphology. *Modern Pathology*, **2**, 306–319.

Roush, G.C., Nordlund, J.J., Forget, B. *et al.* (1988) Independence of dysplastic nevi from total nevi in determining risk for nonfamilial melanoma. *Preventive Medicine*, **17**: 273–279.

Swerdlow, A.J., English, J., MacKie, R.M. *et al.* (1984) Benign naevi associated with high risk of melanoma. *Lancet*, **ii**, 168.

Swerdlow, A.J., English, J., MacKie, R.M. *et al.* (1986) Benign melanocytic naevi as a risk factor for malignant melanoma. *British Medical Journal*, **292**, 1555–1559.

Titus-Ernstoff, L., Duray, P.H., Ernstoff, M.S. *et al.* (1988) Dysplastic nevi in association with multiple primary melanoma. *Cancer Research*, **48**, 1016–1018.

Melanocytic Naevi as Risk Markers for Melanoma

R.M. MACKIE

Melanocytic naevi can be considered as potential precursors to malignant melanoma or as markers of an individual at increased risk of developing malignant melanoma on another site on the skin.

Melanocytic naevi as potential precursors to melanoma

Studies in the literature suggest that between 30 and 50% of all cutaneous malignant melanomas appear to have arisen on a pre-existing acquired naevus. These statements are usually made on the combination of a positive history of a preceding naevus and/or evidence of naevus cells on the excision specimen.

A recent study carried out by Skender-Kalnenas *et al.* (1995) in Perth, Western Australia, looked at 289 cases of cutaneous malignant melanoma measuring <1mm in thickness. They found on the basis of a pathological study that a naevus was associated with the melanoma in 147 (51%) of cases. Sixty-one (41%) of these were associated with common acquired naevi, 82 (56%) with so-called dysplastic or atypical naevi and four (3%) with congenital naevi. In addition, this study suggested that lentiginous melanocytic proliferation was present adjacent to the melanoma in 75% of cases overall, and in 97 (44%) of these a co-existing naevus was also present.

The problem with this kind of study is the impossibility of determining whether or not lentiginous proliferation precedes or follows the development of a malignancy. Provided the cytological criteria for differentiating naevus cells from melanoma cells are reasonably strong, one can assume that a naevus may proceed a melanoma, but the situation with regard to melanocytic proliferation in the basal layer is less clear-cut. Studies such as this, while interesting, do depend on very consistent pathological criteria for distinguishing between melanoma cells and naevus cells. What is needed at the present time are antibodies which will help this task.

This study does, however, confirm the work of others, suggesting that looking at thin relatively early melanomas one can assume that a fairly high percentage may have arisen on the basis of a pre-existing naevus. Thus this may validate the concept of tumour progression. However it must be remembered that the average young European adult has 20–40 benign acquired naevi, and at present the incidence of melanoma is around 10 new cases per 100 000 of the population per year. This emphasizes the fact that the vast majority of benign acquired naevi are not precursors to malignant melanoma.

Congenital naevi are often of concern with regard to malignant change. They are arbitrarily divided into giant, intermediate and small lesions based either on largest diameter or surface area. Studies on giant congenital naevi suggest that the incidence of malignant change over a lifetime is around 6% (Lorentzen *et al.*, 1977), but also emphasize the fact that the malignant change may take place in tissue deep to the skin itself in the central nervous system. Current practice with large congenital naevi is to remove as much as possible of the naevus tissue as early as possible in life, but it must be realized because of the problem of deep nests of naevus cells that this will not entirely remove the risk of malignant change.

Studies of small congenital naevi do suggest that the risk of malignant change is present but this has not been accurately quantitated. In a study carried out in the West of Scotland (MacKie *et al.*, 1991), around 40% of young adults who developed melanoma before the age of 30 years had a history of a congenital or early onset naevus at the site of malignant change and the majority of these clinical histories were verified by pathological examination and observation of the presence of naevus cells. There are no data, at the present time, on the risk of malignant change in intermediate-sized congenital naevi.

Blue naevi can also undergo malignant change but this appears to be excessively rare. However, the author does have personal experience of malignant change supervening on a blue naevus of the naevus of Ota type.

Spitz naevi are a particularly important problem in terms of pathological differential diagnosis. The majority of Spitz naevi occur in children and young adults and a great majority appear to be benign lesions. However, there is a Spitzoid variant (Smith *et al.*, 1989) of malignant melanoma which may be very difficult to differentiate on pathological grounds. It is not yet understood whether or not the Spitzoid melanoma is a progressor lesion from a benign Spitz naevus or whether it arises *ab initio* as a malignancy.

In the past few years there have been a number of case reports of malignant melanoma developing in a naevus spilus (Wagner & Cottel, 1989; Rhodes & Mihm, 1990). The exact frequency with which this event takes place is not yet established, but it underlines the point that patients with naevus spilus should be regarded as an at risk group.

Naevi as markers of melanoma risk

In addition to the above concern about naevi as progressor lesions, studies from the UK (MacKie *et al.*, 1989), North America (Holly *et al.*, 1987) and Germany (Garbe *et al.*, 1994) all confirm the fact that patients with large numbers of acquired naevi have a greater than average risk of developing malignant melanoma. The explanation for this is thought to be the fact that patients who have large numbers of naevi generally have a history of excessive sun exposure in earlier life, and that this in turn has predisposed to the development of malignant melanoma. This leads logically to the study of naevi and factors predisposing to their development. Well-controlled studies carried out in three geographically separate areas of Australia suggest that children aged ≤ 10 years develop larger numbers of naevi in high solar exposure areas (Rivers *et al.*, 1995). Thus the marker of large numbers of banal naevi as a major risk factor for melanoma elsewhere on the body appears to relate to past sun exposure, possibly particularly in childhood. The bulk of studies to date record the total number of any type of naevus, acquired banal, clinically atypical and congenital, as the most statistically significant risk factor. This is logical if one assumes that the risk relates to the relative increase in the total number of melanocytes, and that all melanocytes have the same potential for malignant change. In situations in which differing types of melanocytic naevi have been recorded separately, the greatest risk is associated in the majority of studies with large numbers of banal naevi. At present there are clear gaps in our knowledge concerning both the relative and the absolute risk of progression to melanoma of all types of naevi. This is clearly of major importance in terms of the decisions on the need to excise benign lesions.

References

Garbe, C., Buttner, P., Weiss, J. *et al.* (1994) Risk factors for developing cutaneous malignant melanoma. *Journal of Investigative Dermatology*, **102**, 695–699.

Holly, E.A., Kelly, J.W., Shpall, S.N. & Chiu, S.H. (1987) Number of melanocytic naevi as a major risk factor for malignant melanoma. *Journal of the American Academy of Dermatology*, **17**, 459–468.

Lorentzen, M., Pers, M. & Bretteville Jensen, G. (1977) The incidence of malignant transformation in giant pigmented naevi. *Scandinavian Journal of Plastic and Reconstructive Surgery*, **11**, 163–167.

MacKie, R.M., Freudenberger, T. & Aitchison, T. (1989) Personal risk factor chart for cutaneous melanoma. *Lancet*, **ii**, 487–490.

MacKie, R.M., Watt, D., Doherty, V. & Aitchison, T. (1991) Malignant melanoma occurring in those aged under 30 in the West of Scotland 1979–86. *British Journal of Dermatology*, **124**, 560–564.

Rhodes, A.R. & Mihm, M. (1990) Origin of cutaneous melanoma in a congenital dysplastic naevus spilus. *Archives of Dermatology*, **126**, 500–505.

Rivers, J.K., MacLennan, R., Kelly, J.W. *et al.* (1995) The Eastern Australian childhood nevus study: Prevalence of atypical nevi, congenital nevus-like nevi, and other pigmented lesions. *Journal of the American Academy of Dermatology*, **32**, 957–963.

Skender-Kalnenas, T.M., English, D.R. & Heenan, P. (1995) Benign melanocytic lesions: Risk markers or precursors of cutaneous melanoma? *Journal of the American Academy of Dermatology*, **33**, 1000–1007.

Smith, K.S., Barrett, T.L. Skelton, H.G., Lupton, G.P. & Graham, J.H. (1989) Spindle and epithelioid cell naevi within atypia and metastases—malignant Spitz naevus. *American Journal of Surgical Pathology*, **13**, 931–939.

Wagner, A.F. & Cottel, W.I. (1989) *In situ* melanoma developing in a speckled lentiginous naevus. *Journal of the American Academy of Dermatology*, **20**, 125–126.

Melanocytic Naevi as Precursors for Melanoma

C. GARBE

The relationship between the frequency of melanocytic naevi and risk for melanoma development has been extensively studied during the last decade (Rhodes, 1985; Swerdlow *et al.*, 1986; Garbe *et al.*, 1989; Grob *et al.*, 1990; Weiss *et al.*, 1990; Augustsson *et al.*, 1991b; Holly *et al.*, 1995). It was shown that with a high number of benign melanocytic naevi likewise the relative risk for developing malignant melanoma was increased (Østerlind *et al.*, 1988; MacKie *et al.*, 1989; Garbe & Orfanos, 1992; Garbe *et al.*, 1994). There was nearly a linear relationship between the number of melanocytic naevi and the risk of developing melanoma (Østerlind *et al.*, 1988; Garbe, 1995). Interestingly, the site distribution of melanocytic naevi closely matched that of malignant melanoma with most tumours arising at the trunk in males and at the lower extremity in females (Kelly *et al.*, 1989; Gallagher *et al.*, 1990a; Krüger *et al.*, 1992; Stierner *et al.*, 1992; Rieger *et al.*, 1995). These are also the anatomical locations with the most extensive sun exposure (Gallagher *et al.*, 1990b; Augustsson *et al.*, 1991a; Abadir *et al.*, 1995). Melanocytic naevi seem to be induced by intensive sun exposure in childhood and adolescence. The higher the prevalence of melanocytic naevi is in a population, the higher will be the incidence of melanoma (Rampen *et al.*, 1986; Garbe *et al.*, 1989). It seems to be that the main contribution of UV light to the development of melanoma is the induction of melanocytic naevi as precursor lesions of melanoma.

In addition, the presence of atypical or dysplastic melanocytic naevi contributes to an increased risk for melanoma development as observed in case-control studies (Holly *et al.*, 1987; Garbe *et al.*, 1989, 1994; Augustsson *et al.*, 1991b; MacKie, 1991). The relative risk for melanoma development in sporadic dysplastic naevus syndrome may be increased by a factor of 6–8 (MacKie *et al.*, 1989; Garbe *et al.*, 1994). Several investigators proposed a model of tumour progression in the human melanocytic system in which the melanocyte develops to a benign melanocytic naevus from which a dysplastic melanocytic naevus arises. From there a melanoma can develop over several steps of radial and vertical growth phases (Clark *et al.*, 1984; Kath *et al.*, 1989).

This model has not been proven yet. Therefore, it is an interesting question whether a substantial percentage of melanomas does really develop on the basis of pre-existing naevi. The present view about this model is summarized here from the literature. In addition, the results of a study on naevi as precursors for melanoma in a collective of melanoma patients in Berlin are presented.

Percentage of histologically associated malignant melanomas with melanocytic naevi

There are numerous studies published in the literature on the histological association of melanocytic naevi and melanoma. A review of these studies which were performed during the last 50 years until the end of the 1980s is given by Stolz *et al.* (1989). The findings of more recent studies are summarized in Table 10.2.

Reference	Cases (*n*)	Histological types	Percentage of associations
Crucioli & Stilwell (1982)	129	All types	10.9
Rhodes *et al.* (1982, 1983)	234	All types	27.4
Friedman *et al.* (1983)	557	All types	23.3
Sondergaard (1983)	1916	All types	9
Clark *et al.* (1984)	241	All types	30.7
Kopf *et al.* (1987)	679	All types	26 for < 1.5 mm
			15 for 1.5–3 mm
Stolz *et al.* (1989)	150	All types	22
Stadler & Garbe (1991)	581	All types	23
Sagebiel (1993)	1954	SSM/NM*	57.6

Table 10.2 Results of different studies on the histological association of melanocytic naevi and melanoma in the literature.

* SSM, Superficial spreading melanoma; NM, nodular melanoma.

There is considerable variation in the percentage of naevus-associated malignant melanomas as observed by different investigators. The majority of studies particularly from the United States and from Germany reported that 20–30% of melanomas are found in histological association with melanocytic naevi (Rhodes *et al.*, 1982, 1983; Friedman *et al.*, 1983; Clark *et al.*, 1984; Kopf *et al.*, 1987; Stolz *et al.*, 1989; Stadler & Garbe, 1991). A substantially lower percentage was described by Sondergaard in 1916 patients from Denmark (Sondergaard, 1983). This study, however, was not designed to observe the percentage of associated melanocytic naevi but to identify different prognostic factors in primary melanomas. A clearly higher value of melanomas associated with melanocytic naevi was given by Sagebiel (1993), who found naevus remnants in 57.6% of all melanomas examined. This study, however, was limited to examinations of superficial spreading melanomas and nodular melanomas.

Most studies reported considerable variation between the percentages of naevus-associated melanomas for different histological subtypes of melanoma. The percentages were highest in superficial spreading melanomas (Sondergaard, 1983; Kopf *et al.*, 1987; Stolz *et al.*, 1989). Additionally, the percentages of naevus associations varied by tumour thickness. Sagebiel reported 65% of naevus associations in tumours <0.76 mm thick and 64.5% for those between 0.76 and 1.69 mm thick, whereas in the thickness range 1.70–3.60 mm only 45.6% were found with naevus remnants.

In melanomas thicker than 2.6 mm, there were only 32% noted to have naevus cells (Sagebiel, 1993). Probably, in thicker tumours, naevus remnants may be overgrown by melanoma.

The different percentages of melanomas in association with melanocytic naevi may also be due to different criteria used for the detection of naevus remnants. An improvement of detection is obtained by application of immunohistochemistry. In particular, the monoclonal antibody HMB-45 proved to be useful (Stadler & Garbe, 1991).

Results of the Berlin study on histological associations between melanocytic naevi and melanoma

In the University Medical Centre Steglitz in Berlin, 581 primary melanomas diagnosed during the years 1970 to 1987 have been examined for naevus associations. The 581 melanoma specimens were paraffin embedded and diagnosis was performed on serial sections stained with haematoxylin & eosin. Additionally, patients have been followed up for 5–10 years in intervals of 3–6 months. Relapses and causes of deaths were documented and data were recorded by the databank program DBASE IV. Statistical evaluations have been performed by the statistical program SPSS. Survival rates have been calculated by the method of Kaplan and Meier and statistical differences have been tested by log-rank test.

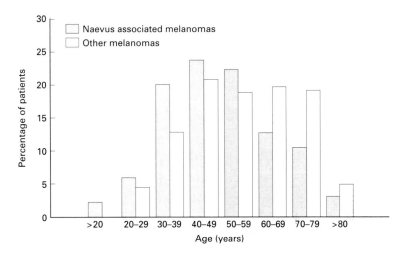

Fig. 10.5 Age distribution of patients with melanoma with histological naevus association (*n* = 135) and without this association (*n* = 374). *P* = 0.004.

Among the 581 primary melanomas 135 (23%) were found to be naevus-associated. In 119 cases (82%) naevus-cell formations were only found in the dermis. Only in a few cases were dermal as well as epidermal naevus nests detected. Patients with naevus-associated melanomas were found to be significantly younger than patients with melanomas without associated naevus (Fig. 10.5). Most naevus associations were detected in melanomas with a medium tumour thickness between 0.76 and 3 mm. Significantly less naevus associations were found in melanomas < 0.76 mm and > 3 mm (Fig. 10.6).

Survival rates of patients with naevus-associated melanomas have been compared to those without associated naevus. No differences in the 5-year overall survival were detected. The examinations have also been performed after stratification for tumour thickness. Differences in survival were neither observed in tumours with < 1.5 mm tumour thickness nor in tumours with > 1.5 mm tumour thickness (Figs 10.7 and 10.8).

Comment

Naevus associations in melanoma are more frequent in younger patients. This fits with the observation that higher naevus counts are obtained in middle-aged persons. The frequency of naevus associations is particularly low in patients with lentigo maligna melanoma or with acrolentigenous melanoma (Crucioli & Stilwell, 1982; Stolz *et al.*, 1989; Stadler & Garbe, 1991).

The diagnosis of naevus association in melanomas is normally based on the presence of dermal remnants of naevus-cell formations. It is rather difficult to establish the association to junctional naevus nests because these are very difficult to distinguish from melanoma-cell formations. The rate of naevus associations in melanoma increases significantly if junctional naevus associations are also evaluated (Sagebiel, 1993). On the other hand, if only dermal naevus-cell formations are validated, it is conceivable that a smaller percentage of thin melanomas is detected with naevus associations. In the Berlin study, we found the highest percentages of naevus associations in tumours with medium tumour thickness between 0.76 and 3 mm. In thicker tumours, naevus remnants may have been already overgrown by the melanoma.

Probably a higher percentage of melanoma develops on the basis of melanocytic naevi than can be detected by histological examinations. If only dermal naevus-cell formations are evaluated, the percentage of naevus associations seems to be between 20 and 30% (Friedman *et al.*, 1983; Kopf *et al.*, 1987; Stolz *et al.*, 1989; Stadler & Garbe, 1991). If, in addition, junctional naevus portions are evaluated, the percentage of naevus associations may be found to be double as high (Sagebiel, 1993). Therefore, it is possible that the majority of melanomas develop from a pre-existing melanocytic naevus. This may be in favour of the hypothesis of Clark and co-workers that tumour progression in malignant melanomas involves melanocytic naevi as one stage of tumour progression (Clark *et al.*, 1984; Kath *et al.*, 1989).

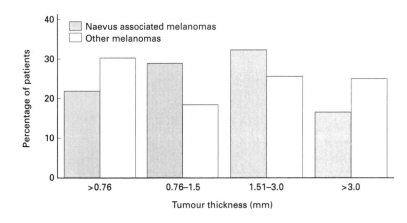

Fig. 10.6 Tumour thickness of naevus-associated melanomas (*n* = 123) in comparison with melanoma without naevus association (*n* = 358). *P* = 0.007.

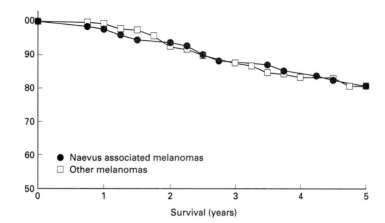

Fig. 10.7 Five-year survival rates for melanoma patients with (*n* = 135) and without (*n* = 374) naevus association. *P* = 0.95.

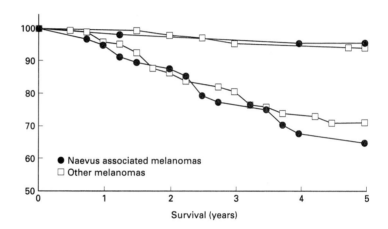

Fig. 10.8 Five-year survival rates for melanoma patients with and without naevus association stratified for tumour thickness.

The results of the Berlin study do not confirm the thesis that naevus association in melanoma is a prognostic factor. It has been proposed by Friedman *et al.* that naevus-associated malignant melanomas have more favourable prognosis than those without this association (Friedman *et al.*, 1983). This hypothesis still cannot be confirmed by any other study. Naevus association is obviously not a prognostic factor in malignant melanoma.

References

Abadir, M.C., Marghoob, A.A., Slade, J., Salopek, T.G., Yadav, S. & Kopf, A.W. (1995) Case-control study of melanocytic nevi on the buttocks in atypical mole syndrome: role of solar radiation in the pathogenesis of atypical moles. *Journal of the American Academy of Dermatology*, **33**, 31–36.

Augustsson, A., Stierner, U., Rosdahl, I. & Suurkula, M. (1991a) Common and dysplastic naevi as risk factors for cutaneous malignant melanoma in a Swedish population. *Acta Dermato-Venereologica*, **71**, 518–524.

Augustsson, A., Stierner, U., Rosdahl, I. & Suurkula, M. (1991b) Melanocytic naevi in sun-exposed and protected skin in melanoma patients and controls. *Acta Dermato-Venereologica*, **71**, 512–517.

Clark, W.H., Jr, Elder, D.E., Guerry, D., IV, Epstein, M.N., Greene, M.H. & Van Horn, M. (1984) A study of tumor progression: the precursor lesions of superficial spreading and nodular melanoma. *Human Pathology*, **15**, 1147–1165.

Crucioli, V. & Stilwell, J. (1982) The histogenesis of malignant melanoma in relation to pre-existing pigmented lesions. *Journal of Cutaneous Pathology*, **9**, 396–404.

Friedman, R.J., Rigel, D.S., Kopf, A.W. *et al.* (1983) Favorable prognosis for malignant melanomas associated with acquired melanocytic nevi. *Archives of Dermatology*, **119**, 455–462.

Gallagher, R.P., McLean, D.I., Yang, C.P. *et al.* (1990a) Anatomic distribution of acquired melanocytic nevi in white children. A comparison with melanoma: the Vancouver Mole Study. *Archives of Dermatology*, **126**, 466–471.

Gallagher, R.P., McLean, D.I., Yang, C.P. *et al.* (1990b) Suntan, sunburn, and pigmentation factors and the frequency of acquired melanocytic nevi in children. Similarities to melanoma: the Vancouver Mole Study. *Archives of Dermatology*, **126**, 770–776.

Garbe, C. (1995) Risikofaktoren für die Entwicklung maligner Melanome und Identifikation von Risikopersonen im deutschsprachigen Raum. *Hautarzt*, **46**, 309–314.

Garbe, C. & Orfanos, C.E. (1992) Epidemiology of malignant melanoma in central Europe: risk factors and prognostic predictors. Results of the Central Malignant Melanoma Registry of the German Dermatological Society. *Pigment Cell Research,* Suppl. **2**, 285–294.

Garbe, C., Krüger, S., Stadler, R., Guggenmoos Holzmann, I. & Orfanos, C.E. (1989) Markers and relative risk in a German population for developing malignant melanoma. *International Journal of Dermatology*, **28**, 517–523.

Garbe, C., Büttner, P., Weiss, J. *et al.* (1994) Risk factors for developing cutaneous melanoma and criteria for identifying persons at risk: multicenter case-control study of the Central Malignant Melanoma Registry of the German Dermatological Society. *Journal of Investigative Dermatology*, **102**, 695–699.

Grob, J.J., Gouvernet, J., Aymar, D. *et al.* (1990) Count of benign melanocytic nevi as a major indicator of risk for nonfamilial nodular and superficial spreading melanoma. *Cancer*, **66**, 387–395.

Holly, E.A., Kelly, J.W., Shpall, S.N. & Chiu, S.H. (1987) Number of melanocytic nevi as a major risk factor for malignant melanoma. *Journal of the American Academy of Dermatology*, **17**, 459–468.

Holly, E.A., Aston, D.A., Cress, R.D., Ahn, D.K. & Kristiansen, J.J. (1995) Cutaneous melanoma in women. II. Phenotypic characteristics and other host-related factors. *American Journal of Epidemiology*, **141**, 934–942.

Kath, R., Rodeck, U., Menssen, H.D. *et al.* (1989) Tumor progression in the human melanocytic system. *Anticancer Research*, **9**, 865–872.

Kelly, J.W., Holly, E.A., Shpall, S.N. & Ahn, D.K. (1989) The distribution of melanocytic naevi in melanoma patients and control subjects. *Australasian Journal of Dermatology*, **30**, 1–8.

Kopf, A.W., Welkovich, B., Frankel, R.E. *et al.* (1987) Thickness of malignant melanoma: global analysis of related factors. *Journal of Dermatology, Surgery and Oncology*,

13, 345–390, 401–420.

Krüger, S., Garbe, C., Büttner, P., Stadler, R., Guggenmoos Holzmann, I. & Orfanos, C.E. (1992) Epidemiologic evidence for the role of melanocytic nevi as risk markers and direct precursors of cutaneous malignant melanoma. Results of a case control study in melanoma patients and nonmelanoma control subjects [see comments]. *Journal of the American Academy of Dermatology*, **26**, 920–926.

MacKie, R.M. (1991) Risk factors, diagnosis, and detection of melanoma. *Current Opinion in Oncology*, **3**, 360–363.

MacKie, R.M., Freudenberger, T. & Aitchison, T.C. (1989) Personal risk-factor chart for cutaneous melanoma. *Lancet*, **ii**, 487–490.

Østerlind, A., Tucker, M.A., Hou Jensen, K., Stone, B.J., Engholm, G. & Jensen, O.M. (1988) The Danish case-control study of cutaneous malignant melanoma. I. Importance of host factors. *International Journal of Cancer*, **42**, 200–206.

Rampen, F.H., van der Meeren, H.L. & Boezeman, J.B. (1986) Frquency of moles as a key to melanoma incidence? *Journal of the American Academy of Dermatology*, **15**, 1200–1203.

Rhodes, A.R. (1985) Acquired dysplastic melanocytic nevi and cutaneous melanoma: precursors and prevention. *Annals of Internal Medicine*, **102**, 546–548.

Rhodes, A.R., Sober, A.J., Day, C.L. *et al.* (1982) The malignant potential of small congenital nevocellular nevi. An estimate of association based on a histologic study of 234 primary cutaneous melanomas. *Journal of the American Academy of Dermatology*, **6**, 230–241.

Rhodes, A.R., Harrist, T.J., Day, C.L., Mihm, M.C., Jr, Fitzpatrick, T.B. & Sober, A.J. (1983) Dysplastic melanocytic nevi in histologic association with 234 primary cutaneous melanomas. *Journal of the American Academy of Dermatology*, **9**, 563–574.

Rieger, E., Soyer, H.P., Garbe, C. *et al.* (1995) Overall and site-specific risk of malignant melanoma associated with nevus counts at different body sites: a multicenter case-control study of the German Central Malignant-Melanoma Registry. *International Journal of Cancer*, **62**, 393–397.

Sagebiel, R.W. (1993) Melanocytic nevi in histologic association with primary cutaneous melanoma of superficial spreading and nodular types: effect of tumor thickness. *Journal of Investigative Dermatology*, **100**, 322S–325S.

Sondergaard, K. (1983) Histological type and biological behavior of primary cutaneous malignant melanoma. I. An analysis of 1916 cases. *Virchows Archives A: Pathology, Anatomy, Histopathology*, **401**, 315–331.

Stadler, R. & Garbe, C. (1991) Navus-assoziierte maligne Melanome — diagnostische Sicherung und Prognose. *Hautarzt*, **42**, 424–429.

Stierner, U., Augustsson, A., Rosdahl, I. & Suurkula, M. (1992) Regional distribution of common and dysplastic naevi in relation to melanoma site and sun exposure. A case-control study. *Melanoma Research*, **1**, 367–375.

Stolz, W., Schmoeckel, C., Landthaler, M. & Braun Falco, O. (1989) Association of early malignant melanoma with nevocytic nevi. *Cancer*, **63**, 550–555.

Swerdlow, A.J., English, J., MacKie, R.M. *et al.* (1986) Benign melanocytic naevi as a risk factor for malignant melanoma. *British Medical Journal: Clinical Research Edition*, **292**, 1555–1559.

Weiss, J., Garbe, C., Bertz, J. *et al.* (1990) Risikofaktoren für die Entwicklung maligner Melanome in der Bundesrepublik Deutschland. Ergebnisse einer multizentrischen Fall-Kontroll-Studie. *Hautarzt*, **41**, 309–313.

11
Melanoma Prevention

Attitudes and Behaviour Towards Sun Exposure: Implications for Melanoma Prevention

J.J. GROB AND J.J. BONERANDI

It has been demonstrated that sun exposure is a risk factor of melanoma, but a number of uncertainties remain. Many campaigns to change sun behaviour have been conducted throughout the world and especially in Australia. However, primary prevention of melanoma is a difficult enterprise since it is based on two risky assumptions: that one can change the behaviour of a population towards the sun and that reducing sun exposure will lower the incidence of melanoma 20 years later.

Knowledge, attitudes and behaviour towards sun in developed countries

In developed countries a number of surveys on sun behaviour have been performed to provide the basis for prevention campaigns. Results show that knowledge about the relation between sun and skin cancer is good in children, teenagers and adults, living not only in countries where many education campaigns have been conducted, such as Australia (Hill *et al.*, 1993; Loescher *et al.*, 1995) and USA (Berwick *et al.*, 1992), but even in countries where less effort has been made to inform the public, such as in Europe (Bourke *et al.*, 1995) and South Africa (Von Schirdning *et al.*, 1991). Although this knowledge can certainly be improved, this finding clearly suggests that transmitting the knowledge is not a limiting factor in prevention.

Sun behaviour and practice of protective measures differs widely from country to country. In Europe and North America there is little relevant data. In France (Grob *et al.*, 1993), 32% of children under 3 years of age and 66% of teenagers reported at least two light sunburns in the previous summer. Forty-eight percent of teenagers and 85% of parents of young children claim to use sunscreens. In 1995, 32% of adults said they always use sunscreens, 27% sunbathed more than 3 hours a day and 15% reported previous severe sunburns (Sanofi & Ipsos, unpublished data). In the UK, 38–60% of children experienced at least one sunburn during the previous year (Bennets *et al.*, 1991; Jarrett *et al.*, 1993; Bourke *et al.*, 1995) and 51% of teenagers who sunbathe reported sunburns (Hughes *et al.*, 1993). In Norway, 90% of teenagers said that they used sunscreens but only 50% applied them effectively and only 25% selected the proper sun-protection factor (SPF) (Wichstrom, 1994). In the USA, a survey conducted among teenagers living in the Washington area showed that < 10% consistently used sunscreens and > 30% never used protection (Banks *et al.*, 1992). According to parents in Canada, 18% of their children had sunburns during the previous summer (Zinman *et al.*, 1995). Twenty-nine percent of young children and 36% of teenagers used sunscreens and 48% of children and 40% of teenagers wore shirts (Zinman *et al.*, 1995). Only 50% of people used protective measures on a regular basis (Campbell & Birdsell, 1994). In Australia in 1992 >80% of teenage boys and 60% of teenage girls living in major cities reported having spent >2 hours at weekends outside during peak times for ultraviolet rays (Fritschi *et al.*, 1992). Only 13% consistently used sunscreens. According to a phone survey conducted before the start of the 'Sunsmart' campaign, 14% of adults reported sunburn during the previous weekend (Hill *et al.*, 1993). The proportion of individuals using sunscreens the previous weekend was low: 10 and 28% in 1988 and in 1990, respectively (Hill *et al.*, 1993). In New Zealand, only 18% of teenagers said that they sunbathed regularly and 54% claimed to use sunscreens regularly (McGee & Williams, 1992). In South Africa, >65% of people surveyed reported going to the beach during the hottest part of the day and 50% of these beachgoers did not use sunscreen (Zinman *et al.*, 1995).

Data from different surveys are fragmentary and difficult to compare because different methods of evaluation (phone questionnaires, interviews) have been used in different populations living in different climatic conditions. However, regardless of the country, it is clear that many subjects are overexposed and do not use proper sun-protective measures. It is also clear that young people are more engaged in activities at high risk for sunburns (Hill *et al.*, 1992).

These data raise two important questions: What is the proportion of people who are actually overexposed in different countries?; and what is their degree of overexposure? These questions are difficult to answer, since a given sun behaviour may be acceptable for an individual with high sun resistance and not for another with low sun resistance, especially in a very sunny area. Obviously, a sunburn can be taken as a rough proof of overexposure, regardless of the skin type. We used another approach, by evaluating exposure not as an absolute measure, but as a relative measure with reference to the constitutional sensitivity of individuals and taking into account their use of effective sun protection. This study was conducted in a population including 3-year-old children and teenagers living on the Mediterranean coast of southern France (Grob *et al.*, 1993). The results conclusively showed that 33% of children and 62% of teenagers were highly overexposed.

Basis for primary prevention of melanoma

Any dermatologist dedicated to primary prevention must bear in mind several facts:

It is difficult to extrapolate data from one country to another. There seem to be three very different zones of sun exposure: zones of intense year-round exposure like Australia; zones of seasonal intense exposure like southern Europe and the United States; and zones of low exposure like northern Europe and Canada. Great differences in the risks of sun exposure, behaviour towards the sun and the adaptation of the population to the climate make it very difficult to compare these zones. People in zones of year-round or seasonal exposure must make sun protection part of their daily routine, whereas people living in zones of low exposure need only take precaution while on vacation. People living in areas deprived of sun often seek the sun during the summer vacation, resulting in mass migrations from the north to south. Conversely, behaviour of people living in more exposed areas is determined by good common-sense. In addition to climate, socio-cultural factors strongly influence attitudes and behaviour towards the sun (Eiser *et al.*, 1995). The number and importance of previous prevention campaigns also account for differences between countries.

Ninety per cent of studies on sun behaviour and 90% of publications on campaigns to change sun behaviour come from Australia, simply because Australians have paid much attention to the disease and as a result authorities began to devote major resources to prevention. The 'Australian bias' consists of considering that studies of behaviour in Australia and the results of information campaigns can be extrapolated to all countries. This is not true because Australia is a specific case for many reasons: intense ambient sun, population with a Celtic phenotype, non-Latin culture and a high degree of awareness of the fatal nature of melanoma.

Tanning is a social phenomenon. This probably began at the turn of the century with heliotherapy for treatment of some diseases such as tuberculosis. The trend expanded in the 1950s under the influence of cinema and exploded in the latter part of the century with the consumer society (Grob & Bonerandi, 1991). Within 60 years, we have gone from a situation in which people in sunny zones instinctively protected themselves by wearing clothes and adapting behaviour (working in the evening and napping in the middle of the day) to a situation in which people painstakingly seek to increase their exposure. A need for sunlight and desire to look attractive and healthy probably account for this tanning fashion in developed countries. The effect of sunlight on mood (Du Laurens, 1599) and psychiatric disorders (Fey *et al.*, 1988; Gerballdo & Thaker, 1991) has long been recognized and the attraction of sunlight is one of the major factors in the southern migration of people living in northern climates during vacation periods. People also place a great value on being tanned (Keesling & Friedman, 1987; Cockburn *et al.*, 1989; Hill *et al.*, 1990, 1993; Broadstock *et al.*, 1992; McGee & Williams, 1992; Grob *et al.*, 1993; Wichstrom, 1994). Teenagers (Fritschi *et al.*, 1992; McGee & Williams, 1992; Lowe *et al.*, 1993), especially girls (Broadstock *et al.*, 1992; Grob *et al.*, 1993), consider that they look more attractive and that it is a sign of good health. The widespread idea that 'sun is good for the health' may also lead many parents to overexpose their young children, as has been shown in France (Grob *et al.*, 1993). In countries where the only way to be tanned is to travel, tanning has become a social status symbol for people who can afford holidays abroad (Grob & Bonerandi, 1991). Thus, it will probably be difficult, or even impossible, to change behaviour without changing fashion (see below) (Arthey & Clarke, 1995).

The risk of melanoma creates a psychological conflict between the desire to be tanned and the dangers of sun exposure. In a psychological conflict, the final decision of individuals depends on how they evaluate the risk and how much effort is required to apply necessary precautions (Janis & Mann, 1977; Robinson, 1992; Eiser *et al.*, 1995). There are several possible choices. Some individuals may consider that the risk (skin cancer) is minor and thus that there is no dilemma. Others may consider the precautions too restrictive or ineffective and thus do not change their behaviour and tend to minimize the risk. Others admit that there is a risk, analyse for and against, but may still consider that the benefits of being tanned outweigh the risks. In this regard, people who placed high value on physical appearance are more likely to overindulge in sunbathing (Wichstrom, 1994). Other people may consider that the precautions can be easily implemented and thus change their behaviour to remove the risk. The response is personal but it is influenced by factors such as age, sex and peer pressure. Young people are more likely to ignore the risk (Marks & Hill, 1988). Women are more likely to value a tan (Broadstock *et al.*, 1992; Lowe *et al.*, 1993).

Psychology is a major factor in prevention campaigns in a number of ways. People tend to underplay long-term risks and overplay short-term risks (Arthey & Clarke, 1995). The trade-off between the immediate denial (no tan) and the long-term risk (cancer, skin-ageing) does not necessarily work in favour of prevention. The short-term risks of sun exposure (heat stroke, sunburn) are more likely to incite individuals to change their behaviour than the long-term risks (cancer, ageing). In this regard, the reason most often given by people for using sunscreens is to avoid sunburn and not to prevent cancer (McDudoc *et al.*, 1992; Grob *et al.*, 1993), except in Australia (Hill *et al.*, 1985). Another factor that must be taken into account is the 'optimistic' or 'it won't happen to me' bias which leads people to greatly minimize the risk and is certainly a major factor in the increasing incidence of sun-induced skin cancer (Arthey & Clarke, 1995). It is known that the arguments most likely to convince people are those which provide causal information (how the sun induces cancer) and not those which are based on statistical probabilities (more cancers in sunbathers) (Ajzen & Fishbein, 1977). In this regard, linking skin cancer with the hole in the ozone layer is probably one of the most effective arguments (Theobald *et al.*, 1991). It should be emphasized that people do not always believe what they are told. A survey of teenagers in France revealed that, although 61% said they were aware of the relationship between sun and cancer, 71% said that they would change their behaviour when 'this relationship was really proven to them' (Grob *et al.*, 1993). The psychological limitations of a prevention campaign have been well summed up in the following truism: any intervention to reduce sun exposure will have limited effects unless the subjects want to decrease their sun exposure (Arthey & Clarke, 1995).

Awareness of one's sun sensitivity is a determinant. Personal delusions about sun sensitivity are widespread. In a study conducted in France, 65% of adolescents considered as highly sensitive on the basis of their phenotype stated they were fairly resistant (Grob *et al.*, 1993). Clearly, sun-sensitive individuals who thinks they are sun resistant will not adopt appropriate sun behaviour. This problem is further complicated by the fact that sun sensitivity may be perceived as a weakness. This perception seems to be less prevalent in English-speaking countries than Latin countries but there are no reliable data. Teaching people the principles of self-assessment should be an important goal of any prevention campaign.

Use of sunscreen is also a social phenomenon. Behavioural changes, adapting one's activities according to the intensity of the sun and wearing proper clothing, are the most effective methods of sun protection. Sunscreens are less efficient but tend to override more effective methods. They are the only hope for people unable to imagine life without roasting half-naked on the beach in the middle of a hot summer's day. In Australia, the reason that most adults give for using sunscreens is to 'avoid cancer and avoid sunburn' (Hill *et al.*, 1985; Pincus *et al.*, 1991). In France and Texas, parents of young people say they use sunscreen to avoid sunburn (McDudoc *et al.*, 1992; Grob *et al.*, 1993). However, knowledge about sunscreens is far from adequate. Even in Australia there are subjects who say they use sunscreens to promote tanning (Hill *et al.*, 1985; Pincus *et al.*, 1991). Similarly, 20% of subjects attending a 'community skin cancer screening' in the USA in 1988 (Berwick *et al.*, 1992) and 14% of teenagers in France (Grob *et al.*, 1993) reported use of sunscreens to promote tanning. Furthermore, many people do not use a sunscreen with an SPF adapted to their phenotype or do not understand the need to re-apply the product. The decision to apply sunscreens is apparently linked more to psycho-social factors than to skin type. Use of sunscreens by children and teenagers depends on prior history of sunburn (McDudoc *et al.*, 1992) and parental behaviour (Banks *et al.*, 1992; Grob *et al.*, 1993), whereas in adults use is dependent on sex (Berwick *et al.*, 1992; Campbell & Birdsdell, 1994), awareness of the risk of cancer (Keesling & Friedman, 1987; Berwick *et al.*, 1992), level of anxiety (Keesling & Friedman, 1987), level of education (Berwick *et al.*, 1992) and age (Berwick *et al.*, 1992). Use of a sunscreen does not appear to be correlated with skin type (Pincus *et al.*, 1991), although fair-skinned people tend to be more frequent users (Berwick *et al.*, 1992; Hill *et al.*, 1993;

Campbell & Birdsdell, 1994). Women tend to use sunscreens more than men, who tend to prefer to wear proper clothing (Berwick *et al.*, 1992; Campbell & Birdsdell, 1994). The cosmetic properties of the products are also important since, before 1990, teenagers reported that sunscreens were sticky and messy (Cockburn *et al.*, 1989).

There is a gap between what people know, what they intend to do and what they do. Knowledge has been shown to affect attitudes and self-reported behaviour (Arthey & Clarke, 1995). However, while behaviour cannot be changed without educating people, it has been shown that even a high degree of awareness does not always lead to appropriate attitude and behaviour (Ajzen & Fishbein, 1977). This is particularly true in adolescents who are generally well informed but do not act accordingly (Cockburn *et al.*, 1989; Grob *et al.*, 1993). Experience in melanoma prevention campaigns demonstrates how quickly people forget good intentions. After the *Goodbye Sunshine* television campaign in Australia, only one-fifth of the people who said they would see a doctor had actually done so 4 weeks later (Theobald *et al.*, 1991). Analysis of efficacy of primary skin-cancer prevention campaigns (Ramstack *et al.*, 1986; Borland *et al.*, 1990; Buller & Buller, 1991; Theobald *et al.*, 1991; Mermestein & Riesenberg, 1992; Hill *et al.*, 1993; Bourke & Graham-Brown, 1995) showed that people's knowledge of the problem increases and that this knowledge sometimes influences attitudes and/or behavioural intentions, but that behaviour seldom changes. Furthermore, it is unclear how long the effects of campaigns last and this constitutes a major uncertainty for the future.

Objective evaluation of primary melanoma prevention campaigns is difficult. Results of prevention campaigns can only be measured in the long term. Because the cancer process is long, a change in behaviour towards the sun will not become evident for 20–30 years. In addition, no one knows how long it will take to change people's behaviour towards the sun. Melanoma prevention is a long-term operation with no guarantee of results and thus is very different from a screening campaign with immediate, easily measured results. This situation is further complicated by the fact that no one is sure about the validity of the information now being given. What is the exact effect of sunburns? Is sun exposure really more harmful during childhood? What are the relative roles of genetic factors and sun exposure? The only reliable way to verify the efficacy of a campaign is to measure actual change in behaviour. However, observation of behaviour is made difficult by the lack of adapted tools (observation at beach, etc.). Failure to tell people that they are observed may be unethical, while informing them that they are being observed may influence their behaviour (Arthey & Clarke, 1995). Simply asking subjects is unreliable because there is often a great difference between what people say they do and what they actually do (Bourke & Graham-Brown, 1995). For example, children's reported sun protection is higher than that observed (Bennets *et al.*, 1991). Evaluation based on people's reported behaviour or, worse, on statements of intention probably over-estimate the efficacy of the campaign. People tend to say what they think is expected rather then their real intentions. Another problem in assessing the results of prevention campaigns is to form a control group since people cannot be isolated from the media. Finally, it must be said that campaigns lead to changes in attitudes and behaviour little by little. These changes are difficult to see from one year to another but may become measurable in terms of decades. In this regard, the tendency to use less tanned models in the Australian press over a 10-year period (Chapman *et al.*, 1992) probably says more about the efficacy of prevention on the public's conceptions than a questionnaire 1 month after a campaign.

Prevention campaigning is resource-intensive. Prevention campaigns have used various approaches: hand-out documentation, media campaigns including newspaper, radio and television, and on-beach and in-school information. They have used a variety of slogans, some funny such as 'Slip! slop! slap!' (Marks, 1990) or 'Beau le soleil, bobo le soleil' (France, 'Vaincre le Mélanome' campaign, unpublished data), some ominous such as 'Are you dying to get a suntan?' (Cameron & McGuire, 1990). Only in Australia have all these methods been used in combination. Since little information is available about the relative efficacy of these approaches (informative versus

ominous versus funny) in different populations, no guidelines have been established for future campaigns. In addition to campaigns, human resources and organizational measures can be used. The most familiar application of human resources consists in using role models, such as well-known sports figures with whom young people can identify, to urge people to change their behaviour. Once again, Australia is the only country to try structural changes including rescheduling sporting activities away from the middle of the day, applying 'no hat–no play' rules at school, erecting canopies and planting trees for shade in school grounds and parks, removing tax from approved sunscreens, encouraging manufacturers to produce attractive and effective clothing and hats, and prohibiting manufacture of ozone layer-depleting substances (Marks, 1990). These measures have probably been very effective and perhaps even more so than information campaigns (Marks, 1995).

Duration, continuity and repetition are also important factors in achieving results. Australia has made the most steadfast national commitment to melanoma prevention. In other countries, campaigns have been mostly sporadic and localized. As for most things, results depend on the resources and determination that are brought into play. It would be interesting, albeit difficult, to evaluate the impact of each method.

Many melanoma prevention campaigns have been conducted in schools for three reasons. The first is that sun exposure during childhood seems to be an important risk factor for melanoma. Second, behavioural patterns are formed during childhood. Third, parents can be reached through their children (Hill *et al.*, 1992). In Australia, skin protection is taught in most schools (Marks, 1990). In the USA (Ramstack *et al.*, 1986; Mermestein & Riesenberg, 1992) several school campaigns have achieved success in raising the level of knowledge and changing attitudes but have had little effect on behaviour. Once again, efficacy probably depends on the resources that are brought to bear. A 4-week training course is more effective in changing behaviour than a single 30-minute lecture (Arthey & Clarke, 1995). A 1-hour talk with a dermatologist improves the level of knowledge but does not change attitude or behaviour (Goldstein & Lesher, 1991). In England

(Hughes *et al.*, 1993), an education package including a colour leaflet, a workbook and a video film was proposed in seven schools. Compared with a control group, there was a difference in knowledge and attitudes but not in behaviour. In several regions of France, we conducted a school-based campaign presented as a game over a 4-week period with elementary school teachers as game hosts (Bastuji-Garin *et al.*, 1997). Comparison of the results of a questionnaire evaluating before and after the campaign indicated a change not only in knowledge and attitudes but also to some extent in reported behaviour (Hill *et al.*, 1992).

An interaction between primary prevention and screening campaigns is inevitable. It is impossible to dissociate screening campaigns aimed at early diagnosis and prevention campaigns aimed at changing sun behaviour. Both enhance awareness of skin cancer. A primary prevention campaign may stimulate a person to consult rather than change his/her behaviour. This attitude provides many people with a way out of the dilemma between the desire to be tanned and the risk of cancer. Obviously, a primary prevention campaign which induces people to consult early is not a failure. The fact that the mean thickness of melanoma at the time of diagnosis has decreased in Australia can probably be attributed to awareness of the disease achieved not only to early diagnosis programmes (Marks, 1995) but also by primary prevention campaigns.

Overview of past worldwide primary melanoma prevention campaigns

In Victoria, Australia, melanoma prevention campaigns, including full media coverage and organizational changes, have been conducted in rapid succession with the 'Slip! slop! slap!' campaign (slip on a shirt, slop on a sunscreen and slap on a hat) and the 'Sunsmart' campaign (Smith, 1979; Rassab *et al.*, 1983; Marks, 1990). These campaigns have achieved a greater awareness with a change in attitudes including pro-tan beliefs and tanning motivation, an increase in the percentage of people using sunscreens and a reduction in the number of sunburns (Borland *et al.*, 1990; Hill *et al.*, 1990, 1992, 1993). These changes have been most notable in women, teenagers and young adults (Hill *et al.*, 1992, 1993). An outstanding part of the 'Sunsmart' campaign was a television documentary entitled *Goodbye Sunshine* which presents the true story of a young man from diagnosis of melanoma to metastasis, chemotherapy and death. The impact of this tragic story was great. Comparison of data from phone surveys conducted before and after the broadcast revealed a clear-cut increase in the number of people who stated an intention to protect themselves after seeing the film. Also, the number of patients consulting for pigmented lesions rose and there was a 167% increase in the number of melanomas diagnosed in the 3 months following this broadcast.

The question can still be asked about how successful these highly resource-intensive Australian campaigns were in achieving prevention. After several years of campaigning from 1988 to 1990, the proportion of people who stated that they had used a sunscreen during the previous weekend rose from 10% to only 28%, the number of people reporting sunburns during the previous weekend decreased from 14% to 5% and the number of people trying to get a dark tan fell from 20% to 12%. Thus, taking into account that many respondents probably did not respond honestly in order to avoid appearing 'stupid' after being informed, the campaigns do not appear to have had spectacular results. In addition, there have been signs of regression (Marks, 1995).

Outside of Australia, campaigns have been much more limited in scope. In America the Sun Awareness Project of Arizona was focused on children, adolescents and the elderly (Buller & Buller, 1991; Loescher *et al.*, 1995). The Rhode Island 'Sunsmart' Project was a pilot operation targeted at beachgoers (Rossi *et al.*, 1994). The Undercover Skin Cancer Program in Texas used a variety of newspapers, television channels and radio stations, and phone surveys suggested some short-term changes in behaviour (Buller & Buller, 1991; Loescher *et al.*, 1995). In the UK a campaign based on the slogan 'Are you dying to get a suntan?' (Cameron & McGuire, 1990) was conducted in 1989 using magazine advertising, leaflets and public relations activities and led to an increased awareness of the problem, but no major change in attitudes. Several campaigns focusing more on screening than primary prevention have also been undertaken and, although results have not been quantified, sun and melanoma awareness have increased (Newman *et al.*, 1988; Melia *et al.*, 1993; Boutwell, 1995). Pilot campaigns have been successfully carried out on beaches in France ('Vaincre le Mélanome', and Sanofi & Ipsos, unpublished data) but we were unable to objectively measure an impact.

Campaigns aimed at primary melanoma prevention by reducing sun exposure are hindered by uncertainties involving the most suitable message, the most effective means of delivery, the actual impact on behaviour, the durability of changes and the difficulty of measuring long-term effects. Experience indicates that, although interesting results have been obtained in countries that have applied intense resources, outcome depends on psychosocial factors.

References

Ajzen, I. (1977) Intuitive theories of events and the effects of base-rate information on prediction. *Journal of Personality and Social Psychology*, **35**, 303–314.

Ajzen, I. & Fishbein, M. (1977) Attitude–behavior relations: a theoretical analysis and review of empirical research. *Psychological Bulletin*, **84**, 888–918.

Arthey, S., & Clarke, V.A. (1995) Suntanning and sun protection: a review of the psychological literature. *Social Science and Medicine*, **40**, 265–274.

Banks, B.A., Silverman, R.A., Scwartz, R.H. & Tunessen, W. (1992) Attitudes of teenagers toward sun exposure and sunscreen use. *Pediatrics*, **89**, 40–42.

Bastuji-Garin, S., Grognard, C., Grosjean, F., Grob, J.J. & Guillaume, J.C. (1997) Melanoma: evaluation of a health campaign for primary schools. Submitted for publication.

Bennets, K., Borland, R. & Swerrisson, H. (1991) Sun protection behaviour of children and their parents at the beach. *Psychology and Heath*, **5**, 279–287.

Berwick, M., Fine, J.A. & Bolognia, J.L. (1992) Sun exposure and sunscreen use following a community cancer screening. *Preventive Medicine*, **21**, 302–303.

Borland, R., Hill, D. & Noy, S. (1990) Being 'Sunsmart': change in the community awareness and reported behaviour following a primary prevention program for skin cancer control. *Behavioural Change*, **7**, 126–135.

Bourke, J.F. & Graham-Brown, R.A.C. (1995) Protection of children against sunburn: A survey of parental practice in Leicester. *British Journal of Dermatology*, **133**, 264–266.

Bourke, J.F., Healsmith, M.F. & Graham-Brown, R.A.C. (1995) Melanoma awareness and sun exposure in Leicester.

British Journal of Dermatology, **132**, 251–256.

Boutwell, W.B. (1995) The Undercover Skin Cancer Prevention Project. *Cancer*, **75**, 657–660.

Broadstock, M., Borland, R. & Gason, R. (1992) Effects of suntan on judgements of healthiness and attractiveness by adolescents. *Journal of Applied Social Psychology*, **22**, 157–172.

Cameron, I.H. & McGuire, C. (1990) 'Are you dying to get a suntan?' The pre- and post-campaign survey results. *Health Education Journal*, **49**, 166.

Buller, D.B. & Buller, M.K. (1991) Approaches to communicating preventive behaviours. *Seminars in Oncology Nursing*, **7**, 53–55.

Campbell, H.S. & Birdsell, J. (1994) Knowledge, beliefs and sun protection behaviours of Alberta adults. *Preventive Medicine*, **23**, 160–166.

Chapman, S., Marks, R. & King, M. (1992) Trends in tans and skin protection in Australian fashion magazines 1982 through 1991. *American Journal of Public Health*, **82**, 1677–1680.

Cockburn, J., Hennrikus, D., Scott, R. & Sanson-Fischer, R. (1989) Adolescent use of protection measures. *Medical Journal of Australia*, **151**, 136–140.

Du Laurens, A. (1599) *A Discourse on the Preservation of the Sight: Of the Melancholike Diseases of Rheuma and Old Age*. Richard Surphlet, London.

Eiser, J.R., Eiser, C., Sani, F., Sell, L. & Casas, R.M. (1995) Skin cancer attitudes: a cross-national comparison. *British Journal of Social Psychology*, **34**, 23–30.

Fey, P., Pflug, B. & Jost, K. (1988) Self-rating of the global state of mood of depressive patients by a bright–dark scale. *Pharmacopsychiatry*, **21**, 410–411.

Fritschi, L., Green, A. & Solomon, P.J. (1992) Sun exposure in Australian adolescents. *Journal of the American Academy of Dermatology*, **27**, 25–28.

Gerballdo, M. & Thaker, G. (1991) A strong preference for darkness in patients with depression. *Canadian Journal of Psychiatry*, **36**, 677–679.

Goldstein, B.G. & Lesher, J.L. Jr (1991) The effect of a school based intervention on skin cancer prevention knowledge and behaviour. *Journal of the American Academy of Dermatology*, **24**, 116.

Grob, J.J. & Bonerandi, J.J. (1991) Nouveau soleil, nouvelle dermatologie. *Annals de Dermatologie et Venereologie*, **118**, 925–929.

Grob, J.J., Guglielmina, C., Gouvernet, J. & Bonerandi, J.J. (1993) Study of sunbathing habits in children and adolescents: application to the prevention of melanoma. *Dermatology*, **186**, 94–98.

Hill, D., Rassaby, J. & Gardner, G. (1985) Determinants of intentions to take precautions against skin cancer. *Community Health Studies*, **8**, 33–34.

Hill, D., Theobald, T. & Borland, R. (1990) Summer activities sunburn attitudes and precautions against skin cancer. Center for Behavioural Research in Cancer. Anticancer Council of Victoria, 13.

Hill, D., White, V., Marks, R., Theobald, T., Borland, R. & Roy, C. (1992) Melanoma prevention: behavioural and non-behavioural factors in sunburn among Australian urban population. *Preventive Medicine*, **21**, 654–669.

Hill, D., White, V., Marks, R. & Borland, R. (1993) Changes in sun-related attitudes and behaviours, and reduced sunburn prevalence in a population at high risk of melanoma. *European Journal of Cancer Prevention*, **2**, 447–456.

Hughes, B.R., Altman, D.G. & Newton, J.A. (1993) Melanoma and skin cancer: evaluation of a health education programme for secondary schools. *British Journal of Dermatology*, **128**, 412–417.

Janis, I.L. & Mann, L. (1977) *Decision-making: A Psychological Analysis of Conflict, Choice and Commitment*. Free Press, New York.

Jarrett, P., Shar, C. & McMelland, J. (1993) Protection of children by their mothers against sunburn. *British Medical Journal*, **306**, 1448.

Keesling, B. & Friedman, H.S. (1987) Psychological factors in sunbathing and sunscreen use. *Health Psychology*, **6**, 477–493.

Loescher, L.J., Buller, M.K., Buller, D.B., Enerson, J. & Taylor, A.M. (1995) Public education projects in skin cancer. *Cancer*, **75**, 651–656.

Lowe, J.B., Balanda, K.P., Gillespie, A.M., Del Mar, C.B. & Gentle, A.F. (1993) Sun-related attitudes and beliefs among Queensland school children: the role of gender and sex. *Australian Journal of Public Health*, **17**, 202–208.

Marks, R. (1990) Skin cancer control in the 1990s: from 'Slip! slop! slap!' to 'Sunsmart'. *Australian Journal of Dermatology*, **31**, 1–4.

Marks, R. (1995) Skin cancer control in Australia. The balance between primary prevention and early detection. *Archives of Dermatology*, **131**, 474–478.

Marks, R. & Hill, D. (1988) Behavioural change in adolescence: a major challenge for skin cancer control in Australia. *Medical Journal of Australia*, **149**, 514–515.

McDudoc, L.R., Wagner, R.F. & Wagner, K.D. (1992) Parent's use of sunscreen on beach-going children. *Archives of Dermatology*, **128**, 628–629.

McGee, R. & Williams, S. (1992) Adolescence and sun protection. *New Zealand Medical Journal*, **105**, 401–403.

Melia, J., Ellmann, R. & Chamberlain, J. (1993) Preventing melanoma. *British Medical Journal*, **307**, 738.

Mermestein, R.J. & Riesenberg, L.A. (1992) Changing knowledge and attitude about skin cancer risk factors in adolescents. *Health Psychology*, **11**, 371–374.

Newman, S., Nichols, S., Freer, C. & Izzartd, L. (1988) How much do the public know about moles, skin cancer and malignant melanoma? The results of a postal survey. *Community Medicine*, **10**, 351–357.

Pincus, M.W., Rollings, P.K., Craft, A.B. & Green, A. (1991) Sunscreen use on Queensland beaches. *Australasian Journal of Dermatology*, **32**, 21–25.

Ramstack, J.L., White, S.E., Hazelkorn, K.S. & Meyskens, F.L. (1986) Sunshine and skin cancer: a school basal skin cancer prevention project. *Journal of Cancer Education*, **1**, 169–172.

Rassab, J., Larcombe, D., Hill, Fr. & Wake, F.R. (1983) 'Slip! slop! slap!' Health education about skin cancer. *Cancer Forum*, **7**, 63–69.

Robinson, J.K. (1992) Compensation strategies in sun protection behaviors by a population with non-melanoma skin cancer. *Preventive Medicine*, **21**, 754–765.

Rossi, J.S., Blais, L.M. & Weinstock, M.A. (1994) The Rhode Island 'Sunsmart' project: skin cancer prevention reaches the beaches. *American Journal of Public Health*, **84**, 672–674.

Smith, A. (1979) The Queensland Melanoma Project—an exercise in health education. (Editorial.) *British Medical Journal*, **253**, 1.

Theobald, T., Marks, R., Hill, D. & Dorevitch, A. (1991) *Goodbye Sunshine*: effects of a television program about melanoma on beliefs, behavior, and melanoma thickness. *Journal of the American Academy of Dermatology*, **25**, 717–723.

Von Schirdning, Y., Strauss, N., Mathee, A., Robertson, P. & Blignaut, R. (1991) Sunscreen use and environmental awareness among beach-goers in Cape Town, South Africa. *Public Health Review*, **19**, 209–217.

Wichstrom, L. (1994) Predictors of Norwegian adolescents sunbathing and use of sunscreens. *Health Psychology*, **13**, 412–420.

Zinman, R., Schwartz Gordon, K., Fitzpatrick, E. & Camfield, C. (1995) Predictors of sunscreen use in childhood. *Archives of Pediatrics and Adolescence*, **149**, 804–807.

Lack of Efficacy of Common Sunscreens in Melanoma Prevention

C.F. GARLAND, F.C. GARLAND AND E.D. GORHAM

Incidence rates of melanoma have risen faster than those of any other cancer in the United States during the past three decades, with an especially rapid rise during the past two decades. It is projected that there will be 40 300 new cases of malignant melanoma diagnosed in the United States in 1997 and 7300 deaths (Parker *et al.*, 1996). Age-adjusted mortality rates in US whites rose from 1.7 to 2.4 per 100 000 during 1973–88 (Parker *et al.*, 1996). As a result of these trends, melanoma is now the second leading cause of cancer death in white men of 15–35 years old in the United States (Gloeckler-Ries *et al.*, 1991) and has emerged as a major public health problem.

Increases in recent decades in age-adjusted incidence and mortality rates of cutaneous malignant melanoma in the United States and other countries where chemical sunscreens are in widespread use led to the proposal that the commonly promoted sunscreens in use since the-mid 1940s do not prevent melanoma and may increase risk by allowing prolonged exposure of susceptible individuals to wavelengths of sunlight that are not effectively absorbed (Garland *et al.*, 1988, 1992, 1993). A review of epidemiological findings and subsequent laboratory research, described below, has provided further support for this hypothesis.

Time trends

One of the most intensely studied areas in the United States for cancer is Connecticut, where cancer has been a legally reportable disease since 1935. Annual age-adjusted melanoma incidence rates in Connecticut tripled from 4 per 100 000 in 1965 to 12 per 100 000 in 1989 (J.T. Flannery Connecticut Tumor Registry, pers. comm., 1991) (Houghton *et al.*, 1980). The trends in age-adjusted incidence rates of melanoma in Connecticut revealed a small increase following introduction in the mid-1940s of commercial chemical suntan lotions containing glyceryl-*p*-aminobenzoate or homosalate, with a much steeper rise following the introduction of sunscreens such as *para*-aminobenzoic acid (PABA) in 1960 and subsequent years (Fig. 11.1).

International comparisons

Worldwide, the countries where chemical sunscreens have been widely promoted and adopted have experienced the greatest rise in cutaneous melanoma, with a rise in death rates following the acceleration in incidence rates by 5–10 years. Differences among countries are apparent when age-adjusted annual mortality rates from malignant melanoma and other skin malignancies are analysed according to year (Fig. 11.2) Data were reported only for all cutaneous

malignancies since many countries do not differentiate among cutaneous malignancies and are shown for men to simplify comparisons. Similar patterns were present for women, but with lower rates (Kurihara *et al.*, 1989). The prominent rise in the age-adjusted mortality rate in the United States following the introduction of commercial UVB sunscreens occurred during the same period when there was little or no increase in death rates in countries at similar latitudes, such as Japan, Italy and France, where sunscreens were less popular than in the United States. Age-adjusted mortality rates from cutaneous malignancies also have risen steeply during the past two to three decades in Australia and Canada, where use of sunscreens has been intensively promoted (Kurihara *et al.*, 1989).

Epidemiological studies

The medical literature beginning in 1966 was searched using the Medline database (National Library of Medicine, Bethesda, MD, USA). This database includes almost all medical research studies published in the United States and most studies from other countries published since 1 January 1966, and covers virtually all the major epidemiological, dermatological and scientific journals likely to publish articles on the epidemiology of melanoma and other skin malignancies, research on biological and clinical effects of chemical sunscreens, and spectral analyses related to ultra-violet carcinogenesis. No epidemiological studies were identified that showed a protective effect of use of chemical sunscreens on risk of melanoma or other cutaneous malignancies in humans. Odds ratios or relative risks of melanoma and basal-cell carcinoma associated with sunscreen use were all ≥ 1.0 (Table 11.1).

Laboratory studies

It has been assumed that PABA and other common UVB-absorbing sunscreens would prevent skin cancer in humans, based mainly on animal studies and the UVB energy absorption spectrum of DNA which peaks in the UVB (Tan *et al.*, 1970). Experimental studies of sunscreens mainly have used artificial sources of irradiation designed to maximize UVB

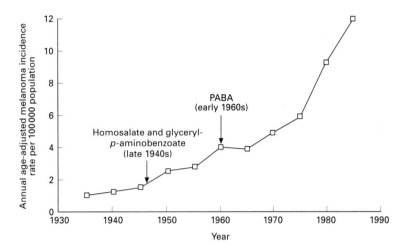

Fig. 11.1 Annual age-adjusted incidence rates of malignant melanoma and dates of introduction of suntan lotions and sunscreens, 1935–85. (Data from J.T. Flannery, Connecticut Tumor Registry, personal communication, 1991.)

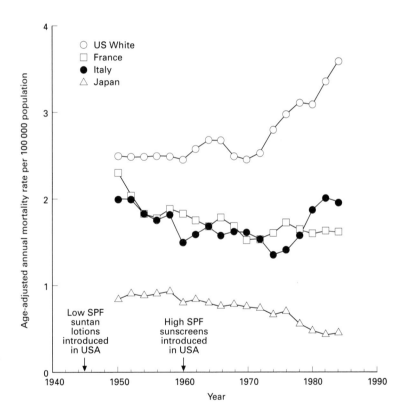

Fig. 11.2 Age-adjusted annual mortality rates for men from skin cancer, including cutaneous malignant melanoma. Data from four countries, 1950–85. SPF, Sun protection factor. (From Kurihara *et al.*, 1989.)

exposures. Most studies have focused exclusively on rodent squamous-cell carcinoma as the outcome, rather than melanoma, as there is no rodent model for melanoma induced solely by sunlight (Pathak *et al.*, 1982).

The association between exposure to particular wavelengths of the ultraviolet spectrum and melanoma recently has been explored (Table 11.2). One found that peak stimulation of melanoma induction in fish occurred in the UVA (maximally at 360–365 nm) (Setlow *et al.*, 1993; Setlow & Woodhead, 1994). Another study found that human melanoma xenografts implanted in rodents grew markedly in response to ultraviolet exposure of the animals from an FS40 source (42% UVA, 58% UVB, 0.5% UVC energy, peak $\lambda = 313$nm), regardless of whether a sunscreen such as *o*-PABA or methoxycinnamate was applied to the skin (Wolf *et al.*, 1994).

No studies were identified that reported reduction in incidence of melanoma in animals for either laboratory model of melanoma, fish (Setlow *et al.*,

1989) or miniature opossum (*Monodelphis domestica*) (Ley *et al.*, 1989).

Spectral aspects of sunlight at ground level, sunscreen absorption and melanoma induction

Spectral data were obtained from standard sources for the terrestrial noon midsummer solar spectrum at 41° North latitude in the United States (Lukiesh, 1946) and for the absorption spectra of commonly used sun-

Table 11.1 Odds ratios or relative risks associated with use of sunscreens in epidemiological studies.

Reference	Location	Type of study	Disease	Sex	Odds ratio or relative risk
Klepp & Magnus (1979)	Oslo	Retrospective	Melanoma	Men	2.8 (1.2–6.7)*
				Women	1.0 (0.4–2.5)**
Graham *et al.* (1985)	Buffalo, NY	Retrospective	Melanoma	Men	2.2 (1.2–4.1)
				Women	1.0**
Holman *et al.* (1986)	Western Australia	Retrospective	Melanoma	Both	1.2 (0.8–1.7)***
Beitner *et al.* (1990)	Stockholm	Retrospective	Melanoma	Both	1.8 (1.2–2.7)†
Hunter *et al.* (1990)	USA	Prospective	Basal-cell carcinoma	Women	1.8 (1.7–1.9)††
Autier *et al.* (1995)	Germany, Belgium, and France	Retrospective	Melanoma	Both	1.5(1.1–2.1)
Westerdahl *et al.* (1995)	Sweden	Retrospective	Melanoma		
			All sites	Both	1.8**
			Trunk	Women	3.7**
			Head, neck, and extremities	Men	3.2**

* 95% confidence intervals was calculated from the data provided.
** 95% confidence interval was not provided.
*** Odds ratio is for 10 years or more duration of use. This odds ratio was adjusted for 'fair pigmentary traits and sensitivity of the skin to sunlight'. According to the authors, 'prior to control of confounding, sunscreen use has been positively associated with all forms of melanoma due to confounding fair pigmentary traits and sensitivity of the skin to sunlight'. The unadjusted odds ratio was not reported.
† Odds ratio for often or very often use of sunscreens was calculated after stratification by age, sex and hair colour. Cases included 240 men and 283 women, with controls matched 1:1 on sex.
†† The relative risk was 1.8 for women who spent ⩾8 hours per week outdoors and used sunscreens, compared to women who also spent ⩾8 hours per week outdoors but did not use sunscreens. There were 377 cases in the 165 784 person-years in women who spent ⩾8 hours per week outdoors without sunscreen; 265 cases in the 65 322 person-years in women who spent ⩾8 hours per week outdoors with sunscreen; and 129 cases in the 42 609 person-years of women who spent <8 hours per week outdoors. Incidence rates used to calculate relative risks were as follows: exposure <8 hours per week outdoors with no sunscreen, 377 cases in 165 784 person-years, i.e. a rate of 227 per 100 000 person-years; exposure ⩾8 hours per week outdoors with sunscreen, 265 cases in 65 322 person-years, i.e. a rate of 406 per 100 000 person-years; exposure <8 hours per week outdoors, 129 in 42 609 person-years, i.e. a rate of 303 per 100 000.

Table 11.2 Experimental studies of ultraviolet radiation and melanoma in animals.

Reference	Animal	Results
Setlow *et al.* (1993)	*Xiphophorus*	Action spectrum for induction of melanoma had peaks at 295 (UVB) and 360 nm (UVA). Only the 360 nm peak is in the terrestrial solar spectrum
Wolf *et al.* (1994)	C3H/HeN mouse	Sunscreens failed to protect against UV radiation-induced increases in melanoma incidence in mice implanted with human melanoma xenografts and irradiated with ultraviolet*

* Sunscreens used were *o*-PABA (8% solution, SPF $\geq$ 8), 2-EHMC (7.5% solution, SPF $\geq$ 8), benzophenone-3 (6% solution, SPF > 4). Incidence was defined as the number of palpable tumours $\geq$ 2 mm divided by the total number of tumour-cell injections.

screens (Sadtler Spectra, 1962). Analysis of the PABA absorption spectrum revealed that PABA absorbed UVB, but provided no absorption in the ultraviolet A (UVA) range, 320–400 nm (Fig. 11.3). The absorption spectra of *o*-PABA and 2-ethylmethoxycinnamate were similar (not shown). Benzophenone-3, another popular compound in sunscreens formulated since 1990, had weaker absorption than PABA in the UVB, and some weak absorption extending into the shorter UVA (not shown).

A possible explanation for the apparent lack of melanoma prevention by sunscreens can be seen when the action spectrum for melanoma induction is convoluted with the terrestrial solar spectrum (Fig. 11.3). This distribution was obtained by multiplying the action spectrum per photon (Setlow *et al.*, 1993) times the terrestrial photon flux for individual wavelengths in the ultraviolet and short visible spectrum (Lukiesh, 1946). Although there is a peak for fish melanoma induction at 295 nm, measurable energy at this and other wavelengths shorter than approximately 300 nm does not occur at sea level due to absorption by the Hartley and Huggins ozone layers (Baker *et al.*, 1982). As a result, UVA and short-wavelength visible energy dominate the terrestrial solar spectrum and, according to the simulation results, may account for more than 95% of melanoma induction (if the data

from fish malignant melanoma can be generalized to human malignant melanoma).

Conclusions

No epidemiological or animal study was identified that supported the assumption that common sunscreens reduce the incidence of melanoma (Tables 11.1 and 11.2). On the contrary, three epidemiological studies found significantly higher risk of melanoma associated with sunscreen use in both sexes combined (Beitner *et al.*, 1990; Autier *et al.*, 1995; Westerdahl *et al.*, 1995), two others reported significantly elevated odds ratios associated with use of sunscreens in men and no favourable association with sunscreen use in women (Klepp & Magnus, 1979; Graham *et al.*, 1985), and one study of a cohort of women reported higher risk of basal-cell carcinoma in women who used sunscreens compared to non-users among women spending $\geq$ 8 hours outdoors. (Hunter *et al.*, 1990). Graham *et al.* (1985) noted that absence of an adverse effect of sunscreens in women might have been a result of more ubiquitous use of sunscreens both by case and control women, regardless of intensity of exposures. If sunlight exposures were less intense in women but sunscreen use was more widespread (despite the less intense exposures) an association of

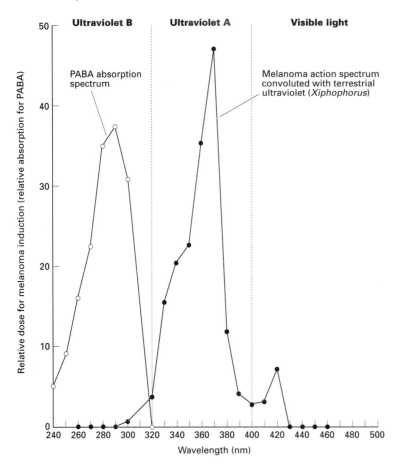

Fig. 11.3 Relative absorption spectrum for *para*-aminobenzoic acid (PABA) sunscreen agent and fish melanoma action spectrum convoluted with terrestrial solar radiation spectrum, midsummer noon, 41° North latitude. If the action spectrum obtained by Setlow *et al.* (1993) from fish is generalizable to humans, the curve suggests that most malignant melanoma is due to ultraviolet A and short-wavelength visible light. [Sources: terrestrial solar radiation (Lukiesh, 1994); PABA action spectrum (Sadtler Spectra, 1962); melanoma (Setlow *et al.*, 1993).]

sunscreens with melanoma use could have been obscured. In the United States, by contrast, women who spent ≥ 8 hours or more per week outdoors and used sunscreens had 1.8-times the incidence rate of basal-cell carcinoma in other women who also spent ≥ 8 hours per week outdoors but did not use sunscreens. It is possible that some of this association represents residual confounding; if so, the study offers no evidence of any protective effect of sunscreen use on risk of basal-cell carcinoma in women.

If the action spectrum for teleost fish melanoma can be generalized to human melanoma, then essentially all melanoma would be due to exposure to wavelengths outside the UVB spectrum. Use of chemical sunscreens that effectively absorb only UVB continues to be recommended for prevention of melanoma and other skin malignancies, despite epidemiological and laboratory data indicating that these chemicals do not

absorb any solar radiation in the parts of the terrestrial solar spectrum most likely to induce malignant melanoma. Fair-skinned individuals who are disproportionately susceptible to melanoma, and who would have been unable to remain for long periods in the sun without sunscreens, may use UVB sunscreens to prolong the skin exposure, preventing accommodation responses by the skin and permitting overexposures.

The findings help to explain some of the paradoxes in the epidemiology of melanoma, particularly its stronger association with skin pigmentation than with latitude. The reason for this is partly that ultraviolet and visible light do not vary with latitude nearly to the extent that UVB varies with latitude. This is to a degree due to the Rayleigh law that states that scattering of light by the atmosphere varies as the fourth power of the reciprocal of the wavelength, λ, making for great increases in scatter with small increases in wavelength (Baker *et al.*, 1982). Some of the energy that is scattered is returned to space. The other reason is that most air contains aerosols that scatter light, mainly sulphate aerosols that scatter UVB more than UVA and short-wavelength visible light. This phenomenon is known as acid haze, and has previously been described (Gorham *et al.*, 1989). Both Rayleigh scatter and aerosol scatter vary exponentially with solar zenith angle (Baker *et al.*, 1982), because low zenith angles are associated with long optical paths through the atmosphere, with more opportunities for photons to be scattered before reaching the ground.

The findings also help to explain why melanoma is more common on the legs of women, which are exposed throughout life to ultraviolet and short-wavelength visible light due to the wearing of skirts. This is true even in women who do not sunbathe. It also helps to explain why melanomas occur rarely on areas of the body that are almost never exposed to light. The addition to sunscreen formulations of relatively weak UVA absorbers such as benzophenone would not be expected to have a great effect on risk of melanoma in the concentrations used (which are necessarily low to reduce the likelihood of irritation).

Arguments against the UVA hypothesis

Latency period

Chemical sunscreens have a history dating to their discovery in 1926. PABA, in particular, was medically advocated for the prevention of sunburn in the *Journal of Investigative Dermatology* in 1942. A popular commercially-promoted tanning lotion containing the ultraviolet absorbing-compound homosalate was introduced by the pharmacist Benjamin Green in 1944 (Packaged Facts, 1988) and glyceryl-*p*-aminobenzoate, a compound related to PABA, soon followed in competitive products. Tanning lotions containing sunscreen compounds were nationally advertised by 1954 (Packaged Facts, 1988) and on billboards by 1958 (Associated Press, 1991). These lotions were promoted mainly as a means of preventing sunburn while allowing tanning, without reference to any role in preventing skin cancer. The assumption implied by advertising of the era appears to have been that reducing the UVB component of sunlight, the lotions

could prevent sunburn and extend by a factor of two to three the duration of exposure without erythema, ostensibly allowing sufficient UVA exposure to permit some degree of tanning as the agents are essentially transparent outside the UVB. The introduction of *para*-aminobenzoic acid sunscreens in 1960 extended the appeal of sunscreens to a wider audience and the agents gained acceptance within a decade as a tool for reducing the incidence of cutaneous malignancies.

Although lotions containing sunscreen compounds had been promoted nationally to the general public since 1954, UVB sunscreens were particularly heavily promoted to physicians, including extensive detailing and sampling programmes, by 1978 (Packaged Facts, 1988). These promotions were followed by introduction of SPF15 formulations in 1980. More than half a century has elapsed since the introduction of the first commercial products containing chemical sunscreens. The median latency period for promotion of cutaneous melanoma in humans has been reported to range from a possible low in the range of 5 years to a possible upper value in the range of 20 years. Mortality rates for skin malignancies in the United States did not rise immediately after introduction of sunscreens (Fig. 11.2), but rather after an appropriate latency period. Increases in incidence earlier are consistent with a short latency period for melanoma. This is logical, as cutaneous melanomas are generally visible on the skin when the tumour mass is smaller than for internal cancers that may have longer latency periods before the mass is clinically evident. The extent that incidence rates were slightly accelerated upward preceding the major rises in age-adjusted incidence rates during the 1960s through to the present may be due to better training of dermatologists and other physicians in detection of the lesions, particularly in the period after the Second World War. Some of the early acceleration in men also might have resulted from unavoidable solar over-exposures while on military duty in regions of high insolation.

Human action spectrum for melanoma compared to fish action spectrum for melanoma

The human action spectrum for melanoma is unknown, and can only be modelled using animals.

However the human spectrum never can be precisely known because humans cannot be subjected to experiments that would be needed to characterize it, even if these were possible. Reliance must instead be placed on temporal trends and epidemiological studies of humans, with some data available from animal models. The research on fish by Setlow *et al.* and on mice by Wolf *et al.* indicate that the relevant chromophore for melanoma promotion apparently is not DNA — at least not directly — since the spectrum does not correspond to that for DNA absorption. In the absence of data on other species, the fish melanoma action spectrum appears to be the most useful model presently available.

Prevention of melanoma

Natural accommodation of the skin to sunlight includes production and oxidation of the pigment eumelanin, which blocks a broad spectrum of energy, including essentially all of the terrestrial ultraviolet and a portion of visible light. Any recommendations concerning sunscreens should at least specify that the sunscreen block transmission to the skin of the entire ultraviolet spectrum and the shorter visible wavelengths, similar to the absorption spectrum of eumelanin. This could be accomplished using compounds that physically scatter or absorb irradiation on the surface of the skin such as various metal oxides which are currently available in a variety of acceptable forms, although some individuals may exhibit sensitivity to these or other compounds placed on the skin, or other as yet undetected negative properties may emerge.

For most individuals, moderate year-round exposure to the sun is desirable to stimulate accommodation and protective pigmentation, as well as for adequate synthesis of vitamin D in the skin. Such moderate year-round exposures would be appropriate for all but those who cannot develop protective pigmentation or who have a history of cutaneous malignancy. Traditional measures for reducing solar overexposures, such as wearing of hats and clothing, would continue to be appropriate for those with unaccommodated skin who must remain in the sun for extended periods.

References

Albert, V., Koh, I.I. Geller, A. *et al.* (1990) Years of potential life lost: another indicator of the impact of cutaneous malignant melanoma on society. *Journal of the American Academy of Dermatology*, **23**, 308–310.

Associated Press (1991) Piece of America Threatened: A Battle is Brewing Over a Proposal to Tear Down a Billboard ... Maintained ... for 33 Years, 1 September 1991.

Autier, P., Dore, J.F., Schifflers, E., *et al.* (1995) Melanoma and uses of sunscreens: an EORTC case-control study in Germany, Belgium and France. *International Journal of Cancer*, **61**, 749–55.

Baker, K. Smith R. & Green, A. (1982) Middle ultraviolet irradiance at the ocean surface: measurements and models. In: *The Role of Solar Ultraviolet in Marine Ecosystems* (ed. J. Calkins), pp. 79–91. Plenum, New York.

Beitner, H., Norell, S., Ringborg, U. *et al.* (1990) Malignant melanoma: aetiological importance of individual pigmentation and sun exposure. *British Journal of Dermatology*, **122**, 43–51.

Garland, F.C., Gorham, E.D. & Garland, C.F. (1988) Sunscreens Increase Risk of Melanoma. Presentation at the National Institutes of Health Consensus Conference, Bethesda, Maryland.

Garland, C., Garland, F. & Gorham, E. (1992) Could sunscreens increase melanoma risk? *American Journal of Public Health*, **82**, 614–615.

Garland, C., Garland, F. & Gorham, E. (1993) Rising trends in melanoma: an hypothesis concerning sunscreen effectiveness. *Animals of Epidemiology*, **3**, 103–110.

Gloeckler-Ries, I. & Hankey, B. (1991) *Cancer Statistics Review 1973–1988* (National Institutes of Health Publication No. 91–2789). National Cancer Institute, Bethesda.

Gorham, E., Garland, C. & Garland, F. (1989) Acid haze air pollution and breast and colon cancer in 20 Canadian cities. *Canadian Journal of Public Health*, **80**, 96–100.

Graham, S., Marshall, J., Haughey, B. *et al.* (1985) An enquiry into the epidemiology of melanoma. *American Journal of Epidemiology*, **122**, 606–619.

Holman, C., Armstrong, B. & Heenan, P. (1986) Relationship of cutaneous malignant melanoma to individual sunlight-exposure habits. *Journal of the National Cancer Institute*, **76**, 403–414.

Houghton, A., Flannery, J. & Viola, M. (1980) Malignant melanoma in Connecticut and Denmark. *International Journal of Cancer*, **25**, 95–104.

Hunter, D., Colditz D., Stampfer, M. *et al.* (1990) Risk factors for basal cell carcinoma in a prospective cohort study of women. *Annals of Epidemiology*, **1**, 13–23.

Klepp, O. & Magnus, K. (1979) Some environmental and bodily characteristics of melanoma patients: a case-control study. *International Journal of Cancer*, **23**, 482–486.

Kurihara, M., Aoki, K. & Hisamachi, S. (1989) *Cancer Mortality Statistics in the World, 1950–1985*, pp. 24–25. University of Nagoya Press, Nagoya.

Ley, R., Applegate, L., Padilla, R. *et al.* (1989) Ultraviolet radiation-induced malignant melanoma in *Monodelphis domestica. Photochemistry and Photobiology*, **50**, 1–5.

Lukiesh, M. (1946) *Germicidal, Erythemal, and Infrared Energy.* Van Nostrand, New York.

Packaged Facts (1988) *Suncare Market, 1988.* Packaged Facts, New York.

Parker, S., Tong, T., Bolden, S. & Wingo, P. (1996) Cancer statistics, 1996. *Cancer Journal for Clinicians*, **46**, 5–27.

Pathak, M., Fitzpatrick, I. & Parrish, J. (1982) Topical and systemic approaches to protection of human skin against harmful effects of solar radiation. In: *The Science of Photomedicine* (eds J. Regan & J. Parrish), pp. 441–473. Plenum, New York.

Sadtler Spectra (1962) *Para-aminobenzoic acid (PABA) Ultraviolet Absorption Spectrum.*

Setlow, R. & Woodhead, A. (1994) Temporal changes in the incidence of malignant melanoma: explanation from action spectra. *Mutation Research*, **307**, 365–374.

Setlow, R., Woodhead, A. & Grist, E. (1989) Animal model for ultraviolet-radiation-induced melanoma: Platyfish–swordtail hybrid. *Proceedings of the National Academy of Science USA*, **86**, 8922–8926.

Setlow, R., Grist, E., Thompson, K. & Woodhead, A. (1993) Wavelengths effective in induction of malignant melanoma. *Proceedings of the National Academy of Science USA*, **90**, 6666–6670.

Tan, E.M., Freeman, R.G. & Stoughton, R.B. (1970) Action spectrum of ultraviolet light-induced damage to nuclear DNA *in vivo. Journal of Investigative Dermatology*, **55**, 439–43.

Westerdahl, J., Olsson, H., Masback, A., *et al.* (1995) Is the use of sunscreens a risk factor for malignant melanoma? *Melanoma Research*, **5**, 59–65.

Wolf, P., Donawho, C. & Kripke M. (1994) Effect of sunscreens on UV radiation-induced enhancement of melanoma growth in mice. *Journal of the National Cancer Institute*, **86**, 99–105.

The Role of Sunscreen Lotions in Melanoma Prevention

M.A. WEINSTOCK

Sun exposure is a cause of melanoma (Elwood, 1992; Armstrong & Kricker, 1995). Furthermore, among the known avoidable causes of melanoma, it is the one associated with the greatest attributable risk. Variations in sun exposure are estimated to account for the majority of melanomas worldwide (Armstrong & Kricker, 1993). These observations present great opportunities for the primary prevention of melanoma, but also present substantial practical problems.

Efforts at primary prevention of melanoma by individuals generally focus on simple sun avoidance, use of sun-protective clothing and use of sunscreen lotions. Sun avoidance is simple, but imposes a substantial burden on individuals by limiting many healthy, enjoyable or otherwise important activities. Furthermore, it may have the hazard of encouraging physical inactivity, which is likely to increase the risk of cardiovascular disease and result in numerous other adverse health effects. Use of sun-protective clothing outdoors is an important strategy, but is sometimes viewed as inconvenient, unfashionable or uncomfortable. Hence the mainstay of sun-protection practices for many individuals has involved the use of sunscreen lotions, despite the expense and bother of their application.

For this reason, the effectiveness of sunscreen use for melanoma prevention remains a particularly important, although controversial issue (Urbach, 1992/93; Garland *et al.*, 1993; Roberts & Stanfield, 1995; Westerdahl *et al.*, 1995b; McGregor & Young, 1996).

Transmission spectra of sunscreens

Sunscreens are primarily marketed and used for the prevention of sun-induced injuries to the skin, of which sunburn is among the most common and painful in the short term. The efficacy of sunscreening agents for sunburn is primarily determined by their effectiveness in blocking ultraviolet B (UVB) and, to a lesser extent, the short-wavelength UVA radiation. There are four types of active agents in common sunscreens: UVB blocks (of which *para*-aminobenzoic acid (PABA) is the best known, although no longer commonly used), short-wavelength UVA blocks (e.g. benzophenones), broader spectrum UVA blocks (e.g. avobenzone) and physical blocks, such as titanium dioxide, which block fairly uniformly throughout the UVB and UVA spectrum. Hence, the transmission of specific wavelengths of UV through sunscreens depends not only on the sun-protection factor (SPF), but also on the specific ingredients.

Action spectrum

The key to understanding the effectiveness of sunscreen use in melanoma prevention is the action spectrum for melanoma, i.e. the relative efficiency of each wavelength of ultraviolet radiation in the genesis of melanoma. Unfortunately, the action spectrum for melanoma in humans is unknown, because the experiments required to define it would be neither practical nor ethical. Hence our inferences must rely on other action spectra that are known.

For disorders of the skin among humans, the action spectrum that has been studied in greatest detail relates to sunburn (the 'erythema action spectrum') (McKinlay & Diffey, 1987). UVB radiation is much more effective in sunburn production than UVA. The advantage for using this action spectrum as a model for melanoma is that sunburns have been repeatedly and consistently linked to melanoma risk in epidemiological data (Weinstock *et al.*, 1989; Marks & Whiteman, 1994; Whiteman & Green, 1994), and that this action spectrum has actually been determined in human beings. However, sunburn is not melanoma, or even neoplasia, so we must examine animal models.

There are no mammalian models of melanoma genesis for which an action spectrum has been determined. However, there is an excellent rodent model for cutaneous carcinogenesis in which ultraviolet radiation causes squamous-cell carcinoma of the skin. The action spectrum for this model is essentially identical to the action spectrum for erythema in humans; UVB is a much more potent inducer of squamous-cell carcinoma than UVA (de Gruijl *et al.*, 1993; de Gruijl & van der Leun, 1994).

The only known action spectrum for an animal model for melanoma relies on experiments with platyfish–swordtail hybrids that have a high frequency of spontaneous melanoma (Setlow *et al.*, 1989). These fish are phylogenetically quite distant from humans, and their melanomas have certain characteristics that may not resemble the human situation, e.g. the hybrids are heavily pigmented and are particularly susceptible to melanoma, and they develop melanomas after induction by a single, relatively small ultraviolet exposure. The data pertaining to the action spectrum for melanoma induction among these fish are displayed in Table 11.3.

For this action spectrum, UVA is more important than UVB, and visible light is also effective in the induction of melanoma. The substantial difference between control groups was apparently due to the different lighting conditions under which they were raised: the first receiving some ambient light in a shaded greenhouse, the second receiving only subdued yellow light. While this model may be helpful in elucidating aspects of the mechanism of melanoma genesis, its usefulness for understanding the human melanoma action spectrum is uncertain (Setlow *et al.*, 1993).

Action spectra for other biological phenomena have been studied, but are less directly relevant to human melanoma.

Human melanoma has been studied for possible association with tanning-booth and sunlamp exposure. Some of these studies have found a direct dose–response relation, but others have not (Weinstock, 1996) (see Chapter 8, pp. 90–95). These studies are of limited assistance in the determination of the action spectrum for melanoma, however, because all are limited by their inability to characterize the wavelengths of ultra-violet to which study participants had been exposed. Some lamps or booths may emit predominantly UVA and others UVB.

The xeroderma pigmentosum model

The rare genetic disease xeroderma pigmentosum may be the most useful human model for understanding the genesis of melanoma (Weinstock, 1992). Patients afflicted by this disorder have specific, well-described defects in DNA repair of UVB-induced pyrimidine dimers. They are particularly susceptible to sunburn and develop sun-induced skin cancers (including melanoma, basal-cell carcinoma and squamous-cell carcinoma) in extraordinarily high numbers at extra-ordinarily early ages. Their melanoma risk is several thousandfold greater than among unaffected individuals, although the distribution by anatomic site is similar (Kraemer *et al.*, 1994). Our understanding of this rare disorder suggests but does not prove that melanoma may be primarily induced by UVB radiation in the general population.

Theoretical effect of sunscreen use on melanoma risk

Regardless of the action spectrum for melanoma, the effectiveness of sunscreen use will depend on how the sunscreens are actually used. If their use does not affect other sun-exposure behaviour (e.g. amount of time spent in the sun), then their use will substantially decrease exposure of the skin to an important portion of the ultraviolet spectrum, and therefore most likely lead to a substantial reduction in melanoma risk. However, one can formulate an alternative hypothesis that individuals will compensate for sunscreen use by increasing their time in the sun or decreasing their use of protective clothing. (Garland *et al.*, 1993). The most extreme form of this 'compensation' hypothesis posits that people expose themselves to the sun until they reach a certain multiple of their minimal erythema dose (such as the dose required for a painful sunburn). Hence if they use a sun-protection factor (SPF) 15 sunscreen, they will expose themselves to 15-fold as much solar

Table 11.3 Melanoma frequency among platyfish–swordtail hybrids after exposure to various wavelengths of light. (From Setlow *et al.*, 1993.)

Wavelength (nm)	Number of fish exposed	Number with melanoma	Percentage with melanoma
Control	124	30	24
302	123	37	30
313	124	46	37
365	85	38	45
Control	20	1	5
405	61	18	30
436	21	5	24

ultraviolet by staying out in the sun longer or using less physical sun protection. Under this hypothesis, those individuals who use a sunscreen with little UVA protection will actually increase their exposure to longer wavelength UVA by using sunscreen. If we further suppose that the long-wavelength UVA radiation is relatively effective in the genesis of melanoma, it is theoretically possible that sunscreen use could increase melanoma risk. Of course, it is quite unlikely that compensation could be complete under realistic circumstances with high SPF sunscreens, since the amount of sunlight available for generating mela-noma is limited, and sunburn is only one of many factors that influences behaviour in the sun.

If melanoma is induced with greater relative efficiency by longer wavelengths in the UV spectrum, then other advice commonly given to the general public may need to be modified. For example, the common recommendation to minimize sun exposure during the hours around solar noon, if followed, will result in a relative increase in exposure to longer wavelengths of ultraviolet radiation, hence functions in a similar manner to many sunscreens. Under the complete compensation hypothesis, an increase in exposure to long-wavelength UVA will result, and hence an increase in melanoma risk.

A further caution regarding the impact of sunscreen use is its effect on the intermittency of ultraviolet exposure to the skin. If sun exposure increases this intermittency because of inconsistent use or missed areas of skin coverage, melanoma risk could be adversely effected. On the other hand, if sunscreens are preferentially used at times of the most intense sun exposures, intermittency may be reduced, with a consequent reduction of melanoma risk. As our understanding of the role of ultraviolet in melanoma incidence improves, we may find the effect of sunscreens on melanoma risk depends on many variables other than the transmission spectrum and the mere fact that the sunscreen is applied.

Epidemiological evidence

For actinic keratoses, the major precursor of squamous-cell carcinoma of the skin, the efficacy of SPF 17 and 29 sunscreens that protect primarily at the UVB and shorter

UVA wavelengths has been demonstrated in randomized trials (Thompson *et al.*, 1993; Naylor *et al.*, 1995). No similar trials have been conducted for melanoma.

Attempts to correlate trends in sunscreen use with melanoma incidence are fraught with difficulty. Until the 1970s, the United States Food and Drug Administration would only allow sunscreens to be promoted for suntanning, and not for avoidance of sunburn or other beneficial health effects (Jass, 1990). Furthermore, until recently, most sun-care products offered relatively little protection. The first year in which sales of sunscreening products (SPF ≥ 5) exceeded those of suntanning products (SPF < 5) was 1987, when sunscreen sales reached approximately $126 million (Jass, 1990). Compared to the United States population of over 200 million, even this level of sales can be expected to have a limited impact on melanoma incidence. In addition, the latent period for melanoma would delay the appearance of any potential effect of these sales on overall population rates, so it may not be noticeable for decades.

Studies of either sunscreens or suntan lotion have been published; some have noted a direct association with melanoma risk (Klepp & Magnus, 1979; Graham *et al.*, 1985; Beitner *et al.*, 1990; Herzfeld *et al.*, 1993; Autier *et al.*, 1995; Westerdahl *et al.*, 1955a), others have noted no association (Klepp & Magnus, 1979; Graham *et al.*, 1985; Holman *et al.*, 1986), and yet another recent study noted an inverse association (Holly *et al.*, 1995). These studies did not include detailed sunscreen use histories, and some are based on single questions regarding 'sun lotions' or even 'suntanning lotions', so the nature of the exposure was not well-defined. The only cohort study of sunscreen use in relation to risk of skin cancer published to date reported that among women who spent at least 8 hours per week outdoors during the summer, sunscreen use was associated with risk of both basal-cell carcinoma and squamous-cell carcinoma after adjusting for age, sun sensitivity and sunburn history (Hunter *et al.*, 1990; Grodskin *et al.*, 1995). The sun exposure and sunscreen history available in this study was quite limited, and the results must be interpreted in light of the well-established action spectrum for squamous-cell carcinoma and well-established efficacy of sunscreens for the prevention of squamous-cell carcinoma precursor lesions described above.

Ultimately, we will rely on epidemiological evidence to verify the effect of changing sunscreen use patterns on melanoma risk. However, epidemiological studies have not been particularly informative to date on this particular point for the following reasons: (a) the most important effects of sun exposure on melanoma risk occur in childhood and early adult years; (b) high SPF sunscreens have only quite recently enjoyed widespread use; (c) recall regarding use in the distant past, particularly at ages when parents are responsible for purchase and application of the lotions, is of limited accuracy; and (d) there are severe potential problems with confounding by sun sensitivity and socio-economic status, both of which are strong risk factors for melanoma and correlates of sunscreen use. In addition, in some countries sunscreens are available that contain psoralen compounds, which are known cutaneous carcinogens.

Conclusion

The effect of sunscreen use on melanoma risk has not yet been established, and may indeed be more complex than is generally appreciated. Present evidence suggests that sunscreens are effective for prevention of melanoma, but several areas of uncertainty must be resolved before this conclusion can be considered established. It would therefore be prudent to recommend to the general public that sunscreens not be used to increase exposure to the sun, that consistent use is preferable, and that broad-spectrum sunscreens are preferable to those that primarily protect against the UVB portion of the spectrum.

Acknowledgements

Dr Barry Rosenstein is thanked for his comments. The author is supported by grants AR43051 and CA50087 from the National Institutes of Health and by the Office of Research and Development, Department of Veterans Affairs.

References

Armstrong, B.K. & Kricker, A. (1933) How much melanoma is caused by sun exposure? *Melanoma Research,* **3**, 395–401.
Armstrong, B.K. & Kricker, A. (1995) Skin cancer, In: *Dermatoepidemiology* (ed. M.A. Weinstock), pp. 583–594.

W.B. Saunders, Philadelphia. (Theirs, B.H. (ed.) *Dermatologic Clinics* **13**(3)).

Autier, P., Doré, J.-F., Schifflers, E. *et al.* (1995) Melanoma and use of sunscreens: an EORTC case-control study in Germany, Belgium and France. *International Journal of Cancer*, **61**, 749–755.

Beitner, H., Norell, S.E., Ringborg, U., Wennersten, G. & Mattson, B. (1990) Malignant melanoma: aetiological importance of individual pigmentation and sun exposure. *British Journal of Dermatology*, **122**, 43–51.

de Gruijl, F.R. & van der Leun, J.C. (1994) Estimate of the wavelength dependency of ultraviolet carcinogenesis in humans and its relevance to the risk assessment of a stratospheric ozone depletion. *Health Physics*, **67**, 319–325.

de Gruijl, F.R., Sterenborg, H.J.C.M., Forbes P.D. *et al.* (1993) Wavelength dependence of skin cancer induction by ultraviolet irradiation of albino hairless mice. *Cancer Research*, **53**, 53–60.

Elwood, J.M. (1992) Melanoma and sun exposure: contrasts between intermittent and chronic exposure. *World Journal of Surgery*, **16**, 157–166.

Garland, C.F., Garland, F.C. & Gorham, E.D. (1993) Rising trends in melanoma: an hypothesis concerning sunscreen effectiveness. *Annals of Epidemiology*, **3**, 103–110.

Graham, S., Marshall, J., Haughey, B. *et al.* (1985) An inquiry into the epidemiology of melanoma. *American Journal of Epidemiology*, **122**, 606–619.

Grodstein, F., Speizer, F.E. & Hunter, D.J. (1995). A prospective study of incident squamous cell carcinoma of the skin in the Nurses' Health Study. *Journal of the National Cancer Institute*, **87**, 1061–1066.

Herzfeld, P.M., Fitzgerald, E.F., Hwang, S.-A. & Stark, A. (1993) A case-control study of malignant melanoma of the trunk among white males in upstate New York. *Cancer Detection Prevention*, **17**, 601–608.

Holly, E.A., Aston, D.A., Cress, R.D., Ahn, D.K. & Kristiansen J.J. (1995) Cutaneous melanoma in women: I. Exposure to sunlight, ability to tan, and other risk factors related to ultraviolet light. *American Journal of Epidemiology*, **141**, 923–933.

Holman, C.D.J., Armstrong, B.K. & Heenan, P.J. (1986) Relationship of cutaneous malignant melanoma to individual sunlight-exposure habits. *Journal of the National Cancer Institute*, **76**, 403–414.

Hunter, D.J., Colditz, G.A., Stampfer, M.J., Rosner, B., Willett, W.C. & Speizer, F.E. (1990) Risk factors for basal cell carcinoma in a prospective cohort of women. *Annals of Epidemiology*, **1**, 13–23.

Jass, H.E. (1990) The sunscreen industry in the United States: past, present, and future. In: *Sunscreens: Development, Evaluation, and Regulatory Aspects* (eds N.J. Lowe & N.A. Shaath), pp. 149–159. Marcel Dekker, New York.

Klepp, O. & Magnus, K. (1979) Some environmental and bodily characteristics of melanoma patients. A case-control study. *International Journal of Cancer*, **23**, 482–486.

Kraemer, K.H., Lee, M.-M., Andrews, A.D. & Lambert, W.C. (1994) The role of sunlight and DNA repair in melanoma and nonmelanoma skin cancer: the xeroderma pigmentosum paradigm. *Archives of Dermatology*, **130**, 1018–1021.

Marks, R. & Whiteman, D. (1994) Sunburn and melanoma: how strong is the evidence? *British Medical Journal*, **308**, 75–76.

McGregor, J.M. & Young, A.R. (1996) Sunscreens, suntans, and skin cancer. *British Medical Journal*, **312**, 1621–1622.

McKinlay, A.F. & Diffey, B.L. (1987) A reference spectrum for ultra-violet induced erythema in human skin. In: *Human Exposure to Ultraviolet Radiation: Risks and Regulations* (eds W.F. Passchier & B.F.M. Bosnjakovic), pp. 83–87. Elsevier Science Publishers, Amsterdam.

Naylor, M.F., Boyd, A., Smith, D.W., Cameron, G.S., Hubbard, D. & Neldner, K.H. (1995) High sun protection factor sunscreens in the suppression of actinic neoplasia. *Archives of Dermatology*, **131**, 170–175.

Roberts, L.K. & Stanfield, J.W. (1995) Suggestion that sunscreen use is a melanoma risk factor is based on inconclusive evidence. *Melanoma Research*, **5**, 377–378.

Setlow, R.B., Woodhead, A.D. & Grist, E. (1989) Animal model for ultraviolet radiation-induced melanoma: platyfish–swordtail hybrid. *Proceedings of the National Academy of Science USA*, **86**, 8922–8926.

Setlow, R.B., Grist, E., Thompson, K. & Woodhead, A.D. (1993) Wavelengths effective in induction of malignant melanoma. *Proceedings of the National Academy of Science USA*, **90**, 6666–6670.

Thompson, S.C., Jolley, D. & Marks, R. (1993) Reduction of solar keratoses by regular sunscreen use. *New England Journal of Medicine*, **329**, 1147–1151.

Urbach, F. (1992/93) Ultraviolet A transmission by modern sunscreens: is there a real risk? *Photodermatology Photoimmunology, Photomedicine*, **9**, 237–241.

Weinstock, M.A. (1992) Human models of melanoma. *Clinical Dermatology*, **10**, 83–89.

Weinstock, M.A. (1996) Controversies in the role of sunlight in the pathogenesis of cutaneous melanoma. *Photochemistry and Photobiology*, **63**, 406–410.

Weinstock, M.A., Colditz, G.A., Willett W.C. *et al.* (1989) Nonfamilial cutaneous melanoma incidence in women associated with sun exposure before 20 years of age. *Pediatrics*, **84**, 199–204.

Westerdahl, J., Olsson, H., Måsbäck, A., Ingvar, C. & Jonsson, N. (1995a) Is the use of sunscreens a risk factor for malignant melanoma? *Melanoma Research*, **5**, 59–65.

Westerdahl, J., Olsson, H. & Ingvar, C. (1995b) The authors' reply. *Melanoma Research*, **5**, 378–379.

Whiteman, D. & Green, A. (1994) Melanoma and sunburn. *Cancer Causes and Contributions*, **5**, 564–572.

Identification and Follow-Up of Populations at High Risk of Developing Melanoma

R.M. MACKIE

Identification of individuals at increased risk of developing melanoma

At present the annual incidence of melanoma ranges from around 10 new cases per 100000 in Europe and North America (Mackie *et al.*, 1992) to over 30 per 100000 in tropical Australian states (MacLennan *et al.*, 1992). Individuals at increased risk should therefore be related to the local risk for the general population. Significantly increased risk may be arbitrarily defined as a risk tenfold greater than that of the local general population, but in some well-recognized situations the level of risk can be over 100-fold. In the individuals at recognized but less dramatically increased risk (for example, tenfold), this risk should be considered in proportion to other commoner cancers. Thus a female with a tenfold increased risk of developing melanoma in the UK will still have a greater annual chance of developing breast cancer. Recommendation of appropriate surveillance measures should take this into account.

Three groups at greatly increased risk of developing melanoma are rare patients with xeroderma pigmentosum, individuals with a positive family history of melanoma and multiple atypical naevi and those who have already had one primary melanoma. In all of these groups, the risk is increased by over 100-fold by comparison with normal individuals, and there is therefore a strong case for regular expert surveillance.

Other well-recognized risk factors for melanoma include large numbers of banal naevi, the presence of large clinically atypical naevi, the presence of freckles, a past history of severe blistering sunburns and a childhood spent in a high ultraviolet environment. An algorithm can be designed to combine these risk factors to give a quantitative estimate of increased risk (MacKie *et al.*, 1989). Individuals with any one of these risk factors are not at greatly increased risk of melanoma but combinations can be used as illustrated

in Fig. 11.4 to select the specific individuals who merit surveillance.

Appropriate follow-up arrangements

Once the population at recognized increased risk of developing melanoma has been identified, appropriate follow-up arrangements, including patient education and advice, must be considered. The usual instrument in papers looking at follow-up is clinical examination coupled, if deemed necessary by the clinician, with biopsy and pathological examination. Although studies in both the USA (Rigel *et al.*, 1989) and Scotland (MacKie *et al.*, 1993) have shown that surveillance by trained dermatologists does lead over 2–5 years to excision of a higher than expected number of thin good prognosis melanomas, no study has yet definitively proved that this type of surveillance saves lives.

Dermatologist surveillance, possibly for life, is time consuming and expensive to any health-care system. A very useful study would be a three-arm randomized trial of dermatologist surveillance compared with primary-care surveillance compared with patient self-inspection to establish whether or not high-risk individuals and their families can be shown how to recognize potentially serious pigmented lesions and take appropriate action. It would also establish the part which should be played by the primary care team in countries where this option is available. This type of assessment coupled with an economic evaluation of the different approaches would be extremely valuable.

In the case of individuals at slightly increased melanoma risk, a current reasonable approach is to show these individuals and their families full-colour illustrations of benign non-serious pigmented lesions such as seborrhoeic keratoses and also pictures of early melanoma. Specific booklets and charts are available and the families should keep them for reference. At-risk individuals should then be examined by an expert and body-mole maps prepared, indicating the site of benign pigmented lesions on their skin. In some centres, pigmented lesions will also be photographed. For this within-family approach to surveillance, it is highly desirable that a family member or friend is present at the consultation. It is very difficult, if not impossible, for individuals to check their own backs.

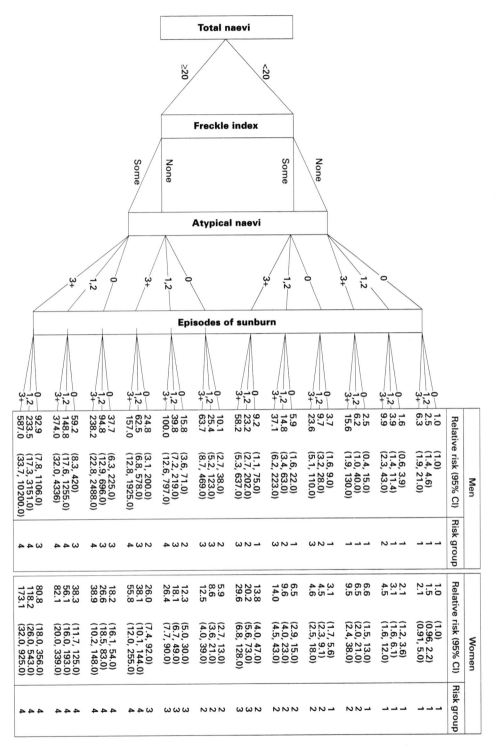

Fig. 11.4 Flow-chart of risk factors for cutaneous malignant melanoma. Risk groups: 1, low risk; 2, average risk; 3, increased risk; 4, worryingly high risk. Relative risk coefficients used (for men/women, respectively): 10:1/5:9 for total naevi; 3:7/3:1 for freckles; 1:6/2:1 for atypical naevi; and 2:5/1:5 for episodes of sunburn.

Families asked to self-survey in this way should be advised that a monthly review of their skin is adequate. Many centres will also give patients and their families a set of baseline photographs for comparison. They must also, however, have rapid access to a specialist centre for expert consultation and treatment if they consider that there is any change in their pigmented lesion pattern.

It is suggested that this type of approach, possibly with an additional annual expert clinical examination, may constitute adequate follow up for those at moderately increased melanoma risk, while more frequent expert review is indicated for the higher risk group with xeroderma pigmentosum, multiple naevi and a family history of melanoma, and a past primary melanoma.

Timing of repeat examinations

The optimal interval between examinations has not been established in any of these groups. For an individual with an apparently unstable and changing naevus pattern, three-monthly review may be indicated, while for a patient with a more stable pattern, six-monthly intervals may be more appropriate. At these reviews, the patient's skin should be examined completely in good light in a warm room, and previous photographs used for comparison if available.

The need for ophthalmological review

In the past some groups have advocated additional regular full ophthalmological examination because of the additional increased risk of ocular melanoma in some patients with multiple naevi. At present, very few centres carry out routine ophthalmological surveillance on the grounds of a low yield of ocular problems, of increased cost and of creating unnecessary anxiety.

Conclusion

The surveillance patterns suggested above all require to be audited to establish their efficacy in recognizing very early treatable melanoma and in time in preventing unnecessary melanoma mortality. The economic cost to both the health-care system and to the individual also require to be evaluated.

References

MacKie, R.M., Freudenberger, T. & Aitchison, T.C. (1989) Personal risk factor chart for cutaneous melanoma. *Lancet*, **ii**, 487–490.

MacKie, R.M., Hunter, J.A. Aitchison, T.C. *et al.* (1992) Cutaneous malignant melanoma in Scotland 1979–89. *Lancet*, **339**, 971–975.

MacKie, R.M., McHenry, P. & Hole, D. (1993) Accelerated detection with prospective surveillance for cutaneous malignant melanoma in high risk groups. *Lancet*, **341**, 1618–1620.

MacLennan, R., Green, A., Martin, N. & McLeod, R. (1992) Increasing incidence of cutaneous melanoma in Queensland. *Journal of the National Cancer Institute*, **84**, 1427–1432.

Rigel, D., Rivers, J.K., Kopf, A.W. *et al.* (1989) Dysplastic naevi, markers for increased risk of melanoma. *Cancer*, **63**, 386–389.

Screening for Melanoma: Methods, Advantages and Limits

F.H.J. RAMPEN AND M.J.M. DE ROOIJ

Incidence and mortality rates of cutaneous melanoma have been rising rapidly during the last few decades. Until recently, prediction of increased rates of melanoma in the near future were based on the belief that the incidence will continue to rise at a rate of >4% annually. Therefore, in recent years, public health bodies and the medical profession have been contemplating and initiating educational programmes directed at primary prevention and early detection.

Currently, screening programmes for skin cancer and melanoma are increasing in number. Screening is thought to be an easy means of secondary prevention. There is the compelling intuitive appeal on the assumption that detection of early stage melanoma will be rewarding. However, screening for cancer is not always simple. This also applies to melanoma and skin cancer. Some critical features relevant to screening for skin cancer in general and melanoma in particular are reviewed here.

Basic principles

The basic principles of screening for disease have been outlined by Wilson and Jungner (1968). These authors distinguished ten prerequisites for a worthwhile screening programme. They presented their criteria for strictly defined large-scale population screenings. However, the same criteria can also be used for selective screening exercises such as skin cancer and melanoma screening based on self-selection. The value of the Wilson and Jungner principles has been critically analysed previously with reference to the skin cancer and melanoma setting (Rampen *et al.*, 1992b). Here we will briefly review this issue.

The condition sought should be an important health problem. Skin cancer is very common, especially in countries with a predominantly white population. In the United States, > 500 000 new non-melanoma skin cancers and approximately 32 000 new melanomas are diagnosed annually (Boring *et al.*, 1994). Melanoma is more common than cervical cancer and leukaemia.

Case fatality rates for non-melanoma skin cancers are low. However, mortality rates are increasing (Glass & Hoover, 1989). About 20% of melanoma patients will eventually die from their disease. Annual mortality from melanoma in the United States is now 6900 (Boring *et al.*, 1994).

The rising incidence of melanoma is worrying. It is one of the principal reasons for the recent emergence of screening exercises. It is worthy of note, however, that levelling off of mortality rates with the more recent birth cohorts has been reported (Scotto *et al.*, 1991). In The Netherlands, no increase of melanoma incidence has been observed in the period 1989–92 (Visser *et al.*, 1995).

There should be an accepted treatment for patients with recognized disease. Treatment for all types of skin cancer, including melanoma, is safe, inexpensive and effective. Management of precursor lesions such as actinic keratoses, and congenital and dysplastic naevi, is more controversial (JAMA, 1984; Marks *et al.*, 1988; Rhodes, 1989).

Facilities for diagnosis and treatment should be available. Most types of skin cancer and melanoma can be managed by simple office procedures that are readily available. In rare instances, hospital admission or referral to a specialized centre is required. It needs emphasizing here that screening for other cancers

is a continuous process; the workload generated by such campaigns is spread over the year. Screening for skin cancer and melanoma so far has involved single-occasion or once-a-year affairs with steep increases in referrals immediately after the campaigns. This may have a marked effect on workload and biopsy rate, especially in countries with a low dermatologist-to-patient ratio (Melia *et al.*, 1995). We found that the extra workload for the general practitioner generated by a skin cancer and melanoma screening clinic was negligible (Rampen *et al.*, 1993).

There should be a recognizable latent or early symptomatic stage. Melanomas and non-melanoma skin cancers have recognizable early stages. Precursor lesions are also easily detectable.

There should be a suitable test or examination. Screening for skin cancer means visual inspection of the skin by, preferably, a dermatologist. Visual examination of skin lesions by the dermatologist constitutes a most reliable screening tool. Koh *et al.* (1990) estimated the validity of a visual examination by dermatologists in a screening setting from 89% sensitivity for squamous-cell carcinoma to 94% for basal-cell carcinoma and 97% for melanoma. In an earlier report we found that the positive predictive value for skin cancer and melanoma in two screening campaigns was 50–60% (Rampen *et al.*, 1991).

Few data are available on the accuracy of visual examination by dermatologists as a screening tool because of the lack of false-negative findings. Sensitivity and specificity of the screening test can only be derived from true-negative and false-negative findings. We obtained follow-up information on 1551 persons with a negative screening result; 15 persons had new skin cancers, three of which had probably been present at the original screening and had been missed (Rampen *et al.*, 1995). The calculated sensitivity of this screening was 93.3%; its specificity was 97.8%.

The accuracy of clinical examination of the skin differs with the observer. In this respect dermatologists score distinctly better than non-dermatologists (Cassileth *et al.*, 1986; Rampen & Rümke, 1988).

The test should be acceptable to the population. A visual examination of skin lesions is painless, non-invasive and has no side effects. Its acceptance to the screenee is high. Full-skin inspection may be embarrassing. However, sufficient data are available confirming the high acceptance of total skin examination (Table 11.4). This applies to patients seen in dermatological practice as well as to persons seen during screening activities. Inconvenience and concern about privacy and modesty seem to be of trivial importance for most patients and screenees, and should not be a barrier to total skin checks.

The natural history of the condition, including development from latent to declared disease, should be adequately understood. Early melanomas, i.e. melanomas with a predominantly radial growth phase, and favourable microstages according to Clark and Breslow, have a good prognosis (Clark *et al.*, 1969; Breslow, 1970). These early stages may last months or even years. Melanoma can be detected far before manifestation of metastatic spread. Accurate prognostication of outcome is possible.

Precursor lesions progress to frank skin cancer very slowly. The lifetime risk of developing melanoma from atypical (dysplastic) naevi ranges from 5 to 100%, according to the personal and family histories of dysplastic naevi or melanoma (Greene *et al.*, 1985). The potential of malignant transformation of congenital naevi is relatively small (Rhodes *et al.*, 1982; Illig *et al.*, 1985). Actinic keratoses evolve into invasive squamous-cell carcinoma only rarely (Marks *et al.*, 1986). The exact value of screening for premalignant skin lesions is subject to controversy. It should be considered that screening tests and programmes indicate that, although some degree of control of skin cancer and melanoma may be achieved at reasonable costs, the costs of higher degrees of control (precursor states) will be disproportionately more.

There should be an agreed policy on whom to treat. In our view, screening must focus on melanoma only (de Rooij *et al.*, 1995). Screening concentrating on melanoma increases the rates of lesions suggestive of melanoma and dysplastic naevi, whereas the proportions of non-melanoma skin cancers and actinic keratoses decrease.

Without doubt, any type of invasive skin cancer detected through screening must be treated appropriately. Whether all precursor lesions discovered at screening should be treated or not, remains debatable. 'Borderline' cases (minor actinic keratoses, vague evidence of dysplastic naevi, small congenital naevi) are preferably left untreated. Depending on definitions and criteria used, the 'borderline' group may be larger than the 'diseased' group, which may disproportionately burden upon the cost-effectiveness of screening.

The cost of screening, including diagnosis and treatment of positive screenees, should be economically balanced in relation to possible expenditures on medical care as a whole. Screening for skin cancer and melanoma is inexpensive. However, the expenditures generated by the screening itself are not final costs. There are many hidden costs such as the follow-up and treatment of positive screenees, and the management of persons who do not wish to attend the screening itself but visit their own family physician or dermatologist. On the whole, however, total costs of screening for skin cancer and melanoma are regarded as relatively cheap in comparison with the costs of similar procedures for other types of cancer.

Screening should be a continuing process and not a single-occasion project. Periodic skin checks have been advocated since 1985 by the American Academy of Dermatology on a nationwide and voluntary basis (Koh *et al.*, 1989). Periodic screening has the advantage

Table 11.4 Patient acceptance of total skin examination.

Reference	Study population	Subjects (*n*)	Acceptance (%)
Boyce & Bernhard (1986)	Office patients	182	94
Rigel *et al.* (1986)	Screening	2239	62
Lookingbill (1988)	New office patients	1157	96
Chiarello (1989)	Office patients	1028	85
Bolognia *et al.* (1990)	Screening	251	98
Lee *et al.* (1991)	New office patients	874	81
de Rooij *et al.* (1996)	Screening	1385	98

of covering more and more of the population at risk. There are no useful data on the ideal frequency of skin cancer and melanoma screening.

Melanoma fulfils, for the most part, all the criteria for screening for disease enunciated by Wilson and Jungner in 1968. For non-melanoma skin cancer the fulfilment of these basic requirements is less clear.

Obvious as the integrity of the screening process for melanoma may sound, a comprehensive and scientifically respectable assessment of its value is not available. Screening has many potential benefits, but also disadvantages (Chamberlain, 1984). The benefits are clear. Some cases detected during screening will have an improved prognosis because of early intervention. Less radical treatment is necessary. This may save health-care resources. Many individuals with negative test results can be reassured and will refrain from seeking medical care. Also this may save costs. Precampaign publicity may elicit changes in knowledge and attitude about skin cancer and melanoma in the target population, with definite primary and secondary prevention effects.

The disadvantages of screening are numerous. There is the longer morbidity of patients whose prognosis is unaltered. The resource costs may be substantial, in terms of the screening itself, the organization and manpower, and the subsequent management and evaluation of positive screenees, including those with precursor lesions and 'borderline' cases. There is the dangerous fallacy of the assumption that if one is screened, all is well: absence of evidence is not evidence of absence of disease. Some persons with false-negative screen results will be given unfounded reassurance, which may occasion undue patient delays. On the other hand, those with false-positive results will be offered unnecessary surgery and, inevitably, many persons with minor or questionable disease will also be unnecessarily treated. Finally, there is the question of needless anxiety in the community in general, and in the screened population in particular.

Feasibility of screening

There are several screening procedures for skin cancer and melanoma. In the 1970s, a number of limited screenings for skin cancer were conducted in the United States at trade fairs, among farmers and rangers, or using mobile house trailers (for review see Koh *et al.*, 1989). Screening programmes of a defined population have also been performed in Australia (Kricker *et al.*, 1990). Screening at the workplace is another means of examining defined populations for skin cancer or melanoma. For example, an active diagnosis programme at the Lawrence Livermore National Laboratory was set up in response to recorded increased melanoma rates and survival after diagnosis of melanoma has been more favourable (Schneider *et al.*, 1990). Screening of sunworshippers on beach locations has been performed in Australia (Elwood, 1991) and The Netherlands (Krol *et al.*, 1991).

Annual melanoma and skin cancer screening on self-selected persons by dermatologists has been conducted in the United States since 1985 (Koh *et al.*, 1989). This national screening programme was initiated by the American Academy of Dermatology. The effort has been received enthusiastically. Similar clinics have been held in The Netherlands (Rampen *et al.*, 1991; de Rooij *et al.*, 1995).

So far, the type of screening according to the American Academy of Dermatology model seems to be the most feasible and ready to organize. However, screening by dermatologists is often hampered by lack of provider time. Especially in countries with a scarcity of dermatologists, like the UK, screening by dermatologists is not practicable. But also in less adverse situations, a proper and rigid type of organization is mandatory. High numbers of attendants necessitate tight schedules in order to examine as many screenees as possible. To that end, we have tried to improve and refine our screenings.

Targeting high-risk persons should enhance the efficiency of skin-cancer screening. Melanoma has a high mortality rate as compared to non-melanoma skin cancer. In terms of health strategy priorities, non-melanoma skin cancers are insignificant. In our view, these cancers should not be screened for. In 1993 we organized a screening concentrating on melanoma and dysplastic naevi only (de Rooij *et al.*, 1995). The rates of lesions suggestive of melanoma and its precursors increased substantially, whereas the proportions of non-melanoma skin cancers, actinic keratoses and benign skin lesions decreased.

We also investigated the effect of additional complete skin examination of persons attending the screening for single lesions. Complete cutaneous examination may result in better melanoma yields than partial examination (Rigel *et al.*, 1986). We assessed the yield of examination of the entire skin, additional to examination of intentionally shown skin lesions. We found no melanomas among 1221 evaluable cases (de Rooij *et al.*, 1996). Thus, total skin exams are probably not worthwhile. Disrobing, gowning, and chaperoning are time-consuming. More screenees can be seen with limited provider time if only partial skin examinations are performed on persons who attend for single lesions. In this way, we have been able to examine 150–200 screenees per dermatologist per day.

There should be sufficient auxiliary personnel and abundant examination rooms (Rampen *et al.*, 1992a). The dermatologist should only operate as the 'screening test', rather than in a physician-to-patient role. The time alloted to each screenee must be restricted. Any set of activities, apart from the visual skin examination, should be performed by auxiliary staff.

In our view, screening clinics should not be held in private offices, in public premises or on the beach. Screening in a hospital setting has distinct advantages. Dermatology out-patient departments are well equipped and properly lighted. Follow-up and patient compliance in the case of suspected melanoma is probably facilitated when the screening session is held at the nearby hospital.

Mass screening on the basis of population registries is impracticable. Access to screening would be inappropriate because of poor availability of the 'screening test'. Only dermatologists should screen. Assessment of skin images by non-dermatologists is, by and large, unreliable (Cassileth *et al.*, 1986; Rampen & Rümke, 1988). This will produce relatively high rates of false-positive and false-negative screens, which will decrease the sensitivity, specificity and predictive values of the screening exercise. Therefore, melanoma screening based on population listings is not recommended. The medical community is not yet sufficiently prepared for embarking upon large-scale systematic and formalized screening. Melanoma screening should be regarded as an experimental procedure with attendant pros and cons. Preferably, randomized studies should be set up to evaluate its benefits (Elwood, 1994). However, the costs of such trial designs may be considerable (Elwood, 1994).

Further considerations

The current situation is that selective and focused screening for skin cancer and melanoma is recommended in many societies without proper evaluation of its benefits and hazards. In the absence of data on population-based screenings, we have to rely upon the results of non-randomized studies offering screening to subjects at high risk only. Interest in campaigns of selective screening is growing. Screening for melanoma only, based on self-assessment of volunteers who come forward to open-access screening opportunities, recruited by appropriate precampaign media publicity, appears rewarding. Such screenings fulfil the critical elements for an ideal secondary prevention approach as recommended by Wilson and Jungner (1968), and meet the necessary practical and organizational requirements if properly planned (Rampen *et al.*, 1992a, b).

A systematic approach to the development and provision of nationwide melanoma screening programmes is a remote goal. There is the issue of disease prevalence. Screening will be more yielding in areas with a high melanoma prevalence such as Australia and the southern parts of the United States. Whether screening for melanoma is justified in areas with lower prevalence is questionable.

There is also the problem of the availability of the screening test, i.e. the dermatologist's eye. Screening is more feasible in countries with a favourable dermatologist-to-patient ratio, such as Germany. Systematic screening is virtually impossible in countries with few dermatologists, such as the UK. Screening by non-dermatologists is unwarranted for the reasons already mentioned.

Volunteer screening campaigns may reach only a small section of the population. If so, the impact on morbidity and mortality is low. From 1985 to 1993, >650 000 persons were screened during the American Academy of Dermatology skin cancer and melanoma detection programmes (Rhodes, 1995). About 7000 presumed melanoma diagnoses were made. Assuming a predictive value of the screening test of 30–40%, the number of confirmed melanomas is only approximately 2500. In the same period, the estimated number of new melanoma cases in the United States was 248 700 (Rhodes, 1995). Thus, only 1% of all melanomas were diagnosed at the American Academy of Dermatology screenings, which appears to be a negligible proportion.

Precampaign publicity may, however, alert many people who consequently seek medical advice beyond the open-access screenings. This secondary effect through education and health promotion can be substantial but is difficult to quantify. Public and professional educational exercises are an inherent ingredient of screening.

Ethical issues merit special attention. Skin cancer and melanoma screening should not be initiated for the benefit of the screener, but for the patient-attender only. In this context it is pertinent to mention the 'borderline' problem. In our view, persons with minimal disease should not be followed. Only attendants with unequivocal malignancies or precursor lesions should be referred. The referral rate in one American study was extremely high, at 31% (Koh *et al.*, 1990). Costs incurred to the health-care system may be considerable. The referral rate in our early studies was about 10% (Rampen *et al.*, 1991). This discrepancy is likely to be related to the extent to which it is thought that follow-up has to be arranged for trivial or 'borderline' lesions.

Programme evaluation is an essential function after implementation. Follow-up data give critical information for feedback, reinforcement and assessment of effectiveness. Non-compliance of positive screenees is a major problem of free-of-charge screenings. In Massachusetts, only 63% of positive screenees responded to repeated inquiries about recommended care (Koh *et al.*, 1990). Compliance with referral in our 1989–90 campaigns was 90% (Rampen *et al.*, 1991).

A final point relates to the cost-effectiveness of skin cancer and melanoma screening. There is the possible strain put on health services. Screening will burden the medical system with a high number of benign lesions. Many of these, however, would be removed anyhow for various reasons (irritation, bleeding, cosmetic reasons). We found an insignificant increase in the general practitioners' workload after screening exercises in Arnhem and Eindhoven (Rampen *et al.*, 1993). On the other hand, the 1987 publicity campaign (which was not a screening campaign) in the UK was not continued in 1988 because of the disproportionate demand on health services (Ellmann, 1991). Total costs of skin cancer and melanoma screening, including follow-up visits, hospital referrals and histopathology, are unknown. Special surveys of economic costs to the participants and the health-care system should be mounted. We need more detailed information on hidden costs.

With regard to the efficacy of skin cancer and melanoma screening, no studies have addressed this issue satisfactorily. Crude numbers of positive screenees are inconclusive. Ideally, one would discover a high proportion of thin good-prognosis melanomas. During our recent campaign in southern Limburg, The Netherlands, most melanomas diagnosed were early lesions (de Rooij *et al.*, 1995). Such intermediate outcome measures, however, should be interpreted cautiously.

Everything possible must be done to enhance the present-day skin cancer and melanoma screening exercises in the United States and elsewhere. Options for maximizing benefits, minimizing adverse effects and lowering costs have been presented here. The key components for success are the following:

1 An organizational forum for programme development, including close cooperation of epidemiologists with experience in this field.

2 An intensive precampaign public education programme.

3 Dedicated personnel and suitable locations.

4 Narrowing the scope of skin cancer screening by focusing on melanoma only.

5 An understanding that complete skin examinations are time consuming and unproductive.

6 Rigorous follow-up of positive screenees.

7 Use of overall outcome measures, such as changes in the Breslow thickness.

8 Assessment of actual and hidden costs.

References

Bolognia, J.L., Berwick, M. & Fine, J.A. (1990) Complete follow-up and evaluation of a skin cancer screening in Connecticut. *Journal of the American Academy of Dermatology*, **23**, 1098–1106.

Boring, C.C., Squires, T.S., Tong, T. & Montgomery, S. (1994) Cancer statistics. *CA: A Cancer Journal for Clinicians*, **44**, 7–26.

Boyce, J.A. & Bernhard, J.D. (1986) Total skin examination: Patient reactions. *Journal of the American Academy of Dermatology*, **14**, 280.

Breslow, A. (1970) Thickness, cross-sectional area, and depth of invasion in the prognosis of cutaneous melanoma. *Annals of Surgery*, **172**, 902–908.

Cassileth, B.R., Clark, W.H., Lusk, E.J., Frederick, B.E., Thompson, C.J. & Walsh, W.P. (1986) How well do physicians recognize melanoma and other problem lesions? *Journal of the American Academy of Dermatology*, **14**, 555–560.

Chamberlain, J.M. (1984) Which prescriptive screening programmes are worthwhile? *Journal of Epidemiology and Community Health*, **38**, 270–277.

Chiarello, S.E. (1989) Complete skin examinations. *Archives of Dermatology*, **125**, 706.

Clark, W.H., From, L., Bernardino, E.A. & Mihm, M.C. (1969) The histogenesis and biological behaviour of primary human malignant melanomas of the skin. *Cancer Research*, **29**, 705–726.

Ellmann, R. (1991) Screening for melanoma in the U.K. In: *Cancer Screening* (eds A.B. Miller *et al.*), pp. 257–266. Cambridge University Press, Cambridge.

Elwood, J.M. (1991) Screening and early diagnosis for melanoma in Australia and New Zealand. In: *Cancer Screening* (eds A.B. Miller *et al.*), pp. 243–255. Cambridge University Press, Cambridge.

Elwood, J.M. (1994) Screening for melanoma and options for its evaluation. *Journal of Medical Screening*, **1**, 22–38.

Glass, A.G. & Hoover, R.N. (1989) The emerging epidemic of melanoma and squamous cell skin cancer. *Journal of the American Medical Association*, **262**, 2097–2100.

Greene, M.H., Clark, W.H., Tucker, M.A. *et al.* (1985) The high risk of melanoma in melanoma-prone families with dysplastic nevi. *Annals of Internal Medicine*, **102**, 458–465.

Illig, L., Weidner, F., Hundeiker, M. *et al.* (1985) Congenital nevi <10 cm as precursors to melanoma: 52 cases, a review, and a new conception. *Archives of Dermatology*, **121**, 1274–1281.

JAMA (1984) Precursors to malignant melanoma: Consensus conference. *Journal of the American Medical Association*, **251**, 1864–1866.

Koh, H.K., Lew, R.A. & Prout, M.N. (1989) Screening for melanoma/skin cancer: Theoretic and practical considerations. *Journal of the American Academy of Dermatology*, **20**, 159–172.

Koh, H.K., Caruso, A., Gage, I. *et al.* (1990) Evaluation of melanoma/skin cancer screening in Massachusetts: Preliminary results. *Cancer*, **65**, 375–379.

Kricker, A., English, D.R., Randell, P.L. *et al.* (1990) Skin cancer in Geraldton, Western Australia: A survey of incidence and prevalence. *Medical Journal of Australia*, **152**, 399–407.

Krol, S., Keijser, L.M.T., van der Rhee, H.J. & Welvaart, K. (1991) Screening for skin cancer in the Netherlands. *Acta Dermato-Venereologica (Stockholm)*, **71**, 317–321.

Lee, G., Massa, M.C., Welykyj, S. *et al.* (1991) Yield from total skin examination and effectiveness of skin cancer awareness program: Findings in 874 new dermatology patients. *Cancer*, **67**, 202–205.

Lookingbill, D.P. (1988) Yield from a complete skin examination: Findings in 1157 new dermatology patients. *Journal of the American Academy of Dermatology*, **18**, 31–37.

Marks, R., Foley, P., Goodman, G., Hage, B.H. & Selwood, T.S. (1986) Spontaneous remission of solar keratoses: The case of conservative management. *British Journal of Dermatology*, **115**, 649–655.

Marks, R., Rennie, G. & Selwood, T.S. (1988) Malignant transformation of solar keratoses to squamous cell carcinoma. *Lancet*, **i**, 795–797.

Melia, J., Cooper, E.J., Frost, T. *et al.* (1995) Cancer Research Campaign health education programme to promote the early detection of cutaneous malignant melanoma. I. Work-load and referral patterns. *British Journal of Dermatology*, **132**, 405–413.

Rampen, F.H.J. & Rümke, P. (1988) Referral pattern and accuracy of clinical diagnosis of cutaneous melanoma. *Acta Dermato-Venereologica (Stockholm)*, **68**, 61–64.

Rampen, F.H.J., van Huystee, B.E.W.L. & Kiemeney, L.A.L.M. (1991) Melanoma/skin cancer screening clinics: Experiences in The Netherlands. *Journal of the American Academy of Dermatology*, **25**, 776–777.

Rampen, F.H.J., van Huystee, B.E.W.L. & Kiemeney, L.A.L.M. (1992a) Practical considerations of melanoma/skin cancer screening clinics. *Dermatology*, **184**, 190–193.

Rampen, F.H.J., Neumann, H.A.M. & Kiemeney, L.A.L.M. (1992b) Fundamentals of skin cancer/melanoma screening campaigns. *Clinical and Experimental Dermatology*, **17**, 307–312.

Rampen, F.H.J., Berretty, P.J.M., van Huystee, B.E.W.L., Kiemeney, L.A.L.M. & Nijs, C.H.H.M. (1993) General practitioners' workload after skin cancer/melanoma screening clinics in The Netherland. *Dermatology*, **186**, 258–260.

Rampen, F.H.J., Casparie-van Velsen, I.J.A.M.G., van Huystee, B.E.W.L., Kiemeney, L.A.L.M. & Schouten, L.J. (1995) False-negative findings in skin cancer and melanoma screening. *Journal of the American Academy of Dermatology*, **33**, 59–63.

Rhodes, A.R. (1989) Congenital nevi: Should these be excised? *Journal of the American Medical Association*, **262**, 1696.

Rhodes, A.R. (1995) Public education and cancer of the skin; What do people need to know about melanoma and nonmelanoma skin cancer? *Cancer*, **75**, 613–636.

Rhodes, A.R., Sober, A.J., Day, C.L. *et al.* (1982) The malignant potential of small congenital nevocellular nevi: An estimate of association based on a histologic study of 234 primary cutaneous melanomas. *Journal of the American Academy of Dermatology*, **6**, 230–241.

Rigel, D.S., Friedman, R.J., Kopf, A.W. *et al.* (1986) Importance of complete cutaneous examination for the detection of malignant melanoma. *Journal of the American Academy of Dermatology*, **14**, 857–860.

de Rooij, M.J.M., Rampen, F.H.J., Schouten, L.J. & Neumann, H.A.M. (1995) Skin cancer screening focusing on melanoma yields more selective attendance. *Archives of Dermatology*, **131**, 422–425.

de Rooij, M.J.M., Rampen, F.H.J., Schouten, L.J. & Neumann, H.A.M. (1996) Total skin examination during screening for melanoma does not increase detection rate. *British Journal of Dermatology*, **135**, 42–45.

Schneider, J.S., Moore, D.H. & Sagebiel, R.W. (1990) Early diagnosis of cutaneous malignant melanoma at Lawrence Livermore National Laboratory. *Archives of Dermatology*, **126**, 767–769.

Scotto, J., Pitcher, H. & Lee, J.A.H. (1991) Indications of future decreasing trends in skin-melanoma mortality among whites in the United States. *International Journal of Cancer*, **49**, 490–497.

Visser, O., Coebergh, J.W.W. & Schouten, L.J. (eds) (1995) *Incidence of Cancer in The Netherlands 1992*. Netherlands Cancer Registry, Utrecht.

Wilson, J.M.B. & Jungner, G. (eds) (1968) *The Principles and Practice of Screening for Disease*. Public Health Papers, No. 34. WHO, Geneva.

Overview of Melanoma Early Diagnosis Campaigns Worldwide

R.M. MACKIE

Early diagnosis campaigns to encourage earlier presentation of patients with melanoma at a stage in the development of the tumour at which cure is more likely began in Queensland, Australia. The Queensland Melanoma Programme was initiated in 1963 by McLeod and others (McLeod *et al.*, 1985). The initial purpose was to gain more information on incidence of and mortality from malignant melanoma. It was observed that the incidence of invasive melanoma increased in Queensland from 15 per 100 000 annually in 1966 to 25 per 100 000 annually in 1977. If non-melanoma skin cancer is excluded, melanoma comprised at that time 10% of all malignancies in Queensland.

A retrospective analysis was carried out in Queensland of melanoma patients treated between 1945 and 1963. A population-based registry of melanoma cases was developed in Queensland between 1963 and 1969, and detailed follow-up carried out on this population for 10 years. This resulted in a valuable database on 1441 patients.

From this background, an early detection programme was developed. The initial aim was to educate physicians about the features of early malignant melanoma. Materials used in the Queensland campaign comprised films, booklets and lectures. These materials were subsequently made available to other appropriate groups including medical students and paramedicals (nurses, physiotherapists, radiographers and podiatrists).

Once the professional education campaign had been established, public education activities were introduced. These took the form of articles in newspapers, public meetings, leaflets and similar methods of disseminating information. Schools were also targeted.

Measures of success of the Queensland campaign included a measure of the change in the proportion of Clark levels of primary melanomas excised in Queensland. Over the period of the Queensland melanoma programme there was a change in pattern, with a reduction in the proportion of Clark level 5 lesions, and an increase in the proportion of Clark level 1, 2 and 3 lesions in both sexes. Throughout the period of the campaign, the incidence of melanoma continued to rise, but mortality rose less rapidly. The comparator used for the Queensland melanoma programme was the situation in other Australian states. In these other states, the rate of rise in incidence was seen to be similar to that observed in Queensland, but the mortality rates rose more steeply in states outside Queensland. This was therefore taken as a measure of success of the Queensland campaign (McLeod, 1988).

Following the lead of the Queensland melanoma programme, other states in Australia have developed extremely effective early detection activities. In a country such as Australia, with a high incidence of melanoma, the policy has been to combine both early detection and primary prevention activities. The extremely successful 'Slip, slop, slap!' campaigns, and now the more sophisticated 'Sun cool' campaigns have both been primarily aimed at prevention of melanoma by encouraging sensible sun exposure (Marks & Hill, 1992). However adjunct material for both campaigns has included high-quality illustrated material aimed at early detection and prompt treatment of thin curable malignant melanoma.

One of the first early detection exercises in Europe was carried out in Italy. This was conducted in the northern province of Trento and led by Cristofolini and colleagues (1986). In 1977, this group began to educate general practitioners concerning the features of early cutaneous malignant melanoma. Thereafter, material was produced for the general public explaining the aspects of self-examination for early malignant melanoma and emphasizing the importance of early diagnosis and prompt treatment. The adjacent areas of the Veneto, Alto Adige and Lombardy were used as control areas. These Italian provinces are at a similar latitude to Trento and contain a population of similar ethnic origin. For the public education section of this campaign, material was disseminated through newspapers, television and radio broadcasts. It is not clear how the adjacent control areas were prevented from access to the materials produced in Trento. Analysis of the northern Italian campaign has been carried out, and has revolved around the number of observed compared with expected melanoma-related deaths in Trento for the period 1977–85 (Cristofolini *et al.*, 1993). Based on past experience, and the experience of the surrounding areas, 40 melanoma-related deaths were expected amongst males and 34 amongst females. The observed number of deaths were 26 for both sexes. The calculation made by Cristofolini and colleagues is that as a result of the campaign, 22 melanoma-related deaths have been prevented. They have further estimated that the cost per year of life saved is around $400. It is of interest to note that the reduction in melanoma-associated mortality in northern Italy appears to have been greater amongst males than females. In most areas where public education activities have been audited, the experience has been that females are more responsive to this education than males.

A further European public education campaign has been conducted in Scotland. This developed following the establishment of the Scottish Melanoma Group in 1979 (MacKie *et al.*, 1992). The aim of this group was to obtain complete information on all aspects of primary cutaneous melanoma presenting in Scotland (having a population of 5.1 million). A detailed database with clinical information, pathological infor-

mation, surgical and other treatment details and follow-up was constructed. By 1985, it was apparent that the proportion of patients presenting with thick, poor prognosis tumours ($\geq 3.5\,mm$) was unacceptably high. An assumption was made that the thick tumours would correlate to a degree with delays in diagnosis. A careful survey was therefore carried out of 110 patients with recently diagnosed melanoma, looking at potential points of delay in receiving treatment (Doherty & MacKie, 1986). These revolved around delay in patient awareness, delay in primary-care awareness, delay after referral to a specialist and delay in receiving appropriate surgical treatment. It was found that in this sample the predominant area of delay lay with the patient. The great majority of patients had recognized that they had a new, changing or growing pigmented lesion on their skin, but 50% of them delayed more than 6 months before seeking medical advice, and 16% delayed more than a year. On this basis it was decided that, in Scotland, a public education campaign was required. However, prior to this public education campaign, primary-care doctors were consulted about their willingness to participate in this activity. The plan from the outset was that the public would be informed about the features of early malignant melanoma and asked to consult their usual primary-care physician (general practitioner with whom they were registered) prior to onward referral to a specialist centre. Thus the activity would be based on normal referral patterns, not on a one-off campaign, that would involve, if successful, a potential rise in workload for doctors working in the primary-care sector. A total of 112 doctors were consulted about their willingness to participate in this activity. The great majority were happy to be involved, but wished an update on the features of early thin melanoma, although the earlier surveys suggested that there had been no significant delay on the part of primary-care physicians.

For these reasons, a 6-month professional education campaign was carried out from January to June 1985. This mainly involved education of primary-care doctors in the Glasgow area (with a population of 900000 and 624 general practitioners), but also involved education of nurses, physiotherapists and others working as members of the primary-care team. Specific booklets on features of early melanoma, features of benign naevi and films were produced, and meetings and discussions held in general practices. The material prepared was prioritized by the primary-care teams who indicated the type of educational material they would find most useful.

The public education campaign was launched in June 1985, and from the outset audit points were established The audit points were as follows:

1 A measure of the increase in interest in pigmented lesions.

2 A measure of the increase in referrals to a dedicated pigmented lesion clinic by general practitioners (patients were not permitted direct access to this clinic other than in unusual circumstances).

3 A measure of the number of pathologically confirmed invasive malignant melanomas seen at the pigmented lesion clinic prior to and after public education activities.

4 A measure of the thickness of primary cutaneous malignant melanomas excised before and after primary education activities.

5 A measure of melanoma-associated mortality before and after primary education activities.

The public education campaign met with a great deal of interest and enthusiasm. In 1985, melanoma was not well-recognized in the UK, and the public education activities were therefore novel. The launching of the campaign coincided with a period of good weather, and 2 weeks after the launch it was reported that the (then) president of the United States, Ronald Reagan, had skin cancer for which he had received surgery. Although President Reagan's lesion was a basal-cell carcinoma, and the Scottish campaign was dedicated purely to early detection of melanoma, this appearance of a public figure with a form of cutaneous malignancy gave the campaign a further boost.

It had initially been planned that the campaign would be confined to the West of Scotland with a population of *c.* 2 million, and that the adjacent area in the East of Scotland would act as a control population who did not receive specific educational material. In the event, the degree of public interest and the wide dissemination of newspapers, television and radio broadcasts made the preservation of an uneducated control group impossible, and the comparisons for audit purposes had to be confined to before and after studies in the West of Scotland.

These studies indicated clearly that, initially, great interest was generated in pigmented lesions in general and melanoma in particular. The number of melanomas diagnosed in the latter part of 1985 was significantly greater than that in the first half of 1985. Following the campaign there was an immediate sharp increase in the number of thin good-prognosis melanomas excised ($\leqslant 1.5$ mm in thickness), with no concomitant rise in thick tumours. This pattern persisted from 1985 to 1995 although no formal secondary campaign has since been conducted. From 1987 onwards, a fall in the absolute number of thick tumours ($\geqslant 3.5$ mm) was noted in females but not in males, and from 1989 onwards a fall in melanoma-associated mortality was observed in females but not in males (MacKie & Hole, 1992). Thus the audit measures available have suggested that the Scottish campaign has succeeded in delivering the message of early detection to females but not as yet to males.

Following the initiation of the West of Scotland Early Detection Campaign, the UK Cancer Research Campaign funded seven centres in other parts of the UK (Edinburgh, London (two), Southampton, Nottingham, Leicester and Exeter). These areas were selected on the basis of individuals with an interest in melanoma, and reasonable precampaign records of numbers of melanomas treated and tumour thicknesses. Funding was provided for local public education activities, for a pigmented lesion clinic and for a rapid surgery service. The results from these centres have been varied. In all centres there has been an initial increase in interest in melanoma and increase in number of referrals to the designated centre, but the relative proportions of thin and thick tumours prior to and after these activities have not shown the same striking change as in the West of Scotland. Similarly, a comparison of tumour thickness in areas covered by the Cancer Research Campaign with those not covered has not shown a clear difference. This may in part be explained by the greater interest in melanoma which was apparent in the UK by 1987, and the blanket coverage of television which we and others have found to be one of the most successful medium's for public education (Melia *et al.*, 1995).

A contrast to the Italian and UK approach through the primary-care physicians has been the activities carried out in both the USA and The Netherlands where the public are encouraged to seek advice directly. These activities may be referred to as 'skin cancer fairs' or 'free melanoma diagnostic clinics'. The system therefore depends on members of the public recognizing new or changing pigmented lesions and seeking help at a specially designated centre, usually just operating for a small part of the year. Many states in the USA now conduct these 'melanoma recognition days', often funded under the aegis of the American Academy of Dermatology or the American Cancer Society. In a country where the health-care system involves a fee for service if a dermatologist is consulted about a pigmented lesion, the offer of a free diagnostic service is clearly attractive. These campaigns have been based on the principle that diagnosis and advice is offered, but treatment is not arranged or given for ethical reasons. The results of the American campaigns have been extensively analysed by Koh and others (1991). Large numbers of Americans have taken advantage of the free screening days. By comparison with the general American population, those who have taken advantage of the screening days have an increased number of melanoma risk factors—fair skin, fair hair and large numbers of naevi. Melanomas recognized and subsequently excised as a result of these screening days are thinner than in the population at large. The structure of these screening days does not however allow for changes in mean thickness or in melanoma-associated mortality to be assessed. An excellent study to confirm the value of the screening-day approach would be a comparison in two American states at similar latitudes and with similar populations, one offering free screening days over a period of 5–10 years, and one depending on conventional referral for suspected melanoma.

The campaigns conducted in The Netherlands and led by Rampen and colleagues (1991) have been very similar to the American campaigns. They have used caravans established on attractive holiday beaches and have offered a free skin check. Melanomas have been recognized at these free skin checks, but the ratio of recognized melanoma to patients examined has indicated that this is a labour-intensive exercise and not cost-effective if carried out on a large scale. Similar activities have been carried out in Germany, where in the town of Bochum a designated clinic was established (Hoffmann *et al.*, 1993). The ratio of melanomas diagnosed to individuals examined was around 1 in 100.

Work carried out in both Austria and Switzerland has suggested that early detection campaigns have an impressive initial impact, but that this impact is short-lived. Thus in Austria (Pehamberger *et al.*, 1993), campaigns carried out in 1988 and 1989 have shown a sharp rise in numbers of melanomas diagnosed during the course of the campaign and a fall in mean thickness from 1.4 to 1.1 mm. However, after 1989 when no further campaigns were conducted, a return to the pre-education pattern of smaller numbers of thicker melanomas was observed. This suggests that regular reminder campaigns are necessary. However, in the canton of Basle in Switzerland (Bulliard *et al.*, 1992), public education activities were carried out in 1986, with a reminder campaign in 1989. The 1986 campaign showed a doubling in the number of newly diagnosed cases immediately after the campaign with a non-significant fall in tumour thickness. The 1989 campaign did not appear to produce any significant changes. Observations of this type have led to the suggestion that the general public can become blasé to repeated messages about early malignant melanoma, and that careful timing of reminder campaigns must be considered, possibly linked to a human interest story about a local personality who has been successfully treated for melanoma.

In summary, worldwide there have been many public education campaigns aimed at early detection of malignant melanoma. The essential features for these include preparation of the medical profession whether or not they are to be integral to the campaign, and clear, sensitive and specific descriptions of early thin cutaneous malignant melanoma. This is vital. Many of the older photographs of melanoma show thick poor-prognosis lesions. The educational material for modern campaigns must confine itself to tumours ≤1mm as these are the object of the exercise. Clear organization, good publicity and good management are essential for the campaigns, as are built-in audit measures of the campaigns' success. In the field of cancer education, it is quite possible to do harm. A poorly designed campaign can initiate fear and delay self-referral for treatment. It can also greatly increase the proportion of patients who attend for reassurance about totally benign pigmented lesions. This influx of the so-called 'worried well' to appropriate referral centres for early melanoma can greatly increase waiting lists and actually delay treatment of true malignant melanoma.

Greater attention needs to be paid to encouraging older males to seek medical advice earlier, as evidence from many centres indicates that this section of the population still presents with a high proportion of thick poor-prognosis tumours.

References

Bulliard, J.L, Raymond, L., Levi, F. *et al.* (1992) Prevention of cutaneous melanoma: An epidemiological evaluation of the Swiss campaign. *Revue Epidemiologie Sante Publique,* **24**, 271–277.

Cristofolini, M., Zumiani, M., Boi, S. & Piscioli, F. (1986) Community detection of early melanoma. *Lancet,* **i**, 18.

Cristofolini, M., Bianchi, R., Sebastiana, B. *et al.* (1993) Analysis of the cost effectiveness ratio of the health campaign for the early diagnosis of cutaneous melanoma in Trentino, Italy. *Cancer,* **71**, 370–374.

Doherty, V.R. & MacKie, R.M. (1986). Reasons for poor prognosis in British patients with cutaneous malignant melanoma. *British Medical Journal,* **292**, 987–989.

Hoffman, K., Kirschka, Th., Shatz, H., Segerling, M., Tiemann, Th. & Hoffmann, A. (1993) A local education campaign on early diagnosis of malignant melanoma. *European Journal of Epidemiology,* **9**, 591–598.

Kohl, H.K., Geller, A.C., Miller, D.R. *et al.* (1991) Who is being screened for melanoma/skin cancer? *Journal of the American Academy of Dermatology,* **24**, 271–277.

MacKie, R.M. & Hole, D. (1992) Audit of public education campaign to encourage earlier detection of malignant melanoma. *British Medical Journal,* **304**, 1012–1015.

MacKie, R.M., Hunter, J.A., Aitchison, T.C. *et al.* (1992) Cutaneous malignant melanoma in Scotland 1978–89. *Lancet,* **339**, 971–975.

Marks, R. & Hill, D. (1992) *The Public Health Approach to Melanoma Control: Prevention and Early Detection.* Australian Cancer Society, Melbourne.

McLeod, G.R. (1988) Control of melanoma in a high risk population. *Pigment Cell,* **9**, 131–140.

McLeod, G.R., Davis, N.C., Little, J.H., Green, J. and Chant, D. (1985) Melanoma in Queensland Australia. Experience of the Queensland Melanoma Project. In: *Cutaneous Melanoma. Clinical Management and Treatment Results Worldwide* (eds C.M. Balch & G.W. Milton), pp. 379–387. Lippincott, Philadelphia.

Melia, J., Cooper, E.J., Frost, T. *et al.* (1995) Cancer Research Campaign health education programme to promote the early detection of malignant melanoma. *British Journal of Dermatology,* **132**, 405–413.

Pehamberger, H., Binder, M., Knollmayer, S. & Wolff, K. (1993) Immediate effects of a public education campaign on a prognostic feature of melanoma. *Journal of the American*
Academy of Dermatology, **29**, 106–109.

Rampen, F.H.J., van Huystee, B.E.W.L. & Kiemeney, L.A.L.M. (1991) Melanoma/skin cancer screening clinics: Experiences in The Netherlands. *Journal of the American Academy of Dermatology,* **25**, 776–777.

Causes for the Delay in Diagnosis of Melanoma

R.G.B. LANGLEY AND A.J. SOBER

A current and significant public health initiative is the early detection (secondary prevention) and prompt excision of primary cutaneous melanoma. The ability to cure *in situ* nearly all early invasive melanomas by surgical excision and the lack of effective therapy for advanced metastatic melanoma have, in part, fuelled this initiative. Early diagnosis and treatment of melanoma is believed to be the principal factor in improving the life expectancy of patients with primary cutaneous melanoma, as reflected by the fall in median primary tumour thickness, the most important prognostic indicator in this malignancy (Day *et al.*, 1981). Despite the trend towards decreasing thickness of the primary melanoma at diagnosis, there is evidence that significant delays in establishing the diagnosis of melanoma currently exist (Temoshok *et al.*, 1984; Doherty & MacKie, 1986; Cassileth *et al.*, 1987, 1988; Hennrikus *et al.*, 1991). This delay may be in the order of 1 year (Doherty & MacKie, 1986; Cassileth *et al.*, 1987, 1988). The data from such studies are not perfect, however, as they suffer recall bias, and fail to account for how long a patient had a melanoma before noticing or becoming suspicious of it.

If this goal of early melanoma detection is to be achieved, it is critical that the factors which cause a delay in the diagnosis be understood so that appropriate interventions are instituted. We will examine some of the salient reasons for the delay in the diagnosis of melanoma and the implications for future public health programmes. In order to understand the reason for delay in diagnosis of melanoma several questions must be addressed:
- Who makes the diagnosis?
- Who is able to make the diagnosis?
- Why the delay? Patient or physician?

Who makes the diagnosis?

Identification of the person who detects, or fails to detect, melanoma is important if we are to decrease the time to diagnosis and to organize educational efforts optimally. A population-based study of 216 cases of melanoma from Massachusetts examined this issue (Koh *et al.*, 1992). Questionnaires were sent to 454 patients diagnosed with primary cutaneous melanoma in 1986. From the 216 responses received, it was determined that 53% (115/216) of melanomas were self-detected, 25% (54/216) were physician detected, 17% (36/216) were detected by family members, 2% were detected by a friend (5/216) and 1% by a nurse (3/216) or other individuals (3/216). Other epidemiological studies have had similar findings. A study of 651 patients in the Western Canada Melanoma Study determined that 61% (384/636) of melanomas were noticed by the patient, 25% (159/636) by a non-physician other than the person and 14% (93/636) by a physician (Elwood & Gallagher, 1988).

In the study by Koh *et al.* (1992), differences in detection rate were noted by sex, as females self-detected more melanomas (66%) than men (42%). This lower detection rate in men may be partly attributed to the increased number of melanomas at sites difficult to visualize (the back is the most frequent site of melanoma in men whereas the lower leg is the most frequent anatomical site in females). The differential anatomical-site predilection, however, does not explain the greater number of melanomas detected by women on their spouses (23% vs. 2%) or that women self-detected most of their own back melanomas compared to men (71% vs. 26%).

A logistic regression analysis was also performed in Koh's (1992) study to determine the role of certain social and demographic factors in the detection of melanoma. It was determined that higher educational status in men led to higher self-detection rates ($P = 0.05$) and men that utilized health-care services in the year prior to diagnosis were more likely to have a medical worker diagnose the melanoma ($P = 0.02$).

Collectively, these studies emphasize the importance of public awareness of melanoma and the need to increase awareness in men.

Who is able to make the diagnosis of melanoma?

The ability of a physician to accurately diagnose or suspect melanoma in a patient and perform a biopsy/excision or make a timely referral is a critical factor in improving the time to diagnosis. Several studies have been published in the past decade which examined the accuracy of diagnosis and comparisons between dermatologists and non-dermatologists (Kopf *et al.*, 1975; Wagner *et al.*, 1985; Cassileth *et al.*, 1986; Rampen & Rumke, 1988; Curley *et al.*, 1989; Grin *et al.*, 1990; Koh *et al.*, 1990; Witheiler & Cockerell, 1991; Bricknell, 1993; McGee *et al.*, 1994). Rigorous data for physician accuracy for the diagnosis of melanoma are, however, lacking as these studies are limited in being retrospective or involve simulated test situations which may not replicate an *in vivo* clinical patient assessment. Studies examining pathology databases retrospectively (Witheiler & Cockerell, 1991) may underestimate physician diagnostic accuracy if physicians fail to record a suspected diagnosis on the requisition. A retrospective study from the extensive database at the New York University Medical Center suggested that the accuracy of diagnosis was perhaps as low as 62–64% (Kopf *et al.*, 1975; Grin *et al.*, 1990). This study, however, underestimates the true diagnostic accuracy as the study design required that no more than a single diagnosis be given.

A summary of the studies which have reported the diagnostic accuracy of clinical examination is presented in Table 11.5. The range in the sensitivity of diagnosis, for which sufficient data are available, was 40–97%, and specificity was in the order of 98–99%. Several of these studies show a higher accuracy rate among dermatologists, especially for the recognition of precursor naevi, than for non-dermatologists (Wagner *et al.*, 1985; Cassileth *et al.*, 1986; Rampen & Rumke, 1988; Bricknell, 1993). Strict comparisons between these studies is not possible as the study designs differ, and different groups of health-care providers and data types are compared (see Table 11.5). Despite these limitations, it is clear that the physicians' diagnostic accuracy is far from perfect and constitutes one basis for delay in the diagnosis of melanoma.

The lower diagnostic accuracy of non-dermatologists in such studies indicates a need for improved pro-

Table 11.5 Diagnostic accuracy of cutaneous melanoma.

Reference	Sensitivity	Specificity	Predictive value
Swerdlow (1952)*	16/22 (73%)	545/556 (98%)	16/27 (59%)
Becker (1954)*	–	–	43%
McMullan & Hubener (1956)*	–	–	44/115 (38%)
Kopf *et al.* (1975)†	76/99 (77%)	5420/5439 (99%)	76/95 (80%)
Rampen & Rumke (1988)	67/120 (56%)†; 45/113 (40%)‡		
Curley *et al.* (1989)†	1/6 (17%)	269/275 (98%)	–
Koh *et al.* (1990)†	97%	–	35–40%
Grin *et al.* (1990)†	81%	99.2%	73%
Witheiler & Cockerell (1991)*	1201/1784 (67%)	–	–
Bricknell (1993)	0/3§, 9/12 (75%)¶	–	–
McGee *et al.* (1994)	81%§, 90%†	–	–

* Physician (specialty not stated); † dermatologist; ‡ surgeon; § general practitioner; ¶ hospital specialist (dermatologist or surgeon).

fessional education given the increasing role of the primary caregiver in the initial assessment of the patient in the United States and their already prominent role in other countries. That education can facilitate the correct recognition and management of pigmented skin lesions, however, was supported by a recent study of general practitioners in New Zealand (McGee *et al.*, 1994). In this study, a self-administered questionnaire and twelve clinical slides were given to 900 general practitioners. A correct decision on the need for biopsy occurred in >80% of this test sample of skin tumours suggesting that, in a high-risk area with a medical-delivery system focused on general physicians, most skin tumours would be diagnosed. In approaching a patient with a suspicious pigmented lesion, it is arguable that rather than having 100% sensitivity, greater importance should be ascribed to the suspicion of melanoma and performing a biopsy of the lesion.

A further physician-related factor contributing to the delay in diagnosis can occur when a primary-care physician or dermatologist fails to screen a high-risk patient for melanoma. A study outlining the utilization of health-care resources in the year prior to diagnosis suggests that such factors are playing a role (Geller *et al.*, 1992). A population-based study of 216 patients with melanoma from Massachusetts determined that 63% of those patients had seen a physician in the year prior to diagnosis, but only 24% had performed self-examination and in only 20% had the physician

examined their skin at the time of the patient–doctor encounter. Although 13% of these patients had seen a dermatologist in the prior year, only 4% were diagnosed at that time. This significant percentage of patients with melanoma that currently have exposure to the health-care system in the year prior to diagnosis provides an opportunity for more aggressive case finding.

Given the importance of early diagnosis, and the difficulties in clinical diagnosis, even among skin-cancer specialists with extensive experience, there has been ongoing research into clinical techniques that may improve diagnostic accuracy. The principal clinical techniques that have been developed include epiluminescence microscopy (ELM) and image analysis. ELM is a non-invasive clinical technique which involves applying immersion oil to the lesion followed by examination with a hand-held scope (dermatoscope) or a stereomicroscope. With ELM, the epidermis becomes translucent making it possible to visualize anatomical structures which are not otherwise visible to the unaided eye. These structures have generated a new set of clinical criteria for the assessment of pigmented lesions (Bahmer *et al.*, 1990; Pehamberger *et al.*, 1993). Certain investigators have attempted to develop a logical system to facilitate the interpretation of these morphological criteria. The principal methods of ELM analysis include: a three-step system (Kenet *et al.*, 1993); the pattern analysis method (Pehamberger *et al.*, 1987; Steiner *et al.*, 1987);

and the ABCD method of dermoscopy (Stoltz *et al.*, 1991; Nachbar *et al.*, 1994).

Computerized image analysis is another non-invasive method used to evaluate pigmented lesions. This technique involves the use of a computer to identify clinical features of a pigmented skin lesion. Current image analysis systems assess parameters such as shape, area, asymmetry, border, colour and infrared reflectance.

One of the more recent developments in the *in vivo* visualization of the skin, with potential applications to pigmented lesion assessment, is the development of confocal scanning laser microscopy. This technique produces high-resolution images of the epidermis and papillary dermis (Rajadhyaksha *et al.*, 1995). We are presently investigating the use of this technique using a Nd:Yag 1064nm laser in the imaging of pigmented lesions, including melanoma, and assessing the clinicopathologic correlation (Langley *et al.*, 1996). It is expected that, with continued development of technology, the *in vivo* imaging of the skin will lead to enhanced diagnostic precision of pigmented skin lesions which should improve physicians' ability to diagnose melanomas, particularly early melanomas, and reduce delay in diagnosis attributable to physician diagnostic accuracy.

Why the delay?

The patient

The major patient-related factors which can lead to a delay in diagnosis relate to a lack of knowledge, inability to see the lesion due to the anatomical site and failure to present to a health-care professional for assessment of a suspicious lesion due to fear, denial or lack of resources.

The importance of a patient's level of understanding for early diagnosis of melanoma has been examined by several studies (Temoshok *et al.*, 1984; Doherty & MacKie, 1986; Cassileth *et al.*, 1988; Hennrikus *et al.*, 1991). In a study from California of 106 patients consecutively diagnosed with melanoma, the patients were dichotomized by prior level of understanding into 'none/little' versus 'substantial' (Temoshok *et al.*, 1984). Patients with no-to-little knowledge had significantly ($P \sim 0.02$) thicker primary lesions than patients with substantial knowledge (2.04mm vs. 1.18mm). The lower level of knowledge was also associated with a delay in seeking medical assessment, as patients with little-to-no knowledge had a mean delay in diagnosis of 4.3 compared to 2.7 months for those with substantial knowledge. A Scottish study also showed that a delay in diagnosis could be related to a lack of patient knowledge of the signs and symptoms of melanoma (Doherty & MacKie, 1986). In this study, 94% (99/105) cited a lack of knowledge of the significance of the melanoma as the reason for delay in presentation for medical assessment, whereas 4% (4/105) were unable to visualize the lesion due to the anatomic site, and 2% (2/105) feared treatment. A public education campaign initiated on the basis of this study documented a favourable trend in preliminary analysis. In the 6 months following, a change in the proportion of melanomas seen in the west of Scotland occurred with an increase in thin (<1.5mm) lesions from 62% compared to 38% before the campaign, and a decrease in thick lesions (>3.5mm) from 34% to 15% was documented (Doherty & MacKie, 1986). Another study of 275 patients with melanoma documented a delay due, in large part, to patient-related failure to recognize the significance of suspicious changes in a pigmented lesion (Cassileth *et al.*, 1988). On average, 6 months had elapsed before patients became suspicious of a changing pigmented lesion, and a further 2.6 months passed before seeking medical attention. A population-based survey of 1344 people in New South Wales, Australia, examined the pre-valence of signs of melanoma, and measured the delay in medical assessment and reasons for this delay (Hennrikus *et al.*, 1991). Of 115 individuals reporting a change in a naevus, only 57% (66/115) had this lesion assessed by a physician. Of those not seeking medical assessment, nearly half (49%) failed to recognize the significance of a changing naevus and believed it was not a serious condition and would resolve spontaneously.

Understanding baseline patient knowledge of the signs and symptoms of melanoma is important to understand the patient-related reasons for a delay in diagnosis and in formulating public education campaigns. Despite extensive public education campaigns through mediasponsored events there is some evidence, from the above studies and from public surveys, that deficiencies remain in the public's knowledge base of melanoma and its early warning signs. An American Academy of Dermatology survey of 1000 adults documented deficiencies in understanding the basic warning signs and risk factors of melanoma, and even in the awareness of melanoma as a type of cancer (*Dermatology World*, 1995). Over one-third (37%) of those interviewed were unable to name any early signs of melanoma and only 57% recognized melanoma as a type of cancer.

Patient denial of a symptom, sign or recognition of melanoma but failing to present for medical assessment due to fear of diagnosis may be an additional patient-related factor causing a delay of diagnosis. Few studies have examined the role that these issues may play in delay. That there is only a relatively minor role for fear or denial is supported by a study by Hennrikus *et al.* (1991). Only 4% (3/77) of those who deferred seeing a physician for a possible sign of melanoma stated they did so because they 'did not want to think about the symptom', and a further 4% (3/77) stated it was due to having 'little faith in physicians'. A UK study of melanoma patients that had a delay in diagnosis found that only 2% (2/105) delayed due to fear of the treatment (Doherty & MacKie, 1986).

From the studies reviewed above, the most frequent reason for delay in diagnosis appears to relate to lack of knowledge. Even in situations where patients are knowledgeable about melanoma, however, there will remain a smaller number of patients who will defer definitive diagnosis due to fear or denial.

The physician

The less-than-perfect diagnostic accuracy of physicians in diagnosing melanoma suggests that physicians play a role in the delay in diagnosis. Doherty and MacKie (1986) found that only 3% (3/105) of patients had a delay in diagnosis attributable to a physician and this delay was approximately 7 weeks. Cassileth *et al.* (1988) found a greater number of patients having delay between the physician visit and establishment of the diagnosis of melanoma, with 21% of the patients having a delay of 2 months, and 13% a delay of 4 months. Factors cited to account for the delay after the initial visit included delays in obtaining pathology reports or in responding to those reports, patient delay

in seeing the physician or seeing multiple physicians. In a study from western Canada, patients with melanomas presenting to the family physician were managed appropriately in most cases. While the majority of melanomas were biopsied or referred to a specialist (dermatologist or surgeon) there was a smaller percentage of patients who suffered a delay in diagnosis due to the physician, as 7% were managed expectantly and 3% were erroneously reassured (Elwood & Gallagher, 1988).

Defining the targets: the messages and strategy of future campaigns

For effective early detection to be achieved, both increased awareness among at-risk members of the public, and a receptive, accessible, skilled health-care force, are required. Different types of programmes are necessary to achieve these separate objectives (MacKie & Cascinelli, 1992).

Public-awareness campaigns are challenging and expensive. An evaluative component should be included in each effort. Before public education programmes can be implemented, an assessment of baseline public knowledge is essential. Factors which need to be addressed include: delay in seeking care; awareness of primary aetiological factors; individual risk assessment; prevention strategies; rudiments of clinical lesion recognition; access to care; and adverse psychological affects resulting from the campaign effort (Brandberg *et al.*, 1993; Rhodes, 1995). Lack of knowledge is the major issue to be addressed in public-directed intervention programmes. Certain groups, such as men, that tend to have longer delays before seeking medical attention may benefit from specific attention in these programmes (Koh *et al.*, 1992). Emphasis should be placed on the relationship between aggressive case finding and subsequent high likelihood of cure.

Professional education programmes must be in place before public education campaigns can be maximally effective (MacKie & Cascinelli, 1992; Marks & Hill, 1992). The importance and cost-effectiveness of examination of the skin must be brought home to all health-care professionals with primary contact to the patient. The skin examination is one more item on the primary-care providers' crowded screening list and must compete for attention with blood-pressure checks, stool guiac, and prostate, breast and gynaecological evaluations. Currently, data from randomized trials or case-control studies on the efficacy of screening in reducing mortality do not exist; however, analyses on the impact of current campaigns are underway (Koh *et al.*, 1995a,b, 1996).

In addition to the recognition of the importance of a cutaneous examination, the health-care provider must have sufficient diagnostic skill to be able to screen for significant lesions (Avril *et al.*, 1994) The basic algorithm has three decision points: (1) lesions which can be safely ignored; (2) lesions which should be followed; and (3) lesions which should be either biopsied or referred to another physician for evaluation. Algorithms and training objectives which help triage appropriate patients may be helpful in this regard (Del Mar & Green, 1995; Weinstock *et al.*, 1996). In addition, patient risk profiles should be assessed (Rhodes *et al.*, 1987; MacKie *et al.*, 1989). Low-risk lesions in a low-risk patient would have a different follow-up strategy than higher risk lesions in a high-risk patient.

More cutaneous education needs to be incorporated into primary-care training and continuing education programmes. Primary prevention education of the patient must also occur along with dietary and substance-abuse advice. That these efforts take time must be recognized by the health-care system, and support for the activities must be provided.

Acknowledgements

Study supported in part by the Marion Gardner Jackson Trust, Bank of Boston, trustee. Dr Langley is the recipient of the Lalia B. Chase Fellowship of the Dalhousie Medical Research Foundation.

References

Avril, M.F., Cascinelli, N., Cristofolini, M. *et al.* (1994) *Clinical Diagnosis of Melanoma* (Publication 3). WHO Melanoma Programme, Milan.

Bahmer, F.A., Fritsch, P., Kreush, J. *et al.* (1990) Terminology in surface microscopy; consensus meeting of the Committee on Analytical Morphology of the Arbeitsgemeinschaft Dermatologische Forschung, Hamburg, Federal Republic of Germany, 17 November 1989. *Journal of the American Academy Dermatology*, **23**, 1159–1162.

Becker, S.W. (1954) Pitfalls in the diagnosis and treatment of melanoma. *Archives of Dermatology and Syphilis*, **69**, 11.

Brandberg, Y., Bolund, C., Michelson, H. *et al.* (1993) Psychological reactions in public melanoma screening. *European Journal of Cancer*, **29A**, 860–863.

Bricknell, M.C.M. (1993) Skin biopsies of pigmented skin lesions performed by general practitioners and hospital specialists. *British Journal of General Practitioners*, **43**, 199–201.

Cassileth, B.R., Clark, W.H. Jr, Lush, E.J. *et al.* (1986) How well do physicians recognize melanoma and other problem lesions? *Journal of the American Academy of Dermatology*, **14**, 555–560.

Cassileth, B.R., Lusk, E.J., Guerry, D. IV *et al.* (1987) 'Catalyst' symptoms in malignant melanoma. *Journal of General Internal Medicine*, **2**, 1–4.

Cassileth, B.R., Temoshok, L., Frederick, B.E. *et al.* (1988) Patient and physician delay in melanoma diagnosis. *Journal of the American Academy of Dermatology*, **18**, 591–598.

Curley, R.K., Cook, M.G., Fallowfield, M.E. *et al.* (1989) Accuracy in clinically evaluating pigmented lesions. *British Medical Journal*, **299**, 16–18.

Day, C.L. Jr, Lew, R.A., Mihm, M.C. Jr *et al.* (1981) The natural break points for primary-tumor thickness in clinical stage I melanoma. (Letter.). *New England Journal of Medicine*, **305**, 1155.

Del Mar, C.B. & Green, A.C. (1995) Aid to diagnosis of melanoma in primary medical care. *British Medical Journal*, **310**, 492–495.

Doherty, V.R. & MacKie, R.M. (1986) Reasons for poor prognosis in British patients with cutaneous malignant melanoma. *British Medical Journal*, **292**, 987–989.

Elwood, J.M. & Gallagher, R.P. (1988) The first signs and symptoms of melanoma: a population-based study. *Pigment Cell*, **9**, 118–130.

Geller, A.C., Koh, H.K., Miller, D.R. *et al.* (1992) Use of health services before the diagnosis of melanoma: Implications for early detection and screening. *Journal of General Internal Medicine*, **7**, 154–157.

Grin, C.M., Kopf, A.W., Welkovich, B. *et al.* (1990) Accuracy in the clinical diagnosis of malignant melanoma. *Archives of Dermatology*, **126**, 763–766.

Hennrikus, D., Girgis, A., Redman, S. *et al.* (1991) A community study of delay in presenting with signs of melanoma to medical practitioners. *Archives of Dermatology*, **127**, 356–361.

Kenet, R.O., Kang, S., Kenet, B.J. *et al.* (1993) Clinical diagnosis of pigmented lesions using digital epiluminescence microscopy. Grading protocol and atlas. *Archives of Dermatology*, **129**, 157–174.

Koh, H.K., Caruso, A., Gage, I. *et al.* (1990) Evaluation of melanoma/skin cancer screening in Massachusetts. *Cancer*, **65**, 375–379.

Koh, H.K., Miller, D.R., Geller, A.C. *et al.* (1992) Who

discovers melanoma? Patterns from a population-based survey. *Journal of the American Academy of Dermatology*, **26**, 914–919.

Koh, H.K., Geller, A.C., Miller, D.R. *et al.* (1995a) The current status of melanoma early detection and screening. *Dermatology Clinics*, **13**, 623–634.

Koh, H.K., Geller, A.C., Miller, D.R. & Lew, R.A. (1995b) The early detection of and screening for melanoma. *Cancer*, **75**, 674–683.

Koh, H.K., Norton, L.A., Geller, A.C. *et al.* (1996) Evaluation of the American Academy of Dermatology's national skin cancer early detection and screening program. *Journal of the American Academy of Dermatology* **34**, 971–978.

Kopf, A.W., Mintzis, M. & Bart, R.S. (1975) Diagnostic accuracy in malignant melanoma. *Archives of Dermatology*, **111**, 1291–1292.

Langley, R.G.B., Rhadyshka, M., Dwyer, P. *et al.* (1996) Confocal scanning laser microscopy in pigmented skin lesions. *Journal of Investigative Dermatology* (Abstract.)

MacKie, R.M. & Cascinelli, N. (1992) *Educational Strategies Designed to Promote Primary and Secondary Prevention of Melanoma* (Publication 1). WHO Melanoma Programme, Milan.

MacKie, R.M., Freudenberger, T. & Aitchison, T.C. (1989) Personal risk factor chart for cutaneous melanoma. *Lancet*, **ii**, 487–490.

Marks, R. & Hill, D. (1992) *The Public Health Approach to Melanoma Screening*. International Union Against Cancer.

McGee, R., Elwood, M., Sneyd, M.J. *et al.* (1994) The recognition and management of melanoma and other skin lesions by general practitioners in New Zealand. *New Zealand Medical Journal*, **107**, 287–290.

McMullan, F.H. & Hubener, L.F. (1956) Malignant melanoma: statistical review of clinical and histological diagnosis. *Archives of Dermatology*, **74**, 618.

Nachbar, F., Stolz, W., Merkle, T. *et al.* (1994) The ABCD rule of dermatoscopy. High prospective value in the diagnosis of doubtful melanocytic skin lesions. *Journal of the American Academy of Dermatology*, **30**, 551–559.

Pehamberger, H., Binder, M., Steiner, A. *et al.* (1993) *In vivo* epiluminescence microscopy: improvement of early diagnosis of melanoma. *Journal of Investigative Dermatology*, **100**, 356S–362S.

Pehamberger, H., Steiner, A. & Wolff, K. (1987) *In vivo* epiluminescence microscopy of pigmented skin lesions. I. Pattern analysis of pigmented skin lesions. *Journal of the American Academy of Dermatology*, **17**, 571–583.

Rajadhyaksha, M., Grossman, M., Esterowitz, D. *et al.* (1995) *In vivo* confocal scanning laser microscopy of human skin: melanin provides strong contrast. *Journal of Investigative Dermatology*, **104**, 946–952.

Rampen, F.H.J. & Rumke, P. (1988) Referral pattern and accuracy of clinical diagnosis of cutaneous melanoma. *Acta Dermato-Venereologica*, **68**, 61–64.

Rhodes, A.R. (1995) Public education and cancer of the skin. What do people need to know about melanoma and nonmelanoma skin cancer? *Cancer*, **75**, 613–636.

Rhodes, A.R., Weinstock, M.A., Fitzpatrick, T.B. *et al.* (1987) Risk factors for cutaneous melanoma: a practical method of recognizing high-risk individuals. *Journal of the American Medical Association*, **258**, 3146–3154.

Steiner, A., Pehamberger, H. & Wolff, K. (1987) *In vivo* epiluminescence microscopy of pigmented skin lesions. II. Diagnosis of small pigmented skin lesions and early detection of malignant melanoma. *Journal of the American Academy of Dermatology*, **17**, 584–591.

Stolz, W., Riemann, A., Przetak, C. *et al.* (1991) Multivariate analysis of criteria given by dermatoscopy for the recognition of melanocytic lesions. In: *Book of Abstracts, Fiftieth Meeting of the American Academy of Dermatology, Dallas, Texas, 7–12 December*, p. 126.

Swerdlow, M. (1952) Nevi: A problem of misdiagnosis. *American Journal of Clinical Pathology*, **22**, 1054.

Temoshok, L., Diclemente, R.J., Sweet, D.M. *et al.* (1984) Factors related to patient delay in seeking medical attention for cutaneous malignant melanoma. *Cancer*, **54**, 3048–3053.

Wagner, R.F. Jr, Wagner, D., Tomich, J.M. *et al.* (1985) Residents' corner: Diagnosis of skin disease: dermatologists vs. nondermatologists. *Journal of Dermatology, Surgery and Oncology*, **11**, 476–479.

Weinstock, M.A., Goldstein, M.C., Dube, C.C. *et al.* (1996) Basic skin cancer triage for teaching melanoma detection. *Journal of American Academy of Dermatology* **34**, 1063–1066.

Witheiler, D.D. & Cockerell, C.J. (1991) Histologic features and sensitivity of diagnosis of clinically unsuspected cutaneous melanoma. *American Journal of Dermopathology*, **13**, 551–556.

Image Analysis and Epiluminescence Microscopy in Early Detection of Cutaneous Melanoma

M. BINDER, H. KITTLER, K. WOLFF AND H. PEHAMBERGER

Introduction

The majority of pigmented skin lesions can be diagnosed correctly on the basis of established clinical criteria, and it is the consensus that the current impressive 5-year survival rates of patients with melanoma are attributable solely to early diagnosis. On the other hand, there remain a surprisingly high number of small melanocytic lesions for which a distinction between benignity and malignancy, and thus between non-melanoma and melanoma, is difficult or even impossible to make on clinical grounds alone. Data indicating that, even in specialized centres, the diagnostic accuracy for early malignant melanoma is only slightly better than 60% may be sobering, but have to be accepted as fact (Grin *et al.*, 1990). Although, theoretically, no melanoma should remain undiagnosed before entering the invasive growth phase, an unbiased assessment of the available pre-operative diagnostic armamentarium indicates clearly that the belief that progressively earlier clinical detection of melanoma eventually will reduce the mortality rate to near zero is highly unrealistic.

Epiluminescence microscopy (ELM) is a non-invasive *in vivo* technique with the potential to correct these diagnostic limitations because it permits the recognition of malignant pigmented lesions much earlier than is possible by clinical inspection alone (Fritsch & Pechlaner, 1981; Pehamberger *et al.*, 1987, 1993; Soyer *et al.*, 1987, 1989; Steiner *et al.*, 1987; Stolz *et al.*, 1987; Kreusch & Rassner, 1990). ELM makes subsurface structures of the skin accessible to visual examination *in vivo* by using surface microscopy and oil immersion (Fritsch & Pechlaner, 1981; Pehamberger *et al.*, 1987, 1993; Steiner *et al.*, 1987). In other words, ELM takes *in vivo* skin microscopy one step further than surface microscopy, because it allows the observer not only to look onto, but also into, the superficial skin layers. The purpose of this review is to describe the principle of, and the procedures employed in, ELM, and to document the significant improvement it offers in the clinical diagnosis of pigmented skin lesions, particularly melanoma.

History

In vivo skin microscopy has been used for decades for nail-bed capillary examination (Gilje *et al.*, 1958). It was recommended for more general dermatological use by Hinselmann in 1933 (Hinselmann, 1933), who proposed the use of a colposcope for high-power examination of skin and mucosal lesions, and by Goldman, who systematically employed surface microscopy as a diagnostic procedure (Goldman & Younker, 1947; Goldman *et al.*, 1948). MacKie first used *in vivo* microscopy in the pre-operative diagnosis of pigmented lesions (MacKie, 1971), and Fritsch and Pechlaner (1981) employed oil immersion in their evaluation, describing the 'pigmented network' that now is widely used as a criterion in distinguishing melanocytic from non-melanocytic lesions. Pehamberger, Steiner, Binder and Wolff (Pehamberger *et al.*, 1987, 1993; Steiner *et al.*, 1987, 1993) systematically applied certain ELM criteria to pigmented skin lesions and created algorithms which were put into test as pattern analysis (Pehamberger *et al.*, 1987; Steiner *et al.*, 1987, 1993). Variously termed 'skin surface microscopy', 'incident light microscopy', 'dermatoscopy' or 'dermoscopy', this technique has gained acceptance as a valuable tool in the pre-operative diagnosis of pigmented lesions and is being used routinely and successfully by a number of centres. The term ELM more specifically describes *in vivo* skin microscopy employing oil immersion, which eliminates reflection from the skin's surface and the air, permitting the investigator to look through the epidermis as far down as the dermal–epidermal junction and, in lesions with little pigmentation, even beyond. A consensus conference on appropriate terminology (Bahmer *et al.*, 1990a,b), several reviews (Kreusch & Rassner 1990; Pehamberger *et al.*, 1993; Sober, 1993; Wolff *et al.*, 1994) and an atlas have been published on this topic (Kreusch & Rassner, 1991).

Principle

The term 'epiluminescence microscopy' describes the non-invasive *in vivo* examination of skin lesions with a microscope using incident light and oil immersion (Pehamberger *et al.*, 1987, 1993). The examination of lesions by ELM is a three-step procedure. The first step is clinical examination, including analysis of the various features of a lesion with the unassisted eye. Next, skin-surface microscopy is performed using a binocular stereomicroscope (Pehamberger *et al.*, 1987) similar to those employed in operative ophthalmology or plastic surgery, or a hand-held microscope which is monocular, small and easily handled (Braun Falco *et al.*, 1990; Pehamberger *et al.*, 1993). A built-in light source and magnifications ranging from 6- to 80-fold provide for a more detailed and subtle analysis of the criteria seen by the unaided eye, including the surface characteristics, configuration, colour and margins of a lesion. Finally, the ELM step employs immersion oil and a glass slide pressed on the lesion if a large stereo-microscope is being employed, or the direct application of the front lens of a hand-held instrument to the lesion. With oil immersion, the incident light is not reflected from the surface of the lesion, but is absorbed, scattered and reflected from structures below the skin's surface. This reveals a new dimension of morphological features, colours and patterns that cannot be detected by clinical examination or skin-surface microscopy.

Analysis

The new dimension opened by ELM required definition of the morphological features that appear regularly in pigmented lesions, to create a terminology for these features and define patterns within which they occur. Three essentially similar, but slightly different, strategies have been developed for ELM interpretation. Kenet suggests the use of overall morphological pigment patterns as basic distinguishing features (Kenet *et al.*, 1993) whereas Nachbar and colleagues employ modified 'ABCD' rules as a starting point (Nachbar *et al.*, 1994). Our group relies on detailed pattern analysis as the most reliable approach to the identification of lesions (Pehamberger *et al.*, 1987; Steiner *et al.*, 1987, 1993). This latter approach is the only one that has been tested in a large number of lesions. Criteria are defined by purely descriptive terms that have been correlated with histopathological features (Pehamberger *et al.*, 1987). Various ELM criteria have been described extensively in the literature (Fritsch & Pechlaner 1981; Pehamberger *et al.*, 1987, 1993; Soyer *et al.*, 1987, 1989; Steiner *et al.*, 1987; Stolz *et al.*, 1987; Kreusch & Rassner, 1990; Kenet *et al.*, 1993). Pattern analysis correlates individual criteria with each other and puts them into the context of a pattern that is typical for a specific pathology and, thus, a lesion.

ELM examination of a lesion involves searching for individual ELM criteria and determining whether they are present or absent. If ELM criteria are found, they are analysed further to whether they are regular or irregular, delicate or prominent, or well defined or ill defined, and their location within the lesion is determined (centre, margin or both). Thus, for each criterion, several variables exist that, taken together and combined in the process of pattern analysis, permit the recognition of patterns that are typical and characteristic for individual lesions. Thus, in pattern analysis, the presence or absence, quality and morphological characteristics of ELM criteria and their distribution with a lesion combine to yield a diagnosis.

Experience based on the analysis of >7000 pigmented skin lesions has permitted the establishment of algorithms defining patterns that are characteristic for different types of lesions. Comparison of these algorithms has revealed that pattern analysis not only permits one to discriminate between melanocytic and non-melanocytic lesions, but also to distinguish between benign and malignant growth pattern (Pehamberger *et al.*, 1993; Steiner *et al.*, 1993).

A study of small (<0.5 cm) pigmented skin lesions that were diagnostically equivocal when examined with the unaided eye revealed that the accuracy of clinical diagnosis can be improved considerably by ELM pattern analysis for practically all types of lesions (Steiner *et al.*, 1987; Pehamberger *et al.*, 1993). This is particularly evident in the improvement observed in the diagnostic score achieved for dysplastic naevi, superficial spreading melanoma *in situ*, superficial spreading melanoma (invasive) and pigmented basal-cell carcinoma (Pehamberger *et al.*, 1993).

Experience with a large number of lesions also has revealed that the ELM technique has a number of limitations. Because pattern analysis is based on the detection and combination of ELM criteria, their presence is more important than their absence. Therefore, the absence or non-visibility of defined criteria, for instance, as a result of heavy overall pigmentation, may render diagnosis by ELM impossible. Because pattern analysis depends on the combination of criteria, a single criterion usually is insufficient for diagnosis, and year-long experience with this technique has revealed that some criteria are more important than others. Pattern analysis does not eliminate diagnostic errors completely, and ELM therefore cannot replace histopathological examination.

The concept of a computer-aided diagnostic system

Although there is no doubt that ELM significantly improves diagnostic accuracy for pigmented skin lesions, particularly for naevi and malignant melanoma, this improvement is restricted to experienced investigators who are familiar with, and trained in, using the technique. ELM diagnosis often is influenced by subjective impression rather than based on objective and reproducible criteria-pattern analysis. A recent study performed in our centre, in which the results of evaluations of ELM images by clinicians experienced in the use of ELM and novices in the field were compared, supported this impression (Binder *et al.*, 1995). Methods are being sought and will have to be found to make pattern analysis more objective. One solution may be computerized imaging of ELM, which also would provide an unlimited capacity for data storage and retrieval. Artificial neural networks (ANN) are computational models based on the principles of neural propagation and processing that are being used increasingly for pattern recognition in various investigative and clinical fields. A recent study attempted to determine whether ELM criteria-pattern analysis can be used in an observer-independent, objective, computerized system, and whether ANN are applicable to the clinical diagnosis of pigmented skin lesions, particularly to discriminating between benign naevi and malignant melanomas (Binder *et al.*, 1994). The basic element in this system is the simulated neuron. This neuron processes a defined number of input patterns (ELM criteria) and, through a learning process, produces an output pattern (using histological diagnosis as the gold standard). Upon completion of learning, the ANN was able to classify correctly a total of 86% of the ELM patterns presented in a test database of 100 pigmented skin lesions. Malignant melanomas were diagnosed correctly 95% of the time, common naevi 87% of the time and dysplastic naevi 73% of the time. In contrast, investigators experienced in the use of ELM correctly recognized 88% of all pigmented lesions, 95% of melanomas, 97% of common naevi and 70% of dysplastic naevi. Thus, the results achieved by the computer using ANN were comparable to those obtained by investigators using ELM pattern analysis in clinical diagnosis. In a dichotomized model comparing compound and dysplastic naevi versus malignant melanomas, the sensitivity and specificity of human diagnosis were 95% and 91%, respectively, and the sensitivity and specificity of ANN diagnosis were 95% and 90%, respectively. In other words, the criteria used for ELM pattern analysis are consistent enough to allow a computerized system to make classifications and yield diagnoses with a high degree of accuracy. In addition, ANN can be interfaced with computerized image analysis systems for texture and colour of pigmented skin lesions that currently are being developed.

Summary

ELM is a new approach to the diagnosis of pigmented skin lesions that holds considerable promise. It reveals a new dimension of *in vivo* morphology that can be used when the diagnostic criteria employed in routine visual diagnosis fail. It does not add to the diagnostic armamentarium available for unequivocal lesions, but has significant value for those equivocal, small, pigmented skin lesions that pose major diagnostic problems even for experienced clinicians. Prerequisites for a sensible approach to ELM include recognition of new morphological ELM criteria and employment of these criteria in an analytical process called 'pattern analysis'. As in clinical dermatology, ELM depends heavily on a learning process and, of course, on experience.

ELM increases diagnostic accuracy for pigmented skin lesions in that it helps to distinguish between melanocytic and non-melanocytic pigmented lesions, and between benign and malignant growth patterns. Thus, ELM has the potential to overcome the diagnostic limitations encountered in clinical dermatology when small, early pigmented lesions are encountered that do not yet express the full complement of diagnostic features needed to arrive at a correct diagnosis. The fact that it is a non-invasive, *in vivo* method makes it even more attractive as a diagnostic tool in clinical practice. ELM already had proven to be of great practical value in several centres by increasing the probability that early melanoma will not be overlooked and by helping determine which lesions need to be removed. Of course, ELM also has limitations. It does not provide 100% diagnostic accuracy and is of little help in small lesions that are pigmented maximally and uniformly because these do not reveal the criteria necessary for ELM pattern analysis. At this stage, therefore, ELM does not replace histopathological examination.

Undoubtedly, ELM can be improved, and continued studies will reveal just how reliable the individual criteria eventually will prove to be in clinical practice. This requires continuing to accumulate and analyse data, and instituting teaching programmes to familiarize dermatologists with ELM criteria and their use in pattern analysis. It is certain, however, that, just as clinicians have learned to employ the 'ABCD' rules in visually recognizing and diagnosing melanoma, they will learn this new and more subtle approach to the previously unknown morphological features that characterize benign and malignant pigmentary lesions on ELM. Finally, ELM criteria and pattern analysis must be made more objective and computerized imaging of ELM may provide the means to achieve this goal.

References

Bahmer, F.A., Fritsch, P., Kreusch, J. *et al.* (1990a) Terminology in surface microscopy. Consensus meeting of the Committee on Analytical Morphology of the Arbeitsgemeinschaft Dermatologische Forschung, Hamburg, Federal Republic of Germany, 17 November 1989. *Journal of the American Academy of Dermatologists*, **23**, 1159–1162.

Bahmer, F.A., Fritsch, P., Kreusch, J. *et al.* (1990b) Diagnostic criteria in epiluminescence microscopy. Consensus meeting of the professional Committee on Analytical Morphology of the Arbeitsgemeinschaft Dermatologische Forschung, Hamberg, Federal Republic of Germany, 17 November 1989. *Hautarzt*, **41**, 513–514.

Binder, M., Steiner, A., Schwarz, M., Knollmayer, S., Wolff, K. & Pehamberger, H. (1994) Application of an artificial neural network in epiluminescence microscopy pattern analysis of pigmented skin lesions: a pilot study. *British Journal of Dermatology*, **130**, 460–465.

Binder, M., Schwarz, M., Winkler, A. *et al.* (1995) Epiluminescence microscopy: A useful tool for the diagnosis of pigmented skin lesions for formally trained dermatologists. *Archives of Dermatology*, **131**, 286–291.

Braun Falco, O., Stolz, W., Bilek, P., Merkle, T. & Landthaler, M. (1990) Das Dermatoskop. *Hautarzt*, **41**, 131–136.

Fritsch, P. & Pechlaner, R. (1981) Differentiation of benign from malignant melanocytic lesions using incident light microscopy. In: *Pathology of Malignant Melanoma* (ed. A.B. Ackermann), pp. 301–312. Masson, New York.

Gilje, O., O'Leary, P.A. & Baldes, E.J. (1958) Capillary micro-

scopic examination in skin disease. *Archives of Dermatology*, **68**, 136–145.

Goldman, L. & Younker, W. (1947) Studies in microscopy of the surface of the skin. *Journal of Investigative Dermatology*, **9**, 11.

Goldman, L., McDaniel, W.E., Younker, W. & Siebentritt, C.R.J. (1948) Clinical microscopy of the surface of the skin. *Interim Session American Medical Association*.

Grin, C.M., Kopf, A.W., Welkovich, B., Bart, R.S. & Levenstein, M.J. (1990) Accuracy in the clinical diagnosis of malignant melanoma. *Archives of Dermatology*, **126**, 763–766.

Hinselmann, H. (1933) Die Bedeutung der Kolposkopie für den Dermatologen. *Dermatologische Wochenschrift*, **96**, 533–545.

Kenet, R.O., Kang, S., Kenet, B.J., Fitzpatrick, T.B., Sober, A.J. & Barnhill, R.L. (1993) Clinical diagnosis of pigmented lesions using digital epiluminescence microscopy. Grading protocol and atlas. *Archives of Dermatology*, **129**, 157–174.

Kreusch, J. & Rassner, G. (1990) Structural analysis of melanocytic pigment nevi using epiluminescence microscopy. Review and personal experiences. *Hautarzt*, **41**, 27–33.

Kreusch, J. & Rassner, G. (1991) *Auflichtmikroskopie pigmentierter Hauttumore*. George Thieme Verlag, Stuttgart.

MacKie, R.M. (1971) An aid to the preoperative assessment of pigmented lesions of the skin. *British Journal of Dermatology*, **85**, 232–238.

Nachbar, F., Stolz, W., Merkle, T. *et al.* (1994) The ABCD rule of dermatoscopy. High prospective value in the diagnosis of doubtful melanocytic skin lesions. *Journal of the American Academy of Dermatology*, **30**, 551–559.

Pehamberger, H., Steiner, A. & Wolff, K. (1987) *In vivo* epiluminescence microscopy of pigmented skin lesions. I. Pattern analysis of pigmented skin lesions. *Journal of the American Academy of Dermatology*, **17**, 571–583.

Pehamberger, H., Binder, M., Steiner, A. & Wolff, K. (1993) *In vivo* epiluminescence microscopy — improvement of early diagnosis of melanoma. *Journal of Investigative Dermatology*, **100**, S356–S362.

Sober, A.J. (1993) Digital epiluminescence microscopy in the evaluation of pigmented lesions: a brief review. *Seminars in Surgery and Oncology*, **9**, 198–201.

Soyer, H.P., Smolle, J., Kerl, H. & Stettner, H. (1987) Early diagnosis of malignant melanoma by surface microscopy. *Lancet*, **2**, 803.

Soyer, H.P., Smolle, J., Hoedl, S., Pachernegg, H. & Kerl, H. (1989) A new approach to the diagnosis of cutaneous pigmented tumors. *American Journal of Dermatopathology*, **11**, 1–10.

Steiner, A., Pehamberger, H. & Wolff, K. (1987) *In vivo* epiluminescence of pigmented skin lesions. II. Diagnosis of small pigmented skin lesions and early detection of malignant melanoma. *Journal of the American Academy of Dermatology*, **17**, 584–591.

Steiner, A., Binder, M., Schemper, M., Wolff, K. & Pehamberger, H. (1993) Statistical evaluation of epiluminescence microscopy criteria for melanocytic pigmented skin lesions. *Journal of the American Academy of Dermatology*, **29**, 581–588.

Stolz, W., Bilek, P., Landthaler, M., Merkle, T. & Braun-Falco, O. (1987) Skin surface microscopy. *Lancet*, **2**, 864–865.

Wolff, K., Binder, M. & Pehamberger, H. (1994) Epiluminescence microscopy: a new approach to the early detection of melanoma. *Advances in Dermatology*, **9**, 45–56.

12
Virus and Skin Cancers

Skin Cancers in Immunocompromised Patients

S. EUVRARD, J. KANITAKIS AND
A. CLAUDY

Immunocompromised patients are prone to develop some cancers, especially those that are associated with viruses. Compared to the general population, the same types of cutaneous malignancies are increased in the course of various immunodeficiencies, and include carcinomas, Kaposi's sarcoma, lymphomas and melanoma. The different frequency of the various tumour types observed in each kind of immunodeficiency highlights the role of other co-carcinogenic factors. Immunosuppression allows activation of oncogenic viruses and potentiates the effects of other carcinogens such as ultraviolet light.

Organ transplantation

The number of organ transplant recipients is growing steadily thanks to the development of transplantation surgery and to improvements in immunosuppressive therapy. The good function of the graft requires patients to be on immunosuppressive treatment during the whole of their life; most of them receive two or three drugs (mainly steroids, azathioprine, cyclosporine or FK 506), inducing long-term immunodeficiency. Organ-transplant recipients are at a high risk to develop cutaneous and extracutaneous tumours. Non-transplant patients receiving immunosuppressive treatment may develop the same malignancies but with a much lower frequency, probably because of the usually smaller dosage of the drugs and the shorter duration of treatment as compared with organ-transplant recipients.

Cutaneous carcinomas

Skin carcinomas, especially squamous-cell carcinomas (SCC), are the most frequent malignancies developing in organ-transplant recipients; they represent a model of viral carcinogenesis where human papillomaviruses (HPV) along with other co-carcinogenic factors such as ultraviolet radiation and immunosuppressive treatment seem to be involved (Barr *et al.*, 1989; Euvrard *et al.*, 1993).

Epidemiology

Skin carcinomas concern mainly fair-skinned patients who are subject to sun exposure. Their frequency increases progressively with time after transplantation: 40–70% of renal transplant patients are involved after 20 years, the highest figures being observed in Australia where both risk factors are important (Sheil, 1992; Bouwes Bavinck *et al.*, 1996). Recipients of non-renal organs show a higher frequency of skin carcinomas as compared with renal transplant recipients (Penn & Brunson, 1988; Euvrard *et al.*, 1995b). The time lapse after transplantation is, on average, 7–8 years in renal-transplant patients and decreases with increasing latitude. This delay is shorter (2–4 years) after heart and liver transplantation (Levy *et al.*, 1993; Espana *et al.*, 1995; Euvrard *et al.*, 1995b). The first carcinomas occur on average 20–30 years earlier than in non-immunosuppressed persons.

189

Clinical features

Carcinomas are chiefly located on sun-exposed areas. They are often associated with warts and various epithelial lesions such as premalignant keratoses, Bowen's disease and keratoacanthomas (KA). The clinical aspects are often misleading since SCC may simulate warts or KA. The differential diagnosis between KA and SCC is sometimes difficult even after histological examination. Carcinomas are predominantly SCC; as compared with the general population the squamous-to-basal-cell carcinoma ratio is reversed and varies from 1.2:1 to 15:1, this reversal being more pronounced in kidney- than in heart- or liver-transplant recipients. The lesions tend to be multiple, and after several years some patients may develop over 100 tumours. SCC sometimes have a very rapid growth and may be complicated by repeated local recurrences. The risk of metastasis per patient (6–8%) (Sheil, 1992; Penn, 1993) appears higher than in control groups. Factors of unfavourable prognosis include clinically an older age, the multiplicity of SCC and the cephalic location, and histologically the thickness of the tumour with involvement of the subcutaneous adipose tissue (Euvrard *et al.*, 1995a).

Pathogenesis

The role of HPV in the development of skin carcinomas is suggested clinically by the presence of warts in the same locations and histologically by a range of intermediate forms from common warts to invasive carcinoma. Most virological studies have shown HPV DNA in at least 50% of premalignant lesions and carcinomas from renal-graft patients. The usual tissue-specific distribution of HPV is switched in transplant recipients, mucosal types being found on skin areas. Oncogenic types are detected in benign lesions and benign types may be found within malignant lesions. Furthermore, epidermodysplasia verruciformis-associated HPV types are frequently detected (Jong Tieben *et al.*, 1995). However, HPV necessitate other co-carcinogenic factors. Immunodepression itself is certainly involved since an increase of cutaneous cancers has been reported in patients undergoing haemodialysis and in acquired immunodeficiency syndrome (AIDS). The specific role of each drug is still debated; because of varying individual sensitivity to immunosuppressive treatment, the role of the mean doses of the drugs is difficult to assess (Bouwes Bavinck *et al.*, 1991). The higher incidence of tumours in heart-transplant recipients is probably due to the greater intensity of the immunosuppressive treatment. The length and the intensity of immunosuppressive treatment are probably more important than the nature of the drug(s) used (Bouwes Bavinck *et al.*, 1996).

The most determinative factor for the development of skin carcinomas is certainly ultraviolet radiation as suggested by the appearance of warts and carcinomas on sun-exposed areas of light-skinned patients. Ultraviolet light induces a local immunodeficiency that may facilitate HPV proliferation and tumour promotion.

Genetic factors could also intervene in the progression towards malignancy. The results of various studies concerning the role of HLA antigens in organ-transplant recipients with skin cancer are contradictory; however, an increased frequency of HLA-DR7 among patients with skin cancers was reported in two independent studies (Czarnecki *et al.*, 1992; Bouwes Bawinck *et al.*, 1993).

Treatment

Most SCC are successfully treated by surgical excision. Topical retinoids can be used to treat multiple premalignant lesions and to prevent the development of carcinomas (Euvrard *et al.*, 1992a). Resurfacing the back of the hands may be useful in patients having multiple lesions over this area (Van Zuuren *et al.*, 1994). When carcinomas become numerous or aggressive, a reduction of the immunosuppressive treatment should be attempted. Systemic retinoids (Shuttleworth *et al.*, 1988; Bouwes Bavinck *et al.*, 1995) slow down the development of carcinomas and dysplastic lesions; unfortunately, their long-term use is often limited by the increase of serum lipids, hepatic intolerance and/or bone side effects. Hence, systemic retinoids should be reserved to the most severe cases either over 1 or 2 years if the immunosuppressive treatment can be substantially reduced or definitively when tapering of immunosuppressive treatment is not feasible. If metastases develop, chemotherapy or interferon-α can be added; however, the risk of interferon-induced graft rejection should be seriously considered

(Magnone *et al.*, 1994). We believe radio-therapy to be ineffective.

Anogenital cancers

Carcinomas of the anogenital region (anus, peri-anal skin and external genitalia) seem to be increased; for instance, vulvar cancer is 30-fold more frequent as compared with control groups (Sheil *et al.*, 1987; Birkeland *et al.*, 1995). The study of Penn (Penn, 1986) reveals an average time interval after transplantation of 7–8 years and a female preponderance. Lymph-node involvement occurs in 11% of patients. Lesions tend to be multiple especially in women who may present simultaneous or successive involvement of the anogenital area, the cervix (30%), vagina or urethra. HPV are probably involved since about one-third of patients have a past history of condylomata acuminata. Studies concerning HPV infection in genitalia performed in cervical and anal lesions showed frequently the presence of oncogenic types (Blessing *et al.*, 1990; Ogunbiyi *et al.*, 1994). Similar to non-immuno-suppressed groups, risk factors include other infections (especially *Chlamydia* and herpes simplex), number of sexual partners and cigarette smoking. Treatment relies on surgery, decrease of the immunosuppressive treatment and topical 5-fluorouracil for *in situ* lesions.

Kaposi's sarcoma (KS)

Epidemiology

Kaposi's sarcoma is the first malignancy to appear after the graft, on average 12 months for patients on cyclosporin and 24 months for those on conventional treatment (azathioprine plus steroids) (Penn & Brunson, 1988); this delay would be shorter (6 months) after liver transplantation (Farge, 1993; Levy *et al.*, 1993; Besnard *et al.*, 1996). KS is 400- to 500-fold more frequent in graft recipients than in control groups (Harwood *et al.*, 1979). In organ-transplant recipients, the ethnic background is decisive: only patients of Mediterranean, Jewish, Arabic or African ancestry are concerned. Thus, the incidence of KS depends on the ethnic origin of the series, varying from 0.4 to 0.5% in Western countries to 4.1% in Saudi Arabia, where this tumour is considered to be the most frequent after renal transplantation (Qunibi *et al.*, 1993). The incidence of KS seems to be higher after liver transplantation. Because of this early appearance, the mean age (40 years) is younger than in the Mediterranean form. There is a male predominance as for other KS groups. HLA antigen distribution in patients with KS is the same as that of control groups of the same ethnic background; poor donor–recipient matching does not seem to be a risk factor (Brunson *et al.*, 1990). KS is a marker of deep immunosuppression: the development of the lesions immediately after rejection episodes treated with an increase of the immunosuppressive treatment and their disappearance within months after reducing the treatment demonstrate the dependence of KS on the level of immunosuppression. Furthermore, KS is the unique cutaneous malignancy that up till now has been reported after FK 506 treatment (Kadry *et al.*, 1993). The viral origin of KS is a still debated hypothesis: herpes simplex virus, cytomegalovirus, Epstein–Barr virus, HPV and hepatitis B virus have been incriminated but definite evidence favouring the role of these viruses in the genesis of KS lesions is as yet lacking. Recently, a new herpes-like virus (HHV-8 or KSHV) has been detected within lesions of KS, in classical, AIDS- and organ-transplantation-associated forms (Chang *et al.*, 1994; Boshoff *et al.*, 1995; Renne *et al.*, 1996). This new agent appears a serious aetiological candidate for the development of KS, but its role remains to be further established.

Clinical features

KS is limited to the skin and/or mucosa in 70–75% of kidney- and 50% of heart- and liver-transplant recipients (Farge, 1993). The cutaneous form is similar to the Mediterranean one, with lesions being much less extensive than in AIDS. The angiomatous plaques or nodules are mainly located on the lower limbs but can spread to the trunk and face. The lesions may appear on scars of various origins. The mucosal involvement especially concerns the upper oral pharynx (nasal mucosa, palate, pharynx and larynx) and the conjunctiva. Visceral involvement mostly concerns the digestive tract and lungs. Purely visceral forms are rare.

Course and treatment

A fatal evolution is observed in one-third of KS cases (Farge, 1993) and is more frequent in liver- and heart- compared with kidney-transplant recipients (Francès *et al.*, 1991). Visceral involvement bears a poor prognosis with a 78% mortality against 11% for purely cutaneous forms. The first treatment step is to reduce immunosuppressive treatment and, if necessary, to stop it completely in the case of kidney transplant recipients who can return to dialysis. If the modification of immunosuppressive treatment is not applicable or ineffective and the lesions are diffuse, it is necessary to resort to cytostatic drugs (vinblastine, vindesine, bleomycin). The use of interferon can lead to rejection and must be avoided except in some liver-transplant recipients. Surgical excision can be useful for single lesions. Radiotherapy should be avoided because of the long-term risk of cutaneous carcinomas.

Lymphomas

Non-Hodgkin's lymphomas occur in 1–2% of graft recipients and are generally of B-cell lineage. They have a predilection for extranodal sites (75%) and are considered to result from excessive immuno-suppression, a reduction in the immunosuppressive treatment often resulting in their regression. Cutaneous locations seem rare but specific lymphomatous involvement may be seen at late stages. Clinically, primary cutaneous B-cell lymphomas present with single or multiple ulcerated nodules of the face (McGregor *et al.*, 1993) and can be successfully treated by surgery or radiotherapy. Epstein–Barr virus is closely associated with all B-cell lymphomas including cutaneous ones. Rare cases of cutaneous T-cell lymphoma have been reported in transplant patients, manifesting as mycosis fungoides (Pascual *et al.*, 1992) or Sézary syndrome (Euvrard *et al.*, 1992b). The delay between transplantation and diagnosis is on average 3 years for B-cell lymphoma and more variable for T-cell lymphoma; T-cell lymphomas may occur after the decrease of the immunosuppressive treatment.

Melanoma

Only a few studies concerning melanoma are available,

the larger series reporting 14 cases. The frequency of melanoma in the transplant population varies from 0.5 to 4/1000 (Greene & Young, 1981; Sheil *et al.*, 1987) and the risk for its development is 1.6–4-fold higher than that of control groups (Sheil *et al.*, 1987; Birkeland *et al.*, 1995). Melanomas appear within 22–40 months after the graft; most lesions occur on unexposed areas, in light-skinned patients, often on dysplastic naevi. Patients having had a melanoma before the graft are prone to develop metastases following transplantation. The development of dysplastic naevi on the back and the palms and soles in children after grafting has recently been reported (Smith *et al.*, 1993). Therefore grafted children seem to have a higher risk for the development of melanoma.

Other rare malignant tumours

These have also been reported: malignant histiocytoma, sweat-gland carcinoma (Blohme & Larkö, 1990), Merkel cell carcinoma (Penn, 1993; Formica *et al.*, 1994), atypical fibroxanthoma (Kanitakis *et al.*, 1996).

Acquired immunodeficiency syndrome (AIDS)

AIDS patients share with transplant recipients a higher risk to various malignancies associated with viruses. The shorter survival time of AIDS patients selects cancers that develop rapidly after the onset of the immunodeficiency, such as KS; cutaneous and anogenital cancers would probably be more increased if the survival of these patients was longer. The occurrence of basal-cell carcinomas at an early stage of human immunodeficiency virus (HIV) infection is puzzling.

Kaposi's sarcoma (KS)

Epidemiology

Kaposi's sarcoma is one of the most common malignancies of HIV infection: the overall risk of KS in patients with AIDS was assessed to be increased 20000-fold as compared with the general population and 300-fold as compared with other immunosuppressed groups (Tappero, 1993). The frequency of KS varies according to the different HIV-transmission groups; KS concerns 20% of homosexual patients and has been reported rarely in haemophilics, mostly homosexual ones (Ragni *et al.*, 1993). The occurrence of KS in HIV-negative homosexual men suggests that it could be a second sexually transmitted disease distinct from HIV. A declining prevalence in high-risk sexual behaviour could explain the decreasing incidence of KS in recent years. Similarly to the organ transplantation-associated form, HHV8 (KSHV) sequences are regularly detected within AIDS-associated KS (Chang *et al.*, 1994; Boshoff *et al.*, 1995).

Clinical features

AIDS-associated KS may develop at any stage of HIV disease but usually appears rather late. It tends to be extensive with widespread cutaneous lesions. Koebnerization occurs at sites of trauma or prior cutaneous disease. Oral lesions (especially palate) occur in about half of the patients with skin lesions. Visceral involvement is observed in 75% of the cases; the most common sites include the gastrointestinal tract, lungs and lymph nodes but KS may also affect the liver, spleen, urogenital tract and brain. Visceral locations without skin involvement are occasionally observed.

Course and treatment

The course of KS is variable and depends on the extent of the lesions, the degree of immunosuppression and the assessment of HIV systemic illness. Local treatments comprise laser, surgery, cryotherapy, radiotherapy, intralesional vinblastine, vincristine or interferon; they are often required for disfiguring or painful lesions. Systemic interferon or chemotherapy may be attempted in disseminated KS; the main agents comprise vinblastine, vincristine, bleomycin and adriamycin in monotherapy or in combination. The various regimens must be given in a dose that will slow the course of the malignancy, but will not further immunosuppress the patient (Conant, 1995).

Cutaneous carcinomas

Cutaneous carcinomas would be the second frequent cutaneous malignancy in HIV-positive patients (Smith *et al.*, 1993). In contrast with organ transplant patients, they are chiefly basal-cell carcinomas (Lobo *et al.*, 1992; Smith *et al.*, 1993; Conant, 1995). The major risks seem to be the same as in the normal population, i.e. fair skin and light-coloured eyes, a positive family history and sun exposure. In the study of Lobo *et al.* (1992) out of 116 carcinomas, 101 were basal-cell carcinomas (mostly superficial multicentric on the trunk) and 15 were SCC of the head and neck. Half of the patients had multiple lesions. Standard treatments were successful except for SCC that had a high recurrence rate (20%). However, the number of carcinomas did not correlate with the degree of immunosuppression, half of the patients being at an early stage of HIV infection. The association of carcinomas with multiple warts seems much rarer than in organtransplant recipients (Milburn *et al.*, 1988) and HPV would only occasionally be involved.

Anogenital cancers

The frequency of anal cancers among homosexual men with AIDS would be increased more than 40-fold compared with the frequency in the general population (Palefsky, 1994). Risk factors include receptive anal intercourse, a history of genital warts and smoking (Daling *et al.*, 1987). The degree to which HIV-associated immunosuppression contributes to this increase beyond the risk associated with homosexual activity *per se* is unknown (Melbye *et al.*, 1994). HPV is currently believed to play a central role in the pathogenesis of both cervical and anal cancer. Several works report an increased incidence of both HPV infection and anal intra-epithelial neoplasia in HIV-positive homosexual men (Kiviat *et al.*, 1993). Data on HIV-positive women also suggest an increased incidence of cervical and anal HPV infection and cytological abnormalities, but anal lesions are more frequent than cervical ones, suggesting that women with HIV infection are also at increased risk of developing anal cancer (William *et al.*, 1994).

The frequency of HPV detection is not related to the level of immunodepression and the finding of a co-localization of HIV-1 and HPV in cervical intra-epithelial neoplasia suggests a possible interaction between the two viruses (Vernon *et al.*, 1994). However, dysplastic lesions are more frequent in patients with lower

CD4 counts. The natural history of anal intra-epithelial neoplasia is not yet understood; only high-grade dysplasia could progress towards malig-nancy but the time for development of invasive cancer from intra-epithelial neoplasia in the setting of HIV infection is not known. In the study of Daling *et al.* (1987) concerning non-immunosuppressed groups, anal warts had been diagnosed at least 10 years before the diagnosis of cancer. HIV-positive women have no higher risk for invasive cervical and anal cancer; this could be explained by the time required for progression of *in situ* towards invasive carcinoma, which is longer than the survival of these patients. The improvement of HIV treatments allowing longer survival will induce higher risks for these cancers.

The absence of external anal lesions does not exclude the presence of internal ones (Palefsky *et al.*, 1990) and anal cytology should be regularly performed in high-risk groups. Anal cancer may have an aggressive course and usually requires radiotherapy.

Similar to organ-transplant recipients, some other rare malignant tumours have been occasionally observed (malignant histiocytoma, Povar Marco *et al.*, 1994; sweat-gland carcinoma, Toi *et al.*, 1995).

Lymphomas

Non-Hodgkin's lymphomas are one of the most common AIDS-associated malignancy, seen mainly in haemophiliacs (Ragni *et al.*, 1993). Similar to the setting of organ transplantion, they are mostly B-cell lymphomas with frequent involvement of extra-nodal sites; cutaneous localizations are rare (Smith *et al.*, 1993), representing a mere 7% of the cases of Ragni *et al.* They are aggressive and seen in advanced disease. Some cases of cutaneous T-cell lymphoma have been reported (Kerschmann *et al.*, 1995). Two forms seem to exist; the first one is that of mycosis fungoides or Sézary syndrome and runs a relatively indolent course. The second presentation is characterized clinically by a single or a few nodules, sometimes with ulceration, arising on the trunk, proximal extremities and head; they correspond to large-cell lymphomas which often harbour CD30[+] cells and Epstein–Barr virus and bear a poor prognosis. The pathogenesis of cutaneous lymphomas in HIV infection is unknown; Epstein–Barr virus could be involved in some cases of both B- and T-cell lymphomas (Dreno *et al.*, 1993) and a role of HIV itself is not excluded.

Melanoma

The association of melanoma with HIV infection has been considered but not yet well established. Some authors have reported the occurrence of eruptive dysplastic naevi (Duvic *et al.*, 1989) and melanomas in the setting of HIV infection (Tindall *et al.*, 1989; Smith *et al.*, 1993). However, homosexual men have often a high-risk lifestyle with heavy sun exposure (Conant, 1995).

Genetic immunodeficiencies

Patients with genetic immunodeficiencies are likely to develop cancers but these are generally extracutaneous. The single disorder showing a high propensity to skin cancers is epidermodysplasia verruciformis (EV). This is a rare genetic disorder (Orth, 1987; Majewski & Jablonska, 1995) generally transmitted as an autosomal recessive trait. The disease begins in childhood and associates multiple flat warts with tinea versicolor-like macules. The course is chronic and 30–60% of patients develop cutaneous carcinomas in adulthood. These are mainly squamous-cell carcinomas, Bowen's disease and occasionally basal-cell carcinomas; a metastatic spread may be observed. Their location on sun-exposed areas suggests an important co-carcinogenic role of ultraviolet light. Most patients have an impaired cell-mediated immunity allowing proliferation of specific HPV types which are not pathogenic in non-immunocompromised people. About 30 different HPV types can be detected within EV lesions but only some of them (mainly types 5 and 8) are involved in the development of carcinomas. A clinical aspect similar to EV (EV-like syndrome) has been observed in the course of other genetic (dyskeratosis congenita, common variable immuno-deficiency) or iatrogenic immunodeficiencies but EV-like syndromes may be complicated by carcinomas only in the setting of organ transplantation.

References

Barr, B., Benton, E., McLaren, K. *et al.* (1989) Human

papillomavirus infection and skin cancer in renal allograft recipients. *Lancet*, **i**, 124–129.

Besnard, V., Euvrard, S., Kanitakis, J. *et al.* (1996) Kaposi's sarcoma after liver transplantation. *Dermatology*, **193**, 100–104.

Birkeland, S., Storm, H., Lamm, L. *et al.* (1995) Cancer risk after renal transplantation in Nordic countries. *International Journal of Cancer*, **60**, 183–189.

Blessing, K., McLaren, K., Morris, R. *et al.* (1990) Detection of human papillomavirus in skin and genital lesions of renal allograft recipients by *in situ* hybridization. *Histopathology*, **16**, 181–185.

Blohme, I. & Larkö, O. (1990) Skin lesions in renal transplant patients after 10–23 years of immunosuppressive therapy. *Acta Dermato-Venereologica*, **70**, 491–494.

Boshoff, C., Whitby, D., Hatziloannou, T. *et al.* (1995) Kaposi's-sarcoma-associated herpesvirus in HIV-negative Kaposi's sarcoma. *Lancet*, **345**, 1043.

Bouwes Bavinck, J., Vermeer, B., Van der Woude, F. *et al.* (1991) Relation between skin cancer and HLA antigens in renal transplant recipients. *New England Journal of Medicine*, **325**, 843–848.

Bouwes Bavinck, J., Gissmann, L., Claas, F. *et al.* (1993) Relation between skin cancer, humoral responses to human papillomaviruses, and HLA class II molecules in renal transplant recipients. *Journal of Immunology*, **151**, 1579–1586.

Bouwes Bavinck, J., Tieben, L., Van der Woude, F. *et al.* (1995) Prevention of skin cancer and reduction of keratotic skin lesions during acitretin therapy in renal transplant recipients, a double-blind, placebo-controlled study. *Journal of Clinical Oncology*, **13**, 1933–1938.

Bouwes Bavinck, J., Hardie, D., Green, A. *et al.* (1996) The risk of skin cancer in renal transplant recipients in Queensland, Australia. *Transplantation*, **61**, 715–721.

Brunson, M., Balakrishnan, K. & Penn, I. (1990) HLA and Kaposi's sarcoma in solid organ transplantation. *Human Immunology*, **29**, 56–63.

Chang, Y., Cesarman, E., Pessin, M.S. *et al.* (1994) Identification of herpesvirus-like DNA sequences in AIDS-associated Kaposi's sarcoma. *Science*, **266**, 1865–1869.

Conant, MA. (1995) Management of human immunodeficiency virus-associated malignancies. *Recent Results in Cancer Research*, **139**, 423–432.

Czarnecki, D., Watkins, F., Leahy, S. *et al.* (1992) Skin cancers and HLA frequencies in renal transplant recipients. *Clinical and Laboratory Investigation*, **185**, 9–11.

Daling, J., Weiss, N., Hislop, G. *et al.* (1987) Sexual practices, sexually transmitted diseases, and the incidence of anal cancer. *New England Journal of Medicine*, **317**, 973–977.

Dreno, B., Milpied-Homsi, B., Moreau, P. *et al.* (1993) Cutaneous anaplastic T-cell lymphoma in a patient with immunodeficiency virus infection. *British Journal of Dermatology*, **129**, 77–81.

Duvic, M., Lowe, L., Rapini, R., Rodriguez, S. & Levy, M. (1989) Eruptive dysplastic naevi associated with human immunodeficiency virus infection. *Archives of Dermatology*, **125**, 397–401.

Espana, A., Redondo, P., Fernandez, A. *et al.* (1995) Skin cancer in heart transplant recipients. *Journal of the American Academy of Dermatology*, **32**, 458–465.

Euvrard, S., Verschoore, M., Touraine, J. *et al.* (1992a) Topical retinoids for warts and keratoses in transplant recipients. *Lancet*, **340**, 48–49.

Euvrard, S., Pouteil-Noble, C., Kanitakis, J. *et al.* (1992b) Successive occurrence of T-cell and B-cell lymphomas after renal transplantation in a patient with multiple cutaneous squamous cell carcinomas. *New England Journal of Medicine*, **327**, 1924–1927.

Euvrard, S., Chardonnet, Y., Pouteil-Noble, C. *et al.* (1993) Association of skin malignancies with various and multiple carcinogenic and non-carcinogenic human papillomaviruses in renal transplant recipients. *Cancer*, **72**, 2198–2206.

Euvrard, S., Kanitakis, J., Pouteil-Noble, C. *et al.* (1995a). Aggressive squamous cell carcinomas in organ transplant recipients. *Transplantation Proceedings*, **27**, 1767–1768.

Euvrard, S., Kanitakis, J., Pouteil-Noble, C. *et al.* (1995b) Comparative epidemiologic study of premalignant and malignant epithelial cutaneous lesions developing after renal and cardiac transplantation. *Journal of the American Academy of Dermatology*, **33**, 222–229.

Farge, D. (1993) Kaposi's sarcoma in organ transplant recipients. *European Journal of Medicine*, **2**, 339–343.

Formica, M., Basolo, B., Funaro, L., Mazzuco, G., Segolini, G. & Piccoli, G. (1994) Merkel cell carcinoma in renal transplant recipient. *Nephron*, **68**, 399.

Francès, C., Farge, D. & Boisnic, S. (1991) Syndrome de Kaposi des transplantés. *Journal des Maladies Vasculaires*, **16**, 163–165.

Greene, M. & Young, T.I. (1981) Malignant melanoma in renal transplant recipients. *Lancet*, **i**, 1196–1199.

Harwood, A., Osoba, D., Hofstader, S. *et al.* (1979) Kaposi's sarcoma in recipients of renal transplants. *American Journal of Medicine*, **67**, 759–765.

Jong-Tieben, L. de, Berkhout, R., Smits, H. *et al.* (1995) High frequency of detection of epidermodysplasia verruciformis-associated human papillomavirus DNA in biopsies from malignant and pre-malignant skin lesions from renal transplant recipients. *Journal of Investigative Dermatology*, **105**, 367–371.

Kadry, Z., Bronsther, O., Van Thiel, D., Randhawa, P., Fung, J. & Starzl, T. (1993) Kaposi's sarcoma in two primary liver allograft recipients occurring under FK 506 immunosuppression. *Clinical Transplants*, **7**, 188–194.

Kerschmann, R., Berger, T., Weiss, L. *et al.* (1995) Cutaneous presentations of lymphoma in human immunodeficiency virus disease. *Archives of Dermatology*, **131**, 1281–1288.

Kiviat, N., Critchlow, C., Holmes, K. *et al.* (1993) Association of anal dysplasia and human papillomavirus with immunosuppression and HIV infection among homosexual men. *AIDS*, **7**, 43–49.

Kanitakis, J., Euvrard, S., Montazeri, A., Faure, M. & Claudy, A. (1996) Atypical fibroxanthoma in a renal graft recipient. *Journal of the American Academy of Dermatology*, **35**, 262–264.

Levy, M., Backman, L., Husberg, B. *et al.* (1993) De novo malignancy following liver transplantation; a single-center study. *Transplantation Proceedings*, **25**, 1397–1399.

Lobo, D., Chu, P., Grekin, R. & Berger, T. (1992) Nonmelanoma skin cancers and infection with the human immunodeficiency virus. *Archives of Dermatology*, **128**, 623–627.

Magnone, M., Holley, J., Shapiro, R. *et al.* (1994) Interferon-α induced acute renal allograft rejection. *Transplantation*, **59**, 1068–1070.

Majewski, S. & Jablonska, S. (1995) Epidermodysplasia verruciformis as a model of human papillomavirus-induced genetic cancer of the skin. *Archives of Dermatology*, **131**, 1312–1318.

McGregor, J., Yu, C., Lu, Qi L., Cotter, F., Levison, D. & MacDonald, D. (1993) Posttransplant cutaneous lymphoma. *Journal of the American Academy of Dermatology*, **29**, 549–554.

Melbye, M., Cote, T., Kessler, L., Gail, M. & Biggar, R. (1994) High incidence of anal cancer among AIDS patients. *Lancet*, **343**, 636–639.

Milburn, P., Brandsma, J., Goldsman, C., Teplitz, E. & Herlman, E. (1988) Disseminated warts and evolving squamous cell carcinoma in a patient with acquired immunodeficiency syndrome. *Journal of the American Academy of Dermatology*, **19**, 401–405.

Ogunbiyi, O., Scholefield, H., Raftery, A. *et al.* (1994) Prevalence of anal human papillomavirus infection and intraepithelial neoplasia in renal allograft recipients. *British Journal of Surgery*, **81**, 365–367.

Orth, G. (1987) Epidermodysplasia verruciformis. In: *The Papovaviridae. 2. The Papillomaviruses* (eds N.P. Salzman & P.M. Howley), pp. 199–243. New York, Plenum.

Palefsky, J. (1994) Anal human papillomavirus infection and anal cancer in HIV-positive individuals: an emerging problem. *AIDS*, **8**, 283–295.

Palefsky, J., Gonzales, J., Greenblatt, R., Ahn, D. & Hollander, H. (1990) Anal intraepithelial neoplasia and anal papillomavirus infection among homosexual males with group IV HIV disease *Journal of the American Medical Association*, **263**, 2911–2916.

Pascual, J., Torrelo, A., Teruel, J., Bellas, C., Marcén, R. & Ortuno, J. (1992) Cutaneous T cell lymphomas after renal transplantation. *Transplantation*, **53**, 1143–1145.

Penn, I. (1986) Cancers of the anogenital region in renal transplant recipients. *Cancer*, **58**, 611–616.

Penn, I. (1993) Tumors after renal and cardiac transplantation. *Hematology and Oncology Clinics of North America*, **7**, 431–445.

Penn, I. & Brunson, M. (1988) Cancers after cyclosporine therapy. *Transplantation Proceedings*, **20** (suppl 3), 885–892.

Povar Marco, J., Alvarez Alegret, R., Arazo Garces, P., Ramos Paesa, C. & Aguirre Errasti, J. (1994) Histiocitoma maligno en un paciente con infeccion por el virus de la immuno-deficienca humana. *Anales de Medicina Interna*, **11**, 150–151.

Qunibi, W., Barri, Y., Alfurayh, O. *et al.* (1993) Kaposi's sarcoma in renal transplant recipients: a report on 26 cases from a single institution. *Transplantation Proceedings*, **25**, 1402–1405.

Ragni, M., Belle, S., Jaffe, R. *et al.* (1993) Acquired immunodeficiency syndrome-associated non-Hodgkin's lymphomas and other malignancies in patients with hemophilia. *Blood*, **81**, 1889–1897.

Renne, R., Zhong, W., Herndier, B. *et al.* (1996) Lytic growth of Kaposi's sarcoma-associated herpesvirus (human herpes virus 8) in culture. *Nature (Medicine)* **2**, 342–346.

Sheil, A. (1992) Development of malignancy following renal transplantation in Australia and New Zealand. *Transplantation Proceedings*, **24**, 1275–1279.

Sheil, A., Flavel, S., Disney, A., Mathew, T. & Hall, B. (1987) Cancer incidence in renal transplant patients treated with azathioprine or cyclosporine. *Transplantation Proceedings*, **19**, 2214–2216.

Shuttleworth, D., Marks, R., Griffin, P. & Salaman, J. (1988) Treatment of cutaneous neoplasia with etretinate renal transplant recipients. *Quarterly Journal of Medicine*, **68**, 717–725.

Smith, C., McGregor, J., Barker, J., Morris, R., Rigden, S. & MacDonald, D. (1993) Excess melanocytic naevi in children with renal allografts. *Journal of the American Academy of Dermatology*, **28**, 51–55.

Smith, K., Skelton, H., Yeager, J. *et al.* (1993) Cutaneous neoplasms in a military population of HIV-1-positive patients. *Journal of the American Academy of Dermatology*, **29**, 400–406.

Tappero, J., Conant, M., Wolfe, S. & Berger, T. (1993) Kaposi's sarcoma. *Journal of the American Academy of Dermatology*, **28**, 371–395.

Tindall, B., Finlayson, R., Mutimer, K., Billson, FA., Munro, VF. & Cooper, D. (1989) Malignant melanoma associated with human immunodeficiency virus infection in three homosexual men. *Journal of the American Academy of Dermatology*, **20**, 587–591.

Toi, M., Kauffman, L., Peterson, L., Golitz, L. &

Myers, A. (1995) Sweat gland carcinoma in a human immunodeficiency virus-infected patient. *Modern Pathology*, **8**, 197–198.

Van Zuuren, E., Posma, A., Scholtens, R., Vermeer, B., van der Woude, F. & Bouwes Bavinck, J. (1994) Resurfacing the back of the hand as treatment and prevention of multiple skin cancers in kidney transplant recipients. *Journal of the American Academy of Dermatology*, **31**, 760–764.

Vernon, S., Zaki, S. & Reeves, W. (1994) Localisation of HIV-1 to human papillomavirus associated cervical lesions. *Lancet*, **344**, 954–955.

William, A., Darragh, T., Vranizan, K., Occhia, C., Moss, A. & Palefsky, J. (1994) Anal and cervical human papillomavirus infection and risk of anal and cervical epithelial abnormalities in human immunodeficiency virus-infected women. *Obstetrics and Gynecology*, **83**, 205–211.

Cutaneous Lymphomas and Retroviral Infection

M. D'INCAN AND P. SOUTEYRAND

Cutaneous T-cell lymphomas (CTCLs) are malignant lymphoproliferations of mature T lymphocytes, with major clinical features in the skin. Three main entities are recognized: mycosis fungoides and Sézary's syndrome, which are epidermotropic lymphomas, and pleomorphic lymphomas, in which proliferation spares the epidermis.

Attempts to find an aetiological factor for CTCLs have been unsuccessful to date (Weinstock & Horm, 1988). Reports of cutaneous pseudolymphomas induced by drugs like phenytoins (see review in Souteyrand & D'Incan, 1990) pointed to the possible role of a chronic antigenic stimulus in the skin. However, their involvement has been ruled out by case-control studies on the incidence of toxic and/or antigenic substances related to the occupation environment of patients with a CTCL (Whittemore *et al.*, 1989).

The birth of the retroviral hypothesis

The discovery of human retroviruses, at the beginning of the 1980s, gave rise to new speculation about the pathogeny and aetiology of CTCLs. The human T-lymphotropic virus type-I (HTLV-I) was first isolated from peripheral blood lymphocytes of a black American male with lymphoproliferation that was clinically and pathologically very close to Sézary's syndrome (Poiesz *et al.*, 1980). Further epidemiological studies demonstrated that HTLV-I was associated with two different diseases: tropical spastic paraparesy, a degenerative neurological disorder; and adult T-cell leukaemia/lymphoma (ATLL). The latter is a malignant lymphoproliferation sharing close clinical, pathological and immunological similarities with mycosis fungoides, pleomorphic T-cell lymphomas or with Sézary's syndrome (D'Incan *et al.*, 1995). At the beginning of the 1980s, there was also a report of retroviral-like particles detected by electron microscopy in Langerhans cells of patients with a mycosis fungoides or Sézary's syndrome (Slater *et al.*, 1983). MacKie (1981) hypothesized that the continuous infection of Langerhans cells by a retrovirus generates a specific T-cell clone whose uncontrolled development could lead to a lymphoma.

Our present aim is not to draw up an exhaustive list of the numerous works that, for more than 10 years, have attempted to detect a retrovirus in CTCLs. Conversely, we should like to review, in the light of certain experimental results, the current state (1995) of knowledge of the subject, and suggest cures for the disease and discuss work in progress.

Methods used and experimental results

Studies of the serological status of patients with a CTCL have yielded conflicting results. In 1986, antibodies against HTLV-I were detected in > 11% of patients with a CTCL in northern Europe and in 1.4% of healthy blood donors (Lange-Wantzin *et al.*, 1986). In view of recent findings concerning the epidemiology of HTLV-I, these results should be treated with caution. Standardized serological tests have shown that the prevalence of HTLV-I in Europe varies from 0.0026% to 0.021% in the blood donor population. Moreover, we and others (D'Incan *et al.*, 1992) found no evidence of such a high prevalence of HTLV-I antibodies in the CTCL population in Europe. This contrasts with results obtained in the United States, where close on 20% of patients with a CTCL have HTLV-I antibodies, albeit at a low level (Srivastava *et al.*, 1990).

The most surprising results have been obtained by

molecular biology techniques, i.e. Southern blotting and polymerase chain reaction (PCR), on fresh samples (skin biopsies, peripheral blood lymphocytes) or on cultured lymphocytes. The first work of this kind was that of Manzari and coworkers (1987), who detected a proviral genome, partially homologous to HTLV-I, that was integrated in a B-cell line established from an Italian patient with a mycosis fungoides. The isolation of this virus and the sequencing of its genome was unsuccessful and hence the existence of HTLV-V — the name given to the virus by the authors — is open to doubt. This pioneering report, however, paved the way, over the following 10 years, for many attempts to detect retroviral genomes in CTCLs. The findings from these various studies suggest that: (1) an HTLV-I-like genome is detected in a significant proportion of true CTCLs but at an incidence that differs greatly between Europe and the USA; (2) the HTLV-I-like genomes detected in CTCLs are usually deleted; (3) CTCL patients with HTLV-I-like sequences are seronegative for HTLV-I; (4) in some cases, an *in vivo* expression of the virus could have been detected. We will discuss each of these points.

Studies of large series of patients with a CTCL have revealed that the incidence of retroviral genomes in CTCLs is much higher in North America than in Europe. Using the PCR on fresh and cultured lymphocytes of 50 patients with a mycosis fungoides, Pancake and coworkers (1995) reported the detection of HTLV-I *pol* and/or *tax* genes in 96% of cases; moreover, in 18 of 20 cases viral-like particles with budding features

were detected on lymphocyte cultures. Table 12.1 gives similar results from other American studies. These unexpected results contrast with those obtained from European patients. As shown in Table 12.1, Southern blot or PCR on fresh and/or cultured lymphocytes or on skin biopsies detected HTLV-I-like sequences in only 0–7.5% of CTCLs. However, the PCR study of peripheral lymphocytes after 10 days culture revealed the presence of HTLV-I *tax* and *pol* genes in 10 of 29 Italian patients with a mycosis fungoides (Manca *et al.*, 1994). One possible explanation of this contradictory result is that *in vitro* cell proliferation increased the number of viral copies and, thereby, made them more easily detectable by PCR. Another possible explanation is that in Italy there exist some small pockets of HTLV-I endemia (Manzari *et al.*, 1985).

Another important finding from viral DNA studies was the detection of deleted HTLV-I viruses from CTCL patients who were seronegative for HTLV-I. One-third of patients with an ATLL are simultaneously infected by complete and deleted HTLV-I strains (Korber *et al.*, 1991). Like the deleted strains observed in ATLL, the deletions in CTCLs were reported at different places in the viral genome but the 3′ region of the genome, mainly encountering the *tax* gene, was generally unaffected (Hall *et al.*, 1991; Ghosh *et al.*, 1994; Manca *et al.*, 1994; Pancake *et al.*, 1995). In contrast, in an Egyptian patient with a mycosis fungoides, an HTLV-I genome was recently detected with no obvious deletions by Southern blot examination and with a great sequence homology with the HTLV-I Japanese

Table 12.1 Incidence of HTLV-I-like sequences in mycosis fungoides and Sézary syndrome.

Reference	Cases (*n*)	Materials	Methods	Incidence (%)	Location
Capésius *et al.* (1991)	24	Cultured PBL	Serology, PCR, SB, EM	0	France, Portugal
D'Incan *et al.* (1992)	51	Fresh PBL and skin biopsies	Serology, PCR	3	France
Lisby *et al.* (1992)	21	Skin biopsies	Serology, PCR	0	Germany, Denmark
Whittaker *et al.* (1993)	40	Skin biopsies	SB	7.5	UK
Manca *et al.* (1994)	29	Cultured PBL	Serology, PCR	30	Italy
Chadburn *et al.* (1991)	27	Fresh PBL	PCR	0	New York (USA)
Chan *et al.* (1993)	15	Skin biopsies	PCR	30	NE, IL (USA)
Ghosh *et al.* (1994)	35	Fresh and cultured PBL, skin biopsies	PCR, RT-PCR	66	PA (USA)
Pancake *et al.* (1995)	50	Cultured PBL	PCR, EM	92	New York (USA)

EM, electron microscopy. PBL, peripheral blood lymphocytes. PCR, polymerase chain reaction. RT-PCR, reverse-transcription PCR. SB, Southern blot.

strains. However, the existence of some slight differences in restriction sites and the inefficient cell-to-cell transmission of the virus *in vitro* indicate that some genomic defects existed in this virus (El-Farrash *et al.*, 1995).

The third salient point is that the HTLV-I serology of CTCL patients with HTLV-I-like sequences, based on serum analysis with several commercially available tests, is always negative. In some cases, however, antibodies against HTLV-I were detected by enzyme-linked immunosorbent assay (ELISA) tests at a low level and with an incomplete pattern on Western blot examination (Srivastava *et al.*, 1990). In other cases, patients lacking antibodies for structural proteins were found positive for antibodies against Tax (Pancake *et al.*, 1995) or Rex protein (Ghosh *et al.*, 1994).

Last, some studies have provided evidence for a viral genome expression *in vivo*. We mentioned above the existence, in some CTCLs, of antibodies against viral proteins. More recently, Ghosh and coworkers (1994), using the PCR after a reverse transcription of whole RNAs extracted from fresh peripheral lymphocytes, demonstrated the expression of the HTLV-I *tax* gene in four of eight patients with Sézary's syndrome.

Comments

The question of the aetiology of CTCLs remains still obscure. The enthusiastic hypothesis of HTLV-V was not confirmed by subsequent data and the situation is much more complex than it was thought to be 10 years ago.

Viral infection is not detected in all cases of CTCLs. When comparing large series of patients studied with similar highly sensitive techniques (PCR on cultured lymphocytes), viral infection is more frequently associated with CTCLs in America than in Europe or the Middle East (Manca *et al.*, 1994; Pancake *et al.*, 1995; El Farrash *et al.*, 1995). Similar geographical differences have previously been reported for viral infections such as Epstein–Barr infection and Burkitt lymphoma.

There are several explanations of the seronegativity of CTCL patients in whom HTLV-I-like sequences are detected. First, the virus is a variant of HTLV-I with differences in the structural protein amino acid sequences so that antibodies are not recognized by HTLV-I-specific serological tests. To date, no complete sequencing of CTCL-associated viral genome has been processed to verify this hypothesis. Second, deletions in the genes encoding for the structural proteins prevent them from being expressed and as a result there is no serological response. Third, the viral proteins are expressed, *in vivo*, at too low a level to induce an immune response. The onset of viral particles in lymphocyte cultures only after a strong long-standing stimulation by haematopoietic growth factors is an argument in favour of the latter hypothesis. Fourth, the virus is only transiently expressed during the course of the disease and so the host loses the immune memory of the infection. Finally, if the infection occurs very early in infancy or during fetal development, the thymus may be affected in such a way that an immunotolerance against the viral proteins develops.

Thus, we could hypothesize that the occurrence of an ATLL or that of a CTCL in an infected patient is determined by the evolutionary events appearing during viral life. If, after the primo-infection, patients have a sufficient number of non-deleted and non-defective for replication viral copies, they will develop an ATLL. Conversely, if genetic events (such as genomic deletions) or host-related factors occur, preventing or restricting both viral expression and replication, the patient will present a form of CTCL. This hypothesis is consistent with the fact that viral-associated CTCLs are more frequent near the HTLV-I and ATLL endemic areas than elsewhere.

Conclusion

More than a century after the first description of mycosis fungoides by Alibert and Bazin, the aetiology of CTCLs is a matter for conjecture. To date, in some cases only, evidence points to a viral origin. However, some questions remains unanswered. First, we do not know how deleted viral strains induce cell transformation. Second the relative incidence of carriers of deleted viral strains among patients with CTCL and healthy subjects is not known, since the former are not included in serological screening because they are seronegative. Finally, the clinical and epidemiological differences between viral-associated and non-associated CTCLs need to be studied.

References

Capésius, C., Saal, F., Maero, E. *et al.* (1991) No evidence for HTLV-I infection in 24 cases of French and Portuguese mycosis fungoides and Sézary syndrome (as seen in France). *Leukemia*, **5**, 416–419.

Chadburn, A., Athan, E., Wieczorek, R. & Knowles, D.M. (1991) Detection and characterization of human T-cell lymphotropic virus type I (HTLV-I) associated T-cell neoplasms in an HTLV-I nonendemic region by polymerase chain reaction. *Blood*, **77**, 2419–2430.

Chan, W.C., Hooper, C., Wickert, R. *et al.* (1993) HTLV-I sequence in lymphoproliferative disorders. *Diagnosis and Molecular Pathology*, **2**, 192–199.

D'Incan, M., Souteyrand, P., Bignon, Y.-J. *et al.* (1992) Retrovirus related sequences in a seronegative patient with a mycosis fungoides and study of 51 cutaneous T-cell lymphomas outside HTLV-I endemic areas. *European Journal of Dermatology*, **2**, 363–371.

D'Incan, M., Antoniotti, O., Gasmi, M. *et al.* (1995) HTLV-I associated lymphoma presenting as a mycosis fungoides in an HTLV-I non-endemic area. A viro-molecular study. *British Journal of Dermatology*, **132**, 983–988.

El-Farrash, M.A., Salem, H.A., Kuroda, M.J. *et al.* (1995) Isolation of human leukemia virus type I from a transformed T-cell line derived spontaneously from lymphocytes of a seronegative Egyptian patient with a mycosis fungoides. *Blood*, **86**, 1822–1829.

Ghosh, S.K., Abbrams, J.T., Terunuma, H. *et al.* (1994) Human T-cell leukemia virus type I *tax/rex* DNA and RNA in cutaneous T-cell lymphoma. *Blood*, **84**, 2663–2671.

Hall, W.W., Liu, C.R., Schneewind, O. *et al.* (1991) Deleted HTLV-I provirus in blood and cutaneous lesions of patients with mycosis fungoides. *Science*, **253**, 317–320.

Korber, B., Okayama, A., Donnelly, R. *et al.* (1991) Polymerase chain reaction analysis of defective human T-cell leukemia virus type I proviral genomes in leukemic cells of patients with adult T-cell leukemia. *Journal of Virology*, **65**, 5471–5476.

Lange-Wantzin, G., Thomsen, K., Nissen, N.I. *et al.* (1986) Occurrence of human T-cell lymphotropic virus type I (HTLV-I) antibodies in cutaneous T-cell lymphoma. *Journal of the American Academy of Dermatology*, **15**, 598–607.

Lisby, G., Reitz, M.S. & Lange-Vejlgaard, G.L. (1992) No detection of HTLV-I DNA in punch biopsies from patients with cutaneous T-cell lymphoma by the polymerase chain reaction. *Journal of Investigative Dermatology*, **98**, 417–420.

MacKie, R. (1981) Initial event in mycosis fungoides of the skin is viral infection of epidermal Langerhans cells. *Lancet*, **ii**, 282–284.

Manca, N., Piacentini, E., Gelmi, M. *et al.* (1994) Persistence of human T cell lymphotropic virus type I (HTLV-I) sequences in peripheral blood mononuclear cells from patients with mycosis fungoides. *Journal of Experimental Medicine*, **180**, 1973–1978.

Manzari, V., Gradilone, A., Barillari, G. *et al.* (1985) HTLV-I is endemic in southern Italy: detection of the first infection cluster in a white population. *International Journal of Cancer*, **36**, 557–559.

Manzari, V., Gismondi, A., Barillari, G. *et al.* (1987) HTLV-V: a new human retrovirus isolated in a Tac-negative T cell lymphoma/leukemia. *Science*, **238**, 1581–1583.

Pancake, B.A., Zuker-Franklin, D. & Coutavas, E. (1995) The cutaneous T-cell lymphoma, mycosis fungoides, is a human T-cell lymphotropic virus-associated disease. A study of 50 patients. *Journal of Clinical Investigation*, **95**, 547–554.

Poiesz, B., Ruscetti, F., Gazdar, A. *et al.* (1980) Detection and isolation of type C retrovirus particles from fresh and cultured lymphocytes of a patient with cutaneous T-cell lymphoma. *Proceedings of the National Academy of Sciences USA*, **77**, 7415–7419.

Slater, D., Bleehen, S., Rooney, N. & Hamed, A. (1983) Type C retrovirus-like particles in mycosis fungoides. *British Journal of Dermatology*, **109**, 120–125.

Souteyrand, P. & D'Incan, M. (1990) Drug-induced mycosis fungoides-like lesions. In: *Cutaneous Lymphoma — Current Problems in Dermatology* (eds W.A. van Vloten, R. Willemze, G. Lange-Veljsgaard & K. Thomsen), pp. 176–182. Karger, Basel.

Srivastava, B.I.S., Gonzales, C., Loftus, R., Fitzpatrick, J.E. & Saxinger, C.W. (1990) Examination of HTLV-I-positive leukemia/lymphoma patients by Western blotting gave mostly negative or indeterminate reaction. *AIDS Research and Human Retroviruses*, **6**, 617–627.

Weinstock, M.A. & Horm, J.W. (1988) Mycosis fungoides in the United States. Increasing incidence and descriptive epidemiology. *Journal of the American Medical Association*, **260**, 42–46.

Whittaker, S. & Luzzatto, L. (1993) HTLV-I provirus and mycosis fungoides. *Science*, **259**, 1470.

Whittemore, A.S., Holly, E.A., Lee, I.M. *et al.* (1989) Mycosis fungoides in relation to environmental exposure and immune response. A case-control study. *Journal of the National Cancer Institute*, **81**, 1560–1567.

Section 3
Inflammatory Dermatoses

13
Psoriasis

Population Genetics of Psoriasis

G. SWANBECK, A. INEROT,
T. MARTINSSON, J. WAHLSTRÖM,
C. ENERBÄCK, F. ENLUND AND
M. YHR

We regard psoriasis as a genetically determined disease with an intense and prolonged inflammatory skin reaction that does not appear to be self-limiting. The inflammatory reaction seems to need a triggering factor like streptococcal throat infection or skin trauma to start. Psoriasis is a highly variable disease between individuals but rather constant after onset within the individual. Some patients are severely affected by psoriasis while others have such minor skin lesions that they are hardly aware of having a skin disease. The age of onset of the disease also varies from earliest infancy to late age, although the most common age at onset is in the second decade of life. These factors impose problems for population genetic studies. The penetrance of the genotype is thus dependent on the age of the individual and a number of external factors. Primarily we assume that there is one specific psoriasis gene but there may be several other genetic factors that influence the severity of the disease, or the age at which it starts.

According to Mendel, we use relatively simple rules to describe the inheritance of different properties, namely autosomal or sex-linked, and dominant or recessive inheritance. These rules makes it possible for us, in a simple and understandable way, to inform patients about the risks of their children getting a disease and explain the distribution of the disease in the family. In the case of psoriasis, however, these simple rules do not appear to describe the inheritance of the disease (Lomholt, 1963; Watson et al., 1972). The main purpose here is to show that this really is not the case.

Lomholt has made an admirable effort to study a large part of the population on the Faroe Islands with respect to the familial occurrence of psoriasis (Lomholt, 1963). His report has to some extent become the 'psoriasis bible', the data of which have been re-evaluated by other investigators (Iselius & Williams, 1984). Hellgren (1967) and Romanus (1945) have also made significant efforts to collect representative Scandinavian data on psoriasis. The mode of inheritance has not come out clearly from these studies. A multifactorial type of inheritance has been suggested (Watson et al., 1972). Lately, a re-evaluation of Lomholt's data has made probable a single major gene for psoriasis (Iselius & Williams, 1984). Other hypotheses on the inheritance of psoriasis with two types of psoriasis vulgaris (Henseler & Christophers, 1985) and genetic imprinting (Traupe et al., 1992) have been put forward. We feel that it is important to look critically at the epidemiology of psoriasis to see how complex genetic models are needed to explain the epidemiological data. On the basis of available information, it is difficult to give information to patients regarding the risk of offspring developing psoriasis.

For a disease with a variable age at onset and different expressions, it is important to get as accurate information as possible about the relationship between the genotype and the phenotype of the disease. By penetrance of the genotype, we mean the quotient between the prevalence of the phenotype and the genotype.

The prevalence of psoriasis in Scandinavia is considered to be slightly >2% (Lomholt, 1963; Hellgren,

1967; Brandrup & Green, 1981). This is the prevalence of the phenotype, which in the case of psoriasis is dependent on the age of the population studied. The prevalence of the phenotype, however, is of course lower than that of the genotype. A lower limit for the prevalence of the genotype can be estimated from the prevalence of the phenotype and data on the age at onset of psoriasis.

When we speak of age at onset, we also have to define what we mean by 'onset'. A person with very minor psoriatic lesions, for instance on the scalp, may not be aware of having psoriasis until he or she gets skin lesions on other body areas, thereby reporting a later age at onset than if the first lesions had been recognized and diagnosed. Our definition of age at onset of psoriasis is the age at which the individual or relatives become aware that the individual has psoriasis.

The age at onset of a disease has to be corrected for the age of the population studied. In a general population, we will have an overrepresentation of younger ages in the age at onset distribution as the older group of the population contributes to onset at a young age while the younger group cannot, of course, contribute to onset at old age. Therefore, the most relevant 'age at onset' curve should be based on data only from the oldest part of the population.

Methods in population genetic studies generally assume random mating with respect to the property or disease being studied. In the case of skin diseases, it is not self-evident that random mating can be assumed. Efforts to check this are therefore important. Reporting of the presence of a skin disease among relatives of the proband may also vary with respect to sex and age.

We should stress that in virtually every human genetic analysis there are imperfections, such as incorrect reporting, lack of random mating, late onset of the disease, incomplete penetrance or too little material. It is important that an analysis of possible errors is made. In data collected on the basis of case findings only, certain parts will have some relevance in differentiating between dominant and recessive inheritance. The study of psoriasis among siblings of probands where no parent has the disease is relevant. Study of the distribution of psoriasis among the parents is also relevant. Study of the children of probands and the other parent of the children is of importance for evaluating if random mating has occurred.

We have tried to get well-defined epidemiological data for testing the simplest possible hypothesis about the inheritance of psoriasis. Some of the results of this study have been published earlier (Swanbeck *et al.*, 1994, 1995).

Methodological considerations

The main purpose of the study is to determine whether an autosomal dominant or an autosomal recessive mode of inheritance is compatible with population genetic data among first-degree relatives. As our data include only first-degree relatives, any discussion concerning multifactorial inheritance is meaningless.

In the present study, only data of psoriasis among first-degree relatives of probands with psoriasis have been analysed, i.e. data about psoriasis among parents, siblings and to some extent children of the probands.

For probands with one or both parents having psoriasis, the risk of the siblings getting the disease does not differ significantly between a dominant and a recessive mode of inheritance. The majority of the probands have no parent with psoriasis. In this situation a dominant inheritance would mean a low penetrance of the genotype. A recessive mode of inheritance can be tested on this group with methods described by Emery (1976). By using the formula $spn_s/(1 - q^s)$, where s is the size of the sibship, n_s the number of sibships of size s and $q = 1 - p$, the number affected in the sibships can be obtained. This formula can also be used to calculate p from the data obtained by solving a polynomial equation. For instance, in autosomal dominant inheritance with one affected parent, p is expected to be 0.5, and for autosomal recessive inheritance with both parents being heterozygotes, p is 0.25. The penetrance values given below are obtained by solving the polynomial equations mentioned above for each sibship size, obtaining an average p value by weighting the calculated p values with the corresponding number of sibships, and dividing by the expected p value (0.25 for recessive mode of inheritance).

For children of affected probands where the other parent is unaffected, there is a 50% risk of the children getting the disease with a dominant mode of inheritance, while with a recessive mode the risk is dependent on the gene frequency in the population.

The distribution of probands with both, one or no parent having psoriasis may give an estimate of the gene frequency in the population. If we have a gene frequency p for psoriasis in the general population, we will have p^2 homozygotes, $2pq$ heterozygotes for the gene and q^2 without the gene according to the Hardy–Weinberg equilibrium. We are now interested in knowing what the distribution of the gene among the parents of the probands will be, assuming a recessive mode of inheritance. In Fig. 13.1, the two bars represent the population of men and women, respectively. The dark grey part of the bars represents those that are homozygotes with respect to psoriasis in each sex. Their part of the population is p^2 where p is the frequency of the psoriasis gene and $p + q = 1$. The light grey bars represent the part that are heterozygotes with respect to the psoriasis gene and they represent $2pq$ of the population according to the Hardy–Weinberg equilibrium. The open part of the bars represents the part of the population without any psoriasis gene.

The frequency of couples that can produce children with psoriasis is indicated in the next level of the diagram (couples). With an equal number of children per family in the different groups, the number of children with psoriasis will then be proportional to the numbers at the level one step down (affected children). When both parents have psoriasis, all children can be expected to get the disease. When one parent has psoriasis in the group that can produce children with psoriasis, half of the children are expected to become affected by psoriasis; therefore, the proportion of

couples in the level above in Fig. 13.1 is divided by two. When no parent has psoriasis among the couples that can produce a child with the disease, one-quarter of the children are expected to be affected and, correspondingly, the proportion in the level above in Fig. 13.1 is divided by four. The numbers obtained may be divided by p^2, giving the numbers in the lowest level. We can thus see that the number of psoriasis sufferers having both parents affected by the disease is proportional to p^2, the number having one parent affected is proportional to $2pq$ and those with no parent affected is proportional to q^2.

For simplicity, the gene frequency has been used above. It is more correct to use the gene frequency multiplied by the lifetime penetrance of the genotype.

Material and methods

Questionnaires were sent to about 22 000 members of the Swedish Psoriasis Association. The members, who practically all have psoriasis, were asked about age at onset of their psoriasis, number of siblings, number of siblings with psoriasis and psoriasis among parents. The response rate was tested for the first 3333 questionnaires sent out; 1578 responded promptly and 1022 after a reminder, giving a response rate of 78%. Among the 3333 first to get a questionnaire, we obtained information on 2434 that reported having psoriasis; 99 did not have psoriasis (for instance, supporting members), 60 had moved to an unknown address and 11 were dead. Of those with psoriasis, 6% did not have reliable information about parents or siblings, for instance adopted persons. The distribution of psoriasis among the parents of those

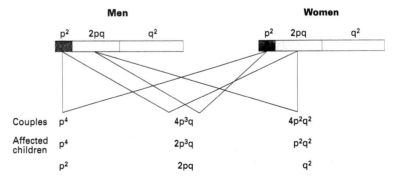

Fig. 13.1 The relation between gene frequency and psoriasis among the parents in the case of an autosomal recessive mode of inheritance. For explanation, see text.

Table 13.1 Comparison of the frequency of reporting psoriasis among parents for male and female probands and for probands older and younger than 40 years of age.

Proband <40 years	Sex (*n*)		Percentage		Proband >40 years	Sex (*n*)		Percentage	
Psoriasis among parents	M	F	M	F	Psoriasis among parents	M	F	M	F
Father	225	480	20.2	23.6	Father	812	1003	19.7	21.9
Mother	212	375	18.9	18.5	Mother	582	716	14.1	15.6
Both	25	44	2.2	2.2	Both	48	78	1.2	1.7
Neither	662	1132	58.7	55.7	Neither	2677	2788	65.0	60.8

responding to the first questionnaire and to the reminder did not differ statistically significantly as judged by the chi-squared test.

In all, data from 14 008 families with psoriasis were collected. In 11 366 families information about psoriasis among parents and siblings could be obtained. Only patients with psoriasis vulgaris have been included. Psoriatic arthritis has not been an exclusion criterion but patients who never had psoriatic skin lesions have not been included, nor have patients with purely pustular diseases like pustulosis palmoplantaris.

To study psoriasis among the children of probands, questionnaires were sent to 1329 probands between the ages of 50 and 70 years to minimize the problem of too young children and late onset of the disease. The response rate was 89.9%.

To check the diagnosis given by the probands, 496 persons from 156 families were examined personally by one of us (A.I.)

The comparisons in Tables 13.1–13.3 with respect to the number of parents with psoriasis (0, 1 or 2) were performed by test for trend in a contingency table (Maxwell, 1961). The chi-squared test with Yates correction was used for comparison of proportions.

Table 13.2 Comparison of the frequency of reporting psoriasis among siblings for male and female probands.

	Male	Female
Number of probands	5375	6696
Number of siblings	13 210	15 962
With psoriasis, *n* (%)	1882 (14.3)	2695 (16.9)
Number of siblings per proband	2.46	2.38

Table 13.3 Comparison of the frequency of reporting psoriasis among children for male and female probands.

	Male	Female
Number of children	1179	1167
With psoriasis, *n* (%)	151 (12.8)	212 (18.2)
Average age of oldest child (years)	32.3	35.4
Children/proband	1.98	1.96

Results

Correctness of diagnosis

Of 149 probands examined, a diagnosis of psoriasis could be verified in 146. Of 293 relatives of probands who were reported not to have psoriasis, 22 could be diagnosed as having psoriasis. In all relatives who were reported to have psoriasis, the diagnosis could be verified.

To get some idea about how probands of different sex and age are reporting, data have been given in Table 13.1 on psoriasis among the parents for male and female probands <40 and >40 years of age.

The tendency for women to report a higher frequency of psoriasis among parents is statistically significant in the older group ($P < 0.001$) but not in the younger group. The younger group reported a higher frequency of parents with psoriasis than the older group among males ($P < 0.001$) and among females ($P < 0.001$).

The difference between males and females in reporting psoriasis among siblings is statistically significant ($P < 0.001$).

For 1329 probands between 50 and 70 years of age, the number of children, the number of children with psoriasis and whether the other parent of the children has psoriasis were requested. In all, 1195 answered the questionnaires.

The data obtained about children of probands (described further below) indicate that women report a higher frequency of psoriasis than men; this also holds for children as shown by Table 13.3 (*P* < 0.01).

Probands

The average age of the probands was 50.8 years with a median of 50 years. The lower quartile was 40 years and the upper 63 years; 55% were women and 45% were men.

Age at onset

Figure 13.2 gives the distribution of age at onset for males and females separately. As there are a number of young individuals contributing to this distribution, there is an overrepresentation of onset at young ages. Figure 13.3 gives the corresponding data for probands >60 years of age. Figure 13.3 thus represents the risk of getting psoriasis at a certain age having the genotype.

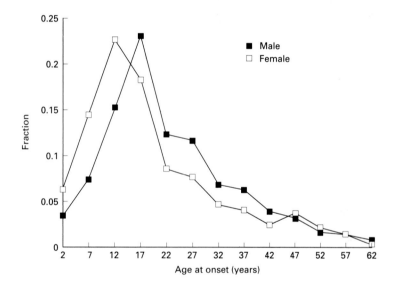

Fig. 13.2 Age at onset for probands.

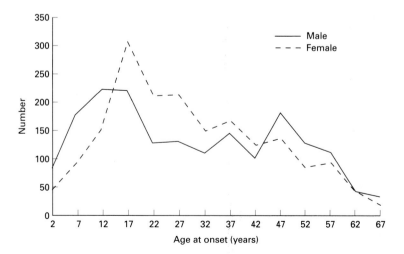

Fig. 13.3 Age at onset for probands over 60 years of age.

Approximately 50% of those getting psoriasis do so before the age of 30 years and 90% before the age of 50 years.

Is a monogenic dominant or recessive inheritance likely?

Psoriasis among parents

As is evident from Table 13.1 nearly two-thirds of the probands have parents that do not have psoriasis. For this to be compatible with a dominant inheritance, the penetrance of the gene must be < 50%. A recessive mode of inheritance is possible if the gene frequency is of the order of 25%.

Psoriasis among siblings

In all studies where the inclusion criterion for probands is having the disease, the families where no child has the disease are not included. This means that the distribution by number of affected children misses the term that corresponds to no affected child. We thus have a truncated binomial distribution. According to Hogben (1931) and Emery (1976), the expected number of affected individuals for different size of sibships can be calculated. When one parent is affected, the probability of the offspring getting the disease is approximately $P = 0.5$ if we have a dominant or a recessive inheritance. Thus, this part of the population differentiates very poorly between these two modes of inheritance.

Table 13.4 gives expected and observed numbers of affected siblings. The definition of penetrance is given above under 'Methodological considerations'. This table tells us nothing about the mode of inheritance. An autosomal dominant and an autosomal recessive inheritance give approximately the same expected number of affected siblings when one parent has the disease and the proband is affected. However, if psoriasis is a monogenic disease, Table 13.4 tells us that the penetrance of the gene in the actual age group is relatively high.

Table 13.5 gives the observed and expected number of affected siblings for male and female probands if none of the parents has psoriasis and the inheritance

Size of sibship (n)	Father with psoriasis		Mother with psoriasis	
	Observed	Expected	Observed	Expected
2	848	908	532	575
3	761	866	593	648
4	578	717	428	506
5	364	470	238	330
Sum	2551	2961	1791	2059
Penetrance (%)	74.1			

Table 13.4 The number of siblings observed to have psoriasis in sibships of different size when one parent has psoriasis compared with the expected number (for $P = 0.5$) as calculated by the method of Emery (1976).

Size of sibship (n)	Male probands		Female probands	
	Observed	Expected	Observed	Expected
2	1026	1055	1280	1278
3	857	932	1130	1187
4	618	689	763	802
5	422	500	489	538
Sum	2923	3176	3662	3805
Penetrance (%)	82.3			

Table 13.5 The number of siblings observed to have psoriasis in sibships of different size when no parent has psoriasis compared with the expected number (for $P = 0.25$) as calculated by the method of Emery (1976).

is recessive, $P = 0.25$. The data of Table 13.5 strongly favour a recessive inheritance for psoriasis.

There are only 160 probands with both parents having psoriasis. If the corresponding calculations in Tables 13.4 and 13.5 are done on these, 52.9% are affected when all siblings are expected to get the disease, as would be the case for a recessive mode of inheritance, while this figure would be about 75% for a dominant mode. The number of probands in this group is small and this material does not differentiate well between the two modes of inheritance.

The mating of probands

For 1329 probands between 50 and 70 years of age, information on the number of children, the number of children with psoriasis and whether the other parent of the children has psoriasis has been requested. In all, 1195 answered the questionnaires: 79 men and 83 women had no children. Of the men with children, 19 had a psoriatic mother for their children and of the women, 25 had a psoriatic father for their children. There were 500 males with children where the mother of the children did not have psoriasis and the corresponding number for females was 489. Of the male probands with children, the mother had psoriasis in 3.7% of cases, and of female probands with children in 4.9% the fathers also had psoriasis. This indicates that mating has been random with respect to having psoriasis or not, as these percentages are very similar to the prevalence of psoriasis in an adult population.

The children of the probands whose other parent does not have psoriasis might in the case of recessive inheritance have one parent with two psoriasis genes and the other parent with either no or one psoriasis gene. We thus have two populations of children, one that will become heterozygotes and cannot get psoriasis and one that has a 50% risk of getting the psoriasis genotype. In Table 13.6 the second population is represented by columns 1–5, while column 0 represents the first population plus children in the second population that belong to sibships without psoriasis.

Using the figures in the columns representing 1–5, children with psoriasis and the formula developed by Hogben (1931) used above with $p = 0.5$, we get a penetrance of the genotype of 82%. Using $p = 0.41$ (0.5×0.82) we can calculate the contribution of the

Table 13.6 Number of families with different numbers of children with psoriasis in sibships of different sizes where one parent has psoriasis (the proband).

Size of sibship (n)	Children with psoriasis (n)					
	0	1	2	3	4	5
1	164	29				
2	356	103	14			
3	150	48	21	3		
4	40	19	9	2	1	
5	12	2	1	1	1	0

above second population to the column representing zero children with psoriasis and thereby also the first population. It turns out that the second population with one heterozygotic parent for psoriasis comprises 42% and the other thus 58%.

With random mating this is approximately what can be expected when we have a gene frequency of 0.25 and the distribution of psoriasis among the parents of the probands reported above.

Two types of psoriasis vulgaris or genetic imprinting

Two types of psoriasis vulgaris have been proposed mainly on the basis of a bump on the age at onset curve at about 50 years of age. In our data (Fig. 13.3) this bump can only be seen for women and coincides with the menopause.

The higher incidence of psoriasis among children from psoriatic fathers than from psoriatic mothers has been the reason for suggesting genetic imprinting in psoriasis (Traupe *et al.*, 1992).

Discussion

Are the members of the Swedish Psoriasis Association representative of psoriasis patients in general? Naturally there is a selection of some kind as with every type of material. The conclusions drawn in this study are therefore valid for this material. As shown below, the present data are very similar to that of Lomholt (1963), which is based on a population study on the Faroe Islands. We believe that psoriasis of very late onset may be slightly underrepresented in our material. Old people getting psoriasis may be less likely to become members of the patient organization.

Among the 149 probands checked, there were three where we could not find sufficient evidence in their skin status or in earlier medical records that they could be regarded as having psoriasis vulgaris. Of the 293 relatives that were reported not to have psoriasis, 22 had clinical signs of the disease and of those reported to have psoriasis, all were correctly diagnosed. Our impression is, therefore, that there is a small number of probands where we cannot be sure of their diagnosis and that there is a slight underreporting about psoriasis among relatives. The underreporting does not seem to be of such a magnitude that it severely disturbs the analysis but it has to be taken into account.

Tables 13.1 to 13.3 and 13.7 indicate that females tend to report a higher frequency of psoriasis among first-degree relatives than do males. The fact that younger probands report a higher frequency of psoriasis among their parents than do older probands does not necessarily mean that there is a difference only in their readiness to report. If age at onset is an inherited property (Swanbeck *et al.*, 1995), the younger group could have a real higher frequency of psoriasis among parents as the young group has an overrepresentation of early onset compared to the old group.

The relation between the number of men and women in our material does not give any information about the same relation in the whole population. However, the relation of psoriasis among the parents may give information on this question, if we assume equal heredity of psoriasis from mothers and fathers. If we believe that women younger than 40 years

of age are the most reliable reporters, 55% of the psoriatics would be men and 45% women. In a large epidemiological study of hand eczema among 20 000 individuals in Gothenburg, Sweden, a question about psoriasis, not only on hands, was also included. The population studied was between 20 and 65 years old and psoriasis was reported among 4.5% of men and 3.7% of women (Meding & Swanbeck, unpublished data). Also, Romanus (1945), Hellgren (1967) and Brandrup and Green (1981) reported a similar relation of psoriasis in the two sexes. We are thus inclined to believe that psoriasis is slightly more common among men. As it is generally accepted that psoriasis is autosomally inherited, this would mean that a smaller fraction of women having the genotype of psoriasis will develop the disease than is the case for men.

The age at onset distribution of Fig. 13.3 reflects the probability of getting psoriasis at a certain age having the genotype. We find this more relevant than using the distribution of Fig. 13.2.

The age at onset curve for men in Fig. 13.3 shows that after the age of 20 years, the number of men getting psoriasis rapidly declines. This could mean that there are fewer individuals left with a psoriatic genotype without having symptoms of psoriasis. In other words, most men with a psoriasis genotype also get the disease. For women, the age at onset curve looks different. There is a considerable number of women between 45 and 55 years of age getting psoriasis. This peak in the age at onset curve coincides with the time for menopause (Swanbeck *et al.*, 1995). This late onset of psoriasis has been interpreted as a special type II psoriasis by Henseler and Christophers (1985).

The fact that as much as > 60% of the probands have

Group	Probands (*n*)	Children (*n*)	Children with psoriasis (*n*)	Percentage with psoriasis
Male probands*				
Mother with psoriasis	19	41	19	46.3
Mother with no psoriasis	500	1132	131	11.6
Female probands†				
Father with psoriasis	25	46	16	34.8
Father with no psoriasis	489	1117	195	17.5

Table 13.7 Psoriasis among children of male and female probands, respectively.

* Father of the children.
† Mother of the children.

both parents unaffected made us compare psoriasis among the siblings of probands with the expected result if a recessive gene was responsible for psoriasis. It is only psoriasis among siblings whose parents do not have psoriasis that can differentiate between dominant and recessive modes of inheritance. The penetrance of the genotype would then be >80%. The penetrance when one parent has the disease is between 70 and 80% and when both parents are affected between 50 and 60%. Further work has shown that a lower degree of penetrance of the genotype when both parents are affected than when one parent is affected, and when one parent is affected compared to when no parent is affected, can be due to a heterogeneity with two or more independently inherited types of psoriasis (Swanbeck *et al.*, unpublished data). Furthermore, the percentage of probands with both parents affected will be lower when there is heterogeneity than with only one gene (Swanbeck *et al.*, unpublished data).

The high frequency of HLA-Cw6 for those with an early onset may be regarded as a modifying factor favouring early onset, and not reflecting the primary gene of psoriasis. We may also look upon menopause as a triggering factor in women. The results of the present report are consistent with two types of non-pustular psoriasis as indicated above.

The data of Table 13.1 are compatible with a recessive inheritance of psoriasis if the gene frequency is about 0.25, taking into account underreporting and incomplete penetrance.

The reason why Lomholt (1963) excluded a recessive mode of inheritance might have been that he was not aware of the effect of high gene frequency on the occurrence of the disease among the parents as shown above. As pointed out above, a gene frequency of 25% in the whole population would be needed. Our material is very similar to that of Lomholt. Table 13.8 gives some overall data comparing the two materials.

The children in our data are older than in Lomholt's;

this can explain the difference in the last column. The lower percentage of psoriasis among the parents in our data may indicate a lower degree of reporting. A comparison between the curves for accumulated age at onset in Lomholt's data and our data shows practically identical values.

The prevalence of psoriasis is generally given for the whole population, children included. The prevalence of psoriasis in a population of old people we estimate as about 1.8-fold that of the whole population. This means around 5% in Scandinavia, which is in good agreement with the frequency found in the hand eczema study mentioned above. The fact that similar figures are obtained among spouses to probands, as given above, indicates that there is a random mating among psoriatics with respect to the partner having psoriasis or not.

Traupe *et al.* (1992) propose a genetic mechanism called 'genetic imprinting' to explain why, in Lomholt's (1963) data, the children seem to have psoriasis more often when the father has psoriasis than when the mother has the disease. Table 13.4 does not give any support for such an effect, but does not exclude it, considering a greater tendency for women to report psoriasis among their relatives than do men.

If we assume that nearly all men having the genotype of psoriasis also get the disease, the genotype frequency in the population is slightly >6%. With an incomplete penetrance and/or a slight underreporting, the frequency will be higher. A frequency for the genotype between 6 and 8% does not, therefore, seem unrealistic. If we have a recessive monogenic inheritance of psoriasis, a gene frequency of 25% would give 6.25% of the population having the psoriasis genotype.

In this study, we have shown that several types of independent data, namely psoriasis among siblings with parents not having psoriasis, the distribution of psoriasis among parents of probands, psoriasis among children to probands and the prevalence of psoriasis

Table 13.8 Comparison of the present material with that of Lomholt's study (1963).	Psoriasis among parents (%)	Psoriasis among siblings	Psoriasis among children
Present material	18	16	15
Lomholt's material	21	16	12

in the general population, are all compatible with the hypothesis that a single recessive gene with a frequency of about 0.25 causes the skin disease psoriasis. However, it is probable that two or more independently inherited forms of psoriasis exist. Such a heterogeneity would only slightly affect the population genetic parameters.

Summary

Epidemiological data for 11 366 families with psoriasis have been presented, and errors in reporting have been analysed. Analysis of the data gives an indication of random mating with respect to the partner's having the skin disease or not. Data on psoriasis among parents, siblings and children have been given. Special attention has been paid to the age at onset of psoriasis. Psoriasis is present among the parents of about 36% of the probands. For families where one or both parents have psoriasis, the occurrence of the disease among the siblings does not give any information that differentiates between a dominant and recessive mode of inheritance but is compatible with both. In families where no parent had psoriasis, provided there was a proband with psoriasis, the probability of the siblings' suffering from psoriasis was close to 0.25, indicating a recessive mode of inheritance. The distribution of psoriasis among the parents of all probands and among the children of probands is also compatible with this mode of inheritance. The prevalence of psoriasis among old people has been estimated to be about 5% and the gene frequency in the whole population 25%.

The findings show that with regard to first-degree relatives, the inheritance of psoriasis can fit an autosomal recessive model. A heterogeneity with two or more independently inherited forms of psoriasis may account for the small deviations found in the epidemiological data from what could be expected for a single autosomal recessive gene.

References

Brandrup, F. & Green, A. (1981) The prevalence of psoriasis in Denmark. *Acta Dermato-Venereologica Stockholm*, **61**, 344–346.

Emery, A.E.H. (1976) *Methodology in Medical Genetics. An Introduction to Statistical Methods*, p. 39. Churchill Livingstone, Edinburgh.

Hellgren, L. (1967) *Psoriasis: The Prevalence in Sex, Age and Occupational Groups in Total Populations in Sweden. Morphology, Inheritance and Association with Other Skin and Rheumatic Diseases.* Almquist & Wiksell, Stockholm.

Henseler, T. & Christophers, E. (1985) Psoriasis of early and late onset: characterization of two types of psoriasis vulgaris. *Journal of the American Academy of Dermatology*, **13**, 450–456.

Hogben, L. (1931) The genetic analysis of familial traits. I. Single gene substitutions. *Journal of Genetics*, **25**, 97–112.

Iselius, L. & Williams, W.R. (1984) The mode of inheritance of psoriasis: Evidence for a major gene as well as a multifactorial component and its implication for genetic counselling. *Human Genetics*, **68**, 73–76.

Lomholt, G. (1963) *Psoriasis: Prevalence, Spontaneous Course and Genetics. A Census Study on the Prevalence of Skin Diseases on the Faroe Islands.* GEC Gad, Copenhagen.

Maxwell, A.E. (1961) *Analysing Qualitative Data*, pp. 63–72. Methuen, London.

Romanus, T. (1945) *Psoriasis from a prognostic and hereditary point of view.* Dissertation, Uppsala University.

Swanbeck, G., Inerot, A., Martinsson, T. & Wahlström, J. (1994) A population genetic study of psoriasis. *British Journal of Dermatology*, **131**, 32–39.

Swanbeck, G., Inerot, A., Martinsson, T. *et al.* (1995) Age at onset and different types of psoriasis. *British Journal of Dermatology*, **133**, 768–773.

Traupe, H., van Gurp, P.J., Happle, R., Boezeman, J. & van de Kerkhof, P.C. (1992) Psoriasis vulgaris, fetal growth, and genomic imprinting. *American Journal of Medical Genetics*, **42**, 649–654.

Watson, E., Cann, H.M., Farber, E.M. & Nall, M.L. (1972) The genetics of psoriasis. *Archives of Dermatology*, **105**, 197–207.

Alcohol, Smoking and Psoriasis

L. NALDI AND L. PELI

In the search for environmental influences on psoriasis, alcohol and smoking have been repeatedly incriminated. Unfortunately, the aetiological role of these factors is difficult to ascertain. Alcohol and smoke are exposures which often go hand by hand, i.e. cigarette smokers are more likely to drink alcoholic beverages than are non-smokers, and, as a consequence, these two factors may confound each other. In addition, stressful life events have been linked with the onset of psoriasis in a few studies (Al'Abadie *et al.*, 1994) and alcohol and smoking may represent behavioural manifestations of stress. Alcohol and smoking may be related to the onset, clinical detection, maintenance and extension of psoriasis. In each circumstance, specific confounding effects and biases are possible. Factors involved in initiating the disease may not be responsible for its progression or chronicity.

The many problems in the area explain why the role of alcohol and smoking remains elusive. Nevertheless, several lines of evidence are worthy of mention. Improvements in this research area are highly desirable considering the widespread use of alcohol and cigarettes, their adverse effects on health, the disabling nature of psoriasis and the lack of effective and safe treatments for the disease.

Disease associations

A first insight into the problem may come from the analysis of disease associations. It has been argued that if two diseases tend to be associated in individuals, they may share one or more common risk factors. In fact, associations may also result from exposures which follow the development of one of the diseases of interest (e.g. iatrogenic factors) or even represent an artifact if the presence of a concomitant disease influences the diagnosis of another disease or its referral (Berkson's bias). Diseases associated with psoriasis have been studied through different methodologies, including cohort studies of psoriatics compared with the general population, record-linkage analyses of hospital discharge diagnoses and cancer registries data. Crucial to these studies is the selection of the control group or the reference population. The use of population figures to compare the experience of selected groups of patients (e.g. PUVA-treated patients) may lead to unreliable results.

A number of diseases which are strongly linked with alcohol consumption and smoking have also been associated with psoriasis (Table 13.9). These include liver cirrhosis, hypertension, cardiovascular diseases and respiratory-tract neoplasms. Unfortunately, negative results also exist and the strength of most associations is rather loosely defined. Interestingly, psoriasis has been, quite consistently, associated with kidney cancer, a tumour for which smoking habits represent the only

fairly well-documented risk factor (US Department of Health and Human Services, 1982).

Analytical studies

Analytical observational studies are a more direct way of addressing the alcohol, smoke and psoriasis issue. It should be noted that mere associations do not indicate possible causal links unless bolstered by specifications on the disease onset–exposure relationship, the strength of the association, the existence of exposure–effect gradients and the degree of control for potential confounders.

The first epidemiological study to draw attention to environmental factors in psoriasis vulgaris was conducted by Kavli *et al.* (1985) in Norway. It was a cross-sectional study based on data from a sample of 14 000 people in the district of Trømso. Factors associated with the prevalence of psoriasis were explored by multiple regression analysis. The occurrence of psoriasis in first-degree relatives contributed to about 90% of the explained variance. In addition, psoriasis was directly associated with smoking and inversely associated with the intake of fruit and vegetables. Unfortunately, no evidence of an exposure–effect relation was observed for smoking. In another cross-sectional population survey, psoriasis prevalence was also associated with a higher frequency of smoking (Braathen *et al.*, 1989). The relation between psoriasis and alcohol consumption was suggested in a hospital-based cross-sectional study examining the prevalence of psoriasis according to daily alcohol consumption (Chaput *et al.*, 1985). The main limitation of these studies is that they were unable to exclude the possibility that the associations were the consequence of the long-term course of the disease itself.

As far as we know, the only incidence study of psoriasis was conducted in Rochester, Minnesota (Bell *et al.*, 1991). Incident cases were defined as cases newly diagnosed at the Mayo Clinic facilities which cover the whole Rochester population. The overall crude incidence rate was 57 per 100 000 people per year. Smoking information was available for 89% of the new cases. Interestingly, the smoking profile for male patients was similar to the profile from a random sample of the Minnesota population while female patients smoked more than women in the population.

Table 13.9 Recent studies concerning the association of psoriasis with non-dermatological diseases.

Country (reference)	Study design	Results
USA (McDonald & Calabresi, 1978)	Comparison of the occurrence rate of occlusive vascular episodes in psoriatic patients and other dermatological controls	Increased occurrence of vascular episodes in psoriatics
Sweden (Lindegård, 1986)	Linkage among hospital discharge diagnoses in a defined population (Gothenburg cohort study)	Association of psoriasis, among others with liver cirrhosis, alcoholism and hypertension and, for women only, lung cancer and myocardial infarction
USA (Stern *et al.*, 1988)	Comparison of mortality in a cohort of PUVA-treated psoriatics with the general population	Increased mortality in psoriatics for cirrhosis, colonic cancer and central nervous system neoplasms. No increased risk for cardiovascular diseases
Sweden (Lindelöf *et al.*, 1990)	Linkage between the Swedish Psoriasis Association's membership registry and the Swedish Cancer Registry	Compared to the general population, increased incidence in psoriatic patients of breast cancer in men and kidney cancer in women
Sweden (Lindelöf *et al.*, 1991)	Linkage between data on 4945 PUVA-treated patients (74% with psoriasis or palmoplantar pustulosis) and the Swedish Cancer Registry	Compared to the general population, increased incidence in PUVA-treated patients of respiratory cancers in both sexes, of pancreatic cancer in men and colon and kidney cancer in women
Denmark (Olsen *et al.*, 1992)	Linkage between the National Hospital Discharge Diagnosis Registry and the Danish Cancer Registry	Compared to the general population, increased incidence in psoriatic patients of lung cancer in both sexes and of cancer of larynx and pharynx in men and colon and kidney cancer in women

More formal analytical observational studies, mainly case-control studies, have also been conducted. Studies which examine the exposure before the reported onset of psoriasis or its incident diagnosis (exposure should be related to the incidence rather than the prevalence of a disease) and control for the correlations among exposure variables, namely alcohol and smoking, offer the most convincing evidence. There are few such studies (Table 13.10).

In a case-control study conducted in Scotland (O'Doherty & MacIntyre, 1985), involving 216 patients with palmoplantar pustulosis and 626 controls with miscellaneous dermatoses, the risk in smokers, calculated from logistic regression analysis, was around 7 (99% confidence limits 3.9–13.2). No association

with alcohol was documented. Stopping smoking in 16 of the 144 patients who smoked did not appear to change the course of the disease, a finding which concurs with other anecdotal reports (Baughman, 1993). The relation of palmoplantar pustulosis to psoriasis is debatable. In another case-control study, limited to male psoriatic patients, information on alcohol consumption and smoking was collected before and after the onset of psoriasis (Poikolainen *et al.*, 1990). An association with alcohol consumption, but not with smoking, was documented before the onset of psoriasis. The odds ratio for psoriasis at an alcohol intake of 100 g/day compared with no intake was 2.2 (95% confidence interval 1.3–3.9). This finding was not confirmed in a subsequent case-control study from

Table 13.10 Summary of epidemiological studies on alcohol, cigarette smoking and psoriasis.

Country (reference)	Study design	Study subjects	Factors analysed and results
UK (O'Doherty & MacIntyre, 1985)	Case-control study (analysis of exposure before onset)	216 cases of palmoplantar pustulosis and 636 controls with other dermatoses	Alcohol: no significant association Smoking: OR 7.2
Finland (Poikolainen *et al.*, 1990)	Case-control study (analysis of exposure before onset)	114 male psoriatics and 285 controls with other skin diseases	Alcohol (>100 g/day): OR 2.2 Smoking: no significant association
USA (Bell *et al.*, 1991)	Survey of newly diagnosed cases	117 cases compared to population-based norms	Smoking: among women, prevalence of current smokers significantly higher than the reference population
UK (Mills *et al.*, 1992)	Case-control study (analysis of exposure before onset)	108 cases of psoriasis and 108 matched community controls	Smoking: OR 3.7 Dose–response relationship
Italy (Naldi *et al.*, 1992)	Case-control study on newly diagnosed cases and controls	215 cases of psoriasis and 267 controls with other skin diseases	Alcohol: no significant association after controlling for smoking Smoking (>15 cigarettes/day): OR 2.1 Dose–response relationship
Australia (Duffy *et al.*, 1993)	Case-control study based on twin registry	60 twins	Alcohol: no significant association
Finland (Poikolainen *et al.*, 1994)	Case-control study (analysis of exposure before onset)	55 women with psoriasis and 108 controls with other skin diseases	Alcohol: no significant association Smoking (≥20 cigarettes/day): OR 3.3

OR, Odds ratio.

Italy which included both sexes (Naldi *et al.*, 1992). In the Italian study, 215 newly diagnosed cases of psoriasis with a history of skin manifestations of no longer than 2 years were selected and compared with controls with new diagnoses of miscellaneous dermatoses. The multivariate estimate of odds ratio in those who smoked ≥ 15 cigarettes per day before diagnosis was 2.1 (95% confidence interval 1.1–4.0). The alcohol risk in this study appeared to be confounded by the association with smoking habits. Two additional case-control studies deserve mention. A group in Cardiff examined smoking habits in a group of psoriasis patients before the onset of the disease and compared the results with matched controls from the community (Mills *et al.*, 1992). There was a significant association between psoriasis and smoking habits with a remarkable dose–response relationship. Alcohol consumption was not assessed. In a case-control study limited to female psoriatic patients, Poikolainen *et al.* (1994), who failed to document an association between smoking and psoriasis in males, found such an association in females before the onset of their disease. In logistic regression analysis, the odds ratio for those smoking 20 cigarettes daily compared with non-smokers was 3.3. No association with alcohol consumption before onset was documented. An important finding of this study was that psoriasis may change women's attitude toward alcohol. In fact, alcohol intake was associated with psoriasis *after* the onset of the disease.

We have recently completed a case-control study involving 471 newly diagnosed cases of psoriasis with a history of skin manifestations of no longer than 2 years and 513 newly diagnosed dermatological controls. Lifetime history of alcohol consumption and smoking was collected through a standardized questionnaire. The exposure preceding the onset of the disease was considered. The study confirmed that smoking is associated with the onset of psoriasis with evidence of an exposure–effect relationship. The risk appeared to be modified by gender. The adjusted odds ratio for smoking ≥ 15 cigarettes was 3.2 in women and 1.6 in men. Interestingly, the risk in 39 patients with pustular lesions was 9.9 (Table 13.11). There was no evidence of an association with alcohol consumption after controlling for smoking habits in women but a risk was documented in men. It is noteworthy that in the study, indexes of stress did not affect the association between alcohol and smoking habits and psoriasis to a significant extent. Moreover, data on coffee consumption were also taken into account, and coffee did not appear to be associated with psoriasis.

In conclusion, the available evidence suggests that smoking is a risk factor for the onset of psoriasis especially in women, while alcohol consumption may represent a risk factor in men. The heterogeneity of the disease or the existence of unmeasured confounding factors may account for the discrepancies among the studies. The role of non-assessed risk modifiers and genetic–environmental interactions are also possible explanations. Heavy drinking may increase the risk of infections and mechanical trauma. Interestingly, Sonnex *et al.* (1988) documented that polymorpho-nuclear leucocytes (PMNs) from psoriatic smokers responded to a significantly greater degree to a stand-ard chemotaxin than did PMNs from psoriatic non-smokers, control smokers and control non-smokers. The gender-dependent risk in smokers points to a possible role of hormonal and reproductive factors since smoking has a well-defined anti-oestrogenic effect (Baron, 1984).

If smoking and alcohol do cause psoriasis, the im-pact on public health could be far from negligible (Williams, 1994). The population attributable fraction, for smoking, calculated from our study, was about 0.2 indicating that about one in five cases of psoriasis may be related to smoking.

A step forward

We have limited our interest to the association between the onset or incidence of psoriasis and alcohol and smoking habits. There is a paucity of data on the prognostic value of alcohol and smoking in established psoriasis. In a clinical study by Gupta *et al.* (1993), alcohol was found to be associated with the chronicity and severity of psoriasis and treatment failures in males but not in females. By contrast, in other studies (Poikolainen *et al.*, 1990, 1994) the relation between alcohol and indexes of severity, i.e. skin area involved, was weak and non-significant in males and stronger and more significant in females. Smoking and alcohol may alter the pattern of distribution (e.g. acral lesions) and affect the clinical variety of psoriasis. Long-term cohort studies of representative samples of newly diagnosed psoriatic patients are clearly needed to as-sess the natural history and prognosis of established

Table 13.11 Odds ratios of psoriasis according to smoking habits and selected covariates. (From L. Naldi *et al.*, unpublished data.)*

Parameter	Cigarettes per day (*n*)			χ^2_1 trend, *P* value
	Non-smokers	< 15	≥ 15	
Sex				
Males	1	0.9	1.6	0.054
Females	1	1.7	3.2	0.003
Age at diagnosis (years)				
≤ 39	1	1.5	2.1	0.001
> 39	1	1.3	1.9	0.056
Clinical variety				
Pustular	1	4.7	9.9	0.001
Others	1	1.3	1.8	0.004

* Odds ratios are adjusted for alcohol consumption and, when appropriate, age and sex.

psoriasis (Naldi, 1995). As already mentioned, scant and largely anecdotal data are available on the effect of stopping smoking and reducing alcohol consumption on psoriasis. The best way to address the issue would be a randomized trial assessing the effect of counselling patients to reduce their consumption of cigarettes and alcohol as part of the routine therapeutic measures.

References

Al'Abadie, M.S., Kent, G.G. & Gawkrodger, D.J. (1994) The relationship between stress and the onset and exacerbation of psoriasis and other skin conditions. *British Journal of Dermatology*, **130**, 199–203.

Baron, J.A. (1984) Smoking and estrogen-related disease. *American Journal of Epidemiology*, **119**, 9–22.

Baughman, R.D. (1993) Psoriasis and cigarettes. Another nail in the coffin. *Archives of Dermatology*, **129**, 1329–1330.

Bell, L.M., Sedlack, R., Beard, M.C., Perry, H.O., Michet, C.J. & Kurland, L.T. (1991) Incidence of psoriasis in Rochester, Minnesota, 1980–1983. *Archives of Dermatology*, **127**, 1184–1187.

Braathen, L.R., Botten, G. & Bjerkedal, T. (1989) Psoriasis in Norway. A questionnaire study of health status, contact with paramedical professions and alcohol and tobacco consumption. *Acta Dermato-Venereologica*, **142** (Suppl.), 9–12.

Chaput, J.C., Poynard, T., Naveau, S., Penso, D., Durrmeyer, O. & Suplisson, D. (1985) Psoriasis, alcohol, and liver disease. *British Medical Journal*, **291**, 25.

Duffy, D.L., Spelman, L.S. & Martin, N.G. (1993) Psoriasis in Australian twins. *Journal of the American Academy of Dermatology*, **29**, 428–434.

Gupta, M.A., Schork, N., Gupta, A.K. & Ellis, C.N. (1993) Alcohol intake and treatment responsiveness of psoriasis: a prospective study. *Journal of the American Academy of Dermatology*, **28**, 730–732.

Kavli, G., Førde, O.H., Arnesen, E. & Stenvold, S.E. (1985) Psoriasis: familial predisposition and environmental factors. *British Medical Journal*, **291**, 999–1000.

Lindegård, B. (1986) Diseases associated with psoriasis in a general population of 159 200 middle-aged, urban, native Swedes. *Dermatologica*, **172**, 298–304.

Lindelöf, B., Eklund, O.D., Lidén, S. & Stern, R.S. (1990) The prevalence of malignant tumors in patients with psoriasis. *Journal of the American Academy of Dermatology*, **22**, 1056–1060.

Lindelöf, B., Sigurgeirsson, B., Tegner, E. *et al.* (1991) PUVA and cancer: a large scale epidemiological study. *Lancet*, **338**, 91–93.

McDonald, C.J. & Calabresi, P. (1978) Psoriasis and occlusive vascular disease. *British Journal of Dermatology*, **99**, 469–475.

Mills, C.M., Srivastava, E.D., Harvey, M. *et al.* (1992) Smoking habits in psoriasis: a case control study. *British Journal of Dermatology*, **127**, 18–21.

Naldi, L. (1995) Psoriasis. *Dermatologic Clinics*, **13**, 635–647.

Naldi, L., Parazzini, F., Brevi, A. *et al.* (1992) Family history, smoking habits, alcohol consumption and risk of psoriasis. *British Journal of Dermatology*, **127**, 212–217.

Naldi, L., Parazzini, F., Peli, L. *et al.* (1995) Dietary factors and risk of psoriasis. Results of an Italian case-control study. *British Journal of Dermatology*, **134**, 101–106.

O'Doherty, C.J. & MacIntyre, C. (1985) Palmoplantar pustulosis and smoking. *British Medical Journal*, **291**, 861–864.

Olsen, J.H., Møller, H. & Frentz, G. (1992) Malignant tumors in patients with psoriasis. *Journal of the American Academy of Dermatology*, **27**, 716–722.

Poikolainen, K., Reunala, T., Karvonen, J., Lauhranta, J. & Karkkainen, P. (1990) Alcohol intake: a risk factor for psoriasis in young and middle aged men? *British Medical Journal*, **300**, 780–783.

Poikolainen, K., Reunala, T. & Karvonen, J. (1994) Smoking, alcohol and life events related to psoriasis among women. *British Journal of Dermatology*, **130**, 473–477.

Sonnex, T.S., Carrington, P., Norris, P. & Greaves, M.W. (1988) Polymorphonuclear leukocyte random migration and chemotaxis in psoriatic and healthy adult smokers and non-smokers. *British Journal of Dermatology*, **119**, 653–659.

Stern, R.S., Lange, R. & members of the Photochemotherapy Follow-up Study (1988) Cardiovascular disease, cancer, and cause of death in patients with psoriasis: 10 years prospective experience in a cohort of 1380 patients. *Journal of Investigative Dermatology*, **91**, 197–201.

US Department of Health and Human Services (1982) *The Health Consequences of Smoking: Cancer. A Report of the Surgeon General of the Public Health Service, US Department of Health and Human Services, Office on Smoking and Health*. US Government Printing Office, Washington.

Williams, H.C. (1994) Smoking and psoriasis. *British Medical Journal*, **308**, 428–429.

Diet and Psoriasis

E. SØYLAND

Psoriasis is an immune-related skin disease affecting approximately 2% of the population in Western countries. This chronic skin inflammation is characterized by hyperkinetic activity of keratinocytes, reduced barrier function with lipid-deficient intercellular space in the stratum corneum, increased number of Langerhans cells, migration of neutrophils from dermis into the epidermis and deposits of autoantibodies and complement components in the cells of the stratum corneum (Miura, 1985; Bos, 1988). Psoriasis is also characterized by abnormal secretion of cytokines, eicosanoids from epidermal cells, infiltration of T cells and macrophages in the dermis, and it is proposed that psoriatic lesions erupt when epidermal influx of antigen-carrying cells and helper T lymphocytes overrides the normal epidermal suppressor mechanism (Baadsgaard *et al.*, 1989; Barker, 1991).

Dietary manipulation in treating psoriasis has primarily been concentrated on vitamin A and *n*-3 polyunsaturated fatty acids. Dietary supplementation with vitamin A was previously used in treating psoriasis. However, because of serious sides effects, vitamin A is now substituted with vitamin A analogues, the retinoids (Fredriksson & Petterson, 1978). Therefore, here it will be mainly focused on the effect of dietary supplementation with *n*-3 polyunsaturated fatty acids and how daily diet may influence this skin disease.

Polyunsaturated fatty acids

Lipids are important constituents of the skin. Lack of polyunsaturated fatty acids promotes dry, scaly and hyperproliferative skin which is normalized by dietary addition of polyunsaturated fatty acids (Burr & Burr, 1929, 1930). As essential components of cell membranes, they may affect receptors, enzymes, ion channels and other messenger systems (Drevon, 1993). In the epidermis, polyunsaturated fatty acids also play an important role as part of the sphingolipids which make up the water barrier (Bowser *et al.*, 1986). The position of the first double bond counted from the methyl group of polyunsaturated fatty acids may be located in the third position, as for *n*-3 fatty acids — or in the sixth position, as for *n*-6 fatty acids. Cells derived from species located high up in the evolutionary hierarchy cannot introduce double bonds in the carbon chain of fatty acids closer to the methyl group C7. Chloroplasts in phytoplankton and plants can synthesize the essential *n*-3 and *n*-6 fatty acids, respectively. This means that mammalian cells cannot

transform *n*-3 into *n*-6 fatty acids, as outlined in Fig. 13.4. *n*-3 and *n*-6 fatty acids share common enzymes for some of their metabolic pathways and they are transferred via the nutrition chain from plankton and plants to higher animals (shrimp, shell, fatty fish, seal, whale and eventually man). In general, the content of the most common very long-chain *n*-3 fatty acids is highest in the marine animals containing the highest amount of fat.

When dietary *n*-3 fatty acids are consumed, they are incorporated into cell membranes and compete with *n*-6 fatty acids as substrates for cyclooxygenase and lipoxygenase pathways. Eicosapentaenoic acid (EPA), dihomo-gamma-linolenic acid (DGLA) and arachidonic acid (AA) are precursors of eicosanoids which affect inflammatory and immunological processes in several ways (Mead & Mertin, 1988). Eicosanoids derived from fatty acids of the *n*-3 series (e.g. leukotriene B_5, thromboxane A_3) are generally less potent than metabolites from the *n*-6 series (leukotriene B_4 and thromboxane A_2) and consequently exert a smaller inflammatory reaction (Ziboh *et al.*, 1986). The biological difference between prostaglandin E_3 (PGE_3) derived from EPA and PGE_2 derived from AA is, however, more uncertain. The type of eicosanoids secreted is dependent on the cell type, e.g. thromboxanes are mainly secreted from thrombocytes, whereas leukotrienes and prostaglandins are secreted from many cell types, including keratinocytes and Langerhans cells.

Dietary supplementation with *n*-3 fatty acids in patients with psoriasis

Eskimos have a low incidence of psoriasis as compared to Danes (Kromann & Green, 1980). On a traditional diet, Eskimos also have a high intake of very long-chain *n*-3 fatty acids, especially EPA and docosahexaenoic acid (DHA) mainly found in seal, whale and fatty fish, whereas Danes have a high intake of *n*-6 fatty acids, especially LA, mainly obtained from vegetable sources and animal fat (Bang *et al.*, 1980). This observation led to a number of reports suggesting that ingestion of several grams per day of very long-chain *n*-3 fatty acids may provide improvement in the clinical state of psoriasis (Ziboh *et al.*, 1986; Maurice

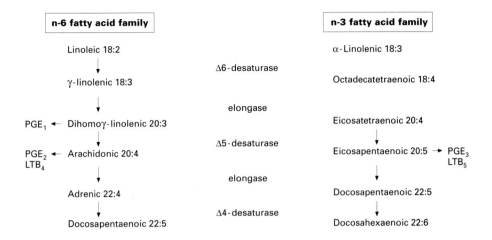

Fig. 13.4 Metabolic pathways for the desaturation and elongation of *n*-3 and *n*-6 fatty acids, which share common enzymes for some of their metabolic pathways.

et al., 1987; Bittiner *et al.*, 1988). However, most of the clinical trials treating psoriatic patients with fish oil are open studies involving <25 patients. Furthermore, the double-blind study reported by Bjørneboe *et al.* (1988) could not demonstrate any significant effect of fish-oil supplementation on the clinical state of psoriasis.

In a double-blind multicentre study, where 145 patients with stable psoriasis were included, dietary supplementation with capsules containing 5.1 g of highly concentrated ethyl esters of EPA and DHA (K85 Pronova Biocare AS) resulted in a significant increase in the EPA/AA ratio of serum phospholipids (Søyland *et al.*, 1993b). This treatment, however, did not significantly improve the clinical state of psoriasis as compared to dietary supplementation with corn oil. Leukotrienes, derived from AA, are elevated in affected skin of psoriatic patients (Brain *et al.*, 1984). Especially leukotriene $B_4(LTB_4)$ is a potent mediator of skin inflammation via its chemotactic and proliferative effect in human skin (Camp *et al.*, 1984; Sperling *et al.*, 1993). One way to inhibit the formation of LTB_4 is to replace the AA in the phospholipids with EPA. EPA is the precursor of LTB_5, which expresses only 3–10% of the chemotactic activity of LTB_4 (Goldmann *et al.*, 1987). Thus, the result of the multicentre study suggests that LTB_4 does not play a major part in affected psoriatic skin, since a highly significant increase in the EPA/AA ratio was not able to improve the clinical state of patients with psoriasis.

Environmental stimuli responsible for inducing cutaneous inflammation promote resident cells of the skin (including fibroblasts, endothelial cells, epidermal keratinocytes and Langerhans cells) to produce various cytokines like interleukin-1 (IL-1), IL-6, IL-8, tumour necrosis factor-α (TNF-α), in addition to eicosanoids and adhesion molecules (Bevilacqua *et al.*, 1987; Griffiths *et al.*, 1989; Kupper, 1990). The consequences are that the resident cells of the skin guide monocytes, lymphocytes and granulocytes through the vessel wall and through dermal tissues along chemotactic gradients (Nickoloff *et al.*, 1990). The activation of T cells takes place when an antigen is presented to the T cells via the major histocompatibility complex (MHC) molecules on antigen-presenting cells, e.g. monocytes, macrophages or Langerhans cells in the skin. The activated T cells become blasts, start to secrete IL-2 and express IL-2 receptors on their cell membrane. When IL-2 binds to their IL-2 receptors, the T cells are able to proliferate. *In vitro* and *ex vivo* studies have shown that *n*-3 fatty acids reduce T-cell proliferation and decrease the synthesis of IL-2 and IL-1β (Espersen *et al.*, 1992; Søyland *et al.*, 1993a; Endres *et al.*, 1993). Since T-cell activation and cytokine production are major features in affected skin in patients with psoriasis (Zachary *et al.*, 1985), it is likely that supplementation with fish oil might possibly have a beneficial effect. However, in the 4-month double-blind multi-centre trial, there was no significant clinical improvement in the experimental group receiving *n*-3 fatty acids, as compared to the control group receiving corn oil (Søyland *et al.*, 1993b). This indicates that *n*-3 fatty acids given as the only treatment does not reduce immunologic parameters responsible for the psoriatic eruptions.

Dietary intake of fish oil combined with UVB light was superior to UVB light alone in the treatment of patients with psoriasis, as demonstrated in a smaller clinical study (Gupta *et al.*, 1989). Thus, dietary intake of *n*-3 fatty acids may potentiate the effect of other antipsoriatic treatments and this possibility needs further investigations.

Dietary habits among patients with psoriasis

Naldi *et al.* (1996) published recently a case-control study where the diets of 316 psoriatic patients were assessed by a semiquantitative food-frequency questionnaire. In this study, psoriasis appeared to be positively associated with body mass index. Furthermore, there was a significant inverse relation between psoriasis and the intake of carrots, fresh fruit and index of beta-carotene intake. Similar results were observed in a Norwegian study, where a decreased prevalence of psoriasis with increased intake of vegetables and fruit was documented (Kavli *et al.*, 1985).

In an unpublished study, the composition of the usual diet among 93 men and 43 women with psoriasis was assessed, and the intake of nutrients was related to their clinical score (Solvoll *et al.*, in press). The diet was assessed by a self-administered quantitative food-frequency questionnaire aiming to cover the whole diet. The results were compared to the diet of a reference group. The patients' intake of energy and nutrients was similar to what was found in the reference group. None of the nutrients gave statistically significant contributions to explain the clinical score values when analysed by correlations and multiple regressions. However, classification of patients in two-by-two tables separated by median values, according to nutrient intake and clinical score, suggested that the diet might have some influence on the skin disease in male patients. Males with high vitamin D intake had better dermatological status as compared to patients with low intake of vitamin D. The same tendency was observed for vitamin A and very long-chain *n*-3 fatty acids. Considering that vitamin D and vitamin A have immunosuppressive and antiproliferative effects on keratinocytes, and that both vitamin D and vitamin A analogues are efficient in treating psoriasis, these are interesting observations. Both vitamin D and vitamin A belong to the steroid superfamily. They act as ligands for nuclear receptors binding to special enhancer regions on DNA (Henry & Cronan, 1992). Recently, fatty acids have been shown to regulate the expression of several genes in a similar way. They do so by acting as a ligand for certain nuclear proteins, like peroxisomal proliferation transcription factors (PPAR), which act as transcription factors and thereby contribute to an altered mRNA synthesis (Göttlicher *et al.*, 1992). PPAR has recently been shown to make dimers with the nuclear receptors for vitamin A as well as vitamin D. One future research area may therefore be to evaluate the effect of dietary fatty acids in combination with fatty acid-soluble vitamins, like vitamin A and D.

Conclusion

n-3 fatty acids do have immunosuppressive effects *in vitro* and dietary supplementation with *n*-3 fatty acids does reduce the chemotactic LTB_4 level in blood. In spite of these findings, dietary intake of high doses of *n*-3 fatty acids as a monotherapy is not able to influence the clinical state of psoriasis (Søyland *et al.*, 1993b).

Epidemiological studies assessing usual dietary habits of psoriatic patients are scarce. Although the results are explorative, the present studies indicate that psoriasis may be influenced by daily dietary intake of fruit and vegetables rich in carotenoids and vitamin A as well as food rich in vitamin D (Kavli *et al.*, 1985; Naldi *et al.*, 1996; Solvoll *et al.*, in press). There is also a potential association of psoriasis and body mass index (Naldi *et al.*, 1996). However, the possible role of usual dietary habits in the development of psoriasis needs further investigations to be verified.

References

Baadsgaard, O., Gupta, A.K., Taylor, R.S., Ellis, C.N., Voorhees, J. & Cooper, K.D. (1989) Psoriatic epidermal cells demonstrate increased numbers and function of non-Langerhans antigen-presenting cells. *Journal of Investigative Dermatology*, **92**, 190–195.

Barker, N.W. (1991) The pathophysiology of psoriasis. *Lancet*, **338**, 227–230.

Bang, H.O., Dyerberg, J. & Sinclair, H.M. (1980) The composition of the Eskimo food in north eastern Greenland. *American Journal of Clinical Nutrition*, **33**, 2657–2661.

Bevilacqua, M.P., Pober, J.S., Mendrick, D.L., Cotran, R.S. & Gimbrone, M.A. (1987) Identification of an inducible endothelial–leucocyte adhesion molecule. *Proceedings of the National Academy of Sciences USA*, **84**, 9238–9242.

Bittiner, S.B., Cartwright, I., Tucker, W.F.G. & Bleehen, S.S. (1988) A double-blind randomised placebo-controlled trial of fish oil in psoriasis. *Lancet*, **i**, 378–380.

Bjørneboe, A., Smith, A.K., Bjørneboe, G.-E.A., Thune, P.O. & Drevon, C.A. (1988) Effect of dietary supplementation with *n*-3 fatty acids on clinical manifestations of psoriasis. *British Journal of Dermatology*, **118**, 77–83.

Bos, J.D. (1988) The pathomechanisms of psoriasis, the skin immune system and cyclosporin. *British Journal of Dermatology*, **118**, 141–145.

Bowser, P.A., White, R.J. & Nugteren, D.H. (1986) Location and nature of the epidermal permeability barrier. *International Journal of Cosmetic Chemists*, **8**, 125–134.

Brain, S., Camp, R., Dowd, P., Black, A.K. & Greaves, M. (1984) The release of leukotriene B_4-like material in biologically active amounts from lesional skin of patients with psoriasis. *Journal of Investigative Dermatology*, **83**, 70–73.

Burr, G.O. & Burr, M.M. (1929) A new defiency disease produced by rigid exclusion of fat from the diet. *Journal of Biological Chemistry*, **82**, 345–367.

Burr, G.O. & Burr, M.M. (1930) On the nature and role of fatty acids essential in nutrition. *Journal of Biological Chemistry*, **86**, 587–589.

Camp, R., Russel Jones, R., Brain, S., Woolard, P. & Greaves, M. (1984) Production of microabscesses by topical application of leukotriene B_4. *Journal of Investigative Dermatology*, **82**, 202–204.

Drevon, C.A. (1993) Sources, chemistry and biochemistry of dietary lipids. Omega-3 fatty acids. In: *Metabolism and Biologic Effect* (eds C.A. Drevon, I. Baksaa & H. Krokan). Birhauser, Basel.

Endres, S., Meydani, S.N., Ghorbani, R., Schindler, R. & Dinarello, C.A. (1993) Dietary supplementation with *n*-3 polyunsaturated fatty acids suppresses interleukin-2 production and mononuclear cell proliferation. *Journal of Leukocyte Biology*, **54**, 599–603.

Esperson, G.T., Grunnet, N., Lervang, H.H. *et al.* (1992) Decreased interleukin-1β levels in plasma from rheumatoid arthritis patients after dietary supplementation with *n*-3 polyunsaturated fatty acids. *Clinical Rheumatology*, **11**, 393–395.

Fredriksson, T. & Petterson, U. (1978) Severe psoriasis — oral therapy with a new retinoid. *Dermatologica*, **157**, 238–244.

Goldmann, D.W., Pickett, W.C. & Goetzl, E.J. (1987) Human neutrophil chemotactic and degranulation activities of leukotriene B_5 (LTB_5) derived from eicosapentaenoic acid. *Biochemical and Biophysical Research Communications*, **117**, 282–288.

Göttlicher, M., Widmark, E., Qiao, L. & Gustasson, J.-Å. (1992) Fatty acids activate a chimera of the clofibric acid-activated receptor and the glucocorticoid receptor. *Proceedings of the National Academy of Sciences USA*, **89**, 4653–4657.

Griffiths, C.E.M., Voorhees, J.J. & Nickoloff, B.J. (1989) Characterization of intercellular adhesion molecule-1 and HLA-DR in normal and inflamed skin: modulation by interferon-gamma and tumor necrosis factor. *Journal of the American Academy of Dermatology*, **20**, 617–629.

Gupta, A.K., Ellis, C.N., Tellner, D.C. *et al.* (1989) Double-blind, placebo-controlled study to evaluate the efficacy of fish oil and low-dose ultraviolet B in the treatment of psoriasis. *British Journal of Dermatology*, **120**, 801–807.

Henry, M.F. & Cronan, J.E. (1992) A new mechanism of transcriptional regulation: release of an activator triggered by small molecule binding. *Cell*, **70**, 671–679.

Kavli, G., Forde, O.H., Arnesen, E. & Stensvold, S.E. (1985) Psoriasis: familial predisposition and environmental factors. *British Medical Journal of Clinical Research*, **291**, 999–1000.

Kromann, N. & Green, A. (1980) Epidemiologic studies in the Upernavik district, Greenland. *Acta Medica Scandinavica*, **208**, 401–406.

Kupper, T.S. (1990) The role of epidermal cytokines. In: *Immunophysiology: The Role of Cells and Cytokines in Immunity and Inflammation* (eds E. Shevach & J. Oppenheim), pp. 285–305. Oxford University Press, New York.

Maurice, P.D.L., Allen, B.R., Barkley, A.S.J., Cockbill, S.R., Stammers, J. & Bather, P.C. (1987) The effect of dietary supplementation with fish oil in patients with psoriasis. *British Journal of Dermatology*, **117**, 599–606.

Mead, J.C. & Mertin, J. (1988) Fatty acids and immunity. *Advances in Lipid Research*, **21**, 103.

Miura, Y. (ed.) (1985) *Current Concepts on Pathogenesis of Psoriasis*. Hokkaido University School of Medicine, Sapporo.

Naldi, L., Parazzini, F., Pali, L., Chatenoud, L. & Cainelli, T. (1996) Dietary factors and the risk of psoriasis. Results of an Italian case-control study. *British Journal of Dermatology*, **134**, 101–106.

Nickoloff, B.J., Griffiths, C.E.M. & Barker, J.N.W.N. (1990) The role of adhesion molecules, chemotactic factors, and cytokines in inflammatory and neoplastic skin disease. *Journal of Investigative Dermatology*, **94** (Suppl.), 151S–157S.

Solvoll, K., Søyland, E., Sandstad, B. & Drevon, C.A. (1997) Dietary habits among patients with psoriasis. *British Journal of Nutrition* (in press).

Søyland, E., Nenseter, M.S., Braathen, L. & Drevon, C.A. (1993a) Very long chain *n*-3 and *n*-6 polyunsaturated fatty acids inhibit proliferation of human T-lymphocytes *in vitro*. *European Journal of Clinical Investigation*, **23**, 112–121.

Søyland, E., Funk, J., Rajka, G. *et al.* (1993b) Effect of dietary supplementation with very-long-chain *n*-3 fatty acids in patients with psoriasis. *New England Journal of Medicine*, **328**, 1812–1816.

Sperling, R.I., Benincaso, A.I., Knoell, C.T., Larkin, J.K., Austen, K.F. & Robinson, D.R. (1993) Dietary omega-3 fatty acids inhibit phosphoinositide formation and chemotaxis in neutrophils. *Journal of Clinical Investigation*, **91**, 651–660.

Zachary, C.B., Allen, M.H. & MacDonald, D.M. (1985) *In situ* quantification of T-lymphocyte subsets and Langerhans cells in the inflammatory infiltrate of atopic eczema. *British Journal of Dermatology*, **112**, 149–156.

Ziboh, V.A., Cohen, K.A., Ellis, C.N. *et al.* (1986) Effect of dietary supplementation of fish oil on neutrophil and epidermal fatty acids: Modulation of clinical course of psoriatic subjects. *Archives of Dermatology*, **122**, 1277–1282.

Psychological Factors and Psoriasis

M.A. GUPTA AND A.K. GUPTA

Psychosocial factors (Gupta *et al.*, 1987) have been implicated as being important in the onset and/or exacerbation of psoriasis in 40% (Farber *et al.*, 1968; Seville, 1977) to 80% (Fava *et al.*, 1980) of patients, and hence are an important factor in the primary, secondary and/or tertiary prevention of psoriasis. Primary prevention is defined as the prevention of the disease process from occurring. A review of the literature suggests that some of the factors that play a role in the primary prevention of psoriasis include stress from major life events, certain personality traits, especially alexithymia or difficulty with the expression of emotions, substance abuse including alcohol and cigarette smoking, and the use of psychotropic agents such as lithium. Secondary prevention includes measures aimed against the progression or recurrence of disease and tertiary prevention is concerned mainly with the effective treatment of disease and prevention of complications. Some of the psychosocial factors of importance in the secondary and tertiary prevention of psoriasis include psoriasis-related daily stress or hassles, stressful major life events, certain personality characteristics such as alexithymia and high interpersonal dependency or the tendency to want the approval of others, depressive disease which may decrease the threshold for pruritus in psoriasis, alcohol consumption of > 80 g daily and the use of psychotropic agents such as lithium.

Here we provide an overview of the literature on the psychosocial factors that may play a role in the primary, secondary and/or tertiary prevention of psoriasis. The literature has focused on four areas: (i) the role of psychosocial stress both originating from major life events and psoriasis-related hassles; (ii) psychopathology such as a major depressive disorder; (iii) use of lithium which is a psychotropic agent and is used largely for the treatment of mood disorders; and (iv) alcohol consumption and cigarette smoking. We will focus mainly on the literature in (i) and (ii), i.e. stress and psychopathology.

Stress and psoriasis

There is a relatively large body of literature implicating the role of stressful life events in the onset and/or exacerbation of psoriasis (Gupta *et al.*, 1987). In contrast to other dermatological disorders such as urticaria, acne, alopecia and non-atopic eczema, there was a greater likelihood that stress predated the onset and/or exacerbation of psoriasis (Al'Abadie *et al.*, 1994). Furthermore, during stressor exposure, psoriasis patients reported greater increase in perceived stress in contrast to atopic dermatitis and control patients (Arnetz *et al.*, 1991). One study reported higher 'strain' levels and higher urinary adrenaline levels during stress-provoking situations among psoriasis patients (Arnetz *et al.*, 1985). However, the overall neuroendocrine reactivity, including growth hormone secretion, was similar among patients with psoriasis, atopic dermatitis and healthy controls (Arnetz *et al.*, 1991). One study has reported the 'incubation time' between a stressful life event and the onset or exacerbation of psoriasis to be between 2 days to 1 month

(Seville, 1977). Prognosis for the psoriasis patients who recollected specific stress 1 month prior to onset of psoriasis was significantly better than the patients who recalled no stress (Seville, 1977).

The literature on stress and psoriasis has focused on two major types of stressors: (i) stressful major life events, and (ii) psoriasis-related daily stress or hassles, arising mainly from the impact of psoriasis on the quality of life. In a recent report, 72% of 179 psoriasis patients reported a stressful life event 1 month before the onset of psoriasis (Polenghi *et al.*, 1994). In an earlier report, 39% of 132 psoriasis patients versus 10% of controls recalled 'specific stress' 1 month before the onset of symptoms (Seville, 1977). Stress was reported to be a provocative factor in 90% of 245 children with psoriasis (Nyfors & Lemholt, 1975). The impact of stressful life events on psoriasis appears to be modulated by other intermediary factors, since monozygotic twins discordant for psoriasis appeared to have the same stress history (Brandrup *et al.*, 1982). Furthermore, no relation has been observed between the *severity* of stress and the time to onset or exacerbation of psoriasis (Al'Abadie *et al.*, 1994). This may be, in part, because of variation in individual coping skills and individual personalities (Al'Abadie *et al.*, 1994) and the fact that the emotional meaning of a particular life event varies from patient to patient (Mazzetti *et al.*, 1994).

The psychosocial impact of psoriasis can result in significant daily stress for the patient, largely secondary to the cosmetic disfigurement and social stigma associated with the disorder (Finlay & Kelly, 1987; Ramsay & O'Reagan, 1988; Ginsburg & Link, 1989; Gupta *et al.*, 1989; Finlay & Coles, 1995; Fried *et al.*, 1995). The effect of psoriasis on the quality of life and the resultant psychosocial disability is usually greater than the physical disability in psoriasis (Finlay & Kelly, 1987; Fried *et al.*, 1995). Comparison of the psychocutaneous characteristics of patients who reported that stress exacerbated their psoriasis (i.e. the high stress reactors or HSR) to the subgroup that reported no significant association between stress and their psoriasis (i.e. the low stress reactors or LSR) revealed that the HSR had more cosmetically disfiguring disease clinically, i.e. they had greater psoriasis severity in their 'emotionally charged' body regions such as the face, neck, scalp, forearms, hands and genitals

(Gupta *et al.*, 1989). Psoriasis in these regions among the HSR is more likely to arouse emotional reactions in the patient because of its effect upon the appearance and close interpersonal relationships including their sexual functioning (Gupta *et al.*, 1989). In contrast to the LSR, the HSR reported greater psoriasis-related stress; however, the stress from major life events did not emerge as being statistically significant when considered along with psoriasis-related daily stress (Gupta *et al.*, 1989). The HSR reported more frequent flare-ups of their psoriasis over the previous 6 months. These findings suggest that the chronic low-grade and often unremitting stress resulting from the psychosocial impact of psoriasis can play a more important role than the typically acute stress resulting from major life events (Gupta *et al.*, 1989). It is possible that, in some cases, the chronic psoriasis-related psychosocial stress in turn exacerbates the psoriasis (Gupta *et al.*, 1989). Aggressive management of cosmetically disfiguring psoriasis may in turn decrease the psoriasis-related stress and result in fewer flare-ups of the psoriasis. In one study, the impact of psoriasis upon the quality of life was the greatest among the 18–45-year age group, a life stage when the individual is expected to be the most productive, both occupationally and socially (Gupta & Gupta, *et al.*, 1995a), in contrast to the older patients. Psoriasis affects socialization of both sexes equally, although men may face more work-related stress as a result of their psoriasis (Gupta & Gupta, 1995a).

The literature suggests that consideration of the psychosocial impact of psoriasis in turn can mitigate the level of psoriasis-related stress, an important consideration in the secondary prevention of psoriasis. Various questionnaires may be used to assess the psychosocial impact of psoriasis. The Psoriasis Disability Index (Finlay & Kelly, 1987) provides an index of the psychosocial disability associated with psoriasis. Ginsburg and Link (1989) have developed a questionnaire that assesses the feelings of stigmatization associated with psoriasis. The Psoriasis Life Stress Inventory (PLSI) (Gupta & Gupta, 1995b) provides an index of the stress the patient perceives secondary to feelings of stigmatization, and the impact of psoriasis upon the quality of life. In this instrument, the patients endorse the degree of stress (using a 0–4-point scale) associated with each of 15 psoriasis-related events,

Table 13.12 The Psoriasis Life Stress Inventory (PLSI) (Gupta & Gupta, 1995b).
Over the past *1 month* how much *stress* have you experienced as a result of the following? Using the following scale write down the number that best describes the degree of stress you experienced (if you did not experience the event, or the event is not applicable in your case, please give the event a rating of 0).
Rating scale: 0 = not at all, 1 = slight degree, 2 = moderate degree, 3 = a great deal

Psoriasis-related event	Over the past 1 month how much stress did this cause you? (Write a number between 0 and 3)
1 Inconvenienced by the shedding of your skin	—
2 Feeling self-conscious among strangers	—
3 Feeling that you have to set aside a large part of your time to take care of your psoriasis	—
4 Not going to a public place (e.g. swimming pool, health club, restaurant) when you would have liked to	—
5 Wearing unattractive or uncomfortable clothes in order to cover certain regions of the body	—
6 Having to avoid sunbathing in the company of others	—
7 Fear of having serious side-effects from medical treatments	—
8 People treating you as if your skin condition is contagious	—
9 Avoiding social situations	—
10 Strangers (children or adults) making rude or insensitive remarks about your appearance	—
11 Not enough money to pay medical bills	—
12 Feeling like an 'outcast' or 'social misfit' a great deal of the time	—
13 People making a conscious effort not to touch you	—
14 Hairdresser or barber appearing reluctant to cut your hair	—
15 People implying that your skin condition may be due to AIDS, leprosy or a venereal disease	—

where a rating of 0 denotes 'not at all' and a rating of 3 denotes 'a great deal' of stress (Table 13.12). In some preliminary studies (Gupta & Gupta, 1995b) involving patients from an American centre, a PLSI score of ≥ 10 (possible range of 0–45) delineated patients with more frequent flare-ups of psoriasis ($P = 0.009$), greater overall psoriasis severity ($P = 0.007$), more cosmetically disfiguring psoriasis ($P < 0.01$) and greater pruritus severity ($P = 0.001$). Delineation of patients who are excessively stressed by their psoriasis can be important in the secondary and tertiary prevention of psoriasis.

Psoriasis and psychopathology

In a recent study (Al'Abadie *et al.*, 1994) no relation was observed between the *severity* of the major life event and time to onset or exacerbation of psoriasis. This suggests that the individual variation in psychological coping mechanisms (Mazzetti *et al.*, 1994) and the presence of psychopathological factors can moderate the effect of psychosocial factors on the course of psoriasis. A review of the literature reveals that psoriasis patients do not have any characteristic personality traits (Gupta *et al.*, 1987); however, certain psychopathological factors, when present, may modulate the course of psoriasis. Some investigators have observed that psoriasis patients have alexithymia or difficulty with the verbal expression of emotion (Rubino *et al.*, 1989; Vidoni *et al.*, 1989). Patients who reported that stress exacerbated their psoriasis had some characteristic personality traits, i.e. difficulty with the expression of angry feelings and had high interpersonal dependency or the tendency to rely upon the approval of others (Gupta *et al.*, 1989). It is important to recognize the presence of depressive disease in psoriasis. In a survey of 217 patients, 9.7% of patients reported a wish to be dead and 5.5% reported active suicidal ideation at the time of the study (Gupta *et al.*, 1993a). Suicidal ideation in psoriasis was associated with higher depression scores and higher patient self-ratings of psoriasis severity (Gupta *et al.*, 1993a).

Pruritus is a very bothersome symptom for many psoriasis patients. For example, in one study (Gupta *et al.*, 1988) 26% of patients rated pruritus as the most bothersome symptom of psoriasis. The degree of depressive psychopathology has been shown to increase with increasing pruritus severity (Fig. 13.5) (Gupta *et al.*, 1988, 1994). The decrease in pruritus pretreatment to post-treatment has been shown to correlate directly with a decrease in depression scores (Gupta *et al.*, 1988). The depressive symptoms may be a primary feature of psoriasis or secondary to the disorder; however the depressed clinical state appears to reduce the threshold for pruritus. Consideration of this factor may be important in the secondary and/or tertiary prevention of psoriasis. Furthermore, treatment of depression may decrease self-excoriative behaviour and exacerbation of psoriasis secondary to the Koebner phenomenon.

Alcohol is recognized as a risk factor for psoriasis especially among men (Monk & Neill, 1986; Poikolainen *et al.*, 1990), and various psychopathological states including depressive disease may predispose the psoriasis patient to drink excessively. In a prospective study, an average daily ethanol consumption of > 80 g

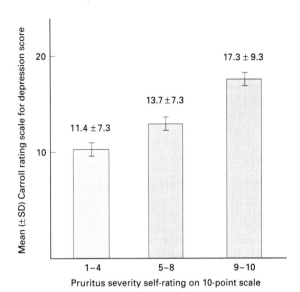

Fig. 13.5 Pruritus severity and depression. $P < 0.005$ by ANOVA. (After Gupta *et al.*, 1988.)

over the previous 6 months was associated with significantly less treatment-induced improvement of psoriasis over the course of in-patient therapy (Gupta *et al.*, 1993b).

Summary

Psychological factors play the most convincing role in the secondary and tertiary prevention of psoriasis. Some of the major psychosocial factors that play a role in psoriasis include stress resulting from both major life events and from the daily hassles arising from the impact of psoriasis upon the quality of life. Personality characteristics such as alexithymia and high interpersonal dependency may contribute toward the stress reactivity of psoriasis. Psoriasis has been associated with depressive illness which may lead to suicidal ideation and a decrease in the threshold for pruritus. Lithium, which is used for the treatment of mood disorders, can further exacerbate psoriasis. Alcohol consumption of > 80 g daily may have an adverse effect on the treatment outcome in psoriasis. These findings suggest that the biopsychosocial model, which assesses the interaction of both biological and psychosocial factors, should be used when managing the psoriasis patient.

References

Al'Abadie, M.S., Kent, G.G. & Gawkrodger, D.J. (1994) The relationship between stress and the onset and exacerbation of psoriasis and other skin conditions. *British Journal of Dermatology*, **130**, 199–203.

Arnetz, B.B., Fjellner, B., Eneroth, P. & Kallner, A. (1985) Stress and psoriasis: psychoendocrine and metabolic reactions in psoriatic patients during standardized stressor exposure. *Psychosomatic Medicine*, **47**, 528–541.

Arnetz, B.B., Fjellner, B., Eneroth, P. & Kallner, A. (1991) Endocrine and dermatological concomitants of mental stress. *Acta Dermato-Venereologica (Stockholm)*, **156** (Suppl.), 9–12.

Brandrup, F., Holm, N., Grunnet, N., Henningsen, K. & Hansen, H.E. (1982) Psoriasis in monozygotic twins: variations in expression in individuals with identical genetic constitution. *Acta Dermato-Venereologica (Stockholm)*, **62**, 229–236.

Farber, E.M., Bright, R.D. & Nall, M.L. (1968) Psoriasis, a questionnaire survey of 2144 patients. *Archives of Dermatology*, **98**, 248–259.

Fava, G.A., Perini, G.I., Santonastaso, P. & Fornasa, C.V. (1980) Life events and psychological distress in dermatologic disorders: psoriasis, chronic urticaria and fungal infections. *British Journal of Medical Psychology*, **53**, 277–282.

Finlay, A.Y. & Coles, E.C. (1995) The effect of severe psoriasis on the quality of life of 369 patients. *British Journal of Dermatology*, **132**, 236–244.

Finlay, A.Y. & Kelly, S.E. (1987) Psoriasis — an index of disability. *Clinical and Experimental Dermatology*, **12**, 8–11.

Fried, R.G., Friedman, S., Paradis, C., Hatch, M., Lynfield, Y., Duncanson, C. & Shalita, A. (1995) Trivial or terrible? The psychosocial impact of psoriasis. *International Journal of Dermatology*, **34**, 101–105.

Ginsburg, I.H. & Link, B.G. (1989) Feelings of stigmatization in patients with psoriasis. *Journal of the American Academy of Dermatology*, **20**, 53–63.

Gupta, M.A. & Gupta, A.K. (1995a) Age and gender differences in the impact of psoriasis on quality of life. *International Journal of Dermatology*, **34**, 700–703.

Gupta, M.A. & Gupta, A.K. (1995b) The Psoriasis Life Stress Inventory: a preliminary index of psoriasis-related stress. *Acta Dermato-Venereologica (Stockholm)*, **75**, 240–243.

Gupta, M.A., Gupta, A.K. & Haberman, H.F. (1987) Psoriasis and psychiatry: an update. *General Hospital Psychiatry*, **9**, 1–16.

Gupta, M.A., Gupta, A.K., Kirkby, S. *et al.* (1988) Pruritus in psoriasis. A prospective study of some psychiatric and dermatologic correlates. *Archives of Dermatology*, **124**, 1052–1057.

Gupta, M.A., Gupta, A.K., Kirkby, S. *et al.* (1989) A psychocutaneous profile of psoriasis patients who are stress reactors. A study of 127 patients. *General Hospital Psychiatry*, **11**, 166–173.

Gupta, M.A., Schork, N.J., Gupta, A.K., Kirkby, S. & Ellis, C.N. (1993a) Suicidal ideation in psoriasis. *International Journal of Dermatology*, **32**, 188–190.

Gupta, M.A., Schork, N.J., Gupta, A.K. & Ellis, C.N. (1993b) Alcohol intake and treatment responsiveness of psoriasis: a prospective study. *Journal of the American Academy of Dermatology*, **28**, 730–732.

Gupta, M.A., Gupta, A.K., Schork, N.J. & Ellis, C.N. (1994) Depression modulates pruritus perception: a study of pruritus in psoriasis, atopic dermatitis, and chronic idiopathic urticaria. *Psychosomatic Medicine*, **56**, 36–40.

Mazzetti, M., Mozzetta, A., Soavi, G.C. *et al.* (1994) Psoriasis, stress and psychiatry: psychodynamic characteristics of stressors. *Acta Dermato-Venereologica (Stockholm)*, **186**, 62–64.

Monk, B.E. & Neill, S.M. (1986) Alcohol consumption and psoriasis. *Dermatologica*, **173**, 57–60.

Nyfors, A. & Lemholt, K. (1975) Psoriasis in children. A short review and a survey of 245 cases. *British Journal of Dermatology*, **92**, 437–442.

Poikolainen, K., Reunala, T., Karvonen, J., Lauharanta, J. & Karkkainen, P. (1990) Alcohol intake: risk factor for psoriasis in young and middle aged men? *British Medical Journal*, **300**, 780–783.

Polenghi, M.M., Molinari, E., Gala, C., Guzzi, R., Garutti, C. & Finzi, A.F. (1994) Experience with psoriasis in a psychosomatic dermatology clinic. *Acta Dermato-Venereologica (Stockholm)*, **186** (Suppl.), 65–66.

Ramsay, B. & O'Reagan, M. (1988) A survey of the social and psychological effects of psoriasis. *British Journal of Dermatology*, **118**, 195–201.

Rubino, I.A., Sonnino, A., Stefanato, C.M., Pezzarossa, B. & Ciani, N. (1989) Separation-individuation, aggression and alexithymia in psoriasis. *Acta Dermato-Venereologica (Stockholm)*, **146** (Suppl.), 87–90.

Seville, R.H. (1977) Psoriasis and stress. *British Journal of Dermatology*, **97**, 297–302.

Vidoni, D., Campiutti, E., D'Aronco, R., De Vanna, M. & Aguglia, E. (1989) Psoriasis and alexithymia. *Acta Dermato-Venereologica (Stockholm)*, **146** (Suppl.), 91–92.

14
Atopic Dermatitis

Defining Atopic Dermatitis in Epidemiological Studies
H.C. WILLIAMS

Why is disease definition so important in epidemiology?

> Developing reliable diagnostic criteria may be as tedious as filling in muddy holes with concrete but both provide the foundation on which all else depends.
>
> Professor R.E. Kendall (1975)

Lack of a disease definition of known validity and repeatability for atopic dermatitis (atopic eczema, or AD) is one of the main reasons why so little is known about the distribution and causes of AD (Williams, 1995). As a result, AD is often ignored in studies of allergic disease, which is a pity, because the determinants of total allergic disease (asthma, hay fever and AD) may be different from the determinants of individual diseases such as asthma. Unlike internal diseases such as asthma where researchers are still grappling with the relationship between symptoms, disease labels and the results of provocation tests, AD is directly visible, which makes the development of an objective definition a realistic goal. Some physicians might regard attempts at defining AD as an imposition because they are perfectly happy about how they diagnose AD in individuals. Therein lies the crux of the problem. Diagnosis by physicians based on many years of clinical pattern recognition is entirely appropriate when dealing with individuals, but problems begin when *groups* of people have to be compared. Whether this be the comparison of different prevalence estimates

from around the world, or comparison of treatments, it is essential to know that researchers all refer to the same entity.

What are the problems with existing definitions?

Although disease definition is perhaps the most fundamental step in any form of medical research, at least ten synonyms for AD were in widespread use up until the late 1970s. This intolerable state of affairs prompted Hanifin, Rajka and Lobitz to propose an extensive list of major and minor diagnostic criteria for AD (Hanifin & Rajka, 1980). These criteria represented an important milestone in describing the clinical syndrome of AD and in ensuring some degree of comparability of individuals in subsequent hospital studies. However, they are less useful in epidemiological studies because of their complexity and unknown validity (Svensson *et al.*, 1985; Seymour *et al.*, 1987; Diepgen & Fartasch, 1991; Schultz Larsen, 1993). They were simply intended as a proposal by a group of leading physicians with a view to further development and testing. They were based largely on experience of AD cases attending hospitals, who by definition are likely to represent a more severe subset of AD.

Various other definitions for AD have been suggested. Svensson *et al.* (1985) examined the discriminatory value of 34 historical, examined and laboratory features in 47 AD hospital subjects and matched controls, and ranked the usefulness of the features according to their statistical significance. Repeatability was not tested, and classification was tested on the same sample from which the scores were derived, a procedure which will overestimate validity. A score-based approach has been scientifically derived and tested by Diepgen and

Fartasch (1991). Such a quantitative approach might be useful in estimating the probability of asymptomatic individuals developing AD, for example in prospective studies of occupational groups such as metalworkers or hairdressers who are exposed to irritants. Schultz Larsen and Hanifin (1992) have proposed a questionnaire method for estimating AD, which includes many features that other workers have considered to be important in the diagnosis of AD. It is written using clear language, although the diagnostic label of 'eczema' (which might have many determinants) is mentioned throughout. Instead of using a binary disease definition (i.e. atopic dermatitis, 'yes/no'), Schultz Larsen and Hanifin have chosen the categories of 'definite AD', 'possible AD' and 'no AD' as the main outcome measures based on an arbitrary points system. Such an approach is an attractive simplification of numerical estimations of the probability of AD in what may well be a disease continuum, but it is not clear how researchers comparing prevalences should deal with the 'possible AD' category, which may form the bulk of cases in community surveys. Defining opposite ends of the AD continuum is easy, but most prevalence or morbidity surveys will require a binary definition which offers a reasonable compromise between specificity of diagnosis and exclusion of asymptomatic disease.

It is also worth pointing out that criteria which work well for individuals in a hospital setting may not be equally good when tested in a community setting. For instance, a clinical feature such as 'dry skin' may be useful in separating cases of AD from other dermatoses in a hospital dermatology clinic, but may be less discriminating in a community setting where dry skin may be generally commoner. Low disease prevalence (Bayes rule) and an increase in borderline cases may also conspire to decrease the predictive value of hospital-derived diagnostic criteria when applied in a community setting (Williams, 1995).

What makes a good epidemiological definition for atopic dermatitis?

Since epidemiological surveys usually involve large numbers of subjects, the choice between different disease definitions is more often governed by practical constraints rather than ideals. Nevertheless it is

Table 14.1 Attributes of a good definition for atopic dermatitis for use in epidemiological studies.

Good epidemiological criteria for AD should be:
1 Valid
2 Repeatable
3 Acceptable to the population
4 Comprehensive
5 Rapid and easy to perform
6 Coherent with the clinical concept of disease phenotype
7 Should reflect some degree of morbidity

---

important to consider what makes a good epidemiological definition for AD (Table 14.1).

1 *Validity.* Clearly, any criteria should measure what they are meant to measure, i.e. they should catch as many cases as possible (sensitivity) and exclude as many non-cases as possible (specificity). The criteria should be sufficiently valid to detect important prevalence differences in groups that are to be compared. Using less valid criteria (e.g. a questions-only model in simple surveys to assess disease burden) is not usually a problem, *providing that the validity is known and tested during the fieldwork.*

2 *Repeatability.* Between-observer and within-observer variation in recording the diagnostic criteria should be kept to a minimum. This aspect can be improved by clear instructions and training of field workers and by clear descriptions in methodology sections of scientific reports.

3 *Acceptable to the population.* Whilst it may be possible for physicians to get away with quite invasive tests to patients in a hospital setting, even relatively non-invasive procedures such as examining the skin may result in a low response rate when conducted in a population setting.

4 *Comprehensiveness.* Criteria need to be applicable to a wide range of subgroups, e.g. criteria which work well in discriminating AD cases amongst white children in the USA may not work so well in Chinese children in Korea. Criteria which work well in children may be less useful in adults with AD. Questions need to be understood and convey the same meaning to people from different socio-economic groups, and when translated to other languages.

5 *Rapid and easy to perform.* Complicated and time-consuming procedures are likely to result in observer fatigue and lower response rates if conducted as part of a large population survey.

6 *Coherence with prevailing clinical concepts.* Criteria should demonstrate a degree of face validity, i.e. they should contain features which leading workers deemed as key elements for the disease syndrome, and they should not include implausible or obscure features.

7 *They should reflect some degree of disease morbidity.* A set of criteria may well pick out all possible cases of AD in a population survey, but many such cases will be extremely mild and asymptomatic. A survey using such criteria will be of little use to those planning appropriate services unless it is accompanied by severity data.

The UK refinement of Hanifin and Rajka's diagnostic criteria

In 1990, a UK working party set about the task of developing a minimum list of reliable discriminators for AD, using the Hanifin and Rajka list of clinical features as the building blocks. The study design shared some similarity to the American Rheumatology Association's study to develop diagnostic criteria for systemic lupus erythematosus (Tan *et al.*, 1982), and the detailed development of these criteria which deal with development of a minimum list of valid discriminators, repeatability and independent validity are published elsewhere (Williams *et al.*, 1994a,b,c). Six criteria were derived and tested by this group as shown in Table 14.2. Five out of the six UK diagnostic criteria are included as major features in a later refinement of the Hanifin and Rajka criteria (Hanifin, 1992), which is a tribute to their original proposal. In order to capture the intermittent nature of AD and to minimize possible seasonal fluctuations in AD activity, the diagnostic criteria are recommended to be used as a 12-month period prevalence measure. A training pack accompanied by further instructions for the use of these criteria in different field settings is available from the author. Potential problems associated with the use of the criteria and how they might be overcome are also discussed in this manual.

The UK criteria have performed well in subsequent independent hospital and community validation

Table 14.2 The UK refinement of Hanifin and Rajka's diagnostic criteria for atopic dermatitis.

In order to qualify as a case of atopic eczema with the UK diagnostic criteria, the child:
Must have:
An itchy skin condition in the last 12 months
Plus three or more of:
1 Onset below age 2 years
2 History of flexural involvement
3 History of a generally dry skin
4 Personal history of other atopic disease or history of any atopic disease in a first-degree relative
5 Visible flexural dermatitis as per photographic protocol

---

studies. In an independent validation study of children attending hospital dermatology out-patients, the criteria were shown to have a sensitivity and specificity of 85% and 96%, respectively, when compared with a dermatologist's diagnosis (Williams *et al.*, 1994c). When used as a 1-year period prevalence measure in a community survey of London children aged 3–11 years of mixed ethnic groups where the prevalence of AD was approximately 10%, sensitivity and specificity was 80% and 97%, respectively (Williams *et al.*, 1996). Positive and negative predictive values in this survey were 80% and 97%, respectively. Acceptable repeatability has been demonstrated for the six features contained within the UK criteria (Williams *et al.*, 1994b). The criteria appear to be equally applicable to children of different ethnic and socioeconomic groups. They have worked well in children down to the age of 3 years, but further evaluation in younger children and adults is awaited. The criteria are easy to ascertain (taking <2 minutes per person including examination for flexural dermatitis), and they have proven to be highly acceptable to children and adults because of their relatively simple and non-invasive nature (Williams *et al.*, 1995). They correspond well to our clinical concept of atopic eczema in that they contain all of the key elements that previous researchers have emphasized. Several groups studying allergic diseases around the world have used the UK criteria without any major problems. Further validation studies of these criteria in developing countries are currently underway.

The future

One must consider the possibility that the newly proposed UK refinement of Hanifin and Rajka's criteria will not last very long. The emergence of many similar 'rival' criteria based on arbitrary arrangements of clinical features alone would not be useful, however, unless they were shown to produce marked benefits over the UK criteria when put to the test in independent validation studies. Even in the absence of 'rival' diagnostic criteria, it is likely that the criteria will produce a number of 'boundary disputes'. Difficulties in establishing international agreement of diagnostic criteria are more likely to be encountered when defining the boundary or outer rim of what separates a condition from other adjacent categories, as opposed to agreeing on what constitutes the core clinical features. Thus one group might insist that all subjects with AD must be atopic as defined by objective tests of immediate hypersensitivity, or that visible 'eczematous' skin changes must be visible in all subjects. Providing these modifications are explicit, and that the individual elements of the diagnostic criteria are recorded separately, then most of these 'boundary disputes' are unlikely to be insurmountable. Indeed, the different nature of the many types of study designs available to researchers means that some modification of the criteria for the purposes of a particular study are inevitable.

The author recognizes that the criteria as proposed today are but a transient step in the process of progressive nosology. Thus if a more rational basis for the classification of atopic eczema is found in the next 20 years, then the current definition based on a clinical syndrome might well lose its value. As Kendall (1975) commented,

> to the contemporary medical research worker, if not to every practising clinician, diseases are little more than convenient working concepts based on a variety of different defining criteria, anatomical, physiological or behavioural, and liable to change their defining characteristics, or even to be abandoned altogether, with advances in knowledge.

References

Diepgen, T. & Fartasch, M. (1991) Stigmata and signs of atopic eczema. In: *New Trends in Allergy*. III (eds J. Ring & B. Pryzbilla), pp. 222–229. Springer-Verlag, Berlin.

Hanifin, J. (1992) Atopic dermatitis. In: *Dermatology* (eds S.L. Moschella & H.J. Hurley), 3rd edn, pp. 441–464. W.B. Saunders, Philadelphia.

Hanifin, J. & Rajka, G. (1980) Diagnostic features of atopic eczema. *Acta Dermato-Venereologica (Stockholm)*, **92**, 44–47.

Kendall, R. (1975) *The Role of Diagnosis in Psychiatry*. Blackwell Scientific Publications, Oxford.

Schultz Larsen, F. (1993) The epidemiology of atopic dermatitis. *Monographs in Allergy*, **31**, 9–28.

Schultz Larsen, F. & Hanifin, J. (1992) Secular change in the occurrence of atopic dermatitis. *Acta Dermato-Venereologica (Stockholm)*, **176** (Suppl.), 7–12.

Seymour, J., Keswick, B., Hanifin, J., Jordan, W. & Milligan, M. (1987) Clinical effects of diaper types on the skin of normal infants with atopic dermatitis. *Journal of the American Academy of Dermatology*, **17**, 988–997.

Svensson, Å., Edman, B. & Möller, H. (1985) A diagnostic tool for atopic dermatitis based on clinical criteria. *Acta Dermato-Venereologica (Stockholm)*, **114** (Suppl.), 33–40.

Tan, E., Cohen, A., Fries, J. *et al.* (1982) The 1982 revised criteria for the classification of systemic lupus erythematosus. *Arthritis and Rheumatism*, **25**, 1271–1277.

Williams, H. (1995) On the definition and epidemiology of atopic dermatitis. *Dermatology Clinics*, **13**, 649–657.

Williams, H., Burney, P., Hay, R. *et al.* (1994a) The UK Working Party's Diagnostic criteria for atopic dermatitis. I: Derivation of a minimum set of discriminators for atopic dermatitis. *British Journal of Dermatology*, **131**, 383–396.

Williams, H., Burney, P., Strachan, D. & Hay, R. (1994b) The UK Working Party's Diagnostic criteria for atopic dermatitis. II: Observer variation of clinical diagnosis and signs of atopic dermatitis. *British Journal of Dermatology*, **131**, 397–405.

Williams, H., Burney, P., Pembroke, A. & Hay, R. (1994c) The UK Working Party's Diagnostic criteria for atopic dermatitis. III: Independent hospital validation. *British Journal of Dermatology*, **131**, 406–416.

Williams, H., Forsdyke, H., Boodoo, G., Hay, R. & Burney, P. (1995) A protocol for recording the sign of visible flexural dermatitis. *British Journal of Dermatology*, **133**, 941–949.

Williams, H., Burney, P., Pembroke, A. & Hay, R. (1996) Validation of the UK diagnostic criteria for atopic dermatitis in a population setting. *British Journal of Dermatology*, **135**, 12–17.

Genetic Epidemiology of Atopy

T.L. DIEPGEN AND M. BLETTNER

Introduction: what is genetic epidemiology?

'Genetic epidemiology' combines the important principles of epidemiology and genetics in the study of human disease. With increasing evidence of the importance of genetic–environmental interactions in the aetiology and pathogenesis of diseases, it was important to integrate research methods of both fields. Before 1977, the term 'genetic epidemiology' was virtually non-existent in titles of published articles. To our knowledge, Morton and Chung (1978) first used the term 'genetic epidemiology' to describe this new field: 'A science that deals with the etiology, distribution, and control of disease in groups of relatives, and with inherited causes of disease in populations.' Therefore it is the study of how and why diseases cluster in families and ethnic groups and of interactions between genetic and environmental factors.

Family history of atopy and twin studies

The influence of hereditary factors in atopic disorders has been established by family and twin studies. A family history of atopy (atopic eczema, allergic rhinitis, allergic asthma) has been reported in 50–68% of individuals with atopic eczema compared with 35% or fewer in children without reported atopic disease (Diepgen & Fartasch, 1992). The inheritability of atopic disorders within families was first proven by Schnyder (1960) who coined the term 'intrafamilial organ constance'. This means that the same organ (bronchial system or skin) is often affected in several family members with atopic diseases. We could demonstrate that the risk for a child to develop atopic eczema is much higher if there is a family history of atopic eczema (odds ratio, OR 6.7) than if there is allergic rhinitis or asthma in the family (OR 1.5) (Diepgen & Fartasch, 1992).

Monozygotic twins run a risk of about 86% of having atopic eczema if the twin partner has the disease, whereas the disease risk of 21% run by dizygotic partners does not differ from the frequency seen in siblings (Schultz Larsen, 1993). However, the increase in the frequency of atopic disorders during less than one generation suggests that time trends in environmental factors play an important role in the manifestation of the disease. In recent years, a model of multifactorial inheritance in combination with a threshold is assumed: for the manifestation of an atopic disease the presence of additional realization factors is required (Fig. 14.1).

Thus, the hypothesis of a multifactorial pathogenesis with polygenetic inheritance has been favoured for the transmission of atopic disorders, i.e. atopic eczema, allergic rhinitis and allergic asthma. The variability of manifestation and severity, however, and the different organ systems (skin, respiratory tract) involved, make it difficult to locate the hereditary base and its molecular genetic mechanisms.

Different loci have been identified as contributing to the atopic state: the first of these was on the long arm of chromosome 11q (Cookson *et al.*, 1989). This linkage was confirmed in families with respiratory atopy and linked to maternal inheritance. The beta-chain of the high-affinity receptor for IgE has been shown to lie on chromosome 11q13. The other loci, the interleukin IL4/IL5 cytokine cluster on chromosome 5 have been shown to influence IgE responses (Marsh *et al.*, 1994). The relevance to eczema is as yet undetermined.

Studies evaluating the genetic role in atopic diseases have differentiated between families with and without atopic diseases and have taken the number of atopic family members into account (Diepgen & Blettner, 1996). They have also distinguished between the genetic risk of different atopic diseases or of combinations of multiple allergies (Dold *et al.*, 1992) or determined risk figures for genetic counselling (Küster *et al.*, 1990; Diepgen & Fartasch, 1992). The results of our study were quite similar to those found by Küster *et al.* (1990): if one child already suffers from atopic disorders, and no parent had atopic manifestations, the risk for the other children in the family to develop atopic eczema was 10% and to develop atopy 16% (Diepgen & Fartasch, 1992). If one parent is healthy and the other affected, the risk for the other

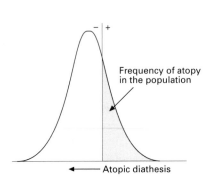

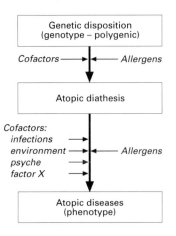

Fig. 14.1 A model of multifactorial inheritance in combination with a threshold is assumed for the inheritance of atopic diseases.

children in the family to develop atopic eczema was between 16% and 47% and for atopy between 19% and 63%, depending on the kind of atopic disease found in the parent. The recurrence risk for atopy was 63% if one parent was suffering from atopic eczema and respiratory atopy, and 48% if from respiratory atopy without eczema. If both parents were affected by atopy and one child has atopic eczema, the recurrence risk for atopy was 70% for other children. According to Kjellmann (1977), the incidence of atopic disease in children is highest (72.2%) when both parents have an identical type of atopic disease, i.e. respiratory or skin.

All these studies, however, are based on positive family history defined as the presence of disease in one or more first-degree relatives of patients with atopic eczema. This has serious limitations because family history depends on many factors, such as the number of relatives, their biological relationship to the index case and the disease frequency in the population. Additionally, observations on family members cannot be considered to be independently distributed. Therefore, the applied statistical approaches used to test for clustering in family studies must be modified (Khoury *et al.*, 1993).

Familial aggregation of atopy

In order to determine the relative importance of genetics and the environment, there is a need for a study examining the aggregation of atopic diseases among classes of relatives within families. This examination of familial aggregation of a disease is an important first step in studying the possible influence of genetic factors and/or shared environmental events contributing to the disease process. The evaluation can be done in an exploratory and descriptive way and will rely on statistical models and methods to quantitate the familial aggregation. This explorative analysis comes before more sophisticated modelling such as segregation and linkage analysis where genetic models are explicitly examined. Recently, a statistical method for detecting interfamilial and intrafamilial aggregation of a binary trait with family data has been proposed (Liang & Beaty, 1991). The methods are based on logistic regression analysis and can incorporate individual covariates while evaluating (measuring) familial aggregation of risk as odds ratio (OR) among classes of relatives. We used this statistical approach and performed an unmatched case-control study on atopic eczema (AE) and respiratory atopic diseases (i.e. allergic rhinitis and allergic asthma) to investigate the familial aggregation for these diseases (Diepgen & Blettner, 1996).

Subjects and statistical methods

In order to determine the relative importance of genetics and the environment on the occurrence of atopic diseases the familial aggregation of atopic eczema, allergic rhinitis and allergic asthma in the relatives of 426 patients with atopic eczema (index cases) and 628 subjects with no history of eczema (index controls) was investigated (in total 5136 family members). Cases were in- and out-patients with a chronically relapsing course of atopic eczema treated in the Department of Dermatology of the University of Erlangen (142 males, 284 females; median age 23 years); controls were subjects with no personal history of eczema from the area surrounding the hospital (353 males, 275 females; median age 24 years). Families were selected through the index subjects. All cases and controls were interviewed by a dermatologist as to whether their first-degree relatives had a history of atopic eczema (itching skin lesions in typical local-izations and relapsing course), allergic rhinitis (hay fever) or allergic asthma which had been previously confirmed by a physician. To analyse the familial aggregation, only data of parents and siblings were included (1054 families comprising 5136 family members).

We used similar methods to those proposed by Liang and Beaty (1991) for the statistical modelling. Details of the statistical models are given elsewhere (Diepgen & Blettner, 1996). Briefly, the associations (correlations) among family members expressed as odds ratios were estimated. The odds ratio describes the association between categorical or binary variables such as presence or absence of a disease. In our context, an odds ratio of 1 means that there is no aggregation within families, while an odds ratio >1 will reflect familial aggregation.

We investigated three different models for the odds ratios:

- OR is the same among any two members of a family (one parameter).
- OR depends on familial relationship, i.e. whether the pairs are parents (pp), siblings (ss) or parent sibling pairs (ps) (three parameters).
- The OR between fathers and children (fs) is not the same as between mothers and children (ms) (four parameters).

All models were calculated for four different outcome variables: atopic eczema (pure atopic eczema or in any combination with allergic rhinitis or asthma), allergic rhinitis (pure allergic rhinitis or in any combination with atopic eczema or allergic asthma), respiratory atopy (pure allergic rhinitis and/or allergic asthma or in any combination with atopic eczema), atopy (atopic eczema and/or allergic rhinitis and/or allergic asthma).

Results: models for familial aggregation

We investigated three different models for familial aggregation of atopic eczema: allergic rhinitis, respiratory atopy and atopy. The results are presented in Table 14.3. Model 1 assumes common risk and constant odds ratios among relatives. The odds ratios are similar for the four atopic diseases and indicate that there is a strong and statistically significant correlation among family members.

In Model 2, three separate odds ratios were esti-mated for different pair constellations: familial aggre-gation between parents (pp), between siblings (ss) and between parents and siblings (ps), respectively. Accord-ing to the results shown in Table 14.3, the odd ratios differ substantially. The odds ratios between parents are low and the 95% confidence intervals of the four different atopic diseases include one indicating only low correlation between the parents. However, there are statistically significant strong associations between parents and siblings (AE ps: OR = 1.97; 95% confi-dence interval 1.13–2.97) and between siblings (AE ss: OR = 3.86; 95% confidence interval 2.10–7.09). The familial aggregation was stronger between sibling pairs compared to parent–sibling pairs. In Model 3, the parent–sibling pairs association is differentiated in father–sibling (fs) pairs and mother–sibling (ms) pairs. For atopic eczema, the familial aggregation be-tween mothers and siblings was stronger compared to the aggregation between fathers and siblings (AE ms: OR = 2.66; fs: OR = 1.29). For other atopic outcome variables (allergic rhinitis, respiratory atopy, atopy) no differences in the familial aggregations of mother–sibling compared to father–sibling for respiratory atopic disorders were seen.

Stronger clustering of atopy within siblings

The results indicate that the familial aggregation of atopic diseases is stronger between siblings than between parents and siblings. This can be a result of shared environment during childhood as effect modi-fiers of atopic diseases. In Danish twins, it was shown that the cumulative incidence rate (in up to 7-year-old children) of atopic eczema has increased in the last decades from 0.03 for the birth cohort 1960–64 to 0.12 for the birth cohort 1975–79 (Schultz Larsen,

Table 14.3 Odds ratio (OR) estimations along with logistic regression adjustment indicating a stronger familial aggregation: (a) between siblings (ss) than between siblings and parents (ps) for all atopic diseases; and (b) between mothers and siblings (ms) than between fathers and siblings (fs) for atopic eczema.

Disease	Model 1* OR⒮	Model 1* 95% CI⒮	Model 2†	Model 2† OR⒮	Model 2† 95% CI⒮	Model 3‡	Model 3‡ OR⒮	Model 3‡ 95% CI⒮
Atopic eczema	2.16	1.58–2.96	pp	1.27	0.63–2.58	pp	1.27	0.63–2.57
			ps	1.97	1.31–2.97	fs	1.29	0.69–1.87
			ss	3.86	2.10–7.09	ms	2.66	1.45–4.88
						ss	3.74	2.04–6.87
Allergic rhinitis	3.53	2.68–4.64	pp	2.01	1.16–3.48	pp	2.01	1.16–3.48
			ps	3.42	2.36–4.96	fs	3.39	2.00–5.74
			ss	5.47	3.10–9.66	ms	3.46	2.04–5.85
						ss	5.47	3.12–9.59
Respiratory atopy	3.10	2.40–4.00	pp	1.51	0.87–2.61	pp	1.51	0.87–2.61
			ps	3.06	2.19–4.27	fs	2.89	1.77–4.72
			ss	5.10	3.06–8.49	ms	3.25	2.03–5.20
						ss	5.10	3.06–8.49
Atopy	2.39	1.93–2.97	pp	1.32	1.00–1.99	pp	1.32	0.87–1.99
			ps	2.44	1.85–3.21	fs	2.48	1.74–3.53
			ss	3.82	2.58–5.65	ms	2.41	1.66–3.50
						ss	3.82	2.58–5.65

* OR is the same among any two members of one family.

† OR depends on familial relationship, i.e. whether the pairs are parents (pp), siblings (ss) or parent sibling pairs (ps).

‡ The OR between the father and the children (fs) is not the same as between the mother and the children (ms) (four parameters).

ⓈThe associations (correlations) among family members expressed as odds ratios (OR) and corresponding 95% confidence intervals (95% CI) were estimated as described by Diepgen and Blettner (1996).

1993). The pairwise concordance rate was 0.72 in monozygotic twins. The genetic background of atopic eczema, however, could not explain the obvious rapidly increasing frequency of the disease in the short time span of three decades. Thus, it seems that other and still unrecognized factors in the environment can affect the occurrence of atopic eczema in genetically susceptible persons. Under the hypothesis of a multifactorial pathogenesis with polygenetic inheritance, it seems plausible that a shift in the whole distribution of latent atopic disease is responsible for the recent changes in disease prevalence (Fig. 14.1). Therefore, it would be interesting to include environmental factors in the analysis of familial aggregation using more complex multiple regression models. This is important because it allows analysis of genetic and environmental factors contributing to the process of atopy.

Higher risk of atopic eczema from maternal than from paternal atopy

In our study we found a higher odds ratio of atopic eczema between mothers and sibling (ms: OR = 2.66) than between fathers and siblings (fs: OR = 1.29). In contrast, similar differences were not observed for the other atopic manifestations like allergic rhinitis and allergic asthma. Family aggregation between mother and child may be explained by shared physical environment at home or environmental events that are passed on to the fetus *in utero*. It can be assumed that environmental factors will be shared more intensively between the mother and the child than between the father and the child. The familial aggregation of atopic eczema can also be explained by stronger maternal heritability and would be consistent with atopic mothers carrying relatively more genes predisposing to disease than atopic fathers. Whether our findings are due to environmental, congenital and/or genetic factors, however, is uncertain.

Küster and coworkers (1990) found in 44 mothers with atopic eczema that 24 (24%) of their 101 children suffered from atopic eczema as opposed to 21 fathers with atopic eczema where only seven (14%) of their 49 children suffered from atopic eczema. This difference, however, was not statistically significant. The authors reported several frequencies of a history of atopy in relatives of patients with atopic eczema without having a control group. Reporting frequencies without a control group has serious limitations because family history depends on the number of relatives and on the disease frequency in the population. In contrast, we analysed the aggregation of atopic disorders in a high number of relatives of index cases and index controls.

A higher risk of infantile atopic eczema from maternal atopy than from paternal atopy was reported by Ruiz and coworkers (1992) in 39 infants from a birth cohort in whom one of the parents had been diagnosed atopic by skin prick testing. Seven of 19 infants with atopic mothers and two of 20 infants with atopic fathers developed atopic eczema during the first year of life (relative risk 4.7, 95% confidence interval 2.5–9.0). Although the numbers were small, the authors compared other potential confounding factors, like breast-feeding, time of starting cows' milk, month of birth, parental atopic eczema and smoking, household pets and other factors, in the group with atopic mothers and fathers and could not find any statistically significant differences.

Happle and Schnyder (1982) investigated the frequency of atopic children of either male or female patients with allergic asthma and were able to demonstrate the so-called 'Carter effect' (Carter & Evans, 1969) for asthma. The Carter effect is present if a disorder determined by polygenic inheritance and with different sex ratios is inherited with a higher frequency by the sex which is affected with a lower frequency in the general population.

Outlook

One important characteristic of the statistical method used is that the interpretation of regression parameters remains the same regardless of the family size. This is an important difference to other proposed methods (Connolly & Liang, 1988), where the interpretation of the conditional log odds ratios will vary with family size. The invariance property of the approach used here is essential for family studies where the size differs (Liang & Beaty, 1991).

Further research is necessary in order to include external covariates and to investigate interactions between genetic and exogenous factors. The methods used in our study could be very helpful in analysing the interrelationship of genetic and environmental factors on atopic diseases.

References

Carter, C.O. & Evans, K.A. (1969) Inheritance of congenital pyloric stenosis. *Journal of Medical Genetics*, **6**, 233–254.

Connolly, M.A. & Liang, K.-Y. (1988) Conditional logistic regression models for correlated binary data. *Biometrika*, **75**, 501–506.

Cookson, W.O.C.M., Sharp, P.A., Faux, J.A. & Hopkin, J.M. (1989) Linkage between immunglobulin E response underlying asthma and rhinitis and chromosome 11q. *Lancet*, **i**, 1292–1295.

Diepgen, T.L. & Blettner, M. (1996) Analysis of familial aggregation of atopic eczema and other atopic diseases by using odds ratio regression models. *Journal of Investigative Dermatology*, **106**, 977–981.

Diepgen, T.L. & Fartasch, M. (1992) Recent epidemiological and genetic studies in atopic dermatitis. *Acta Dermato-Venereologica (Stockholm)*, (Suppl.) **176**, 13–18.

Dold, S., Wist, M., Mutius von, E., Reitmeir, P. & Stiepel, E. (1992) Genetic risk for asthma, allergic rhinitis, and atopic dermatitis. *Archives of Disease in Childhood*, **67**, 1018–1022.

Happle, R. & Schnyder, U.W. (1982) Evidence for the Carter effect in atopy. *International Archives of Allergy and Applied Immunology*, **68**, 90–92.

Khoury, M.J., Beaty, T.H. & Cohen, B.H. (1993) *Fundamentals of Genetic Epidemiology*. Oxford University Press, New York.

Kjellman, N.-I.M. (1977) Atopic disease in seven-year-old children. *Acta Paediatrica Scandinavica*, **66**, 465–471.

Küster, W., Petersen, M., Christophers, E., Goos, M. & Sterry, W. (1990) A family study of atopic dermatitis. *Archives of Dermatology Research*, **282**, 98–102.

Liang, K.-Y. & Beaty, T.H. (1991) Measuring familial aggregation by using odds-ratio regression models. *Genetic Epidemiology*, **8**, 361–370.

Marsh, D.G., Neely, J.D., Breazeale, D.R. *et al.* (1994) Linkage analysis of IL-4 and other chromosome 5q31.1 markers and total serum immunglobulin E concentrations. *Science*, **264**, 1152–1156.

Morton, N.E. & Chung, C.S. (1978) *Genetic Epidemiology*. Academic Press, New York.

Ruiz, R.G.G., Kemeny, D.M. & Price, J.F. (1992) Higher risk of infantile atopic dermatitis from maternal atopy than paternal atopy. *Clinical and Experimental Allergy*, **22**, 762–766.

Schultz Larsen, F. (1993) Atopic dermatitis. A genetic–epidemiologic study in a population-based twin sample. *Journal of the American Academy of Dermatology*, **28**, 719–723.

Schnyder, U.W. (1960) *Neurodermitis, Asthma, Rhinitis, Eine klinisch-allergologische Studie*. Karger, Basel.

Socio-Economic Aspects of Atopic Dermatitis

H.C. WILLIAMS

Introduction

Epidemiology is traditionally concerned with describing the distribution and determinants of disease in human populations. On the other hand, the term 'socio-economic' bears connotations of qualitative research conducted on highly selected individuals. The relevance of this to dermatoepidemiology may therefore seem a little obscure at first. But the socio-economic aspects of atopic dermatitis (AD) are, in their widest sense, as relevant to modern epidemiology as 'harder' randomized controlled intervention studies such as those which examine the efficacy of house-dust mite eradication regimens in reducing AD severity. The study of socio-economic aspects of atopic dermatitis is important from two standpoints: (i) the relationship between socio-economic factors and disease occurrence may provide some useful pointers to specific causes of AD and (ii) socio-economic studies help us to understand why some people with AD choose to seek medical help and why others do not — information which has substantial implications for the delivery of health service.

Socio-economic determinants of the occurrence of atopic dermatitis

Social class

Golding and Peters (1987) studied the occurrence of atopic eczema according to parental report in a national sample of 11 920 children born in 1970 in the UK. They found that the prevalence of reported eczema by the age of 5 years was considerably higher in advantaged socio-economic groups, affecting 17.5% of children from social class I (father's occupation a higher professional) than in class V (father's occupation unskilled), with a statistically significant trend over all social class groupings. Given the imprecise method used in this study to define atopic dermatitis, such a positive social class gradient could easily be due to the fact that parents in higher socio-economic groups were more likely to report the diagnosis of 'eczema' because (i) clinical practice would suggest that the terms 'allergy' and 'eczema' have become more fashionable in wealthier groups in the last 20 years, (ii) wealthier families may be more likely to consult their doctor and receive a diagnosis, (iii) the doctor might have used the term 'eczema' more freely in advantaged families for other minor skin conditions and (iv) recall of eczema in the first years of life might be enhanced in wealthier families. Williams *et al.* (1994) were able to test whether this social class gradient was simply because affluent parents were just more likely to report it by analysing an earlier UK cohort study (the 1958 National Child Development Study or NCDS) where, in addition to reported eczema, children were examined for the presence of skin disease at the ages of 7, 11 and 16 years. This study confirmed the strong positive social class gradient for reported eczema at all ages, but these trends were also present for examined eczema (Fig. 14.2), suggesting that reporting bias was not the main reason for these trends. The positive social class trend for eczema persisted after adjustment for region of residence, ethnic group, breast-feeding, sex of child, parental smoking and family size, and similar trends were not present for examined psoriasis and acne.

There are many possible reasons for these trends. Positive health-related behaviour such as increased immunization rates or underuse of topical cortico-

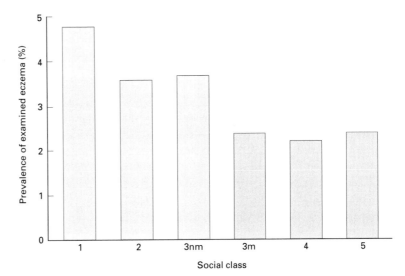

Fig. 14.2 Point prevalence of examined atopic dermatitis and social class according to father's occupation in 8279 children aged 7 years and born in 1958 (χ^2 linear trend 12.6, $P < 0.001$).

steroids might be increased in higher socio-economic groups (Peters & Golding, 1987). Other factors such as differences in the use of carpets, thick continental quilts as opposed to cotton sheets, and reduced ventilation from double glazing could have contributed to higher house-dust mite antigen levels in wealthier homes. Factors which could increase vulnerability to sensitization such as drying the skin through overuse of showers and soaps also need to be considered. Prenatal exposures correlated with higher social class such as higher maternal age and maternal diet may also predispose to higher rates of predisposing atopy (Peters & Golding, 1987; Arshad *et al.*, 1992; Williams, 1995).

Subsequent smaller studies have confirmed these social class findings for AD (Forster *et al.*, 1990; Neame *et al.*, 1995) and for positive skin-prick tests (von Mutius *et al.*, 1994), although it should not be assumed that the constellation of exposures associated with this positive social class gradient will be constant over time. Obesity and heart disease, for example, were once more common in the affluent, but now are more common in poorer social classes.

Other socio-economic correlates

Trends similar to those observed for socio-economic status and AD have also been observed for housing tenure (Williams *et al.*, 1994). The point prevalence of examined eczema at 7, 11 or 16 years in the NCDS

study was 6.1% (222/3622), 5.7% (52/907), 4.5% (146/3254) and 2.0% (4/201) in privately owned, privately rented, council rented and rent-free properties respectively (χ^2 value for owned vs. council-rented property 8.8, $P = 0.003$). Further studies are needed to see whether this association of AD with housing type is due to differences in housing design leading to increased exposure to risk factors such as house-dust mite, or whether it is due to residual confounding by a further factor correlated with social class. Beck *et al.* (1989) have shown that moving AD patients from conventional housing to houses with better indoor climates (high air exchange and low humidity) may be associated with an improvement in symptoms. Collectively, these observations open up the possibility of disease prevention by altering building design, but further work is needed before this can be translated into public-health policy.

The prevalence of AD has also been noted to be higher in smaller families, even after adjusting for social class (Peters & Golding, 1987; Strachan, 1989). Similar observations with number of siblings have been made with more objective measures of atopy such as positive skin-prick tests (von Mutius *et al.*, 1994). Reasons for this finding are still under investigation, but it is possible that frequent minor infections (which would be enhanced in larger families with more children) may have a protective effect in preventing expression of AD in predisposed subjects

(Strachan, 1989), perhaps by stimulating interferon-γ production (Bos *et al.*, 1992).

Ethnicity

Studies of children from Tokelau who migrated to New Zealand (Waite *et al.*, 1980) and Chinese immigrants in Hawaii (Worth, 1962) have shown large increases in the prevalence of atopic eczema in the migrant children when compared with similar genetic groups in their country of origin. London-born black Caribbean children have been shown to be at higher risk of atopic eczema compared with their white counterparts (Williams *et al.*, 1995) and studies examining similar groups in Jamaica are in progress. These migrant studies suggest that environmental factors associated with 'development' and urbanization may be important in the aetiology of atopic eczema. Whether these factors are 'allergic' in nature, such as exposure to new or much higher concentrations of airborne or dietary antigens, or whether they are due to physical factors such as differences in susceptibility to cutaneous irritation and dryness which are unmasked by cooler, less-humid climates, is unknown at present. Since atopic eczema is usually a chronic and intermittent disease, studies of prevalent cases are limited in their ability to separate factors which determine disease incidence from those which determine disease chronicity. Longitudinal studies which record the incidence of atopic eczema with respect to age of migration in those moving from countries with low disease prevalence to high disease prevalence, and follow-up studies of cases moving from countries with high-to-low disease prevalence should help to separate determinants of disease development from trigger factors for established disease.

Secular trends as an indicator of socio-economic factors

Several studies have suggested that the prevalence of eczema has increased two- to threefold over the last 30 years (Williams, 1992). Some of these changes probably reflect secular changes in the use of the label of 'eczema' by parents and doctors, but the magnitude, continuity of the trends, consistency between different studies and reports of similar trends

in asthma symptoms and skin-prick test positivity favour a genuine increase. Reasons for this rise in atopic eczema and other atopic diseases are less clear, but it seems unlikely that genetic factors could account for such a rapid change. Changes in the micro-environment linked with affluence and 'development' favouring increased exposure to allergens are one possible explanation, but it is also feasible that increased vulnerability to sensitization produced by exposure to low-grade primary irritants and atmospheric and indoor pollutants may play a part. Studies from East and West Germany have revealed an inconsistent relationship between urban pollution and atopic eczema so far (Behrendt *et al.*, 1993), but more refined longitudinal studies based on individuals with clearer diagnostic criteria are needed.

Conclusion

These socio-economic observations provide us with a starting point for understanding the epidemiology of AD. Together, they strongly suggest that environmental factors play a strong role in disease expression, which leads onto possible approaches for disease prevention such as alteration of housing design and maternal diet. Social class, family size and ethnicity should be considered as potential confounders in epidemiological studies of atopic dermatitis.

Socio-economic aspects of health-related behaviour

The concept of need, supply and demand for health care for AD sufferers is depicted in Fig. 14.3 (Stevens, 1991). Whilst supply (what is provided in terms of services for AD sufferers) and demand (what people with AD ask for) are relatively easy to understand, the concept of need (defined as the ability to benefit from medical care) for AD sufferers is more difficult. Few would argue that children with severe AD 'need' medical help, but the threshold for different levels of health-service intervention is less clear, especially as so little is known about the differential health gain of specialist versus generalist care. It may be argued that even those with mild AD can benefit from medical care which provides consistent advice on possible protective strategies such as regular application of

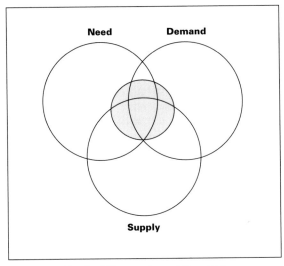

Need	What people would benefit from
Demand	What people ask for
Supply	What the current health service provides
Shaded area	Current provision

Fig. 14.3 Schematic representation of the relationship between need, supply and demand for dermatological health care for atopic dermatitis in the UK.

emollients, avoidance of soaps and woollen garments, ways of reducing house-dust levels at home, avoidance of pets and correct use of topical corticosteroid preparations.

Detailed studies of children with AD suggest that the whole families may endure considerable psychological (Daud *et al.*, 1993) and sometimes large financial burdens because of the disease (Herd *et al.*, 1994). Given the misery caused by constant pruritus, sleep loss and the stigma associated with a visible skin disease, it is not surprising that AD consistently exhibits some of the highest scores on the Dermatology Life Quality Index when compared with other skin diseases (Finlay & Khan 1994). However, it is not known how the disability associated with AD compares with other non-dermatological conditions such as arthritis and heart disease, nor whether it can be compared using conventional quality of life scales which favour health dimensions associated with immobility and mood disturbance. This information is essential if prioritization of health care is to be based on fair and explicit methods.

As Bowker *et al.* (1976) pointed out in their study of sociological factors of eczema in cases referred to hospital, little is known about the factors that determine adherence to prescribed treatment, the degree of tolerance of AD in particular social and ethnic groups and the use of sources of advice such as community pharmacists, health visitors, self-help groups and the 'lay referral system' by different groups. One study in Leicester, UK, showed that Asian children with AD were threefold more likely to present in specialist clinics than white children, whereas no difference in prevalence rates was seen in the community, a finding which might be explained by lack of familiarity with the disease amongst Asian parents (Neame *et al.*, 1995). A large survey of the UK National Eczema Society found that only 12% of eczema sufferers felt that their needs were completely met by consultation with general practitioners (Long *et al.*, 1993), although generalizations from self-help groups are limited since membership of such a group may itself be a determinant of health-service dissatisfaction. A study of 2180 adults in London found that of all those classified as having moderate-to-severe eczema by medical examiners, only 30% made use of medical services, compared with 14% of those with trivial eczema (Rea *et al.*, 1976).

There are thus major gaps in our knowledge on the socio-economic aspects of usage of health services for AD sufferers. Limited reports suggest that AD is characterized by large need, large demand and limited supply as depicted in Fig. 14.3, but more research is needed, especially for evaluating the relative efficacy of different settings for health care such as pharmacies, nurses' clinics and generalist versus specialist medical practitioners.

So what?

The ways in which the study of socio-economic aspects of atopic dermatitis have been helpful in pointing to possible disease causes have been highlighted here. It is true that factors such as social class may appear too nebulous to inform public-health interventions at first. History suggests, however, that socio-economic developments are often responsible for a bigger impact on the burden of disease than discovering any specific 'cause' or 'cure'. For example, improvements in social conditions were responsible for a far greater fall in deaths from childhood infectious diseases in Europe when compared with specific therapies such as vaccination and antibiotics for reasons which are still unclear (McKeown, 1975). A more detailed understanding of the socio-economic factors responsible for the increase in AD prevalence in Western countries may be helpful in preventing similar increases in developing countries undergoing rapid demographic changes.

The importance of understanding more about the factors which determine why some people with AD seek help and why others do not has been high-lighted also, and the urgent need for more research into the optimum delivery of health care for AD sufferers. Even if we are able to identify two or three specific causes for AD within the next 10 years, we are unlikely to progress very far with disease prevention unless we understand the factors which motivate different people to seek and participate in the help that is offered to them.

References

Arshad, S.H., Matthews, S., Gant C. & Hide, D. (1992) Effect of allergen avoidance on development of allergic disorders in infancy. *Lancet*, **339**, 1493–1497.

Beck, H-I., Bjerring, P. & Harving, H. (1989) Atopic dermatitis and the indoor climate. *Acta Dermato-Venereologica* **69** (Suppl 144), 131–132.

Behrendt, H., Krämer, U., Dolgner, R. *et al.* (1993) Elevated levels of total serum IgE in East German children: atopy, parasites, or pollutants? *Allergo Journal*, **2**, 31–40.

Bos, J.D., Wierenga, E.A., Smitt, J.H.S., van der Heijden, F.L. & Kapsenberg, M.L. (1992) Immune dysregulation in atopic eczema. *Archives of Dermatology*, **128**, 1509–1512.

Bowker, N.C., Cross, K.W., Fairburn, E.A. & Wall, M. (1976) Sociological implications of an epidemiological study of eczema in the City of Birmingham. *British Journal of Dermatology*, **95**, 137–144.

Daud, L.R., Garralda, M.E. & David, T.J. (1993) Psychosocial adjustment in preschool children with atopic eczema. *Archives of Disease in Childhood*, **69**, 670–676.

Finlay, A.Y. & Khan, G.K. (1994) Dermatology Life Quality Index (DLQI): a simple practical measure for routine clinical use. *Clinical and Experimental Dermatology*, **19**, 210–216.

Forster, J., Dungs, M., Wais, U. & Urbanek, R. (1990) Atopie-verdächtige Symptome in den ersten zwei Lebensjahren. *Klinische Pädiatrie*, **202**, 136–140.

Golding, J. & Peters, T.J. (1987) The epidemiology of childhood eczema. I. A population based study of associations. *Paediatric and Perinatal Epidemiology*, **1**, 67–79.

Herd, R.M., Tidman, M.J., Hunter, J.A.A., Prescott, R. & Finlay, A.Y. (1994). The economic burden of atopic eczema: a community and hospital-based assessment. *British Journal of Dermatology*, **131** (Suppl 44), 34.

Long, C.C., Funnell, C.M., Collard, R. & Finlay, A.Y. (1993) What do members of the National Eczema Society really want? *Clinical and Experimental Dermatology*, **18**, 516–522.

McKeown, T. (1975) The medical contribution. In: *Health and Disease*, (eds N. Black, D. Boswell, A. Gray, S. Murphy & J. Popay), pp. 107–114. Open University Press, Milton Keynes.

Neame, R.L., Berth-Jones, J., Kurinczuk, J.J. & Graham-Brown, R.A.C. (1995) Prevalence of atopic dermatitis in Leicester: a study of methodology and examination of possible ethnic variation. *British Journal of Dermatology*, **132**, 772–777.

Peters, T.J. & Golding, J. (1987) The epidemiology of childhood eczema. II. Statistical analyses to identify independent early predictors. *Paediatric and Perinatal Epidemiology*, **1**, 80–94.

Rea, J.N., Newhouse, M.L. & Halil, T. (1976) Skin disease in Lambeth: a community study of prevalence and use of medical care. *British Journal of Preventive and Social Medicine*, **30**, 107–114.

Stevens, A. (1991) Needs assessment needs assessment. *Health Trends*, **23**, 20–23.

Strachan, D.P. (1989) Hay fever, hygiene, and household size. *British Medical Journal*, **299**, 1259–1260.

von Mutius, E., Martinez, F.D., Fritzsch, C., Nicolai, T., Reitmeir, P. & Theimann, H-H. (1994) Skin test reactivity and number of siblings. *British Medical Journal*, **308**, 692–695.

Waite, D.A., Eyles, E.F., Tonkin, S.L. & O'Donnell, T.V. (1980) Asthma prevalence in Tokelauan children in two environments. *Clinical Allergy*, **10**, 71–75.

Williams, H.C. (1992) Is the prevalence of atopic dermatitis increasing? *Clinical and Experimental Dermatology*, **17**, 385–391.

Williams, H.C. (1995) Atopic eczema: we should look to the environment. *British Medical Journal*, **311**, 1241–1242.

Williams, H.C., Strachan, D.P., & Hay, R.J. (1994) Childhood eczema: disease of the advantaged? *British Medical Journal*, **308**, 1132–1135.

Williams, H.C., Pembroke, A.C., Forsdyke, H., Boodoo, G., Hay, R.J. & Burney, P.G.J. (1995) London-born black Caribbean children are at increased risk of atopic dermatitis. *Journal of the American Academy of Dermatology*, **32**, 212–217.

Worth, R.M. (1962) Atopic dermatitis among Chinese infants in Honolulu and San Francisco. *Hawaiian Medical Journal*, **22**, 31–36.

Diet and Atopy

E. SØYLAND

Atopic dermatitis, which affects 5–15% of the population in Western countries, is a chronic skin disease where a number of inflammatory and allergic immune reactions take place. The clinical manifestations usually start in the first or second month of life and are characterized by dry, scaly skin as well as pruritus and excoriations. Cellular infiltrates consisting of T-helper lymphocytes, altered interleukin expression and secretion and increased IgE production are some of the factors which indicate profound immunological changes in atopic dermatitis (Zachary *et al.*, 1985; Kapp *et al.*, 1989). The understanding of mechanisms and causal factors underlying the eczematous process is still very limited (de Prost, 1992). The treatment of choice has been corticosteroids, interferon and oral cyclosporin. These interventions all have considerable side effects and are associated with relapse after the therapy has been discontinued (Fradin *et al.*, 1990; David, 1991). Also local treatment with steroids has several side effects such as skin atrophy, development of teleangiectases and depression of the local immune response, and therefore should not be used for longer periods of time (Korting *et al.*, 1992). Because of the chronicity and discomfort of this skin disease, patients are often motivated for changing their lifestyle, including their diet. In 10–20% of the patients, food hypersensitivity is suspected to be an important factor in development of atopic dermatitis. Food allergen avoidance by these patients is a well-recognized, difficult and controversial form of therapy in atopic dermatitis. The rationale and techniques for such allergen avoidance have been well described in reviews (Sampson & McCaskill, 1985; Binkley, 1992; Ortolani, 1995). Less well established are the dietary therapies including oral supplementation with evening primrose oil, fish oil and Chinese tea, which have received increasing interest.

Evening primrose oil

Hansen (1933) first suggested that atopic dermatitis might be related to abnormal essential fatty acid intake or metabolism. He showed that children with atopic dermatitis had a reduced blood level of unsaturated fatty acids, and claimed that addition of linoleic acid (LA) to the diet improved the eczema.

Essential fatty acids are important constituents of the skin. Lack of polyunsaturated fatty acids promotes dry, scaly and hyperproliferative skin which is normalized by dietary addition of polyunsaturated fatty acids (Burr & Burr, 1929, 1930). Dry skin is one of the clinical features in patients with atopic dermatitis. This seems to be partly due to a defect of the epidermal permeability barrier in the stratum corneum, where essential polyunsaturated fatty acids play an important role as part of the sphingolipids which make up the water barrier (Bowser & White, 1985; Elias, 1985; Bowser *et al.*, 1986; Melnik *et al.*, 1988). As essential components of cell membranes, the fatty acids may affect receptors, enzymes, ion channels and other messenger systems (Drevon, 1993).

There are two families of essential fatty acids: the *n*-6 and the *n*-3 fatty acid family (Fig. 14.4). The position of the first double bond counted from the methyl group of polyunsaturated fatty acids may be located in the third position, as for *n*-3 fatty acids — or in the sixth position, as for *n*-6 fatty acids. Cells derived from species located high up in the evolutionary hierarchy cannot introduce double bonds in the carbon chain of fatty acids closer to the methyl group than C7. Chloroplasts in phytoplankton and plants can synthesize the essential *n*-3 and *n*-6 fatty acids, respectively. This means that mammalian cells cannot transform *n*-3 and *n*-6 fatty acids into each other, as outlined in Fig. 14.4. *n*-3 and *n*-6 fatty acids share common enzymes for some of their metabolic pathways and they are transferred via the nutrition chain from plankton and plants to higher animals (shrimp, shell, fatty fish, seal, whale and eventually man).

Dihomo-γ-linolenic acid (DGLA), arachidonic acid (AA) and eicosapentaenoic acid (EPA) are precursors of eicosanoids which affect inflammatory and immunological processes in several ways (Mead & Mertin, 1988). Miller *et al.* (1987) discovered that a metabolite of DGLA inhibits the production of the pro-inflammatory mediator leukotriene B_4 from AA.

Manku *et al.* (1984) reported a somewhat elevated level of LA in plasma phospholipids of adults with atopic dermatitis and reduced levels of its metabolites:

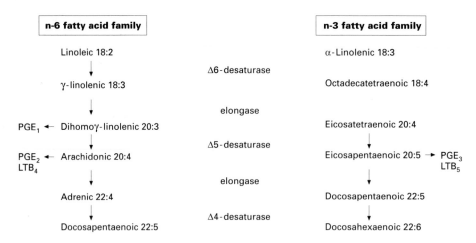

Fig. 14.4 Metabolic pathways for the desaturation and elongation of *n*-3 and *n*-6 fatty acids, which share common enzymes for some of their metabolic pathways.

γ-linolenic acid (GLA), DGLA and AA. This resulted in a hypothesis suggesting that these patients had a defect in the enzyme δ-6 desaturase, which converts LA into GLA (Fig. 14.4). Thus, with a drop in DGLA levels, there would be an increase in leukotrienes, leading to more intense skin inflammation. Melnik and Plewig (1989) postulated that a decrease in levels of another DGLA derivative, prostaglandin E$_1$ (PGE$_1$), may lead to the immunological and clinical signs of atopic dermatitis. There is evidence that E-type prostaglandins inhibit the synthesis of IgE in mononuclear cells *in vitro* (Melnik *et al.*, 1991), and in atopic dermatitis IgE levels are characteristically elevated. This has raised the possibility that the direct administration of GLA, to bypass the apparent metabolic block, would have beneficial effects. Lovell *et al.* (1981) and Wright and Burton (1982) reported that dietary intake of evening primrose oil, which contains large amounts of LA and about 8% of GLA, promoted clinical improvement in patients with atopic dermatitis. Since then, there have been several smaller double-blind, placebo-controlled trials reporting the beneficial effect of oral evening primrose oil supplementation in treating atopic dermatitis (Schalin-Karrila *et al.*, 1987; Morse *et al.*, 1989). However, in two larger placebo-controlled trials no improvement with active

treatment was demonstrated (Bamford *et al.*, 1985; Berthjones & Grahambrown, 1993).

Fish oil

Bjerve *et al.* (1989) reported that dietary intake of *n*-3 fatty acids normalized the dry skin of a patient with *n*-3 fatty acid deficiency. This indicates that *n*-3 fatty acids may be important for a normal skin function. When dietary *n*-3 fatty acids are consumed, they are incorporated into cell membranes and compete with *n*-6 fatty acids as substrates for cyclooxygenase and lipoxygenase pathways. Eicosanoids derived from fatty acids of the *n*-3 series (e.g. leukotriene B$_5$, thromboxane A$_3$) are generally less potent than metabolites from the *n*-6 series (leukotriene B$_4$ and thromboxane A$_2$), and consequently exert a smaller inflammatory reaction (Ziboh *et al.*, 1986). The biological difference between prostaglandin E$_3$ (PGE$_3$) derived from EPA and PGE$_2$ derived from AA is, however, more uncertain.

Furthermore, the very long-chain *n*-3 fatty acids may decrease activation of human T cells *in vitro* (Calder *et al.*, 1992; Søyland *et al.*, 1993). In eczematous skin disorders, activated T cells are a major infiltrating cell type (Zachary *et al.*, 1985). Therefore, *n*-3 fatty acids might reduce clinical symptoms and signs in patients with atopic dermatitis via inhibition of T-cell activation and proliferation.

In a smaller clinical double-blind study, dietary intake of *n*-3 fatty acids given as triacylglycerols to patients with atopic dermatitis significantly improved some of the subjective manifestations (itch, scale and overall severity) as compared to the patients receiving olive oil (Bjørneboe *et al.*, 1987). The study lasted three months; the patients in the fish-oil group received 10 g of Max-Epa/day (30% EPA and dihydroacetic acid (DHA)), whereas the patients in the control group received an equivalent amount of olive oil. Because of this encouraging result, together with the immunosuppressive effect of *n*-3 fatty acids seen *in vitro*, a more extensive randomized double-blind study was carried out using a larger dose, including 145 patients with atopic dermatitis receiving fatty acids for a longer period of time (Søyland *et al.*, 1994). The results showed that 5.1 g of ethyl esters of EPA and DHA (K85 Pronova Biocare AS) caused a significant improvement over 4 months of treatment for all the clinical signs and symptoms evaluated. The patients supplied with corn oil had a similar beneficial effect. Therefore, a placebo effect in both groups is a reliable explanation and cannot be excluded. Corn oil consists of about 60% LA, and LA is a vital constituent of sphingolipids which act as the epidermal permeability barrier in the stratum corneum (Bowser & White, 1985; Elias, 1985). LA has also been shown to reduce T-cell proliferation *in vitro* (Søyland *et al.*, 1993). Thus, the possibility that both corn oil and *n*-3 fatty acids may have some effect in the treatment of atopic dermatitis cannot be excluded.

Chinese herbal tea

In 1992, Atherton *et al.* reported that over one hundred of their patients with atopic dermatitis, who were resistant to convential therapy, improved under the care of a traditional Chinese medical practitioner in London. Although the mixtures prescribed were highly individualized on the basis of characteristics of both the patients and their skin disease, the investigators were able to develop a standardized formula for controlled clinical trials. A daily decoction of the formula containing ten herbs that had been found to be beneficial in open studies was tested in a double-blind, placebo-controlled trial. Forty adult patients with long-standing, refractory atopic dermatitis were randomized into two groups to receive two months' treatment of either the active formulation of herbs or placebo herbs, followed by a crossover to the other

treatment after a 4-week washout period. The study showed a significant difference in both erythema and surface area involved when patients received the Chinese herbal therapy as compared to a placebo herbal solution. There was also a significant subjective improvement in itching and sleep during the Chinese herbal therapy treatment phase (Sheehan *et al.*, 1992). Similar results were found in another smaller study (Sheehan & Atherton, 1992).

The reason for the efficacy of these plant extracts in atopic dermatitis is unknown, but some of the dried plants involved have anti-inflammatory, antimicrobial, immunosuppressive and sedating effects (Sheehan *et al.*, 1992). There have not been any toxicities observed during these studies, but hepatotoxicity has previously been reported to be associated with herbal remedies (Atherton *et al.*, 1992).

Daily diet

When dealing with dietary supplements, it is important to perform dietary recalls to evaluate the dietay habits among patients with atopic dermatitis. In an unpublished large-scale evaluation of dietary intake of foods and nutrients among patients with atopic dermatitis, the dietary ratio of polyunsaturated to saturated fatty acid intake was significantly lower in patients with atopic dermatitis as compared to an age- and sex-matched reference group. However, none of the nutrients gave statistically significant contributions to explain the dermatological score (Søyland *et al.*, unpublished data).

Conclusion

The results of the clinical trials treating patients with atopic dermatitis with evening primrose oil or fish oil are controversial. We know that polyunsaturated fatty acids are important constituents of the lipid barrier in epidermis, and that patients with atopic dermatitis have a defect of this barrier function caused by a reduced amount of especially LA. Furthermore, both *n*-6 and *n*-3 fatty acids do have immunosuppressive effects *in vitro* and *ex vivo* (Esperson *et al.*, 1992; Endres *et al.*, 1993; Søyland *et al.*, 1993). We also know that dietary intake of polyunsaturated fatty acids increases the ratio between polyunsaturated and monounsaturated fatty acids in serum phospholipids (Søyland *et al.*, 1994).

In the two large studies of Bamford *et al.* (1985) and Berthjones and Grahambrown (1993), however, there was no clinical improvement by treating patients with evening primrose oil as compared to liquid paraffin. Also, in the multicentre study by Søyland *et al.* (1994) there was no improvement in the experimental group receiving *n*-3 fatty acids as compared to the control group. In conclusion, neither evening primrose oil nor fish oil seems to have any clinical beneficial effect in treating atopic dermatitis as monotherapies. We do not have any plausible explanation for the discrepancy between the *in vitro* and the clinical result. It may be of interest to investigate if certain subgroups of patients are more responsive to these fatty acids than others, e.g. patients with atopic dermatitis have different types of T-helper cells in their affected skin, dependent on whether they are allergic. Thus, it may be that these subgroups of patients respond differently to dietary intake of very long-chain essential fatty acids.

The clinical results are in correspondence with the data we observed concerning daily dietary habits that do not seem to influence the clinical picture in these patients. However, data dealing with epidemiological studies assessing the usual dietary habits of atopic patients are too scarce and hence it is impossible to make any reliable conclusion.

The clinical results reported on Chinese herbal tea therapy are very positive and may reveal unconsidered avenues. However, the mechanism of action and toxicities of the herbs require further investigation.

Since the standard treatment of chronic immune-related diseases like atopic dermatitis causes unwanted side effects, it is of great interest to evaluate the possible contribution that dietary intake may exert.

References

Atherton, D.J., Sheehan, M.P., Rustin, M.H.A. *et al.* (1992) Treatment of atopic eczema with traditional Chinese medicinal plants. *Pediatric Dermatology*, **9**, 373–375.

Bamford, J.T.M., Gibson, R.W. & Renier, C.M. (1985) Atopic eczema unresponsive to evening primrose oil (linoleic and gamma-linolenic acids). *Journal of the American Academy of Dermatology*, **13**, 959–965.

Berthjones, J. & Grahambrown, R.A.C. (1993) Placebo-controlled trial of essential fatty acid supplementation in atopic dermatitis. *Lancet*, **341**, 1557–1560.

Binkley, K.E. (1992) Role of food allergy in atopic dermatitis. *International Journal of Dermatology*, **31**, 611–614.

Bjerve, K.S., Fisher, S., Wammer, F. & Egeland, T. (1989) Alpha-linolenic acid and long-chain omega-3 fatty acid supplementation in three patients with omega-3 fatty acids deficiency: effect on lymphocyte function, plasma and red cell lipids, and prostanoid formation. *American Journal of Clinical Nutrition*, **49**, 290–300.

Bjørneboe, A., Søyland, E., Bjørneboe, G.E.-A. *et al.* (1987) Effects of dietary supplementation with eicosapentanoic acid in the treatment of atopic dermatitis. *British Journal of Dermatology*, **117**, 463–469.

Bowser, P.A. & White, R.J. (1985) Isolation, barrier properties and lipid analysis of the stratum compactum, a discrete layer of the stratum corneum. *British Jounal of Dermatology*, **112**, 1–14.

Bowser, P.A., White, R.J. & Nugteren, D.H. (1986) Location and nature of the epidermal permeability barrier. *International Journal of Cosmetic Chemists*, **8**, 125–134.

Burr, G.O. & Burr, M.M. (1929) A new defiency disease produced by rigid exclusion of fat from the diet. *Journal of Biological Chemistry*, **82**, 345–367.

Burr, G.O. & Burr, M.M. (1930) On the nature and role of fatty acids essential in nutrition. *Journal of Biological Chemistry*, **86**, 587–589.

Calder, P.C., Bevan, S.J. & Newsholme, E.A. (1992) The inhibition of T-lymphocyte proliferation by fatty acids is via an eicosanoid-independent mechanism. *Immunology*, **75**, 108–115.

David, T.J. (1991) Recent developments in the treatment of childhood atopic eczema. *Journal of the Royal College of Physicians (London)*, **25**, 95–101.

Drevon, C.A. (1993) *Sources, Chemistry and Biochemistry of Dietary Lipids. Omega-3 Fatty Acids. Metabolism and Biologic Effect* (eds C.A. Drevon, I. Baksaa & H. Krokan). Birhauser, Basel.

de Prost, Y. (1992) Atopic dermatitis: recent therapeutic advances. *Pediatric Dermatology*, **9**, 386–389.

Elias, P.N. (1985) The essential fatty acid deficient rodent: evidence for a direct role for intercellular lipid in barrier function. In: *Models in Dermatology* (eds H. Maibach & N. Lowe), pp. 272–285. Basel, Karger.

Endres, S., Meydani, S.N., Ghorbani, R., Schindler, R. & Dinarello, C.A. (1993) Dietary supplementation with *n*-3 polyunsaturated fatty acids suppresses interleukin-2 production and mononuclear cell proliferation. *Journal of Leukocyte Biology*, **54**, 599–603.

Esperson, G.T., Grunnet, N., Lervang, H.H. *et al.* (1992) Decreased interleukin-1β levels in plasma from rheumatoid arthritis patients after dietary supplementation with *n*-3 polyunsaturated fatty acids. *Clinical Rheumatology*, **11**, 393–395.

Fradin, M.S., Ellis, C.N. & Voorhees, J.J. (1990) Management of patients and side effects during cyclosporine therapy for cutaneous disorders. *Journal of the American Academy of Dermatology*, **23**, 1265–1275.

Hansen, A.E. (1933) Serum lipid changes and therapeutic effects of various oils in infantile eczema. *Proceedings of the Society for Experimental and Biological Medicine*, **31**, 160–161.

Kapp, A., Kirnbauer, R., Luger, T.A. & Shopf, E. (1989) Altered production of immuno-modulating cytokines in patients with atopic dermatitis. *Acta Dermato-Venereologica (Stockholm)*, **69** (Suppl 144), 97–99.

Korting, H.C., Kerscher, M.J. & Scafer-Korting, M. (1992) Topical glucocorticoids with improved benefit/risk ratio: do they exist? *Journal of the American Academy of Dermatology*, **27**, 87–92.

Lovell, C.R., Burton, J.L. & Horrobin, D.F. (1981) Treatment of atopic eczema with evening primrose oil. *Lancet*, **i**, 278.

Manku, M.S., Horrobin, D.F., Morse, N.L. *et al.* (1984) Essential fatty acids in plasma phospholipids of patients with atopic eczema. *British Journal of Dermatology*, **110**, 643–648.

Mead, J.C. & Mertin, J. (1988) Fatty acids and immunity. *Advances in Lipid Research*, **21**, 103.

Melnik, B. & Plewig, G. (1989) Is the origin of atopy linked to deficient conversion of omega-6-fatty acids to prostaglandin E_1? *Journal of the American Academy of Dermatology*, **21**, 557–563.

Melnik, B., Hollmann, J. & Plewig, G. (1988) Decreased stratum corneum ceramides in atopic individuals — a pathobiochemical factor in xerosis? *British Journal of Dermatology*, **119**, 547–568.

Melnik, B., Plewig, G. & Tschung, T. (1991) Disturbances of essential fatty acid- and prostaglandin E-mediated immunoregulation in atopy. *Prostaglandins, Leukotrienes, Essential Fatty Acids*, **42**, 125–130.

Miller, C.C., Ziboh, V.A. & Jones, J. (1987) Guinea pig epidermis synthesizes 15-hydroxy-8,11,13-eicosatrienoic acid (15-OH-20:3n-6) from dihomogammalinoleic acid (DGLA): a potent lipooxygenase inhibitor derived from primrose oil. *Journal of Investigative Dermatology*, **88**, 507.

Morse, P.F., Horrobin, D.F., Manku, M.S. *et al.* (1989) Meta-analysis of placebo-controlled studies of the efficacy of Epogam in the treatment of atopic eczema: relationship between essential fatty acid changes and clinical response. *British Journal of Dermatology*, **121**, 75–90.

Ortolani, C. (1995) Atlas on mechanisms in adverse reactions to food. *Allergy*, **50** (Suppl 20), 1–81.

Sampson, H.A. & McCaskill, C.C. (1985) Food hypersensitivity and atopic dermatitis: evaluation of 113 patients. *Journal of Pediatrics*, **107**, 669–675.

Schalin-Karrila, M., Mattila, L., Jansen, C.T. & Uotila, P. (1987) Evening primrose oil in the treatment of atopic eczema: effect on clinical status, plasma phospholipid fatty acids and circulating blood prostaglandins. *British Journal of Dermatology*, **117**, 11–19.

Sheehan, M.P. & Atherton, D.J. (1992) A controlled trial of traditional Chinese medicinal plants in widespread non-exudative atopic eczema. *British Journal of Dermatology*, **126**, 179–184.

Sheehan, M.P., Rustin, M.H.A. & Atherton, D.J. *et al.* (1992) Efficacy of traditional Chinese herbal therapy in adult atopic dermatitis. *Lancet*, **340**, 13–17.

Søyland, E., Nenseter, M.S., Braathen, L.R. & Drevon, C.A. (1993) Very long-chain n-3 and n-6 polyunsaturated fatty acids inhibit proliferation of human T lymphocytes *in vitro*. *European Journal of Clinical Investigations*, **23**, 112–121.

Søyland, E., Funk, J., Rajka, G. *et al.* (1994) Dietary supplementation with very long-chain n-3 fatty acids in patients with atopic dermatitis. A double-blind, multicentre study. *British Journal of Dermatology*, **130**, 757–764.

Wright, S. & Burton, J.L. (1982) Oral evening primrose seed oil improves atopic eczema. *Lancet*, **ii**, 1120–1122.

Zachary, C.B., Allen, M.H. & MacDonald, D.M. (1985) *In situ* quantification of T-lymphocyte subsets and Langerhans cells in the inflammatory infiltrate of atopic eczema. *British Journal of Dermatology*, **112**, 149–156.

Ziboh, V.A., Cohen, K.A., Ellis, C.N. *et al.* (1986) Effect of dietary supplementation of fish oil on neutrophil and epidermal fatty acids: Modulation of clinical course of psoriatic subjects. *Archives of Dermatology*, **122**, 1277–1282.

Overview of Expected Sensitizations in Atopic Dermatitis

M.H. GUILLET AND G. GUILLET

Allergy is among the flare factors of atopic dermatitis (AD), along with aspecific factors (heat, irritant contacts, etc.) that may trigger the disease (Dahl, 1990). When managing atopic dermatitis, it is of great interest to consider the natural history of specific sensitizations in order to prevent cutaneous flares and complications. To this purpose, we carried out systematic allergologic evaluations to assess the course of sensitizations over time and their clinical involvements in children with AD. The aim of these studies was to define both the involvement of IgE-mediated sensitizations and contact dermatitis through prospective studies and comparative analyses (Guillet *et al.*, 1991; Guillet & Guillet, 1992, 1996). These studies were performed on an unselected population of atopic patients, allowing general appraisal of both IgE-mediated and contact sensitizations. Comparative analyses and a short prospective study give an overview of expected sensitizations in childhood according to age and environmental conditions.

Involvement of flare factors in atopic dermatitis

Atopic dermatitis is a multifactorial disease whose manifestations depend on allergic and non-specific environmental factors. The role of specific allergy is clearly supported by clinical observations as well as laboratory data: correlation between global IgE levels and clinical severity of AD undoubtedly confirms the involvement of IgE sensitization in the disease (Clendenning *et al.*, 1973). As for contact dermatitis, although it has been assumed for a long time that AD was little concerned, it is now admitted that contact factors have been underestimated (Blondeel *et al.*, 1987). Therefore, the role of IgE and allergy in atopic dermatitis raises several questions:
• For which patients is allergologic enquiry worthwhile?
• What is the natural history of sensitizations and what evolution may we expect with time?
• Can we understand the switch of cutaneous to respiratory manifestations in atopy?
• Can we predict the risk of asthma or rhinitis in specific groups or at least the date of beginning of respiratory symptoms in childhood?

A survey of allergy in two series of 250 and 252 patients by the use of cross-sectional studies was carried out to answer these questions (Guillet & Guillet, 1992, 1996).

Allergic evaluations of IgE sensitizations according to atopic dermatitis

A first study devoted to AD included minor, moderate and severe patients defined by clinical scores with a standardized method of evaluation (Guillet & Guillet,

Table 14.4 Average level of global IgE (IU/ml) according to age and clinical severity.

Degree OF AD	Age (years)			
	<2	2–7	7–15	>15 and adults
Moderate	10	137	213	683
Severe	407	1030	1487	3315

AD, Atopic dermatitis.

1992): IgE involvement was assessed through skin testing, blood tests and clinical scores after allergen elimination and challenges (with double-blind and open food challenges). This study showed that allergic evaluation of IgE-mediated sensitization was not worthwhile in minor AD.

Dynamic profile of IgE in moderate and severe atopic dermatitis

Focusing on moderate and severe AD, we have pointed out the progressive increase of IgE levels among the different classes of age, with higher levels in the severe AD group compared to the group of moderate AD (Guillet & Guillet, 1996): these data support the idea of a dynamic evolution of IgE production and stimulation in the course of AD (Table 14.4).

Inhalant allergen sensitization

Inhalant allergen sensitizations were evaluated in moderate and severe AD (Table 14.5). These sensitizations were raised to 66% in moderate AD and were higher in severe AD: 93% of patients in the group of 7–15 years with severe AD proved to be concerned with inhalant allergen sensitizations that mainly correlated with respiratory symptoms and seldom with cutaneous flares. In this group of severe AD, symptoms begin earlier (from 18 months) than in moderate AD.

We tried to determine whether the occurrence of respiratory symptoms was selectively predictable in some groups of patients: we developed a prospective study in 29 patients under 2 years of age, followed up from 4 months to 3 years of age (Guillet & Guillet, 1992). This study shows that early food allergy

Table 14.5 Distribution of sensitizations according to age and severity.

Age	Severity	Pneumallergen sensitization (%)	Food allergy with clinical involvement (%)	Contact dermatitis (%)
Group I (<2 years)	MAD = 15	0 ⎫ 7	0	80 ⎫ 24
n = 70	SAD = 55	9 ⎭	98	9 ⎭
Group II (2–7 years)	MAD = 28	53 ⎫ 75	0	82 ⎫ 32
n = 93	SAD = 65	85 ⎭	98	11 ⎭
Group III (7–15 years)	MAD = 9	66 ⎫ 82	0	56 ⎫ 47
n = 23	SAD = 14	93 ⎭	71	43 ⎭
Group IV	MAD = 12	58 ⎫ 89	0 ⎫ 66	100 ⎫ 66
n = 65	SAD = 53	96 ⎭	81 ⎭	58 ⎭
Total children (0–15 years)	MAD = 52	40 ⎫ 51	0 ⎫ 69	77 ⎫ 31
n = 186	SAD = 134	54 ⎭	96 ⎭	14 ⎭
Total population (children and adults)	MAD = 64	44	0 ⎫ 68	81 ⎫ 40
n = 251	SAD = 187	66	91 ⎭	26 ⎭

MAD, Moderate atopic dermatitis; SAD, severe atopic dermatitis.

behaves as a marker of high risk for later respiratory symptoms since 91% of patients with food allergy had inhalant allergen sensitizations. However, these data do not mean that the risk of respiratory symptoms electively concerns children with food allergy: it only means that respiratory complications occur earlier in this group and that infants with food allergy deserve early protection against inhalant allergens.

Food allergy: a marker for severe atopic dermatitis

Food allergy presents as a marker of severity in AD. In a study by Guillet and Guillet (1992), food allergy was demonstrated in 98% of children with severe AD under 2 years of age. This was the earliest sensitization. Food sensitizations are supposed to modify over time (Sampson & Scanlon, 1989): additive sensitizations (for example, superimposed sensitization to eggs and peanuts), or switch between two sensitizations, or sometimes disappear under an elimination diet. The main trophallergens (Table 14.6) differ according to the age and probably to nutritional and cultural habits: in children under 2 years of age, eggs, peanuts, milk and fish are the four major allergens (in our statistics, they were respectively concerned in

77%, 33% 25% and 9% of children under 2 years of age). Later, other trophallergen sensitizations are demonstrated: mainly wheat flour, shellfish and yeast (respectively 20%, 37% and 20%). Although a spontaneous decrease of food allergy is sometimes observed, it must be pointed out that food allergy may still present as a flare factor in adulthood (mainly yeast, shellfish, eggs and pork) in our experience (Guillet & Guillet, 1996).

Table 14.6 Main trophallergens involved in flares of atopic dermatitis according to age (n = 347 patients).

Foodstuff	Global frequency (%)	<2 years (%)	2–7 years (%)	7–15 years (%)	>15 years and adults (%)
Eggs	46	77	55	30	20
Peanut	29	33	37	30	11
Shellfish	24	9	28	30	37
Milk	20	25	25	7	
Wheat flour	14	3	12	20	17
Fish	14	9	14	7	17
Yeast	7.2			20	20
Soybeans	8.9	3	17	20	
Pork	4				10

Respiratory symptoms in moderate and severe atopic dermatitis: sequence of food and respiratory sensitizations

This sequence is a usual finding in the course of severe AD. In a recent study we confirmed that children who develop food allergy should be considered at high risk for early and severe respiratory complications. Of 251 patients (Guillet & Guillet, 1996), 93% of children aged 7–15 years with severe AD and food allergy developed additional inhalant sensitization and respiratory symptoms. In other words, it is likely that food allergy reflects a high potential for other later sensitizations and that severe AD patients will get respiratory symptoms earlier than children with moderate AD.

In moderate AD, the main IgE sensitizations are respiratory with little cutaneous involvement: clinical correlated symptoms were rhinitis or asthma. The incidence was 0% in those under 2 years of age and ranged from 53 to 66% in the other groups.

In severe AD, the rate of respiratory sensitization was much higher in each age class (9% under 2 years, 85% from 2 to 7 years, 93% in the 7–15-year age group and 96% in those >15 years) and respiratory symptoms were preceded by (or associated with) trophallergen sensitization in 81%.

Contact dermatitis

Contact dermatitis is underestimated in AD: systematic patch testing in a series of 251 patients presenting with moderate and severe AD demonstrated that 40% of patients were concerned with contact dermatitis (Guillet & Guillet, 1996). Contact dermatitis was patent in 31% of children and 66% of adults with a progressive increase according to age, as a dynamic process. Contact dermatitis was predominantly observed in moderate AD with a progressive increase. It was estimated to be 11% in children under 2 years, 43% in the group of 7–15 years and 58% in those >15 years of age. Contact sensitizations may begin in the first 2 years with major involvement of nickel, fragrances (cosmetics) and balsam of Peru being the more common allergens. Later sensitizations to other cosmetic and occupational allergens occur in close connection with the specific environment in older children and adults. They often

proved to be correlated with AD exacerbation. Therefore, it must be emphasized that the diagnosis of atopic dermatitis must not lead us to focus on IgE-dependent sensitizations without patch testing: contact dermatitis may be often misdiagnosed as a flare of atopic dermatitis (Guillet & Guillet, 1997).

Since sensitizations progressively increase and may be sometimes statistically predicted, allergic management of AD may be worthwhile. Whether the control of allergens will lead us to observe less allergies is of interest. But in any case, this hypothesis is valuable, considering the short-term benefit on atopic eczema, the efficacy of protection against contact dermatitis (versus occupational and cosmetic environments) and respiratory prevention. Available data indicate that AD may be dependent on allergic factors and that sensitizations are expected to modify and complicate respiratory sensitizations. In this respect, dermatologists and paediatricians should consider the natural history of sensitizations for both cutaneous symptoms and respiratory protection.

References

Blondeel, A., Achten, G., Dooms-Goossens, A., Buckens, P., Broeckse, W. & Oleffe, J. (1987) Atopie et allergie de contact. *Annals of Dermatology and Venereology*, **114**, 203–209.

Clendenning, W., Clack, W., Ogawa, M. & Ishizaka, K. (1973) Serum IgE studies in atopic dermatitis. *Journal of Investigative Dermatology*, **61**, 233–236.

Dahl, M. (1990) Flare factors and atopic dermatitis. *Journal of Dermatological Science*, **1**, 311–318.

Guillet, G. & Guillet, M.H. (1992) Natural history of sensitizations in atopic dermatitis. *Archives of Dermatology*, **128**, 187–192.

Guillet, M.H. & Guillet, G. (1996) Enquête allergologique chez 251 patients atteints de dermatite atopique modérée ou sévère: fréquence et intérêt du dépistage, de l'eczéma de contact, de l'allergie alimentaire et de la sensibilisation aux pneumallergènes. *Annales de Dermatologie et de Venereologie*, **123**, 157–164.

Guillet, M.H., & Guillet, G. (1997) Evolution of contact dermatitis in childhood. Cross-sectional evaluation of 152 children. *European Journal of Dermatology*, **7**, 56–58.

Guillet, M.H., Guillet, G., Nousbaum, B., Sassolas, B. & Ménard, N. (1991) Intérêt de la therapeutique d'éviction sur une série de 86 dermatites atopiques graves. *Revue Française d'Allergologie et Immunologie Clinique*, **31**, 137–144.

Sampson, M. & Scanlon, S. (1989) Natural history of food hyper-sensitivity in children with atopic dermatitis. *Journal of Pediatrics*, **115**, 23–27.

Psychological Factors and Atopic Dermatitis

M.A. GUPTA AND A.K. GUPTA

Psychological factors have been implicated both in the onset and/or exacerbation of atopic dermatitis or eczema, and hence may play a role in the primary, secondary and/or tertiary prevention of atopic dermatitis (AD). Primary prevention is defined as the prevention of the disease process from starting, secondary prevention refers to measures aimed against the progression or recurrences of the disease and tertiary prevention refers to anticipatory care, i.e. effective treatment of the disease and the prevention of complications.

The literature on the psychology of AD has considered three major factors (Gustafsson *et al.*, 1994): (i) the psychophysiological stress model which studies the influence of stressful life events on the course of illness; (ii) psychoanalytical and other psychopathological factors such as the role of repressed emotion and depression, and the role of abnormal psychophysiological reactivity; and (iii) a systems approach, which stresses the interplay between the individual and family members. In this latter model, there may be a primary inherent dysfunction of structure or communication within the family, or alternatively the dysfunction within the family may arise secondary to various environmental factors including the psychosocial impact of AD. Up to 60% of patients have onset of AD in the first year of life, with 85% presenting symptoms before the age of 5 years (Faulstich & Williamson, 1985), therefore a significant body of the literature on the psychology has examined psychosocial factors in the child with AD. The literature suggests that the psychological factors play a role in the primary, secondary and/or tertiary prevention of atopic dermatitis in varying degrees. The most convincing role of psychological factors lies in the secondary prevention, i.e. prevention of the progression or recurrence of AD.

Stress and atopic dermatitis

In a Finnish survey of 801 AD patients, psychological stress was experienced as a major aggravating factor in one-half to two-thirds of patients (Lammintausta *et al.*, 1991). Psychic stress was the most frequently cited factor provoking relapses of AD or aggravating symptoms of AD (Lammintausta *et al.*, 1991). The worsening of AD with stress was less frequently cited by patients with milder skin symptoms; however, 45–67% of patients with severe AD cited stress as being an important factor in the exacerbation of their skin disorder (Lammintausta *et al.*, 1991).

Various investigators have looked at the specific nature of the psychological stressor. Several earlier studies, based on retrospective recall, have associated stress from major life events with the onset or the exacerbation of AD symptoms. An earlier study (Miller & Baruch, 1948) observed that stress from maternal neglect, rejection or separation led to the development of AD. In another study, 55% of 32 AD patients reported that emotional events were related to exacerbations of AD (Greenhill & Finesinger, 1942), and 'severe shock, worry or emotional upset' within 6 months preceding the onset of symptoms was reported by 48% of 82 eczema patients versus 15% of 123 dental controls (Brown, 1972). Studies of the relationship between the severity of stressful life events and AD come up with inconsistent results. No relation was found between the quantity of life change over the previous 2 months and onset of symptoms in AD (Wyler *et al.*, 1971) and no relation was observed between major life events and measures of symptom severity in AD (Gil *et al.*, 1987). However, in a study of 44 AD patients with a mean age of 6.9 years, Gil *et al.* (1987) observed that stress resulting from having a chronic disorder like AD, but not stresses from major life events, correlated significantly with measures of AD severity. The authors propose that when evaluating the role of stress in the AD patients, a focus on stresses specifically related to AD, including possible distress caused by the treatment regimens, must be considered. Gil *et al.* (1987) propose that stress may lead to altered autonomic activity which results in peripheral vascular changes that lower the itch threshold and initiate the itch–scratch cycle. A prospective study employing a daily diary, among 50 adult AD patients with a mean age of 30.6 years, revealed that interpersonal stress and symptom severity in AD were predictive of each other (King & Wilson, 1991). King and Wilson (1991) propose that one explanation for this finding is that interpersonal stress causes an increase in skin symptoms as a result of the physiological consequences of arousal. Alternately, skin symptoms can make sufferers more vulnerable to interpersonal stresses (King & Wilson, 1991).

Psychotherapeutic interventions which help identify life stresses (Brown & Bettely, 1971), and standard medical treatments combined with progressive relaxation and hypnosis (Brown & Bettely, 1971) have been associated with greater improvement of the skin at 14 months' follow-up than standard dermatological treatments alone. Psychotropic drugs such as anxiolytics and major tranquillizers may be used for the acutely stressed AD patient (Gupta *et al.*, 1986).

Psychopathological factors and atopic dermatitis

Consideration of psychopathological factors is important especially in the secondary prevention and to some degree the tertiary prevention of AD. No specific AD-related personality constellation has been discerned. A 15–17-year follow-up of 99 AD patients, first diagnosed in infancy, revealed no characteristic personality patterns or significant similarities of personality in later life (Musgrove & Morgan, 1976). However, various studies have referred to the role of difficulties with the handling of anger (Ginsburg *et al.*, 1993), high levels of anxiety (Garrie *et al.*, 1974; Al-Ahmar & Kurban, 1976; Faulstich & Williamson, 1985; White *et al.*, 1990; Ginsburg *et al.*, 1993) and depressive illness (Gupta *et al.*, 1994) in the onset and/or perpetuation of AD. Therefore, it is possible that while these psychopathological factors are not a primary feature of AD, when present in conjunction with AD, they can affect the clinical course of the disorder. In a study of 61 AD patients (Scheich *et al.*, 1993), individuals with serum IgE levels $> 100\,IU/ml$ had significantly higher scores on excitability and inadequate stress coping than patients with normal (i.e. $< 100\,IU/ml$) IgE levels.

Alexander and French, who had considered atopic dermatitis or 'disseminated neurodermatitis' to be one of the classical psychosomatic disorders, proposed that specific causative emotional conflict in AD was around the child's expression or suppression of anger, which stemmed from maternal rejection (Fritz, 1979).

The earlier psychodynamic formulations considered severe scratching in AD, which is a perpetuating factor in AD, to be reflective of inhibited aggressive urges and restricted sexual expression (Fiske & Obermayer, 1954; Kepecs *et al.*, 1957). Eczema has been described as a 'substitute' psychosomatic symptom for inhibited or suppressed aggressive impulses (Brown, 1967). Eczema patients ($n = 82$) described a significantly greater tendency to bottle up their angry feelings than dental controls ($n = 123$) (Brown, 1972). A recent study reports that AD patients ($n = 34$) were significantly more likely to feel anger but less likely to express their anger than dental controls ($n = 32$) (Ginsburg *et al.*, 1993). The authors observed that the AD patients were less assertive than the dental controls (Ginsburg *et al.*, 1993). Furthermore, depressive illness has been reported to play an important role in the perpetuation of AD, since a direct correlation ($r = 0.21$, $P < 0.05$) was observed between pruritus severity and the severity of depressive symptoms among 143 outpatients with AD (Gupta *et al.*, 1994).

Anxiety has been reported to play a role in the manifestation of AD, since higher anxiety has been associated with a greater tendency to develop a conditioned scratch response in AD patients in comparison to controls (Jordan & Whitlock, 1972). The increased scratching in turn perpetuates the AD. The possible role of psychophysiological overreactivity in AD, however, is inconclusive. In one study (Faulstich *et al.*, 1985), 10 AD patients had higher anxiety scores and greater electromyographical (EMG) and heart-rate reactivity than controls. However, another study (Koehler & Weber, 1992) found no support to the assumption of general psychophysiological overreactivity of several autonomic variables, including blood pressure, heart rate, skin conductance, spontaneous electrodermal fluctuations and the number of active palmar sweat glands, in 20 female AD patients versus 20 controls.

The above findings have important implications in the secondary and tertiary prevention of AD, since global reduction of anxiety and stress for example with EMG biofeedback and progressive relaxation reduces scratching behaviors in AD (Haynes *et al.*, 1979; McMenamy *et al.*, 1988). Eight sessions of EMG biofeedback/relaxation instructions were significantly superior to placebo (bogus biofeedback) and were followed by an approximately 50% reduction in lesion size among eight AD patients (Haynes *et al.*, 1979). EMG biofeedback and home practice of progressive relaxation in five patients was associated with a significant reduction in the severity of eczema and 'irritation' at 2-month and 2-year follow-up (McMenamy *et al.*, 1988). Scratching behaviours have also been reduced with positive reinforcement and extinction procedures and aversive conditioning, especially in children (Ratcliff & Stein, 1968; Bar & Kuypers, 1973). The behavioral method of habit reversal has been shown to be a helpful adjunctive treatment among adults with AD (Melin *et al.*, 1986).

The role of parents and family environment in atopic dermatitis

In 85% of AD patients, the symptoms are present before age 5 years (Faulstich & Williamson, 1985). This explains the relatively large body of literature on the role of parents and family environment in atopic dermatitis. The earlier literature has looked at the role of the 'maternal rejection factor' which was believed to result from two major problems: firstly, the personality traits of the mother and child which lead to a disturbed mother–child relationship, and secondly, a deficiency in the quantity and/or quality of maternal touching and holding of the child (Solomon & Gagnon, 1987). The personality traits of the mother have been variously described as highly anxious, rejecting, hostile and aggressive and those of the child as overactive, anxious, aggressive, insecure and hostile towards the mother, which together culminate in a disturbed mother–child relationship (Miller & Baruch, 1948; Williams, 1951; Rosenthal, 1952; Solomon & Gagnon, 1987). Chronic intractable eczema has been reported to be a sign of an impaired parent–child relationship in a study involving eight cases (Koblenzer & Koblenzer, 1988). The authors propose a psychodynamic formulation wherein the resentment and ambivalence of the parent towards the child manifests as an overcompensation by the parent, who ends up overindulging and overstimulating their child (Koblenzer & Koblenzer, 1988). This in turn leads to emotional overstimulation and anxiety in the child (Koblenzer & Koblenzer, 1988). Some authors maintain that children with eczema have a greater than average need to have skin contact or touch and be held, and that their mothers frustrate this need. A controlled study of 14 mother–child dyads, consisting of seven children with severe eczema and seven controls, revealed no significant difference between the experimental and control mothers with respect to their level of anxiety, negative effect or spontaneous touching or holding of the child (Solomon & Gagnon, 1987). Therefore, there was no support for the contention that mothers of children who have eczema reject them or are cold, hostile or aggressive towards them (Solomon & Gagnon, 1987). However, the mother–infant interactions of the atopic children were different from controls, e.g. mothers of atopic children were less involved unless the child made clear and direct bids for attention, and the mother showed less spontaneous positive reinforcement (Solomon & Gagnon, 1987).

In a study of 44 children with severe AD, Gil *et al.* (1987) have reported that families of atopic children do not foster independence/organization or tend to have a rigid moral/religious emphasis. Those families emphasizing regular routines, self-reliance, independent thinking and clearly designated family responsibilities were associated with reduced symptoms in their children. These family dimensions were important predictors of symptom severity even after taking into consideration non-psychological factors such as serum IgE levels and age at onset of AD (Gil *et al.*, 1987). It is important to consider the observation that a major depressive disorder in the parents should be ruled out before primary family problems are implicated (Allen, 1989). Such parents are likely to benefit from antidepressant drug therapy (Allen, 1989).

In addition to the role of dysfunctional family dynamics in the pathogenesis of AD, the literature suggests that specific parental responses to the symptom of scratching can affect scratching behaviours (Allen & Harris, 1966; Bar & Kuypers, 1973; Gil *et al.*, 1988). This has implications for both the secondary and tertiary prevention of AD, since modification of scratching behaviours can assist in the control of AD by prevention of both the exacerbation of core symptoms and secondary infection of the affected skin. Case studies suggest that social reinforcement in the form of both positive or negative attention from others given in response to scratching may maintain or increase scratching, and withdrawal of attention by ignoring verbalizations and behaviours related to scratching may reduce scratching (Allen & Harris, 1966; Bar & Kuypers, 1973). Controlled videotaped observations of 30 children with chronic atopic dermatitis confirm that social responses from parents when the child is scratching, e.g. by attention or physical contact from the parents, in the form of rubbing or scratching, may reinforce the level of the child's scratching (Gil *et al.*, 1988). Furthermore, social response from the parent when the child is not scratching reinforces the child's involvement in other more appropriate activities and reduces the level of the child's scratching (Gil *et al.*, 1988). Involvement of the child and parent in structured rather than unstructured activities was associated with greater parental involvement and less scratching by the Child (Gil *et al.*, 1988).

Summary

The course of AD in a genetically predisposed individual is affected by an interaction of biological, psychological and social factors. While the psychosocial factors affect any individual patient in varying degrees, it is important to evaluate the role of these factors when assessing the patient. The literature on the role of psychological factors in the primary prevention of AD is inconsistent and inconclusive. Some factors that may play a role in the primary preventive aspects of AD include psychosocial stress both in children and adults with AD, the 'maternal rejection factor', lack of adequate tactile nurturance and repressed emotions including repressed anger resulting in the AD as a 'substitute' psychosomatic symptom. The role of psychological factors in the secondary and tertiary prevention of AD is more definitive. Some of the factors that play a role in the secondary and tertiary preventive aspects of AD include AD-related stress for both the adult patient and the family of the child with AD, stressful major life events, psychological traits associated with high anxiety and difficulty with the expression of anger and assertiveness, major depressive disease which can enhance pruritus severity in AD, 'maternal rejection factor' and lack of adequate tactile nurturance especially in children, social reinforcement of scratching in the child with AD in the form of both positive or negative attention from others and family dynamics that do not foster independence and responsibility in the child, or are lacking in a consistent and structured approach to the child with AD.

References

Al-Ahmar, H.F. & Kurban, A.K. (1976) Psychological profile of patients with atopic dermatitis. *British Journal of Dermatology*, **95**, 373–377.

Allen, A.D. (1989) Intractable atopic eczema suggests major affective disorder: poor parenting is secondary. *Archives of Dermatology*, **125**, 567–568. (Letter.)

Allen, K. & Harris, F. (1966) Elimination of a child's excessive scratching by training the mother in reinforcement procedures. *Behavior Research and Therapy*, **4**, 79–84.

Bar, H. & Kuypers, B. (1973) Behaviour therapy in dermatological practice. *British Journal of Dermatology*, **88**, 591–598.

Brown, D. & Bettely, F. (1971) Psychiatric treatment of eczema: a controlled trial. *British Medical Journal*, **ii**, 729–734.

Brown, D.G. (1967) Emotional disturbance in eczema: a study of symptom-reporting behaviour. *Journal of Psychosomatic Research*, **11**, 27–40.

Brown, D.G. (1972) Stress as a precipitant factor of eczema. *Journal of Psychosomatic Research*, **16**, 321–327.

Faulstich, M.E. & Williamson, D.E. (1985) An overview of atopic dermatitis: toward a biobehavioral integration. *Journal of Psychosomatic Research*, **29**, 647–654.

Faulstich, M.E., Williamson, D.A., Duchmann, E.G., Conerly, S.L. & Brantley, P.J. (1985) Psychophysiological analysis of atopic dermatitis. *Journal of Psychosomatic Research*, **29**, 415–417.

Fiske, C. & Obermayer, M. (1954) Personality and emotional factors in chronic disseminated neurodermatitis. *Archives of Dermatology and Syphilology*, **70**, 261–263.

Fritz, G.K. (1979) Psychological aspects of atopic dermatitis. *Clinical Pediatrics*, **18**, 360–364.

Garrie, E.V., Garrie, S.A. & Mote, T. (1974) Anxiety and atopic dermatitis. *Journal of Consulting and Clinical Psychology*, **42**, 742.

Gil, K.M., Keefe, F.H., Sampson, H.A., McCaskill, C.C., Rodin, J. & Crisson, J.E. (1987) The relation of stress and family environment to atopic dermatitis symptoms in children. *Journal of Psychosomatic Research*, **31**, 673–684.

Gil, K.M., Keefe, F.J., Sampson, H.A., McCaskill, C.C., Rodin, J. & Crisson, J.E. (1988) Direct observation of scratching behaviour in children with atopic dermatitis. *Behaviour Therapy*, **19**, 213–227.

Ginsburg, I.H., Prystowsky, J.H., Kornfeld, D.H. & Wolland, H. (1993) Role of emotional factors in adults with atopic dermatitis. *International Journal of Dermatology*, **32**, 656–660.

Greenhill, M.H. & Finesinger, J.E. (1942) Neurotic symptoms and emotional factors in atopic dermatitis. *Archives of Dermatology and Syphilis*, **46**, 187–200.

Gupta, M.A., Gupta, A.K. & Haberman, H.F. (1986) Psychotropic drugs in dermatology. *Journal of the American Academy of Dermatology*, **14**, 633–645.

Gupta, M.A., Gupta, A.K., Schork, N.J. & Ellis, C.N. (1994) Depression modulates pruritus perception: a study of pruritus in psoriasis, atopic dermatitis, and chronic idiopathic urticaria. *Psychosomatic Medicine*, **56**, 36–40.

Gustafsson, P.A., Bjorksten, B. & Kjellman, N.I.M. (1994) Family dysfunction in asthma: a prospective study of illness development. *Journal of Pediatrics*, **125**, 493–498.

Haynes, S., Wilson, C., Jaffee, P. & Britton, B. (1979) Biofeedback treatment of atopic dermatitis: controlled case studies of eight cases. *Biofeedback and Self-regulation*, **4**, 195–209.

Jordan, J.M. & Whitlock, F.A. (1972) Emotions and the skin: the conditioning of scratch responses in cases of atopic dermatitis. *British Journal of Dermatology*, **86**, 574–585.

Kepecs, J., Rabin, A. & Robin, M. (1957) Atopic dermatitis: a clinical psychiatric study. *Psychosomatic Medicine*, **29**, 67–69.

King, R.M. & Wilson, G.V. (1991) Use of a diary technique to investigate psychosomatic relations in atopic dermatitis. *Journal of Psychosomatic Research*, **35**, 697–706.

Koblenzer, C.S. & Koblenzer, P.J. (1988) Chronic intractable atopic eczema. *Archives of Dermatology*, **124**, 1673–1677.

Koehler, T. & Weber, D. (1992) Psychophysiological reactions of patients with atopic dermatitis. *Journal of Psychosomatic Research*, **36**, 391–394.

Lammintausta, K., Kalimo, K., Raitala, R. & Forsten, Y. (1991) Prognosis of atopic dermatitis, a prospective study in early adulthood. *International Journal of Dermatology*, **30**, 563–568.

McMenamy, C.J., Katz, R.C. & Gipson, M. (1988) Treatment of eczema by EMG biofeedback and relaxation training: a multiple baseline analysis. *Journal of Behavior Therapy and Experimental Psychiatry*, **19**, 221–227.

Melin, L., Frederiksen, T., Noren, P. & Swebilius, B.G. (1986) Behavioral treatment of scratching in patients with atopic dermatitis. *British Journal of Dermatology*, **115**, 467–474.

Miller, H. & Baruch, D.W. (1948) Psychosomatic studies of children with allergic manifestations. I. Maternal rejection: a study of sixty-three cases. *Psychosomatic Medicine*, **10**, 274–278.

Musgrove, K. & Morgan, J.K. (1976) Infantile eczema: a long-term follow-up study. *British Journal of Dermatology*, **95**, 365–372.

Ratcliff, R. & Stein, N. (1968) Treatment of neurodermatitis by behavioral therapy: a case study. *Behavioral Research and Therapy*, **6**, 397–399.

Rosenthal, M.H. (1952) Psychosomatic study of infantile eczema. I. Mother–child relationship. *Pediatrics*, **10**, 581–592.

Scheich, G., Florin, I., Rudolph, R. & Wilhelm, S. (1993) Personality characteristics and serum IgE level in patients with atopic dermatitis. *Journal of Psychosomatic Research*, **37**, 637–642.

Solomon, C.R. & Gagnon, C. (1987) Mother and child characteristics and involvement in dyads in which young children have eczema. *Developmental and Behavioral Pediatrics*, **8**, 213–220.

White, A., Horne, D.J. & Varigos, G.A. (1990) Psychological profile of the atopic eczema patient. *Australasian Journal of Dermatology*, **31**, 13–16.

Williams, D. (1951) Management of atopic dermatitis in children: control of the maternal rejection factor. *Archives of Dermatology and Syphilology*, **63**, 545–547.

Wyler, A.R., Masuda, M. & Holmes, T.H. (1971) Magnitude of life events and seriousness of illness. *Psychosomatic Medicine*, **33**, 115–122.

Is Contact Dermatitis to Aeroallergens Involved in Atopic Dermatitis?

M. CASTELAIN

Aeroallergens

Some allergens may elicit positive tests in 20 minutes in atopic dermatitis (AD). They are essentially extracts of dust mites, hair, skin scales, feathers or antigens from animal saliva, pollens and moulds.

The correlation between these tests and the pathology encountered is evident in allergies of the respiratory mucosae; therefore, these allergens are called 'aeroallergens'. From the dermatological point of view, we have suspected that aeroallergens may also affect the cutaneous condition of AD since 1930.

In 1986, Bruijnzeel-Koomen *et al.* demonstrated the presence of IgE receptors on the surface of Langerhans cells (LC) in the epidermis. This discovery has entailed an important renewal of interest concerning the connection between the skin and aeroallergens.

During the 1980s, several authors studied the eventual responsibility for aeroallergens to induce dermatological lesions in AD (Platts-Mills *et al.*, 1983; Burges & Lang, 1987; Barnetson *et al.*, 1987; Beck & Korsgaard, 1989; Wühtrich, 1989). These authors have particularly emphasized, in some cases, the benefit of cleaning houses, aspiration of dust and removal of the patient from the allergenic domestic environment (Roberts, 1984).

Contact dermatitis specificities in atopic dermatitis

Bieber (1994) demonstrated that LC express three different receptors for IgE:
• High-affinity IgE receptor (FcεRI), usually found on mastocytes and basophils.
• Low-affinity IgE receptor (CD23/FcεRII).
• A lectin:IgE-binding protein (εBP).
In AD, the IgE high-affinity receptor is present in great quantity on LC. This is partly specific to AD and correlates with blood IgE. These receptors are present but included in the cytoplasm in normal LC; the LC in AD are unable to express these surface receptors.

Tanaka *et al.* (1989, 1990) have shown that aeroallergens such as dust mites are capable of penetrating the skin, using double immunolabelling, with immunofluorescence and electron microscopy. They traced the mite allergens during their penetration into the tissues. These allergens were found after 6 h in the epidermis, especially on the surface of LC (CD1+) which carry surface IgE. Then, after 24 and 48 h, mite allergens were found in the dermis, where they were captured by macrophages and so brought into close contact with T lymphocytes. This seemed to happen in the same way as in the inductive phase of contact eczema, but with one difference, namely the presence of IgE on the LC. The significant participation of polynuclear eosinophils should also be noted.

Bruijnzeel-Koomen *et al.* (1994) demonstrated that a positive patch test to an aeroallergen in AD is really a specific allergic reaction to an antigen. Culture of T lymphocytes extracted from skin biopsies of AD lesional skin reveals the presence of specific T lymphocytes for aeroallergens. After antigenic stimulation, these T lymphocytes produce interleukin-4 (IL-4) and interleukin-5 (IL-5) and only little or no γ-interferon (IFNγ), like TH2-type lymphocytes. The presence of aeroallergens in the skin initiates, in 12 h, an influx

of allergen-specific TH2 lymphocytes. They persist for at least 48 h at the site of the allergen application. The epidermal LC of injured skin cannot present aeroallergens to T lymphocytes unless they have surface-bound IgE. Clinically, there is a significant correlation between the presence of LC with surface IgE in the epidermis and the induction of positive patch tests to aeroallergens. In the first 24 h after the reaction, the lymphocytes produce IL-4 in particular, suggesting that they are a TH2 subgroup, but most also produce IFNγ showing that they are instead of a TH0 type. Around 48 h, the IL-4 reduces; the response tends towards TH1, and the production of cytokines approaches that found in AD-damaged skin. This was confirmed by Kubota *et al.* who showed that, in 23 AD with positive dust mite patch tests, at 72 h, T lymphocytes incubated with dust mites are of the TH1 type, producing IL-2 and IFNγ but no IL-4 (Kubota *et al.*, 1994).

Patch testing with aeroallergens in atopic dermatitis

After an initial study on delayed skin reactions to mite antigens (Castelain *et al.*, 1993), the GERDA (Groupe d'Etudes et de Recherches en Dermato-Allergologie) evaluated delayed patch tests with a panel of aeroallergens in AD (Castelain *et al.*, 1994), fulfilling Hanifin and Rajka's criteria (Hanifin & Rajka, 1980), versus a control population of non-atopic patients. The aim and the method of this study were to perform patch tests with the European standard procedure, and with current allergen dosage used for prick tests. We wanted thereby to prove the cutaneous allergenicity of aeroallergens in AD, in a relatively low concentration, comparable with those existing in the environment of atopic patients. We did not use any scratch or stripping test, to avoid technical difficulties and to let the dermatologist use the method he or she is trained in.

Our patch-test series included nine inhalant allergens known for their frequent involvement in respiratory allergy in France and Belgium:
• *Dermatophagoïdes pteronyssinus* (Dp) and *farinae* (Df), cat epithelial extract, pollen extracts of *Dactylis glomerata* and *Phleum pratense* at a concentration of 200 IR (*in vivo* reactivity index of aeroallergens) in Vaseline.
• Pollen extracts of *Artemisia vulgaris*, *Plantago*, park

tree mix and wet countries' tree mix, at a concentration of 1/20 (w/v). We performed prick tests with the same, but half-concentrated, products.

All the allergens were provided by Laboratoire Stallergènes (7 Allée des Platanes, F-94264 Fresnes Cedex, France).

We tested 450 AD patients fulfilling Hanifin and Rajka's criteria and 225 control subjects without AD.

One hundred and twelve AD patients (24.9%) had one or more patch tests positive with our AD series versus six of the controls (2.7%). We did not consider weak or doubtful reactions. The two mites totalled 122 of the 214 positive patch tests. We observed, moreover, 10 'angry backs' which we could not include in our results, and immediate reactions in a few cases.

There was no correlation between positive patch and prick tests in > 50% of cases. Moreover, there was no significant difference of positivity in AD between children and adults, except for the predominance of 'angry back' in children (9/10).

Two readings are necessary; 29.4% of positive tests are lost if only one reading is performed. The relevance of this kind of test is mostly difficult to ascertain and requires a follow-up of several years.

In a recent paper (Castelain, 1995), the present author pointed out the absence of standardization of material, methods and patients in former studies:

• Antigens for patch tests were very different in form, concentration, source and vehicle.

• The patch tests were often performed with additional artefacts such as stripping or repeated open application tests. Times of reading and duration of test application were exposed to great variations. Reading criteria were sometimes not specified.

• Some authors did not specify the inclusion criteria of AD patients. Some added restrictive inclusion criteria such as positive prick tests or radio-allergosorbent test (RAST) to dust mite or other aeroallergens.

• Some performed comparative tests on a healthy control population or control patients with contact allergy but without AD. Others did not perform any control.

• Some performed associated prick tests and/or evaluation of blood specific IgE level.

All these differences make for a very uneasy and unclear comparison of the results. From the epidemi-

ological point of view, it is very difficult to come to a definite conclusion for these studies. More recent studies (Castelain *et al.*, 1994; Gaddoni *et al.*, 1994; Darsow *et al.*, 1995; Manzini *et al.*, 1995) try to establish a new standardization of patch tests with aeroallergens. They use commercial preparations from known laboratories, incorporated in petrolatum, and perform patch tests on the normal skin of the back, with ICDRG standard procedures and reading criteria. The patients are included into the study by fulfilling specific criteria of AD and compared with non-atopic control subjects. The most studied allergens are dust mites. The number of tested AD vary from 36 to 313, and the percentage of positive results to mites from 28 to 72%, with a mean score of 39%. The percentage of positive results seems to be correlated with the concentration of allergens, but irritative results are rare for some authors or exist but are not taken into account for others.

There is no evident correlation between positive patch tests and corresponding prick tests or RAST. Moreover, Imayama *et al.* (1992) establish several clinical profiles according to the positivity of patch tests alone, RAST alone or both.

Conclusion

Aeroallergen-delayed hypersensitivity exists in some patients with atopic eczema and this can be shown by patch tests.

The involvement of delayed hypersensitivity in the elicitation of skin lesions is not yet obvious, but seems to be probable, from the induction of syndrome reactions by the tests, the worsening of some patients in the presence of allergens like pollens and the improvement of patients who are sensitive to dust or its allergenic fractions by removal of dust from the habitat.

The great problem is now the definition of a new standard of aeroallergens for patch tests. Because of regional variations, it does not seem to be possible to define a standard series of inhalant allergens for patch tests. However, recent results are corroborative and encourage the exploration of this type of allergic study in AD.

References

Barnetson, R.S.C., McFarlane, H.A.F. & Bentone, C. (1987) House dust mite allergy and atopic eczema: a case report. *British Journal of Dermatology*, **116**, 857–860.

Beck, H.I. & Korsgaard, J. (1989) Atopic dermatitis and house dust mites. *British Journal of Dermatology*, **120**, 245–251.

Bieber, T. (1994) FcεRI on human Langerhans cells: a receptor in search of new functions. *Immunology Today*, **15**, 52–53.

Bruijnzeel-Koomen, C.A.F.M., van Wichen, D.F., Toonstra, J., Berrens, L. & Bruijnzeel, P.L.B. (1986) The presence of IgE molecules on epidermal Langerhans cells in patients with atopic dermatitis. *Archives of Dermatological Research*, **278**, 199–205.

Bruijnzeel-Koomen, C., van Reijsen, F., Langeveld-Wildschut, E. *et al.* (1994) Allergens and atopic eczema. In: *Postgraduate Course in Allergological Aspects of Dermatology, Proceedings of ICACI XV EAACI '94 Stockholm*, 26 June–1 July 1994, pp. 89–99.

Burges, C.E. & Lang, P.G. (1987) Atopic dermatitis exacerbated by inhalant allergens. *Archives of Dermatology*, **123**, 1437–1438.

Castelain, M. (1995) Atopic dermatitis and delayed hypersensitivity to dust mites. *Clinical Reviews in Allergy and Immunology*, **13**, 161–172.

Castelain, M., Birnbaum, J., Castelain, P.-Y. *et al.* (1993) Patch-test reactions to mite antigens: a GERDA multicenter study. *Contact Dermatitis*, **29**, 246–250.

Castelain, M., Barbaud, A., Dooms-Goossens, A. *et al.* (1994) Patch test reactions to aeroallergens and *Staphylococcus*: results of a GERDA multicentre study. In: *Second Congress of the European Society of Contact Dermatitis, Barcelona, 6–8 October 1994*. Programme abstract book, p. 69.

Darsow, U., Vieluf, D. & Ring, J. (1995) Atopy patch test with different vehicles and allergen concentrations: An approach to standardization. *Journal of Allergy and Clinical Immunology*, **3**, 677–684.

Gaddoni, G., Baldassari, L. & Zucchini, A. (1994) A new patch test preparation of dust mites for atopic dermatitis. *Contact Dermatitis*, **31**, 132–133.

Hanifin, J.M. & Rajka, G. (1980) Diagnostic features of atopic dermatitis. *Acta Dermato-Venereologica (Stockholm)*, **92** (Suppl.), 44–47.

Imayama, S., Hashizume, T., Miyahara, H. *et al.* (1992) Combination of patch test and IgE for dust mite antigens differentiates 130 patients with atopic dermatitis into four groups. *Journal of the American Academy of Dermatology*, **27**, 531–538.

Kubota, Y., Koga, T., Imayama, S. & Hori, H. (1994) Mite-antigen-stimulated cytokine production by peripheral blood mononuclear cells of atopic dermatitis patients with positive mite patch tests. *Contact Dermatitis*, **31**, 217–219.

Manzini, B.M., Motolese, A., Donini, M. & Seidenari, S. (1995) Contact allergy to *Dermatophagoides* in atopic dermatitis patients and healthy subjects. *Contact Dermatitis*, **33**, 243–246.

Platts-Mills, T.A.E., Mitchell, E.B., Rowntree, S. *et al.* (1983) The role of dust mite allergens in atopic dermatitis. *Clinical and Experimental Dermatology*, **8**, 233–247.

Roberts, D.L.L. (1984) House dust mite avoidance and atopic dermatitis. *British Journal of Dermatology*, **110**, 735–736.

Tanaka, Y., Tanaka, M., Anan, S. & Yoshida, H. (1989) Immunohistochemical studies on dust mite antigen in positive reaction site of patch test. *Acta Dermato-Venereologica (Stockholm)*, **69** (Suppl. 144), 93–96.

Tanaka, Y., Anan, S. & Yoshida, H. (1990) Immunohistochemical studies in mite antigen-induced patch test sites in atopic dermatitis. *Journal of Dermatology (Tokyo)*, **1**, 361–368.

Wühtrich, B. (1989) Atopic dermatitis flare provoked by inhalant allergens. *Dermatologica*, **178**, 51–53.

Can We Prevent Atopic Dermatitis?

A. TAÏEB

Introduction

Heredity and environment are closely associated in the pathogenesis of atopic diseases. Among these, atopic dermatitis (AD), the first objective marker of atopy, is increasing steadily in Western countries, especially within the paediatric age group. Mild cases are very common and current figures for prevalence in population-based studies are ≥15% in northern European countries. If AD may just precede respiratory involvement which causes more morbidity and mortality, AD by itself represents a real burden for affected children and their families. Thus, several arguments for prophylaxis (reviewed in Björkstén, 1991) may be put forward. However, there are major reasons hindering carrying out such a policy.

Population-based prevention

Heredity is clearly demonstrated in AD but its striking increase in incidence over the past decades is probably more linked to environmental or sociocultural changes, and some agents or behavioural modifications have been pointed out, such as irritancy due to more hygiene and washing, urban dwelling and air pollution, changes in feeding practices especially breast-feeding, delayed aged for pregnancies, attendance at day-care centres and season of birth. However, epidemiological studies have not so far designed one culprit amenable to reasonable preventive measures at the population level. On the genetic side, discouraging atopics to have children together, a real factor of increased risk, could be termed, at the very least, unethical.

Family-based prevention

Affected individuals should be made aware of the risks for their children by their physicians. Passive smoking should be especially targeted for prevention (Cogswell *et al.*, 1987). There is an agreement to reduce critical household aeroallergen exposure especially for mites and domestic animals (Platts-Mills *et al.*, 1993, Anonymous, 1994) mostly with respect to respiratory symptoms. The strategy to reduce the level of mite allergen to $<2\,\mu g/g$ of dust has been clearly delineated (Platts-Mills *et al.*, 1993). Aeroallergens, like mites, may contribute significantly to skin symptoms as contact allergens and this could be demonstrated by patch testing even in very young children (Taïeb & Ducombs, 1996). Information concerning the prevention of allergic disorders through feeding habits remains more controversial, if not biased, by conflicts of interest. Infant-milk companies have intensively marketed so-called 'hypoallergenic products' which provide no clear short- or long-term benefit for children. Data concerning extensive hydrolysates of casein have shown a slight benefit in terms of prevalence of eczema for hydrolysates when compared to adapted formula in patients receiving this regimen for the first 4 months; however, the number of patients was small (Mallet & Henocq, 1992). Data concerning soy protein formulas are even more controversial (reviewed in Businco *et al.*, 1992). Breast-feeding as a prophylaxis for atopic disease has been the subject of much debate. In a recent long-term Finnish prospective study, breast-feeding was found to be protective against atopic dermatitis but also other atopic manifestations up to the age of 17 years old. Surprisingly, the differences due to breast-feeding were more pronounced than those due to heredity at the age of 17 years (Saarinen & Kajosaari, 1995). There is further evidence to suggest that avoidance of cows' milk, eggs and fish during the first 3 months of lactation may reduce the prevalence of AD (Arshad *et al.*, 1992; Sigurs *et al.*, 1992). There are also data indicating that early feeding of solids predisposes susceptible children to recurrent or chronic childhood eczema (Fergusson *et al.*, 1990). However delayed introduction of allergens without associated breast-feeding may simply postpone, and not prevent, food allergy and AD. On the contrary, a recent prospective study in children followed from birth to the age of 7 years failed to demonstrate any long-term benefit on AD and other atopic symptoms of a combined approach using breast-feeding with a hypoallergenic diet by the mother plus a casein hydrolysate in the first year of life and delayed introduction of food allergens (Zeiger & Heller, 1995). However, a confounding factor might be that the control group had also prolonged breast-feeding.

The future of prophylaxis in atopic dermatitis

A more targeted policy for prevention may be available in the future if sensitive and specific probes for atopy are available at birth, or even before. Current data indicate that antenatal IgE-mediated sensitization exists. Early immunomodulation when lymphocytes undergo thymic education may be helpful to down-regulate TH2 pathways (Tang *et al.*, 1994; Warner *et al.*, 1994). Candidate immunomodulatory molecules already exist, especially interferon-γ, eicosanoids and unsaturated fatty acids. Later in established lesions of AD, interleukin-10 (IL-10) seems to be the predominant cytokine and IL-12 might be a valuable antagonist (Ohmen *et al.*, 1995).

The other possibility for prevention which has not been well developed so far concerns the epithelial barriers, either mucous or cutaneous. The irritant and allergenic load from the environment may be lowered if we can implement specific protective measures. For skin, emollients which increase the impaired barrier function of atopic individuals (Tupker *et al.*, 1990) could be used on a preventive basis in association with the usual measures to avoid irritancy and non-specific reactivity. A particularly prudent approach is needed to avoid sensitization to contact allergens which is a most prevalent problem in AD patients (Uehara & Sawai, 1989; De Groot, 1990; Cronin & McFadden, 1993).

Interventional epidemiological studies are needed to establish whether such a strategy can only delay the onset of atopic symptoms or induce long-term tolerance.

Conclusion

The current medical guidelines for nursing at-risk babies should be given more publicity, especially those for prolonged breast-feeding (6 months) and the delayed introduction of solid foods. The modification of the mother's feeding habits is not supported by enough data to be advocated. For most items, like skin care and irritancy, general hygiene, smoking and inhalant allergens such as mites and pets, more family-oriented information should be available to high-risk individuals. It would be also of interest to release information to the general population through appropriate media campaigns because of the magnitude of the problem. Gynaecologists, midwives, general practitioners, paediatricians and paediatric nurses should be primarily involved in such a programme. Dermatologists who frequently attend infants should be aware of the continued spectrum of atopy, of which AD is in most cases the first clinical marker. Their impact in managing AD should not be limited to prescribe emollients, topical steroids and anti-histamines, but they should implement prophylactic measures concerning aeroallergens and contact allergy, together with other physicians, namely allergists, paediatricians and general practitioners (Cooper & Taïeb, 1988). Drug prophylaxis of asthma is currently being studied in large-scale studies like the ETAC (Early Treatment of the Atopic Child) study with cetirizine and early intervention on air-way non-specific inflammation might be proposed in AD infants if convincing data appear. Later in life, counselling concerning professional occupation should be systematically given to AD patients, especially with hand dermatitis.

References

Anonymous (1994) *Workshop Report: Environmental Measures in the Prevention of Allergy. The UCB Institute of Allergy*, St Mary's Hospital, Newport, Isle of Wight, UK.

Arshad, S.H., Matthews, S., Gant, C. & Hide, D.W. (1992) Effect of allergen avoidance on development of allergic disorders in infancy. *Lancet*, **339**, 1493–1497.

Björkstén, B. (1991) Atopic prophylaxis. In: *Handbook of Atopic Eczema* (eds J. Ring & B. Przybilla), pp. 339–344. Springer, Berlin.

Businco, L., Bruno, G., Giampietro, P.G. & Cantani, A. (1992) Allergenicity and nutritional adequacy of soy protein formulas. *Journal of Pediatrics*, **121**, S21–S28.

Cogswell, J.J., Mitchell, E.B. & Alexander, J. (1987) Parental smoking, breast feeding and respiratory infection in development of allergic disease. *Archives of Disease in Childhood*, **62**, 338–344.

Cooper, K.D. & Taïeb, A. (1988) Atopic dermatitis. In: *Current Therapy in Allergy, Immunology and Rheumatology* (eds L.M. Lichenstein & A.S. Fauci), pp. 177–182. Dekker, Toronto.

Croner, S. & Kjellman, N.I.M. (1990) Development of atopic diseases in relation to family history and cord blood IgE levels. Eleven-year follow-up in 1654 children. *Pediatric Allergy and Immunology*, **1**, 14–20.

Cronin, E. & McFadden, J.P. (1993) Patients with atopic eczema do become sensitized to contact allergens. *Contact Dermatitis*, **28**, 225–228.

De Groot, A. (1990) The frequency of contact allergy in atopic patients with dermatitis. *Contact Dermatitis*, **22**, 273–277.

Fergusson, D.M., Horwood, J. & Shannon, F.T. (1990) Early solid feeding and recurrent childhood eczema: a 10-year longitudinal study. *Pediatrics*, **86**, 541–546.

Mallet, E. & Henocq, A. (1992) Long-term prevention of allergic diseases by using protein hydrolysate formula in at-risk infants. *Journal of Pediatrics*, **121**, S95–S100.

Ohmen, J.D., Hanifin, J.M., Nickoloff, B.J. et al. (1995) Overexpression of IL-10 in atopic dermatitis. Contrasting cytokine patterns with delayed-type hypersensitivity reactions. *Journal of Immunology*, **154**, 1956–1963.

Platts-Mills, T.A.E., Thomas, W.R., Aalberse, R.C. et al. (1993) Dust mite allergens and asthma: report of a second international workshop. *Journal of Allergy and Clinical Immunology*, **89**, 1046–1060.

Saarinen, U.M. & Kajosaari, M. (1995) Breastfeeding as prophylaxis against atopic disease: prospective follow-up study until 17 years old. *Lancet*, **346**, 1065–1069.

Sigurs, N., Hattevig, G. & Kjellman, B. (1992) Maternal avoidance of eggs, cow's milk, and fish during lactation: effect on allergic manifestations, skin prick tests, and specific IgE antibodies at age 4 years. *Pediatrics*, **89**, 735–739.

Taïeb, A. & Ducombs, J. (1996) Aeroallergen contact dermatitis. *Clinical Reviews in Allergy and Immunology*, **14**, 209–223.

Tang, M.L.K., Kemp, A.S., Thorburn, J. & Hill, D.J. (1994) Reduced interferon-γ secretion in neonates and subsequent atopy. *Lancet*, **344**, 983–985.

Tupker, R.E., Pinnagoda, J., Coenraads, P.J. & Nater, J.P.

(1990) Susceptibility to irritants: role of barrier function, skin dryness and history of atopic dermatitis. *British Journal of Dermatology*, **123**, 199–205.

Uehara, M. & Sawai, T. (1989) A longitudinal study of contact sensitivity in patients with atopic dermatitis. *Archives of Dermatology*, **125**, 366–368.

Warner, J.A., Miles, E.A., Jones, A.C., Guint, D.J., Colwel, B.M. & Warner, J.O. (1994) Is deficiency of interferon gamma production by allergen triggered cord-blood cells a predictor of atopic eczema? *Clinical and Experimental Allergy*, **24**, 423–430.

Zeiger, R.S. & Heller, S. (1995) The development and prediction of atopy in high-risk children: follow-up at age seven years in a prospective randomized study of combined maternal and infant food allergen avoidance. *Journal of Allergy and Clinical Immunology*, **95**, 1179–1190.

15
Fungal Skin Diseases

Epidemiology of Fungal Diseases

E.L. SVEJGAARD

Introduction

The mycoses include the superficial, the subcutaneous and the systemic mycoses. Some mycoses are limited to restricted geographical areas due to the organism's demand for a special environment (plants, animals) or to a warm, humid climate, while others are found all over the populated world. Some are caused by primary pathogenic organisms, for instance *Cocciodioides immitis* and the dermatophytes, while opportunistic less-virulent saphrophytes, which may find a niche in a compromised host, are responsible for a growing number of all three groups of mycoses. The new trends in the epidemiology of mycoses are often found in the latter group. Generally speaking, three factors are responsible for the changes we see in developed countries during the last decades. First, life expectancy has improved for both the newborn and elderly. Newborns with very low birthweight and an immature immune system are kept alive artificially, often with intravenous lipid nourishment, which may establish a substrate for fungal growth. In old people, a natural ageing of normal defence mechanisms physically and immunologically disposes for fungal invasion. Diseases related to old age like diabetes mellitus also increase the risk for mycotic infection.

Second, from the beginning of the 1980s, the acquired immune deficiency syndrome (AIDS) has been an essential factor. The gradually decreasing number of T lymphocytes during the course of the disease predisposes the patient to many inflammatory skin diseases, including superficial mycoses and, more rarely, systemic.

Third, iatrogenic factors play a role. Many autoimmune, malignant, immunodeficiency and endocrine diseases can now be kept under control for years due to medical progress, resulting in better and longer lives. However, the use of corticosteroids, cytostatics, hormones, antibiotics and, in addition, antimycotics inevitably results in various unwanted effects like depressed T-cell-dependent immune responses, neutropenia, a selection of other infections and a selection of resistant strains. This review largely includes experiences and reports from Western countries and does not pretend to be a global overview.

The superficial mycoses

These include dermatophytosis, candidosis, pityrosporosis, *Hendersonula/Scytalidium* infections, tinea nigra and black-and-white piedra.

Piedra is caused by *Trichosporum* species and is a benign disorder with nodular elements on axillary and genital hair but this genus is also able to cause systemic infection in the immunocompromised host and, in addition, is found in onychomycosis. *Hendersonula/Scytalidium* species produces tinea-like infections and is seen with increasing frequency in the UK, related to immigrants from the West Indies (Gueho *et al.*, 1994; Clayton, 1977).

The distribution of dermatophytes and dermatophytosis has been followed closely in many countries for nearly 100 years, especially those countries with former colonies in Africa and the Far East. The distribution, as well as the clinical picture, has changed and is still changing (Rippon, 1985). In Europe, tinea capitis was very frequent in both children and adults at the beginning of the century and was caused by anthropophilic species, especially *Trichophyton schoenleini*. Later, during the Second World War, epidemics were due to *Microsporum audouini* in the west, *Trichophyton violaceum* in the east and *T. megnini* in various parts of Europe (Binazzi *et al.*, 1983). Thanks to griseofulvin, introduced in the 1950s, control of these infections was achieved. Actually, these old anthropophilic species have nearly vanished but have been replaced by *T. rubrum*, first identified in Europe in 1937. It is generally considered to have been introduced into Europe and the United States from the Far East during the Second World War. It is noteworthy that the clinical picture in the temperate zones gradually has changed from inflamed tinea corporis in the original tropical area to the usually less inflammatory disorders of the feet, groin and nails, along with a change in morphology which became less sporulating and downy (English, 1980). *T. rubrum* is now, worldwide, the most common cause of tinea pedis, cruris and unguis, being the most common dermatophyte infections in European countries such as the UK and Denmark (Fig. 15.1), France, Germany and Switzerland. Apart from *T. rubrum*, other anthropophilic species like *T. mentagrophytes* and *E. floccosum* are usually isolated from these mycoses (Clayton, 1977; Foged & Nielsen, 1982; Svejgaard, 1986; Colomb

et al., 1987; Knoll & Reinert, 1989; Monod *et al.*, 1992). It is generally agreed that sport activities, extensive use of athletic shoes and communal bathing are essential epidemiological factors for the spread of tinea pedis and unguis. The incidence of dermatophyte infections in immunocompromised patients does not seem to be higher than in normal individuals, but the course of the disease is often altered to a more widespread, deep or clinically unusual picture (Torssander *et al.*, 1988; Odom, 1994).

During the 1970s and 1980s, the most frequently isolated zoophilic species has become *M. canis* which causes tinea capitis and corporis, mainly in children. In some East European countries the increase of this infection has been substantial, e.g. Slovenia (Fig. 15.2) (Lunder & Lunder, 1992), Poland (Wiekowska & Nawiecki, 1990) and Armenia (Danielan & Mokrousov, 1992). In the big cities of Italy (Caprilli *et al.*, 1986; Difonzo *et al.*, 1986; De Silverio *et al.*, 1989; Sberna *et al.*, 1993), *M. canis* is responsible for most cases of tinea capitis and corporis, and is the dominant species followed by *T. rubrum*, *E. floccosum* and *T. mentagrophytes*. The epidemiological source of *M. canis* is stray cats, inadequately controlled, combined with overpopulation, poverty and poor hygienic standards. Often preventive procedures have been unsuccessful.

Local factors may, in a big country, give a varied distribution pattern. In Spain, *M. canis* is frequent in Madrid, *T. mentagrophytes* in Catalonia (due to rabbits) and *T. verrucosum* is nearly exclusively confined to the

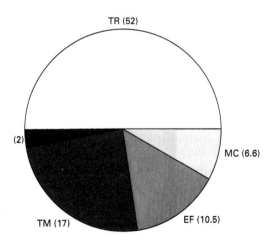

Fig. 15.1 Distribution of dermatophytes in Denmark 1969–80. TR, *Trichophyton rubrum*; TM, *T. mentagrophytes*; EF, *Epidermophyton floccosum*; MC, *Microsporum canis*; Tviol, *T. violaceum*.

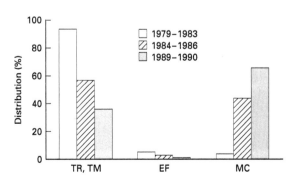

Fig. 15.2 Distribution of dermatophytes in Slovenia, 1979–90. TR, *Trichophyton rubrum*; TM, *T. mentagrophytes*; EF, *Epidermophyton floccosum*; MC, *Microsporum canis*.

Salamanca area where cattle are common (Velasco Benito *et al.*, 1979; Torres-Rodriquez *et al.*, 1986; Palacio Hernanz *et al.*, 1989; Pereiro Miguens *et al.*, 1991).

Tinea capitis due to anthropophilic species, however, has not been eradicated at all. *T. tonsurans* is now the most frequent cause of the disease in North America (Sinski & Kelley, 1991; Rippon, 1992) and is usually seen in Iceland and Australia. In North Africa and other Mediterranean countries, *T. violaceum* is a frequent cause of tinea capitis. Immigrants from these zones seem to be the source of a growing number of cases of tinea capitis due to anthropophilic species in northern countries, often spread through infant schools. In Denmark, the number of isolated *T. violaceum* cases has doubled during the last few years (Stenderup, 1994; pers. commun.). In the big cities of the UK, Holland and France, the impact of immigration is expressed   in an increasing number of patients with tinea capitis due to imported exotic anthropophilic species (Clayton & Midgely, 1977; van der Willingen *et al.*, 1990, Dardé, 1992).

Changes in the pattern of dermatophytoses caused by anthropophilic dermatophytes can thus be explained by the increase in migration and other forms of travel activity, change in life habits, including sport activities, environmental factors and the use of griseofulvin. For zoophilic infections, animal contacts, rural environment, low hygienic standards, overpopulation and, in addition, virulence factors play a role. The virulence of zoophilic species is generally considered higher than that of anthropophilic species due to a more extensive proteolytic activity (Table 15.1).

Pityrosporosis is caused by *Pityrosporum ovale* or *Malassezia furfur*, a lipophilic yeast, which is a member of the natural skin flora and present in the skin from early childhood in seborrhoic areas. Pityriasis versicolor and *Pityrosporum* folliculitis are the primary *Pityrosporum*-related diseases. For some years, however, interest in this organism has increased and it has been found to be related to other skin diseases like seborrhoic dermatitis, atopic dermatitis and psoriasis. Its role as the aetiological factor in seborrhoic dermatitis is still under discussion (Groisser *et al.*, 1989; Schechtman *et al.*, 1995). In atopic dermatitis, it seems able to trigger exacerbations (Kieffer *et al.*, 1990). *Pityrosporum*-related skin disorders are often seen in immunocompromised patients such as AIDS patients and organ-transplanted individuals under immunosuppressive therapy (Odom, 1994). *Pityrosporum* has been found to have inflammatory properties related to specific and non-specific immune-defence mechanisms. Finally, *M. furfur* has been identified as the cause of systemic infection in patients receiving intravenous lipids (Walsh *et al.*, 1994).

Superficial candidosis: the yeasts, *Candida albicans* and *C. glabrata*, are often found as part of the normal microflora of the mucosal membranes. The gastrointestinal tract is considered the main reservoir, but not all are colonized with *Candida*. A suggestion built on published data is that 14% of carriers have yeast in the mouth, 24% in the lower bowel and 10% in the vagina. In most carriers, 60–75%, the yeast is *C. albicans*, while *C. glabrata* is the second most frequent (Roberts *et al.*, 1984). The predisposing factors for developing an infection with *Candida* species are listed in Table 15.2.

In HIV-infected individuals, the appearance of candidosis of the oral, oesophageal or vaginal mucosal membranes is closely related to the number of CD4 T cells in the blood. Thus, the degree of morbidity due to candidosis may be considered a significant marker

Table 15.1 Epidemiological factors in dermatophytosis.

Anthropophilic	Zoophilic
Migration	Animal contacts
Sports activities	Environment (rural)
Immune incompetence	Poor hygiene
Environment (urban)	Overpopulation
Griseofulvin	Virulence

Table 15.2 Predisposing factors in superficial candidosis.

Host factors	Iatrogenic factors
Age (infancy/old age)	Antibiotics
Obesity	Immunosuppressives
Alcoholism	Cytostatics
Atopy	
Epithelial defects	
Malnutrition	
Endocrine disorders	
HIV infection	

of the patient's immune function. In HIV-infected patients, superficial candidosis rarely develops into invasive disease. On the other hand, superficial candidosis may, rarely, be secondary to systemic mycoses in otherwise immunosuppressed patients (Dupont *et al.*, 1994).

Subcutaneous mycoses

These are also called the mycoses of implantation (Table 15.3) because it is believed that the causative fungi enter the skin through contaminated plant material, e.g. thorns. Clinically, these infections are characterized by invasion of the dermis, the subcutaneous tissues and lymph nodes. They are geographically restricted to tropical zones, but may appear sporadically everywhere. In immunocompromised patients, there seems to be a risk for dissemination of these diseases.

Systemic mycoses

These may be divided into two groups (Table 15.4): one group is caused by primary pathogenic organisms like *Histoplasma capsulatum*, *Blastomyces dermatitis* and *Coccidioides immitis*, and are seen in normal immuno-

competent individuals, as well as in the immunocompromised hosts, such as AIDS patients. These infections occur predominantly in certain areas in North and South America. The mycoses of the second group are caused by opportunistic agents and occur worldwide in immunocompromised hosts. Candidosis is the most common invasive mycosis in patients with neoplastic disorders, in patients receiving cytostatics and immunosuppressive treatment and in organ-transplanted, especially bone-marrow transplanted, patients. Lack of neutrophils for shorter or longer periods disposes for invasive infection (Table 15.5). In patients with a T-cell deficiency, such as in AIDS, disseminated candidosis is rare, while superficial *Candida* infection is a major problem. The reason for this diversity is that cell-mediated immunity is the primary host defence against superficial candidosis and neutrophils are the essential host-defence mechanism against disseminated candidosis. *Cryptococcus meningitis* is seen relatively often in AIDS patients and, in addition, a number of other unusual yeast infections have been reported (Table 15.6). These include fungaemia with *Saccharomyces cerevisiae* and *Rhodotorula rubra*, osteomyelitis due to *Candida glabrata* and meningitis due to *Cryptococcus clavatus*. In addition to *Aspergillus*, mould infections, superficial and systemic, with *Rhizopus*, *Absidia*, *Fusarium*, *Alternaria curvularia* and many others are reported, often with unusual clinical

Table 15.3 Subcutaneous mycoses.

Sporotrichosis
Chromomycosis
Phaeohyphomycosis
Rhinosporodiosis
Lobomycosis
Mycetoma

Table 15.4 Systemic mycoses.

Primary	Opportunistic
Histoplasmosis	Candidosis
Coccidioidomycosis	Aspergillosis
Cryptococcosis	Cryptococcosis
Paracoccidioidomycosis	Zygomycosis
Blastomycosis	Hyalohyphomycosis
	Phaeohyphomycosis
	Penicilliosis

Table 15.5 Neutropenic patients: predisposing diseases and mycoses.

Predisposing diseases
Malignant disorders
Lymphoma
Myelodysplastic syndrome
Bone-marrow transplantation

Most common mycoses
Candidosis
Aspergillosis

New trends in pathogens
Fusarium sp.
Dematiaceous fungi
Trichosporon
Cryptococcus neoformans
Zygomycetes
Resistant strains of *Candida*

Table 15.6 Mycoses in T lymphocyte deficiency/HIV infection.

Cryptococcal meningitis
Invasive candidosis rare
Penicillium marneffei infection
Aspergillosis
Sporotrichosis
Paracoccidioidomycosis
Blastomycosis
Unusual mycoses

---

manifestations (Dupont *et al.*, 1994). Special interest has been devoted to infections caused by *Penicillium marneffei*. This organism, which was first isolated in Vietnam in 1956 from a bamboo rat, may cause skin infections or disseminated mycoses. Only a few cases were seen before the AIDS epidemic in Thailand and other areas of South-East Asia, the first in 1973 in a patient with Hodgkin's disease. HIV-related infection with *P. marneffei* has been reported since 1987. The first was diagnosed in Chicago, but most cases have been reported from Thailand, while a few HIV-positive individuals from USA, Australia and European countries were infected when visiting the endemic area. The geographical distribution of the organism is believed to be wide throughout South-East Asia. It is not yet clear whether bamboo rats are an important reservoir for *P. marneffei* or whether the organism is to be found in some environmental source. Most likely, soil could be a reservoir, from which fungal spores might be transmitted to animals or humans by inhalation, analogous to other pathogenic dismorphic fungi, like *Histoplasma capsulatum* and *Coccidioides immitis*. The epidemiology, pathogenesis and natural history of *P. marneffei* infections are still partly unclear, and more information is needed about this new HIV-related pathogen (Dupont *et al.*, 1994).

Conclusion

Several host factors such as lifespan, lifestyle, migration and HIV infection are responsible for the change in incidence and the clinical manifestations of mycotic disease. Also, parasitic factors play a role. New opportunistic pathogens causing new characteristic diseases have emerged. And finally, the development

of resistant strains of certain *Candida* species (Odds, 1987) along with the intensive use of broad-spectrum antifungal agents in immunosuppressed patients may lead to new patterns in the epidemiology of fungal infections.

References

Binazzi, M., Papini, M. & Simonetti, S. (1983) Skin mycoses — geographic distribution and present-day pathomorphosis. *International Journal of Dermatology*, **22**, 92–97.

Caprilli, F., Mercantini, R., Polamava, G. *et al.* (1986) Distribution and frequency of dermatophytes in the City of Rome between 1978 and 1983. *Mykosen*, **30**(2), 86–93.

Clayton, Y.M. (1977) Epidemiological aspects of dermatophyte infections. *Current Therapeutic Research*, **22**(1), 2–9.

Clayton, Y.M. & Midgeley, G. (1977) Tinea capitis bei Schulkindern in London. *Der Hautartzt*, **28**, 32–34.

Colomb, D., Battesti, M.R. & Cognot, Th. (1987) Evolution des epidermomycoses et de leurs agents en region Lyonnaise. *Annales Dermatologie et Venereologie*, **114**, 515–521.

Danielan, E.E. & Mokrousov, M.S. (1992) Epidemiology of trichophytosis, microsporosis, and favus in Armenia over 36 years (1955–90). *Vestnik Dermatologie et Venereologie*, **2**, 58–60.

Dardé, M.L. (1992) Epidemiologie des dermatophytics. *Annales Dermatologie et Venereologie*, **11**, 99–100.

Dupont, B., Denning, D.W., Marriott, D., Sugar, H., Viviani, M.S. & Sirisanthana, T. (1994) Mycoses in AIDS patients. *Journal of Medical and Veterinarian Mycology*, **32** (Suppl 1), 65–77.

De Silverio, A., Mosca, M., Gatti, M. *et al.* (1989) Superficial mycoses observed at the Department of Dermatology of the University of Pavia. *Mycopathologia*, **105**, 11–17.

Difonzo, E.M., Palleichi, G.M., Guadagni, R. *et al.* (1986) Epidemiology of the dermatophytoses in the Florence area: 1982–1984. I. *Microsporum canis* infections. *Mykosen*, **29**(11), 519–525.

English, M.P. (1980) Ecological aspects of dermatophytes regarded essentially as anthropophilic. In: *Medical Mycology*, Vol. 261, Bacteriology Suppl 8, pp. 53–58. Gustav Fischer Verlag, Stuttgart.

Foged, E.K. & Nielsen, T. (1982) Etiology of dermatophytosis in Denmark based on material of 1070 cases. *Mykosen*, **25**(3), 121–125.

Groisser, D., Bottone, E.F. & Lebwohl, M. (1989) Association of *Pityrosporum orbiculare (Malassezia furfur)* with acquired immunodeficiency syndrome (AIDS). *Journal of the American Academy of Dermatology*, **20**, 770–773.

Gueho, E., Faergemann, J., Lyman, D. & Anaissie, E.J. (1994)

Malassezia and *Trichosporon*: two emerging pathogenic basidiomycetous yeast-like fungi. *Journal of Medical and Veterinary Mycology*, **32** (Suppl 1), 367–378.

Kieffer, M., Bergbrant, I.-M., Faergemann, J. *et al.* (1990) Immune reactions to *Pityrosporum ovale* in adult patients with atopic and seborrheic dermatitis. *Journal of the American Academy of Dermatology*, **22**, 739–742.

Knoll, R. & Reinert, D. (1989) Dermatophyte flora in a catchment area of the Hamburg Military Hospital. *Zeitschrift für Hautkrankheiten*, **64**(8), 670–676.

Lunder, M. & Lunder, M. (1992) Is *Microsporum canis* infection about to become a serious dermatological problem? *Dermatology*, **184**, 87–89.

Monod, M., Baudraz-Rosselet, F., Porchet, S. *et al.* (1992) Dermatophytes isolated in Switzerland: proposal of a simple key for identification. *Der Hautarzt*, **43**(5), 294–297.

Odds, F.C. (1987) Resistance of yeasts to azole-derivative antifungals. *Journal of Medical and Veterinarian Mycology*, **25**, 29–37.

Odom, R.B. (1994) Common superficial fungal infections in immunosuppressed patients. *Journal of the American Academy of Dermatology*, **31**, 56–59.

Palacio Hernanz, A. del, Gonzalez Lastra, F. & Moreno Palancar, P. (1989) Survey of dermatophytosis in Madrid during a decade (1978–1987). *Revista Iberica de Micologia*, **6**(2), 86–101.

Pereiro Miguens, M., Pereiro, M. & Pereiro, Jr M. (1991) Review of dermatophytoses in Galicia from 1951 to 1987, and comparison with other areas of Spain. *Mycopathologia*, **113**, 65–78.

Rippon, J.W. (1985) The changing epidemiology and emerging patterns of dermatophyte species. *Current Topical Medical Mycology*, **1**, 208–234.

Rippon, J.W. (1992) Forty four years of dermatophytes in a Chicago clinic (1944–1988). *Mycopathologia*, **119**, 25–28.

Roberts, S.O.B., Hay, R.F. & Mackenzie, D.W.R. (1984) The superficial mycoses. In: *A Clinician's Guide to Fungal Disease*, pp. 44–45. Marcel Dekker Inc., New York.

Sberna, F., Farella, F., Geti, V. *et al.* (1993) Epidemiology of the dermatophytoses of the Florence area of Italy: 1985–1990. *Trichophyton mentagrophytes, Epidermophyton floccosum* and *Microsporum gypseum* infections. *Mycopathologia*, **122**(3), 153–162.

Schechtman, R.C., Midgley, G. & Hay, R.J. (1995) HIV disease and *Malassezia* yeasts: a quantitative study of patients presenting with seborrhoeic dermatitis. *British Journal of Dermatology*, **133**, 694–698.

Sinski, J.T. & Kelley, L.M. (1991) A survey of dermatophytes from human patients in the United States from 1985–1987. *Mycopathologia*, **114**(2), 117–126.

Stenderup, J. (1994) *Reports from the Danish Society of Mycopathology 1994*. Danish Society of Mycopathology, Copenhagen.

Svejgaard, E. (1986) Epidemiology and clinical features of dermatomycoses and dermatophytoses. *Acta Dermato-Venereologica (Stockholm)*, (Suppl 121), 19–26.

Torres-Rodriguez, J.M., Balaguer-Meler, J., Ventin-Hernandez, M. *et al.* (1986) Multicenter study of dermatophyte distribution in the metropolitan area of Barcelona (Catalonia, Spain). *Mycopathologia*, **93**, 95–97.

Torssander, J., Karlsson, A., Morfeldt-Manson, L. *et al.* (1988) Dermatophytosis and HIV infection. A study in homosexual men. *Acta Dermato-Venereologica*, **68**(1), 53–56.

van der Willingen, A.H., Orange, A.P., de Weerdt van Ameijden, S. & Wagenvoort, J.H. (1990) Tinea capitis in The Netherlands (Rotterdam area). *Mycoses*, **33**(1), 46–50.

Velasco Benito, J.A., Martin-Pascual, A. & Garcia Pérez, A. (1979) Epidemiologic study of dermatophytoses in Salamanca (Spain). *Sabouraudia*, **17**, 113–123.

Walsh, T.J., Pauw, B. De., Anaissie, E. & Martioro, P. (1994) Recent advances in the epidemiology, prevention and treatment of invasive fungal infections in neutropenic patients. *Journal of Medical and Veterinary Mycology*, **32** (Suppl 1), 33–51.

Wiekowska, A. & Nawiecki, R. (1990) *Microsporum* infections in patients treated at the Dermatological Clinic Medical Academy, Gdansk 1984–1988. *Przegl Dermatology*, **72**(2), 111–117.

The Influence of Environmental Factors on Superficial Fungal Infections

CH. DE VROEY

Mycoses, i.e. infections caused by a still growing variety of microfungi, may be subdivided on the basis of aetiological, nosological or epidemiological criteria. In an overview of the influence of factors such as climate, lifestyle and occupation, it may seem appropriate to use a grouping based on the sources of superficial mycoses.

Superficial mycoses may be acquired from propagules of parasitic origin (group 1) shed by infected individuals or of saprobic sources, which may be exogenous/environmental (group 2) but which may also be epi- or endogenous (group 3) since the human body is the normal habitat of certain 'commensal' microfungi.

Group 1: superficial mycoses from parasitic origin

Dermatophytoses (ringworm, tinea) caused by anthropophilic or zoophilic dermatophytes (for a recent review, see Weitzman and Summerbell, 1995) are the only contagious mycoses: the infective particles of parasitic origin are usually transmitted directly, but also indirectly, from one host to another (De Vroey, 1985). Infective propagules are shed by infected individuals; however carriage of pathogenic dermatophytes by healthy animals has been repeatedly demonstrated, and the same carriage, such as agents of tinea capitis on the human scalp, has also been well documented (Mariat *et al.*, 1967).

Tinea capitis, caused by anthropophilic species, is a clear example of a dermatophytosis where socio-economic status and hygiene are probably the most important factors. Isolated cases of tinea capitis in schoolchildren should not be treated solely with orally active antifungal drugs but also with topical agents to prevent further spreading to other individuals.

In Europe, tinea capitis due to imported anthropophilic dermatophytes (such as *Trichophyton violaceum* and *T. soudanense*) is apparently increasing. As noticed, for example, by Badillet (1988) and by Viguié *et al.* (1992), other members of the family including the mothers should be examined to detect other active scalp lesions and to prevent spreading or re-infections (Leeming & Elliott, 1995). The emergence of *Trichophyton tonsurans* tinea capitis in some cities in the UK is a further example of import pathology.

In countries where tinea capitis is still highly prevalent among schoolchildren, prevention could include the use of an azole-containing shampoo. This should be applied to all the children since healthy carriage, mainly when a species such as *Microsporum langeroni* (*M. audouini*) is the main agent in a school, is probably 100%.

Tinea imbricata (tokelau), geographically restricted mainly to the Pacific Islands of Oceania and to some places in Latin America, is caused by one anthropophilic species, *T. concentricum*. It is another example of the role of hygiene and washing facilities in the prevention of certain dermatophytoses caused by anthropophilic species. Evidence for genetic susceptibility to this dermatophytosis has been demonstrated

in Papua New Guinea (Hay *et al.*, 1983).

Skin, particularly tinea pedis, and (toe)nail infections caused by *T. rubrum* or *T. interdigitale* are, by contrast, examples of infections connected with our way of life including well-known factors such as clothing and occupational or recreational activities. Outbreaks of tinea gladiatorum in wrestling teams are examples of direct transmission (Stiller *et al.*, 1992; Beller & Gessner, 1994). The role of swimming baths, showers and other communal life in the indirect transmission has been repeatedly demonstrated. This includes not only recreational but also professional activities (use of protective clothing and footwear in some industries together with the use of common bathing facilities). De Vroey and Meysman (1980) introduced the use of contact plates which not only allow direct sampling from, for example, floors of swimming pools, but also give quantitative results. With this technique, on average, 110 colonies/m^2 of dermatophytes (*Epidermophyton floccosum*, *Trichophyton interdigitale*, *T. rubrum*) were isolated in various public swimming baths in Belgium (Norland & Detandt, 1988).

Prevention may be achieved by various, often inexpensive means. Individual measures should include thorough drying of feet and application of foot powder (with an antifungal), avoiding the wearing of clothing which favours moisture and the sharing of towels. Infected individuals should also be educated not to put themselves in direct contact with others. Wearing disposable sandals in synthetic fabric could also help to prevent contagion in places where people, for professional or recreational reasons, use common showers.

The use of foot dips with 'wonder' products in communal swimming baths is generally considered of little benefit as an environmental measure: effective water spraying and scrubbing of the floors will eliminate most of the scales and other infective propagules. The use of (wooden) duckboards, e.g. in showers, should be discouraged since fungal propagules remain stuck to these substrates (Martinet, 1988).

Zoophilic dermatophytes are responsible for familial (e.g. *M. canis*), recreational or occupational (e.g. *M. persicolor*, *M. mentagrophytes*, *T. verrucosum*) infections. *M. canis* is transmitted essentially from cats directly, or probably more often indirectly, to individuals. Using our direct isolation procedure, numerous *M. canis* isolates have been obtained not only from infected, cured or healthy cats, but also from many different sites in the owner's homes, including bedding, furniture, carpets and clothing. Using an air sampler, Symoens *et al.* (1989) isolated >1000 colonies/mm³ of *M. canis* in the rooms of a house in which one infected cat lived! Similar results are recorded with *T. mentagrophytes* in laboratory animals or pet rodents.

Formolization or spray, smoke or dipping with antifungals (e.g. enilconazole, Janssen-Cilag) are effective ways to eliminate this inoculum. Enilconazole, the use of which is restricted to veterinary practice, not only disinfects premises, cages and other items but also eliminates or diminishes the carriage, since it may be used in the presence of animals or applied to the animals directly.

Group 2: superficial mycoses from environmental saprobic origin

This group includes dermatophytoses caused by geophilic species and onychomycoses caused by 'moulds'.

Microsporum praecox and *M. gypseum* are examples of dermatophytes which are responsible for recreational or occupational infections of saprobic origin. Transmission from infected individuals probably never occurs.

Dermatophytoses caused by *M. praecox* are commonly seen in patients with a history of horse-riding and are clearly due to exposure to high numbers of spores of saprobic origin in stables (De Vroey *et al.*, 1983; Phelippot *et al.*, 1988; Degeilh *et al.*, 1994). It should be noticed that, thus far, clinical infections by *M. praecox* have only been reported in humans. *M. gypseum* skin infections in gardeners and in cucumber growers have been traced to occupational exposure to soil enriched with powdered bovine keratin which had enhanced the growth of this geophilic dermatophyte (Alsop & Prior, 1961; Klokke, 1962; Bensch & Gemeinhardt, 1966).

Probably no more than 5% of onychomycoses are caused by non-dermatophytic filamentous fungi or moulds, most commonly *Scopulariopsis brevicaulis*. It is widely accepted that 'altered keratin' explains why *Scopulariopsis* onychomycosis (mainly the big toe) is more frequent in elderly people. Although this species is usually considered 'of widespread occurrence' it is not impossible that nail infections result from contact

with a well-defined but still undiscovered source.

Hendersonula toruloidea (*Nattrassia mangiferae*) is a plant pathogen in tropical and subtropical countries. Onychomycosis, athlete's foot and palmar infections caused by this exotic species in Western countries are almost exclusively seen in immigrants from certain tropical areas (Hay & Moore, 1984). It is generally accepted that these imported infections have been acquired, sometimes several years before, from soil and plant detritus. Intrahuman transmission seems to not occur. Wearing shoes that are too tight could explain the evolution from a latent to an active infection.

Group 3: superficial mycoses from epi- or endosaprobic origin

Superficial mycoses acquired from the autochtonous human skin flora consist mainly of pityriasis versicolor and other skin disorders (folliculitis, seborrhoeic dermatitis pro parte?) due to one (or more than one?) species (or a variety) of a commensal lipophilic yeast of the genus *Pityrosporum* (*Malassezia*).

Several factors may be responsible for this change from a harmless skin inhabitant to a pathogen, most of them being still putative but clearly patient linked. External factors (sun exposure, warmth and humidity) may be incriminated but still in relation with individual susceptibility. The possible role of body lotions, sun oils and bath oils (Roed-Peterson, 1980; Gründer & Mayer, 1991; Mayer & Gründer, 1991) should be further investigated.

Superficial candidoses are also mostly caused by our own mucosal or skin yeast flora. Infections due to *Candida albicans* or other *Candida* species are quick to develop when there is any imbalance in the host–commensal relationship. Increased moisture leading to maceration may be considered as an environmental factor predisposing to *Candida* intertrigos. However, the several well-known factors are not really environmental but patient linked or iatrogenic and concern mainly invasive candidosis.

Conclusion

Environmental factors are clearly involved in the transmission of some superficial mycoses such as tinea

Table 15.7 List of fungi discussed and some of their epidemiological characteristics.

Agent	Genus and species	Main pathological implication
Dermatophytes		
Anthropophilic species	*Epidermophyton floccosum*	Tinea cruris
	Microsporum langeroni	Tinea capitis
	Trichophyton concentricum	Tinea imbricata
	Trichophyton interdigitale	Tinea pedis/onychomycosis
	Trichophyton rubrum	Tinea pedis/onychomycosis
	Trichophyton soudanense	Tinea capitis/onychomycosis
	Trichophyton tonsurans	Tinea capitis/corporis
	Trichophyton violaceum	Tinea capitis
Zoophilic species	*Microsporum canis*	Tinea corporis/capitis
	Microsporum persicolor	Tinea corporis
	Trichophyton mentagrophytes	Tinea corporis/kerion
	Trichophyton verrucosum	Kerion/sycosis
Geophilic species	*Microsporum gypseum*	Tinea corporis
	Microsporum praecox	Tinea corporis
Moulds		
Environmental/saprobic		
	Hendersonula toruloidea	Onychomycosis
	(Nattrassia mangiferae)	
	Scopulariopsis brevicaulis	Onychomycosis
Yeasts		
Episaprobic	*Pityrosporum/Malassezia* spp.	Pityriasis versicolor
Endosaprobic	*Candida albicans*	Candidiasis

capitis, tinea pedis and tinea unguium. However, the role of patient-linked factors is more important in most superficial mycoses.

References

Alsop, J. & Prior, A.P. (1961) Ringworm infection in a cucumber greenhouse. *British Medical Journal,* **i**, 1081.

Badillet, G. (1988) Dermatophytes et immigration. *Annales de Biologie Clinique,* **46**(1), 37–43.

Beller, M. & Gessner, B.D. (1994) An outbreak of tinea corporis gladiatorum on a high school wrestling team. *Journal of the American Academy of Dermatology,* **31**(2), Part 1, 197–201.

Bensch, G.J. & Gemeinhardt, H. (1966) Über weiter Fälle von Gärtnerei-Mikrosporie durch *Microsporum gypseum*. *Berufsdermatosen,* **14**, 250–254.

Degeilh, B., Contet-Audonneau, N., Chevrier, S. & Guiguen, C. (1994) A propos de trois nouveaux cas de dermatophytie à *Microsporum praecox*. Revue de la littérature des cas humains. *Journal de Mycologie Médicale,* **4** (3), 175–178.

De Vroey, Ch. (1985) Epidemiology of ringworm (dermatophytosis). *Seminars in Dermatology,* **4**(3), 185–200.

De Vroey, Ch. & Meysman, L. (1980) Direct isolation of dermatophytes from floors of an indoor swimming pool. *Zentralblatt für Bakteriologie, Mikrobiologie und Hygiene,* **170**, 123–125.

De Vroey, Ch., Wuytack-Raes, C. & Fossoul, F. (1983) Isolation of saprophytic *Microsporum praecox* Rivalier from sites associated with horses. *Sabouraudia,* **21**, 255–257.

Gründer, K. & Mayer, P. (1991) *Malassezia furfur* und die medizinischen Ölbäder. *Aktuelle Dermatologie,* **17**, 213–216.

Hay, R.J. & Moore, M.K. (1984) Clinical features of superficial fungal infections caused by *Hendersonula toruloidea* and *Scytalidium hyalinum*. *British Journal of Dermatology,* **110**, 677–683.

Hay, R.J., Reid, S., Talwat, E. & Macnamara, K. (1983) Immune responses of patients with tinea imbricata. *British Journal of Dermatology,* **108**, 581–586.

Klokke, A.H. (1962) *Microsporum gypseum* infectie bij kom-

kommerkwekers. *Nederlands Tijdschrift voor Geneeskunde*, **106**, 1892–1895.

Leeming, J.G. & Elliott, T.S.J. (1995) The emergence of *Trichophyton tonsurans* tinea capitis in Birmingham, UK. *British Journal of Dermatology*, **133**(6), 929–931.

Mariat, F., Adan-Campos, C., Gentilini, M. & Gaxotte, P. (1967) Présence de dermatophytes chez l'homme en l'absence de lésions cliniques. *Bulletin de la Société Française de Dermatologie et de Syphilographie*, **74**, 724–729.

Martinet, F. (1988) Isolement de dermatophytes dans les installations sanitaires de collectivités. Etude comparative de deux méthodes de prélèvements: 'Rodac' et 'carré de tapis'. *Revue de l'Association belge des Technologues de Laboratoire*, **15**(4), 243–251.

Mayer, P. & Gründer, K. (1991) Wachstumsverhalten von *Malassezia furfur* in handelsüblichen Sonnenölen. *TW Dermatologie*, **00**, 131–137.

Nolard, N. & Detandt, M. (1988) Dermatophytes and swimming pools: seasonal variations. *Mycoses*, **31**(10), 495–500.

Phelippot, R., Feuilhade de Chauvin, M., Michel, Y. *et al.* (1988) *Microsporum praecox*: à propos de quatre observations. *Annales de Dermatologie et de Vénéréologie*, **115**, 11, 1154–1156.

Roed-Petersen, J. (1980) Tinea versicolor and body lotions. *Acta Dermato-Venereologica*, **60**, 439–440.

Stiller, M.J., Klein, W.P., Dorman, R.I. & Rosenthal, S. (1992) Tinea corporis gladiatorum: an epidemic of *Trichophyton tonsurans* in student wrestlers. *Journal of the American Academy of Dermatology*, **27**(4), 632–633.

Symoens, F., Fauvel, E. & Nolard, N. (1989) Evaluation de la contamination de l'air et des surfaces par *Microsporum canis* dans une habitation. *Bulletin de la Société Française de Mycologie Médicale*, **18**(2), 293–298.

Viguié, C., Ancelle, T., Savaglio, N., Dupouy-Camet, J. *et al.* (1992) Enquête épidémiologique sur les teignes à *Trichophyton soudanense* en milieu scolaire. *Journal de Mycologie Médicale*, **2**(3), 160–163.

Weitzman, I. & Summerbell, R.C. (1995) The dermatophytes. *Clinical Microbiology Reviews*, **8**(2), 240–259.

The Influence of Internal Factors on Superficial Fungal Infections

Y.M. CLAYTON

The superficial fungal infections are the commonest of human mycoses and include pityriasis versicolor, candidosis and dermatophytosis. Pityriasis versicolor is caused by the lipophilic yeast, *Malassezia furfur*, which is a normal inhabitant of the skin and the yeast, *Candida albicans*, the most frequent cause of superficial candidosis, is resident in the gastrointestinal tract of healthy subjects. These infections are therefore endogenous, almost always arising from organisms present in the normal flora. The filamentous dermatophytes which infect man and cause dermatophytosis belong to three genera, *Microsporum*, *Trichophyton* and *Epidermophyton*, and may be divided into those which are spread from man to man (anthropophilic), from animal to man (zoophilic) and from soil to man (geophilic). In contrast to the yeasts, dermatophytes are not part of the normal human flora and infections are acquired by transfer of fungal elements in keratin shed from lesions on infected humans or animals. These differences are relevant to the consideration of the influence of internal factors on these infections.

Age

Pityriasis versicolor

The incidence of the yeast phase of *M. furfur* on the chest and back of healthy adults has been reported to be 92% (Roberts, 1969). However, in a study of clinically normal skin from the backs of newborn infants and those aged 6 months to 15 years old, *M. furfur* was not found in children under 1 year old; the highest prevalence (93%) was in the 15-year-old children (Faergemann & Fredriksson, 1980). This study reflects the comparative rarity with which this infection, resulting from the conversion of the yeast to a mycelial phase, occurs in children under 10 years of age, and suggests that physiological changes in skin lipids during puberty could enhance fungal pathogenicity. The disease itself is most commonly seen in young adults with a lower incidence in the elderly.

Superficial candidosis

Since the most important source of *Candida* in human disease is endogenous, many studies have been carried out on the yeast flora of the mouth, rectum and vagina of healthy subjects. Odds (1988) has calculated from published data that carriage rates of *C. albicans* in the mouths of healthy subjects ranged from 2 to 41%.

Oral *Candida* carriage also varies according to age; the mean carriage rate in neonates (up to 7 days old) was 17.3%, in infants aged 1 week to 18 months it was 46.3% and in children over 18 months 15.1%; the mean carriage rate in adults was 25.1% (Odds, 1988). The high frequency of oral candidosis in neonates is well known, probably reflecting their immature immune mechanism. The occlusive effects of diapers are a cause of superficial candidosis in babies and thumb sucking may lead to maceration of the nail-fold and subsequent infection by *Candida*.

The elderly are also more susceptible to candidosis, possibly due to senescence of immune responsiveness. However, factors such as the presence of other diseases and their associated therapies (such as antibiotics and corticosteroids) may be implicated and the presence of an oral prosthesis is known to favour the development of oral candidosis.

Dermatophytosis

The vast majority of dermatophyte infections are seen in healthy individuals and affect all age groups. However, tinea pedis, tinea unguium and tinea cruris are uncommon before puberty and tinea capitis is rarely seen in adults. Surveys of tinea pedis in school children in the UK have recorded prevalences ranging from 2.2% in 7–10-year-old boys to 6.6% in 11–14-year-old boys (English & Gibson, 1959). A study of adult office and shop workers revealed a 14.8% prevalence of tinea pedis (Howell *et al.*, 1988). The reason for the difference in prevalence in children and adults is not known. Tinea unguium is also uncommon in children, the prevalence increasing with age. In a UK study, only one case of tinea unguium was found in a survey of 494 schoolchildren aged from 5 to 10 years, an overall prevalence of 0.2% (Philpot & Shuttleworth, 1989). As distinct from adults, most cases of tinea unguium in children show no sign of infection in adjacent skin sites. However, the parents of infected children are frequently also found to be infected and therefore are the most likely source of infection.

Tinea capitis infections are unusual after puberty when there is generally spontaneous resolution even in untreated cases, suggesting that some protective factor then becomes operative. Tinea capitis in adults is uncommon. In London, between 1990 and 1993,

only ten cases of tinea capitis were seen in adults compared to 360 cases in children. The majority of adult cases reported are in elderly females. For example of 27 cases reported in Milan, 14 were over 60 years old and 24 were women (Terragni *et al.*, 1989). The preponderance of females is unexplained. Infection in the elderly may reflect poor physiological defences due to qualitative and quantitative differences in sebum. However, other immunological factors which have not been elucidated are also thought to play a role, as tinea capitis has been reported in patients with systemic lupus erythematosus, transplant recipients and other patients on immunosuppressive drugs. Tinea capitis has also been reported in patients with diabetes.

Genetic factors

Pityriasis versicolor and candidosis

There is no firm evidence to date that predisposition to either of these conditions is determined by genetic factors, although it has been suggested that epidemiological studies might reveal subtle genetically-based variations in individual susceptibility to *Candida* invasion (Odds, 1988). In the rare condition chronic mucocutaneous candidosis, many patients show clear evidence of a hereditary linkage. Most familial cases involve more than one autosomal recessive gene (Wells *et al.*, 1972) but a few have been associated with an autosomal dominant gene (Sams *et al.*, 1979).

Dermatophytosis

There is little evidence that susceptibility to dermatophytosis is genetically determined. However, one form of tinea, tinea imbricata, which has a very restricted geographical distribution (found only in the Western Pacific area, South-East Asia and Amazonia), is an example where genetic susceptibility may explain the pattern of disease. A report from one area in Papua New Guinea suggested that the expression of disease in the community fitted the hypothesis that susceptibility was inherited as an autosomal recessive trait (Ravine *et al.*, 1980). This does not, however, appear to be the case in all endemic areas. A study from a different part of Papua New Guinea did not support the involvement of an autosomal recessive trait but could not exclude genetic susceptibility on the basis of autosomal dominant transmission with incomplete penetrance (Hay, 1992).

Immune status

There is evidence of acquired immune reactions to many fungal diseases, primarily through demonstrating serum antibodies. There is also evidence of cell-mediated immune reactions, most obviously apparent through the presence of delayed hypersensitivity reactions to antigenic preparations from the causative organism. However, evidence is often lacking that immune reactions demonstrable in the laboratory or in skin tests actually affect the course of the disease, rather than being simply a marker of infection with a particular fungus. For example, it is useful to have evidence of a correlation between antibody titre and the patient's clinical status and to show that patients known to be immunocompromised are more severely ill. These circumstances would indicate that immune mechanisms play a discernible role in controlling the disease. When this is the case, monitoring immune reactivity to the causal fungus or, in the case of immuno-compromised patients, monitoring immune competence will be valuable in assessing the patient's progress. Reliable assessment of immune function may require monitoring an antibody which could affect the course of the disease, for example a neutralizing antibody.

Pityriasis versicolor

Immunological studies have not yet provided an explanation for the susceptibility of some patients to the development of this infection. The decreasing prevalence of this infection in subjects over 30 years old could reflect an acquired immunity to the disease although the mechanism is unclear. For example, humoral antibody levels against *M. furfur* are often higher in patients with pityriasis versicolor, although T-cell function (as expressed by lymphocyte migration tests using *M. furfur* antigens) may be reduced (Roberts, 1986).

Pityriasis versicolor most commonly occurs in healthy subjects with no evidence of immunosuppression. However, immunosuppressive therapy may predispose patients to infection, particularly in the case of renal transplant patients, although no increased incidence of pityriasis versicolor has been reported in AIDS patients.

Candidosis

Normal healthy adults have a high innate immunity to infection by *Candida*, and disease is uncommon unless there is alteration of host defences or environmental conditions. Immune defects, particularly in T-lymphocyte function, predispose to superficial forms of candidosis. Over 80% of AIDS patients have oral candidosis at some stage of their illness and the development of this condition is often the initial clinical manifestation in asymptomatic HIV-1 positive individuals.

Chronic mucocutaneous candidosis is often associated with defects in cell-mediated immunity (Sams *et al.*, 1979). Patients may also have humoral immune abnormalities. The patient's immune status in any form of candidosis is of major importance in determining the course and severity of the disease. When, as in AIDS, candidosis is a major factor in the patient's illness or is life-threatening, immunostimulation may be employed as therapy. In such circumstances, monitoring immune reactivity to *Candida* may be a key factor in assessing results of such therapy. This could be equally true when immunostimulation is employed as a form of prophylaxis against development of florid disease in HIV-1-infected individuals.

Dermatophytosis

Humoral antibodies are produced by patients with active dermatophyte infections, their presence and levels depending on the site, extent and nature of the infection. However, since uninfected subjects may also have antibodies to dermatophyte antigens, their role is doubtful. There may be cross-reactivity between dermatophyte and host antigens or there may be natural antibodies to these organisms. Dermatophyte infections, although confined to superficial and fully keratinized parts of the body, elicit and are regulated by cell-mediated immunity responses. Cell-mediated immunity may play an important role in defence against dermatophyte infection since both cure and resistance to re-infection correlate well with the development of delayed-type hypersensitivity to trichophytin (Jones *et al.*, 1974). Persistence of infection has been associated with absence of delayed hypersensitivity reaction or poor *in vitro* response to dermatophyte antigens or to T- and B-cell mitogens, the latter indicating generalized depressed immune reactivity (Calderon, 1989). It is unclear how extensively immunosuppression increases susceptibility to dermatophyte infections. However, AIDS patients may have extensive and atypical presentations of infections and a characteristic form of rapidly spreading proximal subungual onychomycosis has been described which may be a marker for HIV-1 infection.

Intercurrent disease

Pityriasis versicolor

This infection is often associated with Cushing's syndrome and increased susceptibility occurs in patients receiving systemic corticosteroid therapy.

Candidosis

Diabetes mellitus, which increases levels of available sugar in tissues and reduces phagocytic activity, is a condition that predisposes to superficial candidosis. Endocrine disorders such as hypothyroidism, hypoparathyroidism and hypoadrenocorticism are also conditions associated with *Candida* infections, particularly chronic mucocutaneous candidosis. Malignant disease predisposes patients not only to systemic *Candida* infection but also to superficial and oral candidosis. This in turn may be a function of the immunosuppression associated with malignant disease. *Candida* carriage is common among cancer patients, particularly those with leukaemia, and it is exacerbated by chemotherapy and radiotherapy, the highest risk of infection being associated with neutropenia (Odds, 1988). Any intercurrent disease requiring antibiotics or corticosteroids places the patient at potential risk of developing candidosis. Antibacterial antibiotics, by eliminating the bacterial competition, allow commensal yeasts to increase in numbers and give rise to invasive infection. Corticosteroids with their anti-inflammatory and immunosuppressive effects may reduce host resistance to *Candida* infection. The association of oral candidosis and AIDS has already been mentioned.

Dermatophytosis

Persistent dermatophyte infections are associated with palmoplantar keratoderma or tylosis where abnormal keratinization favours fungal colonization. Patients with ichthyosis may have an increased susceptibility to dermatophytosis. Patients with chronic mucocutaneous candidosis may have an associated dermatophyte infection. An association between respiratory atopy and persistent *Trichophyton rubrum* infection has been found in many studies with as many as 40% of patients having a personal or family history of asthma or hay fever (Hay & Brostoff, 1977).

Although these internal factors have been considered under four separate headings, clearly many are interrelated. For example, age, immunosuppression and intercurrent disease may all play a role in determining susceptibility to superficial candidosis. The interplay of these various internal factors has to be determined by clinical studies.

References

Calderon, R.A. (1989) Immunoregulation of dermatophytosis. *CRC Critical Reviews in Microbiology*, **16**, 339–368.

English, M.P. & Gibson, M.D. (1959) Studies in the epidemiology of tinea pedis. I. Tinea pedis in schoolchildren. *British Medical Journal*, **i**, 1442–1446.

Faergemann, J. & Fredriksson, T. (1980) Age incidence of *Pityrosporum orbiculare* on human skin. *Acta Dermato-Venereologica (Stockholm)*, **60**, 531–533.

Hay, R.J. (1992) Genetic susceptibility to dermatophytosis. *European Journal of Dermatology*, **8**, 346–349.

Hay, R.J. & Brostoff, J. (1977) Immune responses in patients with chronic *Trichophyton rubrum* infections. *Clinical and Experimental Dermatology*, **2**, 373–380.

Howell, S.A., Clayton, Y.M., Phan, Q.C. & Noble, W.C. (1988) Tinea pedis: the relationship between symptoms, organisms and host characteristics. *Microbial Ecology in Health and Disease*, **1**, 131–135.

Jones, H.E., Reinhardt, J.H. & Rinaldi, M.G. (1974) Acquired immunity to dermatophytes. *Archives of Dermatology*, **109**, 840–848.

Odds, F.C. (1988) *Candida and Candidosis*, 2nd edn. Baillière Tindall, London.

Philpot, C.M. & Shuttleworth, D. (1989) Dermatophyte onychomycosis in children. *Clinical and Experimental Dermatology*, **14**, 203–205.

Ravine, D., Turner, K.J. & Alpers, M.P. (1980) Genetic

inheritance of susceptibility to tinea imbricata. *Journal of Medical Genetics*, **17**, 342–348.

Roberts, S.O.B. (1969) *Pityrosporum orbiculare*: incidence and distribution in clinically normal skin. *British Journal of Dermatology*, **81**, 264–269.

Roberts, S.O.B. (1986) Pityriasis versicolor. In: *Superficial Fungal Infections* (ed. J. Verbov). MTP, Lancaster.

Sams, W.M., Jorizzo, J.L., Snyderman, R. *et al.* (1979) Chronic mucocutaneous candidiasis: immunological studies of three generations of a single family. *American Journal of Medicine*, **67**, 948–959.

Terragni, L., Lasagni, A. & Oriani, A. (1989) Tinea capitis in adults. *Mycoses*, **32**, 482–486.

Wells, R.S., Higgs, J.M., MacDonald, D. *et al.* (1972) Familial chronic mucocutaneous candidiasis. *Journal of Medical Genetics*, **9**, 302–310.

Causes and Prevention of Recurrent Candidal Vulvovaginitis

E. SEGAL AND H. SANDOVSKY-LOSICA

Introduction

Candidal vaginitis is a common disease caused by the opportunistic fungi of the genus *Candida*, primarily *C. albicans*. *Candida albicans* is the most frequently reported species from unselected groups of women, as well as from patients with vaginitis. It is estimated that up to 75% of women have an episode of candidal vaginitis during their lifetime. The yeast *C. albicans* is considered part of the normal oral, gastrointestinal and vaginal flora. The carriage rate of yeasts has been studied extensively. Most studies showed that the vaginal yeast-carriage rate in normal females is < 30% (Sobel, 1992, 1993; Edwards, 1995). A significant association was found between the number of yeasts isolated and symptoms of pruritus and signs of abnormal discharge. Candidal vaginitis poses a serious problem because the infections tend to be recurrent, are not always eradicated by the standard treatments and are often unexplained. The rate of recurrence, depending on the criteria for definition, is estimated by some investigators to be as high as 20% of the afflicted women (Sobel, 1992, 1993; Edwards, 1995).

Causes of the infection

As depicted in Table 15.8, antibiotic pretreatment, use of hormonal contraceptives, diabetes mellitus and certain stages of the menstrual cycle are traditionally viewed as predisposing factors to *Candida* overgrowth in the vagina. The vaginal carriage of yeasts is more prevalent in pregnant females with a higher prevalence during the third trimester of pregnancy. Among the physiological factors that predispose to candidal colonization and overgrowth during pregnancy are progesterone and oestradiol concentration, and vaginal pH. Availability or presentation of receptor(s) for binding of *Candida* on the vaginal epithelial surfaces may be considered a possible factor (Sobel, 1992, 1993; Edwards, 1995).

Adhesion of a pathogen to host tissues is currently an established attribute contributing to the initial step in the evolution of infection by allowing the pathogen to evade from host defence forces (Ofek & Doyle, 1994). For *Candida* spp. to colonize the vaginal mucosa, yeasts must first adhere to the vaginal epithelial cells (VEC). Thus, differences in adhesive ability might present possible causes for differential tendency for infection. Here we will focus on candidal adhesion to VEC as a virulence attribute involved in the pathogenesis of vaginitis and on factors affecting this process. This will be followed by a description of attempts to interfere in the process of adhesion as a possible means for prevention of infection.

Adhesion can be studied in quite simple *in vitro* systems such as incubation of mixtures of the micro-organism and host cells, and quantitative evaluation by microscopic counts of the number of epithelial cells with attached yeasts. Using such *in vitro* systems (Segal *et al.*, 1982, 1984) we assessed whether vaginal epithelial cells from non-infected women of groups known by epidemiological data for increased susceptibility to develop vaginitis, such as diabetic or pregnant females, reveal increased potential for binding of *Candida*. The results showed that the highest values of *in vitro* adherence were obtained with VEC from pregnant diabetic women, and that each of these factors in itself, e.g. pregnancy or diabetes, also contributed to high adhesion values. To affirm the implication of these results pointing to a hormonal influence on adhesion, the data were analysed in respect to the hormonal

Table 15.8 Possible causes of recurrent vulvovaginal candidiasis.

Host-associated factors
Pregnancy
Uncontrolled diabetes mellitus
Oestrogen, corticosteroids and oral contraceptives
Antibiotics
Adhesion capacity of host cells
Immune deficiency

Candida-associated factors
Adhesion capacity of *Candida*
Switching phenomenon

Table 15.9 Detection of fibronectin on subpopulations of vaginal epithelial cells and the adherence level of each subpopulation.

Fraction (% Percoll)	Superficial cells (%)	Fluorescent cells (%)	Adherence (%)
Control (before separation)	42.1 ± 5.4	41.4 ± 11.9	30.7 ± 8.4
20	79.0 ± 9.8	6.3 ± 4.9	7.5 ± 6.1
30	37.8 ± 8.6	49.2 ± 8.6	37.5 ± 8.2
40	37.5 ± 12.6	52.3 ± 10.6	29.8 ± 14.0

The results are mean values (± S.D.) from ten experiments, each in duplicate.

status, as expressed by cytology of vaginal smears (Kalo & Segal, 1988). Specifically, the ratio between the superficial (S) and the intermediate (I) VEC, namely the karyopyknotic index (KPI) in women of fertility age, and the ratio of S:I:P (parabasal), the maturation index (MI) in postmenopausal females, was determined. Evaluating the adherence data of the various groups in relation to the KPI index revealed that high adherence is seen at low KPI, namely low numbers of S cells and high number of I cells, which would suggest that the intermediate cells possess more marked adhesive ability.

The following study revealed that separated subpopulations of VEC had different adherence ability, i.e. subpopulations enriched in I cells had higher adhesion values than those enriched in S cells. As S cells appear under high oestrogen levels, while I cells appear under high progesterone levels, the effect of external addition of various sex hormones was assessed, revealing that addition of progesterone caused an increase in adhesion.

All these data suggesting the higher adhesive ability of the I cells led to a search for putative receptors on these cells (Kalo *et al.*, 1988). As it was known from previous studies by use of fluorescent antifibronectin antibodies that human VEC possess on their surface fibronectin (FN), a glycoprotein known for its role in cell–cell interactions, we investigated whether the different VEC types differ in FN level. Fluorescence-activated cell sorter (FACS) analysis of VEC subpopulations labelled with antifibronectin antibodies revealed that fractions enriched in S cells have lower

fluorescence, indicating that the level of FN is lower in these cells than in the I cells. Concurrently it was shown that those cells with high FN level have higher adherence values (Table 15.9) and that FN binds to *C. albicans*.

Thus the *in vitro* adhesion data indicated correlative relationships between the following:
1 Adhesion capacity of VEC and predisposition to vaginal infection.
2 Effect of sex hormones, particularly progesterone, on adhesion.
3 The intermediate (I) type of VEC, which predominate under high levels of progesterone, have increased adhering capacity.
4 Fibronectin, found at higher level in I-cell subpopulations, acts as a receptor for binding of *Candida*. *In vivo* studies to corroborate the *in vitro* data have been initiated in experimental animal models (Lehrer *et al.*, 1983; Segal *et al.*, 1988; Segal & Josef-Lev, 1995). The studies included three murine vaginal models:
1 Infection in naive animals (Lehrer *et al.*, 1983).
2 A model of constant oestrus induced by pretreatment with hormones (Segal *et al.*, 1988). This model is analogous to human situations with high predisposition for candidal infection when subjects are under hormonal influence.
3 Diabetic mice (Segal & Josef-Lev, 1995).

In all models, infection was induced by intravaginal inoculation of *C. albicans*. As for naive mice, if the inoculation is done at the oestrus stage, it is possible to see in vaginal smears yeasts adhering to mucosa a few hours after inoculation, followed by development of hyphae thereafter. Comparison of infection rate as assessed by microscopy, or enumeration of colony-forming units, in the different models 24 h post-fungal inoculation shows that in naive mice only about half were infected, while among hormone-treated and particularly among diabetic mice, almost all inoculated animals developed infection. Moreover, in diabetic mice, a much lower dose of *C. albicans* was sufficient to induce infection in a high percentage of animals. Furthermore, while in naive animals infection was short lived in animals with constant oestrus or with induced diabetes, the infection was persistent and lasted for a considerable period.

Prevention

As indicated above, recurrence of infection is a principal problem associated with candidal vaginitis, therefore attempts for prevention by prophylactic treatment with antifungals have been undertaken (Fang, 1994). However, this did not lead to solution of the problem.

It is known from various microbial systems that adhesion can be inhibited by analogues of the adhesin(s) — the microbial cell-wall component(s) involved in adherence — or by analogues of the receptor on the host-cell surface, respectively (Ofek & Doyle, 1994). Out of the analogues of the *Candida* cell-wall polysaccharides and their monosaccharides, only chitin and *N*-acetylglucosamine had an inhibitory effect on the *in vitro* adhesion of *C. albicans* to VEC. Later it was found that an aqueous extract of chitin (chitin-soluble extract; CSE), whether when prepared from chitin isolated from *C. albicans*, or when prepared from chitin purchased commercially, was active in reducing the adhesion of *C. albicans* (Lehrer *et al.*, 1983, 1988; Segal *et al.*, 1988; Segal & Josef-Lev, 1995).

The effect of CSE was also assessed *in vivo* in the murine models (Fig. 15.3). The mice were treated intravaginally prior to fungal inoculation and in some cases shortly thereafter. CSE was effective in all models in preventing development of infection, however with a much lower efficacy in the models with massive persistent infection. Nevertheless, even in these animals, the infection cleared more rapidly among the treated than non-treated.

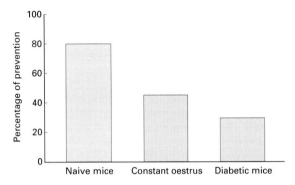

Fig. 15.3 Effect of CSE *in vivo* in experimental murine candidiasis. Percentage prevention represents the ratio of number of mice without infection among CSE-treated animals to those of untreated controls. In each column the ratio relates to a corresponding non-treated control.

Conclusion

It is possible to conclude that, based on the understanding of the pathogenesis of the infection, it is feasible to undertake prevention which is based on the interaction of the fungus with the host and thereby interfere in the development of infection.

References

Edwards, J.E. (1995) *Candida* species. In: *Principles and Practice of Infectious Diseases* (eds G.L. Mandell, J.E. Bennett & R. Dolin), Vol. 2, 4th edn, pp. 2289–2306. Churchill Livingstone, New York.

Fang, I.W. (1994) The value of prophylactic (monthly) clotrimazole versus empiric self-treatment in recurrent vaginal candidiasis. *Genitourinary Medicine*, **70**, 124–126.

Kalo, A. & Segal, E. (1988) Interaction of *Candida albicans* with genital mucosa: Effect of sex hormones on adherence of yeasts *in vitro*. *Canadian Journal of Microbiology*, **34**, 224–228.

Kalo, A., Segal, E., Sahar, E. & Dayan, D. (1988) Interaction of *Candida albicans* with genital mucosal surfaces: Involvement of fibronectin in adherence. *Journal of Infectious Diseases*, **157**, 1253–1256.

Lehrer, N., Segal, E. & Barr-Nea, L. (1983) *In vitro* and *in vivo* adherence of *Candida albicans* to mucosal surfaces. *Annals of Microbiology*, **134**, 293–306.

Lehrer, N., Segal, E., Lis, H. & Gov, Y. (1988) Effect of *Candida albicans* cell wall components on the adhesion of the fungus to human and murine vaginal mucosa. *Mycopathologia*, **102**, 115–121.

Ofek, I. & Doyle, R.J. (1994) *Bacterial Adhesion to Cells and Tissues.* Chapman and Hall, New York.

Segal, E. & Josef-Lev, A. (1995) Induction of candidal vaginitis in diabetic mice and attempts to prevent the infection. *Journal of Medical and Veterinary Mycology*, **33**, 1–8.

Segal, E., Lehrer, N. & Ofek, I. (1982) Adherence of *Candida albicans* to human vaginal epithelial cells: Inhibition of amino sugars. *Experimental Cell Biology*, **50**, 13–17.

Segal, E., Soroka, A. & Schechter, A. (1984) Correlative relationship between adherence of *Candida albicans* to human vaginal epithelial cells *in vitro* and candidal vaginitis. *Sabouraudia*, **22**, 191–200.

Segal, E., Gottfried, L. & Lehrer, N. (1988) Candidal vaginitis in hormone treated mice: Prevention by a chitin extract. *Mycopathologia*, **102**, 157–163.

Sobel, J.D. (1992) Pathogenesis and treatment of recurrent vulvovaginal candidiasis. *Clinical Infectious Diseases*, **14** (Suppl 1), S148–S153.

Sobel, J.D. (1993) Genital candidiasis. In: *Candidiasis: Pathogenesis, Diagnosis and Treatment* (ed. G.P. Bodey), pp. 225–247. Raven Press, New York.

Onychomycosis

R. BARAN

Incidence

There are no exact figures regarding the incidence of onychomycosis since studies have involved at-risk groups of individuals who regularly use communal bathing facilities. Roberts (1992) estimates that up to 5% of the general population in the UK may have fungal nail infection. In France, the Sofres Medical Survey (1991) found that toenails are affected in 84% of cases of onychomycosis, with the highest prevalence in the 36–45-year-old age group; this is in contrast to Roberts' findings with the highest prevalence in patients aged ⩾ 55 years. According to Haneke (1990), the incidence of onychomycosis is as summarized in Table 15.10.

Pathogenesis

Interestingly, the transmissibility of fungal organisms does not seem to play a significant part in determining the prevalence of tinea pedis and distal lateral subungual onchomycosis (Zaias, 1992) and there is a

Table 15.10 Incidence of onychomycoses (after E. Haneke).

18–40% of all nail disorders
30% of all dermatomycoses
43% of the 72 abnormal toenails
37% of nail lesions in podiatric patients
43% of the 183 subungual keratoses

Table 15.11 Biological normal host.

Occupation (sport activities, miners)
Climate (hot and humid)
Environmental factors (tennis shoes)
Walking barefoot
Inherited host susceptibility

Table 15.12 Individuals exposed at risk.

Sewer workers
Dustmen
Excavation workers
Steel and furnace workers
Employees of indoor swimming pools
Mine workers
Athletes
Soldiers

Table 15.13 Pathological predisposing factors.

Peripheral vascular disease
Peripheral neuropathies
Major or repeated trauma
Diabetes mellitus
Other endocrine diseases
Metabolic disorders
Immunological disorders

lack of transmission among married couples.

In a normal host (Table 15.11) emphasis should be given on occupational activities such as sport, the military and miners (Haneke, 1992). We have listed, as examples, individuals exposed to risk (Table 15.12); incidentally, coalminers have the highest prevalence (Roberts, 1992).

Host susceptibility for *Trichophyton rubrum* infection may probably be considered an autosomal dominant condition (Zaias *et al.*, 1993).

Pathological predisposing factors should be looked for. Most of them are noted in Table 15.13. Whatever the predisposing factors, many recurrent bouts of onychomycosis are caused by the re-infection of tinea pedis reaching the nail bed from the stratum corneum of the foot, this layer harbouring a reservoir of spores (Elewski, 1994).

Many publications stress the frequency of mycoses and maceration of the feet in occupations which fulfill the following conditions:
• Those which require wearing hermetic security shoes which create a confined, damp and warm atmosphere that facilitates the development of dermatophytic mycoses and bacterial infections.
• Those which do not provide sufficient information to workers about the importance of foot hygiene.
• Those which provide communal showers, which can lead to recurrent fungal contamination.

Collective preventive measures

These are generally ineffective because they are difficult to apply and/or are not sufficiently respected (Nardi, 1995). Ideally the following situations are desirable:
• Tiled shower floors should be inclined to allow sufficient drainage and non-stagnation of wastewater (*Trichophyton rubrum* survives 25 days in stagnant water at 23–25°C).
• Wooden shower-floor grids should be replaced by plastic ones to limit the adhesion of scales shed by infected feet.
• Floors of communal showers must be washed and disinfected at least once daily with, for example, sodium hypochlorite, if possible after use by each group of workers.

Individual preventive measures

These have to be added to the collective preventive measures. Recommended methods of disinfection are as follows:
• Discard or treat old shoes.
• Preventive disinfection of safety shoes with 3–5% formaldehyde is theoretically possible but presents the risk of allergic reaction (Feuilhade, 1990). A cotton swab soaked in 40% formaldehyde solution is placed inside the tip of the shoes which are stored for 24–48 h in a plastic bag which is sealed and put in a warm place. The formaldehyde vapour will permeate the inside of the shoes, killing all fungal organisms. The shoes are then removed from the plastic bag and left to air for 4 days (Haneke, pers. commun., 1994).
• Socks are indispensable (Steigleder & Klenk-Pfeufer, 1994) and must be sterilized. If they are made of cotton, which is highly recommended, they can be sterilized by boiling. If made of synthetic material, socks must be sterilized with disinfectants.
• Daily washing of the feet at home is essential.

An important aspect of *recurrent infection* is that most antifungal therapy involves drugs that are primarily fungistatic. Therefore, the new antifungals (Allylamine, Amorolfine, Ciclopirox) which are fungicidal offer the promise of prolonged remission through eradication of the causative dermatophyte (Leyden, 1993). In addition, we advise intermittent conventional topical antifungal application to the soles of the feet and between the toes, and transungual antifungal delivery system use twice a month indefinitely.

References

Elewski, B.E. (1994) Onychomycosis. *Fitzpatrick's Journal of Clinical Dermatology*, **2**, 48–54.

Feuilhade, M. (1990) Pied et mycoses, aspects épidémiologiques. *Le Pied*, **6**, 5–6.

Haneke, E. (1990) Epidemiology and pathology of onychomycoses. In: *Onychomycoses. Local Antimycotic Treatment* (eds S. Nolting & H.C Korting), pp. 1–11. Springer, Berlin.

Leyden, J. (1993) Progression of interdigital infections from simplex to complex. *Journal of the American Academy of Dermatology*, **28**, S7–S11.

Nardi, L. (1995) Onchomycose des orteils: aspects diagnostiques et stratégies thérapeutiques. *Revue de Médecine du Travail*, **22**, 83–86.

Roberts, D.T. (1992) Prevalence of dermatophyte onychomycosis in the United Kingdom: Results of an omnibus survey. *British Journal of Dermatology*, **126** (Suppl 39), 23–27.

Sofres Medical Survey (1991) *Patients with Onychomycosis and their Dermatology*. Roche Laboratories,

Steigleder, G.K. & Klenk-Pfeufer, E. (1994) Reinfections Prophylaxie von Fussmykosen. *Deutsche Medizinische Wochenschrift*, **119**, 1744.

Zaias, N. (1992) Clinical manifestations of onychomycosis. *Clinical and Experimental Dermatology*, **17** (Suppl 1), 6–7.

Zaias, N., Tosti, A., Baran, R. *et al.* (1993) Distal subungual onychomycosis in an inherited autosomal dominant disease. Poster 126 presented at the American Academy of Dermatology meeting, 4–9 December 1993. American Academy of Dermatology, Washington, DC.

16
Viral and Bacterial Skin Diseases

Hepatitis Virus and Skin Diseases

B. CRIBIER, O. CHOSIDOW, N. DUPIN
AND C. FRANCES

Among all the viruses causing hepatitis, hepatitis B virus and hepatitis C virus are most frequently associated with cutaneous disease symptoms, rather than hepatitis A virus infection, which is rarely encountered. Up to now, hepatitis E virus and other newly discovered hepatitis viruses have not been associated with skin diseases. Many isolated cases of unusual cutaneous symptoms associated with hepatitis virus infection have been reported. However, in the present review, we only consider associations with documented epidemiological data.

Hepatitis A, B and C viruses

Hepatitis A virus (HAV)

HAV is classified within the genus hepatovirus of the family Picornaviridae. Oral ingestion is the major route of transmission of HAV and modes of transmission other than oro-faecal are uncommon. HAV can cause an acute hepatitis with or without jaundice, but mortality is rare and chronic infection does not occur. HAV infection induces life-long protection against clinical disease, and an effective formalin-inactivated vaccine is available.

Hepatitis B virus (HBV)

HBV is a hebnavirus and is the smallest DNA virus known. HBV infection is one of the major causes of chronic hepatitis, cirrhosis and hepatocellular carcinoma worldwide. The risk of developing a chronic infection is high and varies inversely with the age of infection, since chronic infection occurs in 90% of infants infected at birth, and in 5–10% of persons infected as older children. The transmission of the virus occurs by percutaneous and mucous membrane exposition, including blood transfusion and intravenous drug use. HBV infection is frequent among hospital or medical workers and can also be sexually transmitted. Perinatal transmission is due to exposure to infectious body fluids. Recombinant hepatitis B vaccine provides excellent protection and is used for both pre- and post-exposure protection.

Hepatitis C virus (HCV)

HCV was discovered in 1989 and is classified in the family Flaviviridae. It is the major cause of non-A, non-B hepatitis and since serological tests are available, the risk of post-transfusional hepatitis due to HCV has now strongly declined. Chronic infection is extremely frequent (50–60% of cases) and 30–60% of patients with a chronic infection develop chronic active hepatitis. Cirrhosis is frequently observed and HCV is also involved in hepatocellular carcinoma. The most efficient mode of transmission of HCV is blood percutaneous exposure. Blood transfusion, intravenous drug use and health-care work are the main risk factors for being infected by HCV. The other routes of transmission may include materno-fetal transmission and sexual contacts with HCV-positive individuals; 30–40% of patients infected by HCV have no risk factors.

Cutaneous diseases and hepatitis virus

Urticaria

During the pre-icteric phase of HBV infection, cutaneous symptoms are observed in 14–42% of cases (Lewis *et al.*, 1973; Steigman, 1973). Acute urticaria is the most frequent symptom and can be associated with arthralgia and headache. Angioedema occurs in 4% of patients (McElgunn, 1983). Urticaria is rarely observed simultaneously with jaundice or in the chronic phase of infection. The cutaneous lesions of urticaria associated with the acute phase of HBV infection are not different from those of the common form of urticaria. Chronic urticaria is only rarely associated with the presence of hepatitis B markers (Doutre *et al.*, 1987), since HBV markers were found in only 9% of 100 patients with chronic urticaria in this series, and none had hepatitis B surface antigen (HBs antigen). Immune complexes and HBs antigen deposits were demonstrated in the small vessels of the skin in patients with urticaria and acute phase of HBV infection (Neumann *et al.*, 1981).

HAV infection is more rarely associated with urticaria or maculopapulous exanthema at the acute phase (Routenberg *et al.*, 1979) and only sporadic cases of urticaria associated with HCV infection were observed (Pawlotsky *et al.*, 1995).

Vasculitis of the small vessels

HBV infection is a classic cause of necrotizing vasculitis (Popp *et al.*, 1981). Characteristic histopathological changes of leucocytoclastic vasculitis were noted in patients with palpable purpura. Immune complexes made of HBs antigen and anti-HBs antibodies were shown in the serum of these patients. Moreover, HBs antigen was demonstrated in the cutaneous vessels, associated with complement deposits. Cutaneous vasculitis can be associated with immune complex deposits in the kidneys, muscles and in other organs. Leucocytoclastic vasculitis can occur in both the acute and chronic phases of HBV infection.

Leucocytoclastic vasculitis is very rare in HAV infection, and the occurrence of vasculitis of the small blood vessels independently of the presence of cryoglobulinaemia seems to be exceptional in HCV infection, since only rare case reports were published (Pawlotsky *et al.*, 1995).

Cryoglobulinaemia

The role of HBV in mixed cryoglobulinaemia is controversial. HBV markers were found in high proportions of patients with type II or type III cryoglobulinaemia during the 1970s (Levo *et al.*, 1977) and the presence of HBs antigen was demonstrated in the cryoprecipitate in some patients. However, in more recent studies, the link between HBV and cryoglobulinaemia was discussed (Popp *et al.*, 1980) and HBV DNA seems to be only rarely demonstrated in these patients. HCV is now considered to be the major cause of 'essential' cryoglobulinaemia. HCV markers were found in about 85% of these patients, and the presence of HCV RNA in the serum was clearly demonstrated (Agnello *et al.*, 1992; Lunel *et al.*, 1994). Conversely, the presence of cryoglobulinaemia is very frequent in patients with HCV infection, but it is only rarely symptomatic. The role of HCV in cryoglobulinaemia is reinforced by the fact that HCV RNA was demonstrated in the cryoprecipitate (Agnello *et al.*, 1992); moreover, the concentration of HCV RNA and HCV antibodies is 10- to 100-fold higher in the cryoprecipitate than it is in the serum. It was shown that under interferon therapy, the cryoglobulinaemia disappeared in patients that were good responders, but not in poor responders (Misiani *et al.*, 1994).

The comparison of HCV-positive and -negative patients that had cryoglobulinaemia showed that the frequency of palpable purpura was higher in cases of HCV infection and that it was related to the level of serum cryoglobulin (Dupin *et al.*, 1995). Since current assays for the detection of cryoglobulinaemia may often lead to false-negative results, the most sensitive test is serological detection of rheumatoid factors in patients infected by HCV and presenting with signs of cutaneous vasculitis (Karlsberg *et al.*, 1995). In the latter study, the frequency of cutaneous vasculitis in a group of 408 HCV-positive patients was 2.5%.

Polyarteritis nodosa (PAN)

The link between HBV infection and polyarteritis was

established in 1970. The prevalence of HBV markers in patients with PAN is generally estimated to be 30–40% (Trepo, 1989), but can be up to 69% in certain series (Cacoub *et al.*, 1994). The HBV infection rate is probably underestimated when HBs antigen is detected by polyclonal antibody (Marcellin *et al.*, 1991). The results of HBV detection in patients with PAN are better when immunohistochemistry is performed on hepatic fragments in order to find HBc antigen (Cacoub *et al.*, 1994). These patients are older than those having PAN without HBV infection, but the cutaneous symptoms of PAN are similar in the two groups of patients. It seems that in the case of HBV infection, the pulmonary manifestations of PAN are less frequent. The prognosis of PAN associated with HBV infection is controversial. In the first series, the mortality of HBV-positive patients was increased, whereas the response to steroids was better in the other series. More recently, data showed that mortality is not different (Guillevin *et al.*, 1989). It was also suggested that those forms of PAN with HBV infection must be treated in a different way than PAN without HBV infection. Protocols using plasma exchange and antiviral agents seem to be effective (Guillevin *et al.*, 1993). HBV infection probably plays a major role in the pathogenesis of PAN since HBs antigen was demonstrated in the affected vessels.

High prevalence of HCV markers was noted in at least three studies, showing that 5–20% of patients with PAN were infected with HCV (Cacoub *et al.*, 1992; Deny *et al.*, 1992; Carson *et al.*, 1993). HCV infection could therefore be also involved in the pathogenesis of PAN, but is clearly less frequent than HBV infection. The detection of HCV RNA is extremely important in order to assess a true association between the viral infection and PAN, since studies using serological tests of the first and second generation can lead to false-positive results, especially in patients with PAN.

Gianotti–Crosti syndrome (GCS)

The role of HBV infection in GCS was discovered in 1973. In the first publications, the HBV subtype ayw was demonstrated in association with the disease. Other subtypes of HBV can be involved, such as adr (Lee *et al.*, 1985). The eruption of GCS is associated with an anicteric hepatitis and occurs during the acute phase of HBV infection. It is now established that many other viruses can be associated with this eruption (Draelos *et al.*, 1986; Caputo *et al.*, 1992), but HBV remains the major cause of GCS. In the large series of 308 patients published by Caputo *et al.* (1992), 22.4% of cases were caused by HBV. There is no distinction between HBsAg-positive and HBsAg-negative forms of GCS. Since detailed virological studies were routinely performed, the frequency of HBsAg-positive forms showed a sharp decrease.

Lichen planus

The link between lichen planus and chronic hepatitis has been well established since the 1980s (Rebora & Rongioletti 1984; GISED, 1990). The high rate of chronic active hepatitis and other liver diseases was demonstrated initially in Italy, but also in the USA (Korkij *et al.*, 1984). The frequency of HBV infection markers is between 4.6% and 42% in the various published series of lichen planus, but the replication of HBV in these patients was generally not demonstrated (Rebora *et al.*, 1985; Divano *et al.*, 1992). Lichen planus has also been reported after HBV vaccination in isolated cases. The link between lichen planus and HBV infection is difficult to establish because: (i) most series originated from Italy, where the prevalence of HBV markers in the general population can be up to 34%, especially in the north of the country and the few rigorous case-control studies are not convincing; (ii) the distinction between HBS antigen and other markers of past HBV infection is often unclear in some of these studies; and (iii) all series were published when serological detection of HCV was not available. The results are controversial even in Italy. In a study of 62 patients from Sassari, Italy, 13 patients were found to have HBV markers (Cottoni *et al.*, 1988) whereas in another study from Italy, the prevalence of HBs antigen was not different in patients with erosive lichen planus than in the general population (Ayala *et al.*, 1986). The pathogenesis of the association between lichen planus and HBV is unclear: HBV infection could induce antibodies directed against the basal cells from keratinizing epithelia. It was also hypothesized that lichen planus can be a cutaneous and hepatic disease, with predominantly cutaneous manifestations.

The association of lichen planus with HCV infection has become more controversial since the early 1990s. Since 1991, many cases of lichen planus associated with HCV antibodies have been reported (Pawlotsky *et al.*, 1995). It seems that HCV infection is more frequent in patients with erosive lichen planus. No particular HCV genotype was associated with lichen planus (Pawlotsky *et al.*, 1995). The prevalence of HCV infection among patients with lichen planus was shown to be very different in several European studies, ranging from 3 to 35%. Nevertheless, most of these studies used only anti-HCV detection and the HCV RNA was not investigated. All these data must be carefully interpreted, since many of the series do not comprise a control group.

The frequency of the association between lichen planus and HCV infection could be related to the prevalence of HCV in the general population: the high frequency of HCV positivity was published mainly in Italy and in Spain. In a large case-controlled study in the east of France, no difference of prevalence of HCV was found between 52 patients with lichen planus and 112 controls (3.8% vs. 2.6%) (Cribier *et al.*, 1994). Moreover, the prevalence of HCV infection among 72 patients with oral lichen planus was not significantly higher than in a group of 5216 controls from the same Paris hospital (5.5% vs. 3.7%) (Dupin *et al.*, 1994). In Italy, the prevalence of HCV infection among 46 patients was 23% (Divano *et al.*, 1992) and 14% among 87 patients in another study (Rebora, 1992), and it is 13% in the experience of Pawlotsky *et al.* (1995) in Paris. Nevertheless, these studies did not comprise a control group. The highest prevalence was noted in a small group of 30 patients from Florida (23% vs. 4.8% in 41 controls) (Bellman *et al.*, 1995).

Large and controlled epidemiological studies are therefore needed in order to determine the exact prevalence of HBV and HCV infection in patients with lichen planus in different parts of the world. It remains to be established whether this association is fortuitous or not.

Porphyria cutanea tarda (PCT)

HBV markers are frequently associated with PCT, as shown in two large series of patients (Rocchi *et al.*, 1986; Valls *et al.*, 1986). The frequency of HBV markers was 50–70% in these studies, but HBs antigen was present in only 17% of the patients reported by Rocchi *et al.* (1986) and 12% of the patients reported by Valls *et al.* (1986). This was, nevertheless, higher than the incidence of HBV markers in the general population of these countries. These series were published before the serological tests for HCV were available and the exact role of HBV infection in PCT was never established. HBV was considered to be a triggering factor along with alcohol or drugs. In a recent series, the genomes of both HBV and HCV were found in 40% and 65% of patients, respectively (Navas *et al.*, 1995). Co-infection by HBV and HCV is a frequent event in these patients.

The link between PCT and HCV infection was established by a large series of studies, in which the prevalence of HCV infection ranged between 50 and 91% in the south of Europe (Fargion *et al.*, 1992; Herrero *et al.*, 1993; Lacour *et al.*, 1993; Cribier *et al.*, 1995; Navas *et al.*, 1995). In the north of Europe, the prevalence of HCV infection in PCT patients was lower, being 8% in Germany (Stölzel *et al.*, 1995), 10% in Ireland (Murphy *et al.*, 1993) and 18% in The Netherlands (Siersema *et al.*, 1992). It is important to note that in these countries, the prevalence of HCV among the general population was much lower. These data suggest a strong epidemiological link between HCV infection and PCT.

A detailed virological study (Cribier *et al.*, 1995) showed that there was no correlation between the viral disease and PCT, therefore suggesting that the link between viral hepatitis and the cutaneous disease is indirect. It was recently demonstrated by the present authors that in patients without PCT, HCV infection was not sufficient to induce significant changes in the metabolism of porphyrins. It is likely that PCT occurs in genetically predisposed individuals and that HCV infection plays the role of a major triggering factor of the disease along with other exogenous factors.

Conclusion

Cutaneous diseases associated with HAV infection are rare, probably because of the absence of chronic infection by this virus. HBV infection is strongly associated with polyarteritis nodosa and Gianotti–Crosti syndrome, and is significantly associated with small-vessel vasculitis, including urticaria, leucocytoclastic vasculitis and some cases of cryoglobulinaemia, and with porphyria cutanea tarda. The link between HBV and lichen planus remains controversial. Since the discovery of HCV, it was shown that HCV infection is strongly associated with cryoglobulinaemia and porphyria cutanea tarda. HCV can be the cause in polyarteritis nodosa, but far less frequently than HBV. The association between lichen planus and HCV infection remains to be confirmed. Serological detection of HBV and HCV antibodies must therefore be frequently carried out in dermatological studies.

References

Agnello, V., Chung, R.T. & Kaplan, L.M. (1992) A role for hepatitis C virus infection in type II cryoglobulinemia. *New England Journal of Medicine*, **327**, 1490–1495.

Ayala, F., Balato, N., Tranfaglia, A., Guadagnino, V. & Orlando, R. (1986) Oral lichen planus and chronic liver disease. *Journal of the American Academy of Dermatology*, **14**, 139–140.

Bellman, B., Reddy, R.K. & Falanga, V. (1995) Lichen planus associated with hepatitis C. *Lancet*, **346**, 1234.

Cacoub, P., Lunel-Fabiani, F. & Le Thi Huong, D. (1992) Polyarteritis nodosa and hepatitis C virus infection. *Annals of Internal Medicine*, **116**, 605–606.

Cacoub, P., Valla, D., Chemlal, K. *et al.* (1994) Atteintes hépatique et biliaire associées aux maladies systémiques. *Gastroenterologie Clinique et Biologique*, **18**, 414–423.

Caputo, R., Gelmetti, C., Ermacora, E., Gianni, E. & Silvestri, A. (1992) Gianotti–Crosti syndrome: a retrospective analysis of 308 cases. *Journal of the American Academy of Dermatology*, **26**, 207–210.

Carson, C.W., Conn, D.L., Czaja, A.J., Wright, T.L. & Brecher, M.E. (1993) Frequency and significance of antibodies to hepatitis C virus in polyarteritis nodosa. *Journal of Rheumatology*, **20**, 304–309.

Cottoni, F., Solinas, A. & Piga, M.R. (1988) Lichen planus, chronic liver disease and immunologic involvement. *Archives of Dermatological Research*, **280** (Suppl), S55–S60.

Cribier, B., Garnier, C.,Laustriat, D. & Heid, E. (1994) Lichen planus and hepatitis C virus infection: an epidemiological study. *Journal of the American Academy of Dermatology*, **31**, 1070–1072.

Cribier, B., Petiau, P., Keller, F., Schmitt, C., Heid, E. & Grosshans, E. (1995) Porphyria cutanea tarda and hepatitis C virus infection: a clinical and virological study. *Archives of Dermatology*, **131**, 801–804.

Deny, P., Bonacorsi, S., Guillevin, L. & Quint, L. (1992) Association between hepatitis C virus and polyarteritis nodosa. *Clinical and Experimental Rheumatology*, **10**, 319–324.

Divano, M.C., Parodi, A. & Rebora, A. (1992) Lichen planus, liver kidney microsomal (LKM1) antibodies and hepatitis C virus antibodies. *Dermatology*, **185**, 132–133.

Doutre, M.S., Beylot, C., Beylot, J. & Bioulac, P. (1987) Marqueurs du virus de l'hépatite B chez les sujets ayant une urticaire chronique. 100 observations. *Presse Médicale*, **16**, 1009–1010.

Doutre, M.S., Beylot, C., Beylot-Barry, M., Couzigou, P. & Beylot, J. (1995) Les manifestations cutanées associées au virus de l'hépatite C. *Revue de Medicine Interne*, **16**, 666–672.

Draelos, Z.K., Hansen, R.C. & James, W.D. (1986) Gianotti–Crosti syndrome associated with infections other than hepatitis B. *Journal of the American Medical Association*, **256**, 2386–2388.

Dupin, N., Chosidow, O., Lunel, F. *et al.* (1994) Lichen buccal et infection par le virus de l'hépatite C: étude épidémiologique préliminaire. *Annals de Dermatologie et de Venereologie*, **121**, S52–S53.

Dupin, N., Chosidow, O., Lunel, F. *et al.* (1995) Essential mixed cryoglobulinemia. A comparative study of dermatologic manifestations in patients infected or noninfected with hepatitis C virus. *Archives of Dermatology*, **131**, 1124–1127.

Fargion, S., Piperno, A., Cappellini, M.D. *et al.* (1992) Hepatitis C and porphyria cutanea tarda: evidence of a strong association. *Hepatology*, **16**, 1322–1326.

Gruppo Italiano Studi Epidemiologici in Dermatologia (1990) Lichen planus and liver diseases: a multicentre case control study. *British Medical Journal*, **300**, 227–230.

Guillevin, L., Le Thi Huong, D., Gayraud, M. *et al.* (1989) Systemic vasculitis of the polyarteritis nodosa group and infection with hepatitis B virus: a study in 98 patients. *European Journal of Internal Medicine*, **1**, 97–105.

Guillevin, L., Lhote, F., Leon, A., Fauvelle, F., Vivitski, L. & Trépo, C. (1993) Treatment of polyarteritis nodosa related to hepatitis B virus with short term steroid therapy associated with antiviral agents and plasma exchanges. A prospective trial in 33 patients. *Journal of Rheumatology*, **20**, 289–298.

Herrero, C., Vicente, A., Brugera, M. *et al.* (1993) Is hepatitis C virus a trigger of porphyria cutanea tarda? *Lancet*, **341**, 788–789.

Karlsberg, P.L., Lee, W.M., Casey, D.L., Cockerell, C.J. & Cruz, P.D. (1995) Cutaneous vasculitis and rheumatoid factor positivity as presenting sign of hepatitis C virus-induced mixed cryoglobulinemia. *Archives of Dermatology*, **131**, 1119–1123.

Korkij, W., Chuang, T.Y. & Soltani, K. (1984) Liver abnormalities in patients with lichen planus: a retrospective case-control study. *Journal of the American Academy of Dermatology*, **11**, 609–615.

Lacour, J.P., Bodokh, J.M., Schaeffer, A., Bekri, S. & Ortonne, J.P. (1993) Porphyria cutanea tarda and antibodies to hepatitis C virus. *British Journal of Dermatology*, **128**, 121–123.

Lee, S., Kim, K.Y., Hahn, C.S., Lee, M.G. & Cho, C.K. (1985) Gianotti–Crosti syndrome associated with hepatitis B surface antigen (type adr). *Journal of the American Academy of Dermatology*, **12**, 629–633.

Levo, Y., Gorevic, P., Kassab, H.J., Zucker-Franklin, D. & Franklin, E.C. (1977) Association between hepatitis B virus and essential mixed cryoglobulinemia. *New England Journal of Medicine*, **296**, 1504–1507.

Lewis, J.H., Brandon, J.M., Gorenc, T.J. & Maxwell, N.G. (1973) Hepatitis B. A study of 200 cases positive for the hepatitis B antigen. *Digestive Diseases*, **18**, 921–929.

Lunel, F., Musset, C., Cacoub, P. *et al.* (1994) Cryoglobulinemia in chronic liver diseases: role of hepatitis C virus and liver damage. *Gastroenterology*, **106**, 1291–1300.

McElgun, P.S.J. (1983) Dermatologic manifestations of hepatitis B infection. *Journal of the American Academy of Dermatology*, **8**, 539–548.

Marcellin, P., Calmus, Y., Takayashi, H. *et al.* (1991) Latent hepatitis B infection virus infection in systemic necrotizing vasculitis. *Clinical and Experimental Rheumatology*, **9**, 23–28.

Misiani, R., Bellavita, P., Fenili, D. *et al.* (1994) Interferon alpha-2a therapy in cryoglobulinemia associated with hepatitis C virus. *New England Journal of Medicine*, **330**, 751–756.

Murphy, A., Dooley, S., Hillary, I.B. & Murphy, G.R. (1993) HCV infection in porphyria cutanea tarda. *Lancet*, **341**, 1534–1535.

Navas, S., Bosch, O., Castillo, I., Mariotte, E. & Carreno, V. (1995) Porphyria cutanea tarda and hepatitis C and B viruses infection: a retrospective study. *Hepatology*, **21**, 279–284.

Neumann, H.A., Berretty, P.J.M., Reinders Folmer, S.C.C. & Cormane, R.H. (1981) Hepatitis B surface antigen deposition in the blood vessel walls of urticarial lesions in acute hepatitis B. *British Journal of Dermatology*, **104**, 383–388.

Pawlotsky, J.M., Dhumaux, D. & Bagot, M. (1995) Hepatitis C virus in dermatology. A review. *Archives of Dermatology*, **131**, 1185–1193.

Popp, J., Dienstag, J.L., Wands, J.R. & Bloch, K.J. (1980) Essential mixed cryoglobulinaemia without evidence for hepatitis B virus infection. *Annals of Internal Medicine*, **92**, 379–383.

Popp, J.W., Harrist, T.J., Dienstag, J.L. *et al.* (1981) Cutaneous vasculitis associated with acute and chronic hepatitis. *Archives of Internal Medicine*, **141**, 623–629.

Rebora, A. (1992) Lichen planus and the liver. *International Journal of Dermatology*, **31**, 392–395.

Rebora, A. & Rongioletti, F. (1984) Lichen planus and chronic active hepatitis. *Acta Dermato-Venereologica (Stockholm)*, **64**, 52–56.

Rebora, A., Rongioletti, F. & Grosshans, E. (1985) Le syndrome lichen-hépatite. Revue générale à propos d'un cas. *Annales de Dermatologie et de Venereologie*, **112**, 27–32.

Rocchi, E., Gibertini, P., Casanelli, M. *et al.* (1986) Hepatitis B virus infection in porphyria cutanea tarda. *Liver*, **6**, 153–157.

Routenberg, J.A., Dienstag, J.L., Harrison, W. *et al.* (1979) Foodborne outbreak of hepatitis A: clinical and laboratory features of acute and protracted illness. *American Journal of Medical Science*, **278**, 123–137.

Siersema, P.D., Ten Kate, F.J.W., Mulder, P.G.H. & Wilson, J.H.P. (1992) Hepatocellular carcinoma in porphyria cutanea tarda: frequency and factors related to its occurrence. *Liver*, **12**, 56–61.

Steigman, A.J. (1973) Rashes and arthropathy in viral hepatitis. *Mount Sinaï Journal of Medicine (New York)*, **40**, 752–757.

Stölzel, U., Köstler, E., Koszka, C. *et al.* (1995) Low prevalence of hepatitis C virus infection in porphyria cutanea tarda in Germany. *Hepatology*, **21**, 1500–1503.

Trépo, C. (1989) Virus de l'hépatite B et périartérite noueuse. *Gastroenterologie Clinique et Biologique*, **13**, 117–119.

Valls, V., Enriquez de Salamanca, R., Lapena, L. *et al.* (1986) Hepatitis B serum markers in porphyria cutanea tarda. *Journal of Dermatology*, **13**, 24–29.

HIV-Associated Dermatoses: Prevalence and Prognostic Marker Function

C. GARBE

HIV-associated dermatoses have significantly enlarged the spectrum of dermatological diseases since the early 1980s (Table 16.1). In HIV infection, infectious dermatoses with unusual widespread manifestations and severe courses were observed, rare tumours like Kaposi's sarcoma were found in new variants and classical dermatoses like seborrhoeic dermatitis and psoriasis developed in a higher prevalence and were more difficult to treat (Friedman-Kien, 1981; Berger *et al.*, 1988; Coldiron & Bergstresser, 1989; Berger & Green 1991; Cockerell, 1991a,b; Dover & Johnson, 1991a,b). Investigation of diseases associated with HIV infection increased our knowledge and the aetiology

Table 16.1 Classification of HIV-associated dermatoses.

Infections
Viral
Bacterial
Mycotic
Protozoal

Tumours
Kaposi's sarcoma
Lymphoma
Carcinoma
Melanoma

Dermatoses
Seborrhoeic dermatitis
Psoriasis
Pruritic papular dermatosis
Eosinophilic folliculitis
Vasculitis
Hair/nail disorders
Pigmentary disorders
Others

Table 16.2 Prevalence of HIV-associated dermatoses among 456 HIV-infected patients in the Berlin study.

Disease	Prevalence (%)
Oral candidosis	44.5
Seborrhoeic dermatitis	38.6
Folliculitis	32.9
Kaposi's sarcoma	23.5
Xeroderma	22.8
Herpes zoster	20.6
Tinea unguium	20.2
Tinea pedis	20.0
Herpes genitoanalis	19.3
Condylomata acuminata	18.4
Oral hairy leucoplakia	15.6
Herpes labialis	13.6
Anal eczema	13.2
Pyoderma	11.8
Verrucae vulgares	11.2
Drug eruptions	10.7
Mollusca contagiosa	8.6
Contact dermatitis	7.5
Tinea corporis	6.6
Psoriasis	6.4
Atopic dermatitis	5.9
Erythrasma	3.9
HIV exanthema	3.9

of certain diseases like Kaposi's sarcoma has been better elucidated.

The present study examines the prevalence of HIV-associated dermatoses and their relationship to the immune status of the patient. In particular, it is interesting to see whether HIV-associated dermatoses can be taken as a marker for an early diagnosis of HIV infection and whether they have a prognostic significance.

Patients and methods

In the Department of Dermatology, University Medical Center Benjamin Franklin in Berlin, all HIV-infected patients were documented over the years 1982 to 1992 (Garbe *et al.*, 1994). The data were recorded with the databank program DBASE IV and statistically evaluated. Altogether, 456 HIV-infected patients were included in the present study. These patients were seen in the Department of Dermatology as out-patients or in-patients. They were followed up in a special HIV clinic in the Department, and the course of the disease was documented. During the course of HIV infection, certain diseases may have been documented several times.

The diagnosis of HIV infection was confirmed in all patients by enzyme-linked immunosorbent assay (ELISA) and Western blot analysis. Additionally, CD4$^+$ and CD8$^+$ T-lymphocyte counts were performed regularly, every 6–8 months. The occurrence of dermatological diseases could, therefore, be related to the immune status over the same period. Several patients died during the follow-up. Causes of death were likewise recorded and evaluated.

The median follow-up time of the patients was 27 months. The cumulative follow-up time was 1026 years of observation. Survival rates were calculated by the method of Kaplan and Meier. Differences in survival rates were tested by the log-rank test and $P < 0.05$ values were regarded as statistically significant.

Demographic data

The patients consisted of 91% males, 8% females and 1% transsexuals. The medium age of the patients was 33 years. HIV infection occurred mainly within the homosexual or bisexual risk groups. This was true for

Table 16.3 Prevalence of dermatoses in HIV-infected individuals in the Berlin study and in a military population in the USA.

Disease	Percentage in Berlin study	Percentage in US study
Oral candidosis	45	24
Seborrhoeic dermatitis	39	53
Folliculitis	33	25
Kaposi's sarcoma	24	6
Xeroderma	23	75
Herpes zoster	21	6
Tinea unguium	20	
Tinea pedis	20	64
Herpes genitoanalis	19	17
Condylomata acuminata	18	19
Oral hairy leucoplakia	16	19

Table 16.4 Median and 75% percentile values of CD4$^+$ T lymphocytes/µl blood at diagnosis of different skin diseases in HIV-infected patients. The diagnoses are given in the order of their 75% percentile value.

Disease	CD4$^+$ counts	
	Median	75% Percentile
Tinea corporis	232	588
Contact dermatitis	330	571
Verrucae vulgares	321	571
Pyoderma	217	486
Tinea pedis	274	483
Condylomata acuminata	320	476
Folliculitis	259	448
Herpes zoster	288	432
Herpes labialis	242	431
Seborrhoeic dermatitis	244	413
Xeroderma	112	397
Psoriasis	133	390
Atopic dermatitis	241	371
Tinea unguium	156	369
Erythrasma	169	364
Oral hairy leucoplakia	224	354
Oral candidosis	142	346
Herpes genitoanalis	139	327
Mollusca contagiosa	113	246
Drug eruptions	95	226
Kaposi's sarcoma	82	213

78% of all patients. In 13% of patients, drug abuse was noted. Only 7% of the patients belonged to the heterosexual group. In 2% of the patients, an infection by blood transfusion was supposed and in 1%, the routes of infection remained unclear.

Immune status

The mean number of CD4$^+$ T lymphocytes at the first dermatological presentation was 310/µl; the median number was 239/µl. The first diagnosis of HIV infection was made in about 25% of patients in the Department of Dermatology. Among those patients with a pre-existing diagnosis of HIV positivity, the CD4$^+$ T-lymphocyte values from previous medical examinations at the first diagnosis were known in 139 patients. These were only slightly higher than at the first dermatological presentation with a mean value of 324/µl and a median value of 264/µl, respectively. The proximity between the CD4$^+$ T-lymphocyte values at first diagnosis and that at the first dermatological presentation indicates that dermatological disorders belong to the earliest symptoms in HIV infection.

Of all patients, 41% were diagnosed in CDC stages I–III, even before manifestation of AIDS (CDC, 1987); 59% were diagnosed only in the stages of full-blown AIDS. Among these patients, 17% had AIDS-defining infections, 18% had other infections and 22% were diagnosed as having Kaposi's sarcoma.

Prevalence

Table 16.2 summarizes the prevalence of HIV-associated dermatoses in the present study. Infectious dermatoses represented the majority of disease manifestations. Oral cand idosis was found in 45% of patients, seborrhoeic dermatitis in 39% and folliculitis in 33% (Goodman *et al.*, 1987; Alessi *et al.*, 1988). This was followed by Kaposi's sarcoma which was diagnosed in 24% of all patients (Smith *et al.*, 1993c). Other frequent diseases were viral infections like herpes zoster (21%), herpes genitoanalis (19%), condylomata acuminata (18%) and oral hairy leucoplakia (15%) (Friedman-Kien *et al.*, 1986; Feigal *et al.*, 1991; Schwartz & Myskowski, 1992). Mycotic infections were also among the most frequent disease manifestations, like tinea pedis (20%) and tinea unguium (20%). Relatively rare were classical dermatoses like psoriasis (6%) and atopic dermatitis (6%) (Cockerell, 1991a; Smith *et al.*,

1993a,b). However, the prevalence of psoriasis in HIV-positive individuals is, at 6%, clearly higher than in the general population (2–3%) (Coldiron & Bergstresser, 1989; Arnett *et al.*, 1991; Obuch *et al.*, 1992).

Comparisons of the prevalence evaluated in the Berlin study to examinations of the prevalence in other studies are interesting. Recently, Smith *et al.* published a study in 912 military employees who have been followed up for a medium time of 42 months (Smith *et al.*, 1994). All these military employees were obliged to attend an HIV test. A considerable percentage of these subjects, therefore, were already diagnosed in the asymptomatic stages. This study also consisted of 91% males, and the medium age was comparable, at 42 years. The values of this American study were quite close to those found in our Berlin study (Table 16.3).

Interestingly, the American study presented with clearly higher values of tinea pedis, which might be related to the work of soldiers. On the other hand, Kaposi's sarcoma and herpes zoster were less common. This may be due to the fact that the immune status was more favourable at the first diagnosis in the American study, with obligatory HIV tests.

Relation to the immune status

To analyse the relationship between manifestation of the diseases and the immune status, the median CD4$^+$ T-lymphocyte counts and their 75% percentiles were evaluated (Table 16.4). The 75% percentile indicates an immune value for the detection of early manifestations of the disease; 25% of the patients had already developed their specific diseases with immune values above the 75% percentile.

The earliest manifestations of HIV infection were tinea corporis, contact dermatitis, verrucae vulgaris, pyoderma, tinea pedis, condylomata acuminata and folliculitis (Berger *et al.*, 1988; Berger & Greene, 1991). These infectious diseases are not specific for HIV infection and may, in part, be likewise present in healthy individuals or in homosexuals. Nevertheless, they are much more frequent in immune-suppressed HIV-infected persons.

Several HIV-associated dermatoses occur only during the late stages of HIV infection and in advanced immunosuppression. This is mainly true for Kaposi's sarcoma with median CD4$^+$ T-lymphocyte counts of 82/μl for oral hairy leucoplakia (Greenspan *et al.*, 1984), oral candidosis, persistent herpes genitoanalis and for mollusca contagiosa (Fleischer *et al.*, 1992; Koopman *et al.*, 1992). Interestingly, drug eruptions occur likewise rather late in the course of HIV infection (Saiag *et al.*, 1992; Coopman *et al.*, 1993). The reason may be that multiple drugs are often prescribed in the late stages for the treatment of opportunistic infections.

Prognostic significance

The CD4$^+$ T-lymphocyte counts are presently regarded as the most important prognostic factor in HIV infection. For example, in the Berlin study, the median survival time was 96 months for patients with CD4$^+$ T-lymphocyte counts > 300/μl at their first diagnosis, whereas it decreased to 72 months in patients with 100–300/μl and to 42 months in patients with CD4$^+$ T-lymphocyte counts < 100/μl.

We looked for the prognostic significance of different dermatoses separately for the subgroups with > 300 or < 300 CD4$^+$ T lymphocytes/μl by survival calcu-lations according to Kaplan and Meier and by the log-rank test. The manifestation of Kaposi's sarcoma was associated with a significantly poorer prognosis in both the more immunocompetent as well as the immunosuppressed subgroups. The manifestation of oral hairy leucoplakia was also associated with a poorer prognosis only in the subgroup with > 300 CD4$^+$ T lymphocytes/ml. None of the other dermatological disorders showed any prognostic marker function.

References

Alessi, E., Cusini, M. & Zerboni, R. (1988) Mucocutaneous manifestations in patients infected with human immunodeficiency virus. *Journal of the American Academy of Dermatology*, **19**, 290–297.

Arnett, F.C., Reveille, J.D. & Duvic, M. (1991) Psoriasis and psoriatic arthritis associated with human immunodeficiency virus infection. *Rheumatic Diseases Clinics of North America*, **17**, 59–78.

Berger, R.S., Stoner, M.F., Hobbs, E.R., Hayes, T.J. & Boswell, R.N. (1988) Cutaneous manifestations of early human immunodeficiency virus exposure. *Journal of the American Academy of Dermatology*, **19**, 298–303.

Berger, T.G. & Greene, I. (1991) Bacterial, viral, fungal, and parasitic infections in HIV disease and AIDS. *Dermatology Clinics*, **9**, 465–492.

CDC (1987) Leads from the MMWR. Revision of the CDC surveillance case definition for acquired immunodeficiency syndrome. *Journal of the American Medical Association*, **258**, 1143–1154.

Cockerell, C.J. (1991a) Noninfectious inflammatory skin diseases in HIV-infected individuals. *Dermatology Clinics*, **9**, 531–541.

Cockerell, C.J. (1991b) Human immunodeficiency virus infection and the skin. A crucial interface. *Archives of Internal Medicine*, **151**, 1295–1303.

Coldiron, B.M. & Bergstresser, P.R. (1989) Prevalence and clinical spectrum of skin disease in patients infected with human immunodeficiency virus. *Archives of Dermatology*, **125**, 357–361.

Coopman, S.A., Johnson, R.A., Platt, R. & Stern, R.S. (1993) Cutaneous disease and drug reactions in HIV infection. *New England Journal of Medicine*, **328**, 1670–1674.

Dover, J.S. & Johnson, R.A. (1991a) Cutaneous manifestations of human immunodeficiency virus infection. Part I. *Archives of Dermatology*, **127**, 1383–1391.

Dover, J.S. & Johnson, R.A. (1991b) Cutaneous manifestations of human immunodeficiency virus infection. Part II. *Archives of Dermatology*, **127**, 1549–1558.

Feigal, D.W., Katz, M.H., Greenspan, D. *et al.* (1991) The prevalence of oral lesions in HIV-infected homosexual and bisexual men: three San Francisco epidemiological cohorts. *AIDS*, **5**, 519–525.

Fleischer, A.B. Jr, Gallagher, P.N. & van der Horst, C. (1992) Mucocutaneous abnormalities predicted by lymphocyte counts in patients infected with the human immunodeficiency virus. *Southern Medical Journal*, **85**, 687–690.

Friedman-Kien, A.E. (1981) Disseminated Kaposi's sarcoma syndrome in young homosexual men. *Journal of the American Academy of Dermatology*, **5**, 468–471.

Friedman-Kien, A.E., Lafleur, F.L., Gendler, E. *et al.* (1986) Herpes zoster: a possible early clinical sign for development of acquired immunodeficiency syndrome in high-risk individuals. *Journal of the American Academy of Dermatology*, **14**, 1023–1028.

Garbe, C., Husak, R. & Orfanos, C.E. (1994) HIV-assoziierte Dermatosen und ihre Prävalenz bei 456 HIV-Infizierten. *Hautarzt*, **45**, 623–629.

Goodman, D.S., Teplitz, E.D., Wishner, A., Klein, R.S., Burk, P.G. & Hershenbaum, E. (1987) Prevalence of cutaneous disease in patients with acquired immunodeficiency syndrome (AIDS) or AIDS-related complex. *Journal of the American Academy of Dermatology*, **17**, 210–220.

Greenspan, D., Greenspan, J.S., Conant, M., Petersen, V., Silverman, S. Jr & de Souza, Y. (1984) Oral 'hairy' leucoplakia in male homosexuals: evidence of association with both papillomavirus and a herpes-group virus. *Lancet*, **ii**, 831–834.

Koopman, R.J., van Merrienboer, F.C., Vreden, S.G. & Dolmans, W.M. (1992) Molluscum contagiosum; a marker for advanced HIV infection. (Letter.) *British Journal of Dermatology*, **126**, 528–529.

Obuch, M.L., Maurer, T.A., Becker, B. & Berger, T.G. (1992) Psoriasis and human immunodeficiency virus infection. *Journal of the American Academy of Dermatology*, **27**, 667–673.

Saiag, P., Caumes, E., Chosidow, O., Revuz, J. & Roujeau, J.C. (1992) Drug-induced toxic epidermal necrolysis (Lyell syndrome) in patients infected with the human immunodeficiency virus. *Journal of the American Academy of Dermatology*, **26**, 567–574.

Schwartz, J.J. & Myskowski, P.L. (1992) Molluscum contagiosum in patients with human immunodeficiency virus infection. A review of twenty-seven patients. *Journal of the American Academy of Dermatology*, **27**, 583–588.

Smith, K.J., Skelton, H.G., Yeager, J. *et al.* (1993a) Clinical features of inflammatory dermatoses in human immunodeficiency virus type 1 disease and their correlation with Walter Reed stage. Military Medical Consortium for Applied Retroviral Research. *Journal of the American Academy of Dermatology*, **28**, 167–173.

Smith, K.J., Skelton, H.G., Yeager, J. *et al.* (1993b) Histopathologic and immunohistochemical findings associated with inflammatory dermatoses in human immunodeficiency virus type 1 disease and their correlation with Walter Reed stage. Military Medical Consortium for Applied Retroviral Research. *Journal of the American Academy of Dermatology*, **28**, 174–184.

Smith, K.J., Skelton, H.G., Yeager, J., Angritt, P. & Wagner, K.F. (1993c) Cutaneous neoplasms in a military population of HIV-1-positive patients. *Journal of the American Academy of Dermatology*, **29**, 400–406.

Smith, K.J., Skelton, H.G., Yeager, J. *et al.* (1994) Cutaneous findings in HIV-1-positive patients: A 42-month prospective study. *Journal of the American Academy of Dermatology*, **31**, 746–754.

Rickettsia, Borrelia and Bartonella Skin Infections

PH. BROUQUI AND D. RAOULT

Introduction

Rickettsioses, borrelioses and bartonelloses are vector-borne diseases of humans acquired after contact with arthropods such as ticks, lice and fleas. Rash and 'tache noire' (tick bite) is one of the most frequent clinical symptoms of most rickettsioses, while erythema chronicum migrans and acrodermatitis chronica atrophians are common in Lyme diseases. More recently, great interest has been shown in the cutaneous manifestations of bartonelloses, especially in bacilliary angiomatosis and verruga peruana. The epidemiology of these skin diseases is dependent on the ecology of their vectors and we have therefore separated them into tick-transmitted rickettsioses, louse-transmitted rickettsioses, tick-transmitted borrelioses and louse-transmitted borrelioses and bartonelloses.

Tick-transmitted rickettsioses

These rickettsioses are caused by the spotted fever group rickettsiae with *Rickettsia rickettsii* being the agent of Rocky Mountain spotted fever (RMSF), *R. conorii* the agent of Mediterranean spotted fever (MSF) and *R. africae* the agent of African tick-bite fever (ATBF). Cutaneous expression of these disease includes both 'tache noire' and a febrile rash. However, the frequencies of both symptoms are very different between the diseases; RMSF patients rarely present with 'tache noire', ATBF patients rarely present with a rash but frequently multiple 'tache noire' and MSF patients usually present both symptoms.

Description of pathogen

The three causative agents are taxonomically very close and all are strict intracellular bacteria which preferentially invade endothelial cells, leading to the classical rickettsial vasculitis (Walker & Raoult, 1995). They can be identified in the laboratory by immunostaining of either cutaneous biopsy or circulating endothelial cells (Drancourt *et al.*, 1992). However, the diagnosis is more usually confirmed serologically by indirect microimmunofluorescence.

Epidemiology

Rocky Mountain spotted fever

This is transmitted by *Dermacentor variabilis* ticks (the American dog tick) in the eastern United States and

D. andersonii (the Rocky Mountain wood tick) in the western states. Thus, RMSF is as likely to be an occupational disease for woodcutters in Montana as an infection of a dog owner in the city of Baltimore. RMSF occurs in both North and South America, having been reported in the United States, Brazil and Mexico. *R. rickettsii* is transmitted trans-stadially (stage to stage) and transovarially in ticks, which are thus both the vector and the main reservoir of *R. rickettsii*. Of the three tick stages, larva, nymph and adult, only the last bites humans. Most cases of RMSF occur during late spring and the summer when this stage is most prevalent. The prevalence of *R. rickettsii* in ticks is usually low. However, variation in infection rates among tick populations exists. What influences this variation is not clear, although humidity, climatic variation, human activities altering vegetation and fauna and the use of insecticides have been suspected to play a role in the fluctuation of the prevalence of human rickettsioses. Although the prevalence of *Rickettsia* in ticks is low, the frequent contact between man and tick means the prevalence of the disease may be as high as 14.9 per 10 000 inhabitants (mean of 3 per 10 000). Incubation time ranges from 2 to 14 days with a median of 7 days. Unlike *Rhipicephalus* tick bites, those of *Dermacentor* rarely lead to cutaneous symptoms at the site of the bite, thus 'tache noire' are only very seldom encountered in RMSF.

Mediterranean spotted fever

This is also named 'boutonneuse fever' or 'Marseilles fever' and is transmitted by *Rhipicephalus sanguineus* ticks (the brown dog tick). This tick is widely distributed throughout the world and MSF has been reported in southern Europe, Morroco, South Africa, Kenya, Ethiopia, the Ukraine, Georgia, Russia, Israel, Pakistan and India (Walker & Raoult, 1995). The epidemiology of MSF is closely related to the ecology of ticks. The frequent absence of apparent tick bites in patients with MSF is due to transmission by immature larvae and nymphs which often go unnoticed. Transmission has also been reported via the conjunctival mucosae following contact with bacterial-contaminated fingers. *R. conorii* is transmitted transovarially through the tick *R. sanguineus*. Thus, as with *R. rickettsii*, the arthropod is both the vector and the reservoir of the bacterium. It is estimated that 10% of *R. sanguineus* are infected with *R. conorii* which is a higher rate than for *R. rickettsii* (see above). However, as *R. sanguineus* bite humans less frequently than *Dermacentor* ticks, the prevalence of MSF is closer to that of RMSF. Transmission of the disease to humans is only possible if the tick adheres to the body for more than 20 hours. Cases occur mainly in warm months with the peak incidence in July, August and September. A substantial number of imported cases occur in travellers returning to the United States and to northern Europe from Africa and southern Europe.

African tick-bite fever

This is a disease of southern Africa. The main clinical expression of the disease is febrile eschars related to multiple bites. The vector of *R. africae* is the tick *Amblyomma hebraeum* which bites humans and other mammals frequently. Geographical repartition of the disease is closely related to the distribution of *A. hebraeum*. African tick-bite fever is an underestimated cause of febrile 'tache noire' in travellers returning to the United States from southern Africa.

Other spotted fever group rickettsia include *R. japonica*, *R. sibirica* and *R. australis*. Their epidemiology depends upon the ecology of their vectors, which are *Haemaphysalis longicornis* for *R. japonica*, *Dermacentor nuttalli* for *R. sibirica* and *Ixodes holocyclus* for *R. autralis*.

Prevention

A well-organized and carefully implemented programme can successfully control medically important ticks in a limited geographical area. Such programmes include the widespread use of acaricides on domestic animals or the breeding of domestic animals that are resistant to tick infestation. However, the use of insect repellents on domestic animals should be done with care, as such practice could lead to ticks feeding more often on humans. Spraying of an area with appropriate chemicals may temporarily reduce the tick population.

Persons who risk exposure to ticks should wear protective clothing, use insect repellents and examine themselves carefully for ticks. Children should be examined periodically by their parents during the tick season in endemic areas (mid-spring to late summer).

The immediate removal of ticks obviously reduces the risk of transmission of the disease. Periodic removal of ticks from household pets is also important and should help to prevent the spread of ticks within the household. However, when doing this, gloves should be worn in order to prevent fingers becoming contaminated by crushed ticks. Antibiotic chemoprophylaxis fails to prevent the development of the disease after a tick bite, and merely delays its onset until the treatment is ceased. Antibiotic therapy should only be prescribed once the symptoms have appeared.

Lice-transmitted rickettsioses (epidemic typhus) (Saah, 1995)

Lice infestation has been observed in virtually every inhabited area of the world. At times of war, overcrowding or widespread inattention to personal hygiene resulted in major epidemics. Lice are medically important not only because they can cause significant cutaneous disease, but also because they may serve as vectors for infectious diseases.

Description of pathogen

Epidemic typhus is caused by *R. prowazekii*, a species of the typhus group, closely related to the agent that causes murine typhus, *R. typhi* (see below). The major clinical manifestations are a febrile eruptive disease with neuropsychiatric dysfunction. The rash consists of non-confluent, pink macules that fade on pressure and became maculopapular, darker, petechial and confluent, covering all the body within a few days. Pathogenesis of the rash is based upon the rickettsial vasculitis due to infection of vascular endothelial cells.

Epidemiology

Louse-borne typhus is transmitted from person to person by the body louse, *Pediculus humanus corporis*. The cycle is thought to be initiated by the louse feeding on an infected rickettsiaemic person. The organism infects the alimentary tract of the louse, resulting in large numbers of organisms being excreted in its faeces. The irritation caused to the host by the louse leads to scratching, thereby contaminating the bite wound with louse faeces. *R. prowazekii* is also pathogenic to its louse vector, which dies of its infection within 3 weeks. No transovarial transmission of *R. prowazekii* therefore occurs. Human conditions that foster the proliferation of lice are especially common during the winter and during times of war or natural disasters when clothing is not changed, overcrowding occurs and bathing is very infrequent. A reservoir of *R. prowazekii* other than in humans exists in the flying squirrel, *Glaucomys volans*, in the United States and zoonotic cases have been reported.

Prevention

Control of the human body louse and the conditions that foster its proliferation is the mainstay in preventing louse-borne typhus. Delousing should be done with a suitably effective insecticide. Usually dichlorodiphenyltrichloroethane (DDT) or lindane in powder form is effective. If the lice are not susceptible to these insecticides, then malathion or carbaryl may be used. As the louse lives in dirty clothes, delousing the affected population may also be easily done by removing contaminated clothes and replacing them frequently. Contaminated clothes may be treated by insecticides or boiled. However, because lice do not survive, without feeding, for more than 24 hours, removing clothes for 48 hours is an efficient way to kill the arthropod. Typhus vaccine is prepared from formaldehyde-inactivated whole bacteria. This vaccine is recommended only for special risk groups, such as scientific investigators, or medical and laboratory personnel who work with the pathogen.

Flea-transmitted rickettsioses (murine typhus) (Dumler & Walker, 1995)

The rat flea, *Xenopsylla cheopis*, is the primary vector of murine typhus. The aetiological agent of this disease is *Rickettsia typhi*, an obligate intracellular bacterium that shares common antigens with *R. prowazekii*.

Description of pathogen

Murine typhus is characterized by headaches, myalgia and fever. A macular rash is observed in 60–80% of cases, becoming evident between the third and the fifth day of illness. The rash subsequently becomes maculopapular and typically remains for 4–8 days; however, it may vary greatly in duration and intensity and may be quite evanescent. Diagnosis is usually serologically confirmed.

Epidemiology

Murine typhus is found in all parts of the world, among people whose occupation or living conditions brings them into close contact with rats. Ilness in humans is a peripheral occurrence to the natural transmission of *R. typhi* in rodents. In the rat, the disease is non-fatal. It is transmitted by the rat flea (*X. cheopis*) and possibly by the rat louse, *Polypax spinulosis*. In the flea, the organism multiplies in the cells of the digestive tract. *R. typhi* is now also thought to be transmitted transovarially. As for epidemic typhus, human infection follows contamination of the bite wound with *R. typhi*-infected flea faeces by scratching of the irritating bite.

Prevention

The occurrence of murine typhus indicates the failure of effective ectoparasite and rodent control. Public health officials should be alerted when the disease is suspected. The occurrence of murine typhus implies a situation that would facilitate the transmission of other flea- and rodent-borne diseases if introduced (e.g. plague). However, killing of rats without first destroying their ectoparasites can also lead to epidemics in humans.

Tick-transmitted borrelioses (Lyme disease and tick-borne relapsing fever)

The most common tick-borne disease in the United States is Lyme disease. The known vectors of Lyme disease include *Amblyomma americanum* and several species of *Ixodes*, the most well known of which is *I. dammini*.

Description of pathogen

Lyme disease is a multisystemic disorder caused by

the spirochaete *Borrelia burgdorferi*. At the site of the tick bite, an erythematous papule may develop and expand into an erythematous annular lesion with a central clearing, an eruption known as erythema chronicum migrans (ECM). Patients with Lyme disease may also have late internal involvement, primarily of the cardiovascular system, nerves and joints. Acrodermatidis chronica atrophians (ACA) is a late cutaneous manifestation of Lyme disease which can occur years after ECM. It is characterized by red violacious lesions that become sclerotic or atrophic. This lesion may be the presenting manifestation of Lyme disease, and may last for 20 years. Cutaneous manifestation of Lyme disease, especially ACA, is more frequent in female patients.

Epidemiology (Stanek *et al.*, 1993)

In the north-eastern and mid-western United States, *Ixodes dammini* is the main vector of *B. burgdorferi*, whereas *I. pacificus* is the vector of Lyme disease on the west coast. Other ticks are involved in the infectious cycle of *B. burgdorferi*, including *A. americanum*, *I. scapularis* and *R. sanguineus*. In Europe, *I. ricinus* is the primary vector. In the United States, 10–50% of ticks are infected with *B. burgdoferi*. The nymphal stage of ticks is responsible for transmission of the disease. As the peak period for nymphs is May to July, the peak incidence of ECM occurs in June and July (May to November). *Borrelia burgdorferi* seems to be transmitted by regurgitation of mid-gut contents or by injection of infected tick saliva during feeding. As in MSF, tick attachment for more than 24 hours is necessary before significant transmission of the spirochaete can occur. *Borrelia burgdorferi* is transmitted trans-stadially in the tick; however, these acarians act as vectors rather than reservoirs of the disease. Deer appear to play an important role in the life cycle of *I. dammini*, and deer are abundant in endemic areas of Lyme disease in the United States. In Europe, it is generally assumed that mice (*Apodemus* spp.) and voles (*Clethrionomys* spp.) serve as spirochaetal reservoirs. Some species of ground-frequenting birds have also demonstrated their reservoir competence for *B. burgdorferi*. Although forestry workers and cross-country hikers have been shown to be groups significantly at risk for Lyme disease, it is likely that risk is

really represented by all outdoor activities and tick exposure. Data on seroprevalence in humans suggest an infection rate of between 3% and 40% in Europe. Such a range may be due to geographical variation in the number of *B. burgdorferi*-infected ticks.

Prevention

Prevention of Lyme disease requires the same measures as other tick-borne diseases (see above). Removal of ticks should be performed as soon as possible, certainly before attachment for 24 hours. The following method has been proposed for removal of ticks (Weber & Burgdorfer, 1993):

1 Use blunt forceps or tweezers; pointed forceps are not recommended because they readily puncture partially or fully engorged ticks.

2 Grasp the tick as close as possible and repeatedly pull upward with increasing pressure. Do not jerk, as this may cause the hypostome to break off.

3 Do not squeeze, crush or puncture the attached tick, as its fluids may be infected with *B. burgdorferi* or other infectious agent (see above).

4 Do not attempt removal of a tick with bare hands, as spirochaetes and other agents may enter the body via mucous membranes or skin.

5 Do not use, oil, petroleum jelly, fingernail polish, alcohol or other chemicals, because they do not effect proper detachment of ticks and may even induce the tick to salivate.

After removal, the bite wound should be thoroughly disinfected. The tick should be kept in a box with the date of removal for at least four weeks as a reminder of potential source of infection. Prophylactic antibiotics are usually recommended only if the removed tick has been examined and proven to be infected. In this case either doxycycline (200 mg/day) or amoxycillin (500 mg three times daily) for 5–7 days is given. Treatment should only be prescribed after consultation with the patient and only if clinical symptoms compatible with Lyme disease have been noted.

Tick-borne relapsing fever

This is caused by at least 15 *Borrelia* species and is transmitted to man by soft ticks of the genus *Ornithodoros*. This disease is characterized by several onsets of high fever with severe headaches, myalgia, arthralgia, photophobia and cough. A truncal skin rash of 1–2 days' duration is common at the end of the primary febrile episode. The rash can be macular, petechial or papular (Johnson, 1995).

Many rodents and small animals serve as reservoirs for these borreliae. Infection of humans occurs when saliva or excrement is released by the tick while feeding. Transovarial transmission of borreliae to progeny is important for perpetuation of the spirochaete population. The distribution of the disease is governed by the ecology of ticks. *Ornithodoros* prefer warm and humid environments and altitudes of 1500–6000 feet. They are distributed worldwide, inhabiting caves, decaying wood, rodent burrows and animal shelters. The ticks have a range of movement of less than 50 yards, although they may be carried into human dwellings by rodents. Their presence often passes unnoticed as they are typically night feeders, lack a painful bite and complete their blood feeding in 5–20 minutes. Tick-borne relapsing fever usually occurs sporadically, although a large outbreak has been reported among campers residing in log cabins (Arizona) (Center for Disease Control and Prevention, 1973). Prevention of tick-borne relapsing fever requires the avoidance or elimination of the arthropod vectors by methods similar to those cited above.

Louse-transmitted borrelioses (louse-borne relapsing fever)

The clinical manifestation of louse-borne relapsing fever is quite similar to that of tick-borne relapsing fever, except that it is usually associated with only a single relapse and that its prognosis is much more severe, with death occurring in 40% of untreated cases.

Louse-borne relapsing fever is caused by a single species, *Borrelia recurrentis*, and is transmitted by the human body louse (*Pediculus humanus*). Thus, as described above with epidemic typhus, the distribution and ocurrence of epidemic relapsing fever is largely determined by socio-economic and ecological factors (Johnson, 1995). Following ingestion of infected human blood, the spirochaete multiplies in the haemolymph of the louse. As louse tissues are not invaded by borreliae, disease cannot be transmitted via louse excreta or saliva, nor transovarially. The disease is acquired when infected lice are crushed, releasing borreliae, which are capable of penetrating intact skin or mucous membranes. Humans are the only host for this organism. Louse-borne relapsing fever usually occurs in epidemics that are associated with catastrophic events, such as war or famine. Under such conditions, a lack of hygiene and overcrowding facilitate dissemination of body lice. The last large-scale epidemic was observed during the Second World War in North Africa and Europe and caused an estimated 50 000 deaths (Bryceson *et al.*, 1970). The disease remains endemic in central and east Africa and the South American Andes. Prevention of louse-borne relapsing fever requires measures similar to those used in the prevention of epidemic typhus (see above).

Sandfly-transmitted bartonellosis (verruga peruana)

Cutaneous manifestation of *Bartonella bacilliformis* infection is more commonly referred to as 'verruga peruana', and has been known in Peru since before Columbus.

Description of pathogen

Verruga peruana is characterized by haemangiomatous nodules which develop in the skin and subcutaneous tissues with minor variations in histological characteristics and evolution depending on location (Roberts, 1995). These lesions consist of numerous newly formed small vessels with proliferation of endothelial cells that may contain the causative organism, *Bartonella bacilliformis*. The nodules develop over a period of 1–2 months usually following an acute onset of Oroya fever which is the primary manifestation of *Bartonella bacilliformis* infection, consisting of an acute febrile haemolytic anaemia. The verrugas appeared mostly on the exposed part of the body. They may vary from red to purple, and may be sessile, miliary, nodular pedunculated or confluent.

Epidemiology

Oroya fever and verruga peruana have a strictly limited regional occurrence that is likely due to the limited habitats of its sandfly vector, *Lutzomyia*.

Phlebotomus verrucatum, other species of sandfly and possibly other arthropods, propagate and transmit this infection in the inter-Andean valleys of Peru, Ecuador and Columbia at altitudes of between 1000 and 3000 metres. In these regions, the disease is endemic, with asymptomatic cases and long-term carriers serving as reservoirs of infection.

Prevention

Prevention of infection requires control of the sandfly. For the community, this consists of spraying interiors of dwellings with DDT; for the individual, protection may be obtained by the use of insect repellents and bed netting.

Louse-transmitted bartonellosis (*Bartonella quintana* infections)

Description of pathogen

Bartonella (Rochalimaea) quintana is a small Gram-negative bacterium capable of causing several different clinical diseases in humans, including bacillary angiomatosis, lymphadenopathy, endocarditis in homeless patients and trench fever which was encountered in vast epidemics among troops during the First World War (Byam *et al.*, 1919). Bacillary angiomatosis is the main skin manifestation of the disease. Bacillary (epithelioid) angiomatosis is a neovascular proliferative disorder originally described involving the skin and regional lymph nodes of HIV-infected persons (Slater *et al.*, 1990). These lesions are remarkably similar to those of verruga peruana. However, in HIV-infected individuals, the main differential diagnosis is atypical Kaposi sarcoma. Lesions can be subcutaneous or dermal nodules and/or single or multiple dome-shape, skin-coloured or red-to-purple papules, any of which may display ulceration, serous or bloody drainage and crusting. Their number may vary from a few to hundreds and size from millimetres to centimetres in diameter. Histologically, they consist of lobular proliferation of small blood vessels containing plump, cuboidal endothelial cells interspersed with mixed inflammatory-cell infiltrates having a predominance of neutrophils. Warthin–Starry staining or electron microscopy demonstrates these to be clusters of bacilli.

Epidemiology

Bartonella quintana is believed to be globally endemic and trench fever has been reported in many countries. Most outbreaks of the disease have been associated with conditions of poor sanitation and personal hygiene, such as war. Under such conditions, people are more likely to be infested by the arthropod vector of *Bartonella quintana*, the body louse. *Bartonella quintana* has no known non-human vertebrate reservoir. Infection is transmitted to humans by the excreta of infected lice, which may enter the body through broken skin or intact conjunctivas. Very recently, trench fever has been encountered among the homeless populations of American and European cities. As the number of homeless people continues to rise, the incidence of trench fever may again increase, and the disease should be considered to be potentially a significant public-health problem.

Prevention

Prevention of louse-transmitted *B. quintana* infections is achieved using the same methods as used for other louse-transmitted infectious diseases. However, as it is likely that homeless people are today the main reservoir of the bacteria, preventative measures should be focused on this group. Delousing should be encouraged and, clearly, access to better sanitation facilities provided.

Cat and cat flea-associated bartonellosis (*Bartonella henselae* infection)

Description of pathogen

The newly recognized species, *Bartonella (Rochalimaea) henselae*, has now been associated with a range of diseases in both immunocompetent and immuno-compromised patients. Among the latter (especially patients with HIV infection), *B. henselae* infection often presents with symptoms identical to those of *B. quintana* infection, including bacillary angiomatosis. However, its most common presentation among immunocompetent patients is cat-scratch disease (CSD). Chronic regional lymphadenopathy is the most common clinical feature of CSD. An inoculation site (a scratch, a primary lesion, or both) is detected in over two-thirds of patients. Whether or not there is a local cutaneous lesion, lymphadenitis becomes the major manifestation of CSD. Enlarged, tender lymph nodes are most commonly found in the head or neck area. The axillary nodes are also frequently involved. Transient exanthema (maculopapular, petechial or erythema multiforme or nodosum) have been observed in CSD patients usually lasting for less than 2 weeks (Fischer, 1995).

Epidemiology

Cat-scratch disease occurs worldwide, and in temperate climates it is seasonal, with most cases occurring between August and January. Most cases are observed in children. About 90% of patients have been exposed to cats and a bite or a scratch had occurred in 75% of patients. The infectious agent is transmitted through the skin lesion. In the United States, studies have demonstrated that 30–41% of cats are infected with *B. henselae*. Moreover, the cat can be chronically bacteraemic (Kordick *et al.*, 1995). Thus it is likely that the cat is the main reservoir of the bacterium. *Bartonella henselae* has also been recovered from cat fleas collected from infected cats (Koehler *et al.*, 1995), suggesting CSD to be a vector-borne disease. Such a hypothesis may explain the occurrence of disease in the 25% of patients who do not suffer a cat bite or scratch.

Prevention

Prophylactic antibiotic therapy after cat scratches or bites has not yet been evaluated nor has diagnosis and treatment of chronically infected cats. The only recommended prophylaxis is to avoid contact with cats.

References

Bryceson, A.D.M., Parry, E.H.O. & Perine, P.L. (1970) Louse-borne relapsing fever. A clinical and laboratory study of 62 cases in Ethiopia and a reconsideration of the literature. *Quarterly Journal of Medicine*, **39**, 129–170.

Byam, W., Carroll, J.H., Churchill, J.H. *et al.* (1919) *Trench Fever: A Louse-Borne Disease*. Oxford University Press, London.

Center for Disease Control and Prevention (1973) Relapsing fever. *Mortality Morbidity Weekly Record*, **22**, 242–246. (Abstract.)

Drancourt, M., George, F., Brouqui, P., Sampol, J. & Raoult, D. (1992) Diagnosis of Mediterranean spotted fever by indirect immunofluorescence of *Rickettsia conorii* in circulating endothelial cells isolated with monoclonal antibody-coated immunomagnetic beads. *Journal of Infectious Diseases*, **166**, 660–663.

Dumler, J.S. & Walker, D.H. (1995) Murine typhus. In: *Principles and Practice of Infectious Diseases* (eds G.L. Mandell, J.E. Bennett & R. Dolin), Vol. 4, pp. 1737–1739. Churchill Livingstone, New York.

Fischer, G.W. (1995) Cat scratch disease. In: *Principles and Practice of Infectious Diseases* (eds G.L. Mandell, J.E. Bennett & R. Dolin), Vol. 4, pp. 1310–1312. Churchill Livingstone, New York.

Johnson, Jr W.D. (1995) *Borrelia* species (relapsing fever). In: *Principles and Practice of Infectious Diseases* (eds G.L. Mandell, J.E. Bennett & R. Dolin), Vol. 4, pp. 2141–2143. Churchill Livingstone, New York.

Koehler, J.E., Glaser, C.A. & Tappero, J.W. (1995) *Rochalimaea henselae* infection. A new zoonosis with the domestic cat as reservoir. *Journal of the American Medical Association*, **271**, 531–535.

Kordick, D.L., Wilson, K.H., Sexton, D.J., Hadfield, T.L., Berkhoff, H.A. & Brettschwerdt, E.B. (1995) Prolonged *Bartonella* bacteremia in cats associated with cat-scratch disease in patients. *Journal of Clinical Microbiology*, **33**, 3245–3251.

Roberts Jr, N.J. (1995) *Bartonella bacilliformis* (bartonellosis). In: *Principles and Practice of Infectious Diseases* (eds G.L. Mandell, J.E. Bennett & R. Dolin), Vol. 4, pp. 2209–2210. Churchill Livingstone, New York.

Saah, A.J. (1995) *Rickettsia prowazekii* (epidemic or louse-borne typhus). In: *Principles and Practice of Infectious Diseases* (eds G.L. Mandell, J.E. Bennett & R. Dolin), Vol. 4, pp. 1735–1737. Churchill Livingstone, New York.

Slater, L.N., Welch, D.F., Hensel, D. & Coody, D.W. (1990) A newly recognized fastidious Gram-negative pathogen as a cause of fever and bacteremia. *New England Journal of Medicine*, **323**, 1587–1593.

Stanek, G., Satz, N., Strle, F. & Wilske, B. (1993) Epidemiology of Lyme borreliosis. In: *Aspects of Lyme borreliosis* (eds K. Weber & W. Burgdorfer), pp. 358–367. Springer-Verlag, Berlin.

Walker, D.H. & Raoult, D. (1995) *Rickettsia rickettsii* and other spotted fever group rickettsiae (Rocky Mountain spotted fever and other spotted fevers). In: *Principles and Practice of Infectious Diseases* (eds J.L. Mandell, J.E. Bennett & R. Dolin), Vol. 4, pp. 1721–1727. Churchill Livingstone, New York.

Weber, K. & Burgdorfer, W. (1993) Therapy of tick bite. In: *Aspect of Lyme Borreliosis* (eds K. Weber & W. Burgdorfer), pp. 350–351. Springer-Verlag, Berlin.

Sexually Transmitted Diseases: Syphilis, Gonorrhoea, Chancroid and Lymphogranuloma Venereum

D.C.W. MABEY

The epidemiology of sexually transmitted diseases (STDs) is intimately tied up with human sexual behaviour. STDs are most prevalent in adolescents and young adults, in those with many sexual partners, in commercial sex workers and their clients and in mobile population groups who are often separated from their families such as sailors, truck drivers and soldiers. Historically, STD control in Europe and North America has focused on these groups, with STD clinics being set up in ports and by the military authorities. However, the explosive growth in the tourist industry in the past 30 years means that holidaymakers are now by far the largest group of international travellers, making STD control a truly global issue.

The prevalence of the bacterial STDs described here is also greatly influenced by access to medical services, since their early and effective treatment will prevent further transmission in addition to preventing sequelae. They are, therefore, very much more prevalent in developing countries and in impoverished and marginalized groups in the inner cities of developed countries (De Schryver & Meheus, 1990; Mabey, 1996). Poverty and population pressure in developing countries has also led to vast human migrations in recent years, with rural villagers moving to cities in search of work, with a consequent increase in casual and commercial sex and therefore of STD rates (Horton, 1996).

The incidence and prevalence of an infectious disease depends on its basic reproductive rate, R_0, which is the average number of subjects infected by an index case. For an STD, this in turn depends on the rate of change of sexual partner, the duration of infectivity and the probability of transmission per sexual contact. The first of these parameters is susceptible to interventions which influence behaviour; the second can be reduced by early and effective treatment; and the third is an intrinsic biological attribute of the particular infection which can, however, be reduced by the

use of condoms. In a large proportion of the population in many developed countries, a combination of behaviour change and easy access to treatment has reduced R_0 to <1. In these circumstances, the disease would be expected to disappear, and indeed chancroid and lymphogranuloma venereum (LGV), which are usually symptomatic and are not easily transmissible, are now very rare in many countries.

Even when $R_0 < 1$ in the general population, however, an STD can be maintained in that population by the existence of a 'core group', who change their sexual partners more frequently than the general population. The 'core group' concept was originally put forward by Hethcote and Yorke, who used it to model the transmission dynamics of gonorrhoea (Hethcote & Yorke, 1984). It has been used to predict the theoretical impact and cost-effectiveness of control strategies targeted towards high-risk groups versus those delivered to the general population, and has provided some valuable insights (Over & Piot, 1991). But targeting of groups perceived to be at high risk is all too likely to lead to stigmatization in the real world, which drives the target group (e.g. sex workers, or men who have sex with men) underground, making it difficult or impossible to gain access to them. The control of STDs has assumed higher priority due to the HIV/AIDS epidemic, since there is now considerable evidence that the bacterial STDs facilitate the heterosexual transmission of HIV infection (Cameron *et al.*, 1989; Laga *et al.*, 1993; Grosskurth *et al.*, 1995). It is no coincidence that the populations hardest hit by AIDS are also those with the highest STD rates. Since no vaccines are yet available for the bacterial STDs, prevention strategies depend on health education to modify risky sexual behaviour and on the provision of condoms (primary prevention), and on early and effective treatment, including the treatment of sexual partners of index cases, to prevent further transmission (secondary prevention). Since syphilis and gonorrhoea may be asymptomatic, especially in women, passive case detection is often supplemented by active screening and case finding, for example for syphilis in pregnant women. In some countries, screening programmes have been implemented for certain high-risk groups, e.g. sex workers, which may be mandatory. Unfortunately, screening tests for syphilis and gonorrhoea are not widely available in developing countries.

Syphilis

Syphilis is a systemic disease caused by the spirochaete *Treponema pallidum*. After an incubation period of 7–70 days (median 21 days) an ulcer (the primary chancre) appears at the site of inoculation. At 6–8 weeks after the appearance of the primary chancre, which is usually self-limiting, dissemination of the infection is marked by the appearance of secondary lesions affecting the skin and mucous membranes. These lesions are teeming with organisms and the patient is highly infectious at this stage. Other organs, e.g. the lymph nodes, eyes, liver or kidneys, are also frequently involved. In the absence of treatment, secondary lesions usually regress after a few weeks, though relapses may occur over the subsequent 1–2 years. The patient then enters a latent stage. At this stage he or she is much less infectious, though infection may still be transmitted transplacentally or through blood transfusion. A proportion of individuals with latent syphilis will develop tertiary lesions, which usually affect the cardiovascular or central nervous systems. The disease is eminently treatable, a single intramuscular dose of benzathine penicillin being sufficient in the primary, secondary and early latent stages. Late latent and tertiary syphilis require three doses at weekly intervals.

Syphilis is diagnosed by the demonstration of *T. pallidum* in lesions from cases of primary or secondary syphilis by dark field microscopy, or serologically. A positive rapid plasma reagin (RPR) or venereal disease research laboratory (VDRL) test is confirmed by a specific treponemal test, usually the absorbed fluorescent treponemal antibody (FTA-Abs) or *T. pallidum* haemagglutination assay (TPHA) test. Latent cases are diagnosed serologically, and tertiary cases are diagnosed on clinical grounds with confirmatory serology. The response to treatment is monitored by repeated serological testing to ensure a falling RPR or VDRL titre.

Since *T. pallidum* is highly susceptible to drying, it can only be transmitted by direct contact between skin or mucous membranes, transplacentally or via blood transfusion. In industrialized countries, it is essentially only transmitted by sexual contact or from mother to infant. Among rural populations living under poor hygienic conditions in developing countries, it may be transmitted from skin to skin where the climate is hot and humid, giving rise to yaws, or from mucous membrane to mucous membrane where the climate is dry, causing endemic syphilis. There is close DNA homology between *T. pallidum* subsp. *pertenue*, which causes yaws, and *T. pallidum*, which causes venereal and endemic syphilis, and the two organisms are morphologically and antigenically indistinguishable. Cross-protection undoubtedly occurs, subjects with untreated treponemal infection being resistant to superinfection; this so-called 'chancre immunity' was well known to syphilologists in the nineteenth century (Hutchinson, 1887). Unfortunately, immunity appears not to persist after effective treatment.

The non-venereal treponematoses were virtually eliminated by the mass treatment campaigns organized by the World Health Organization in the 1950s and 1960s, but are now resurgent in parts of Africa, Asia and South America (Meheus & Antal, 1992). Yet venereal syphilis, which has replaced them in many parts of the developing world, especially in the burgeoning cities, is of greater public health importance, since it is more likely to be transmitted from mother to infant, and more likely to cause tertiary lesions (Schulz *et al.*, 1987).

Syphilis is now a rare disease in many industrialized countries, especially in northern Europe. In 1993, only 312 cases were reported in England and Wales. The USA continues to report the highest incidence in the developed world. The incidence in 1990 was 20 per 100 000 total population — the highest reported since 1952 — but had declined to 12 per 100 000 by 1993 (Centers for Disease Control and Prevention, 1993). Risk factors for syphilis in the USA are poverty, chronic unemployment, illicit drug use and low education. The incidence is 60-fold higher in black people than in white, and is similar in males and females. The incidence of congenital syphilis was 107 per 100 000 live births in 1991. In developing countries, it is not uncommon to find that >10% of antenatal clinic attenders have serological evidence of syphilis. In one African city, congenital syphilis was shown to be the most common cause of hospital admission in infants aged under 3 months (Hira *et al.*, 1990). The high prevalence of syphilis in women of child-bearing age results in high rates of stillbirth and perinatal mortality. Tertiary syphilis is now hardly seen in industrialized countries, and is surprisingly uncommon in developing countries, even those with a high prevalence of early and latent disease. It is not clear to what extent this is due to underascertainment or to the use of antibiotics for intercurrent diseases.

Syphilis was controlled in industrialized countries through the provision of accessible, acceptable, affordable and effective treatment for symptomatic cases, accompanied by the tracing and treatment of their sexual partners and by widespread screening programmes for pregnant women. The RPR test is cheap, and single-dose treatment with benzathine penicillin costs less than $1; yet there are few developing countries in which more than a small minority of pregnant women are screened for syphilis. In Zambia, where >10% are infected, such screening programmes have been shown to be among the most cost-effective health interventions available in terms of cost per healthy life-year saved (Hira *et al.*, 1990; Temmerman *et al.*, 1993).

Gonorrhoea

Gonorrhoea is caused by the Gram-negative bacterium *Neisseria gonorrhoeae*. In males, it gives rise to an acute purulent urethritis, with an incubation period of 3–5 days. Complications include epididymitis and, after repeated or inadequately treated infections, urethral stricture. In women, *N. gonorrhoeae* infects the cervix, urethra and rectum; the acid environment of the vagina does not support its replication. Pharyngeal infections are occasionally seen in persons of both sexes who practise oral sex. Characteristic symptoms in women include vaginal discharge and dysuria, but many infections are asymptomatic; asymptomatic infections are also not uncommon in men (Grosskurth *et al.*, 1996). Important complications in women include pelvic inflammatory disease, which has a spectrum of clinical presentations, ranging from acute peritonitis to mild lower abdominal discomfort, and may result in infertility or ectopic pregnancy following irreversible damage to the fallopian tubes, and ophthalmia neonatorum, a potentially blinding disease which affects approximately 30% of infants born to an infected mother. Ocular infection also occurs sporadically in adults as a result of auto-inoculation. Disseminated infections are sometimes seen, particularly in women,

which give rise to a febrile illness accompanied by a rash and/or an arthritis, typically an asymmetric arthritis affecting one or more large joints.

The definitive diagnosis of gonorrhoea depends on the isolation of *N. gonorrhoeae* from the site of infection. Urethritis in males and ocular infection can be diagnosed fairly reliably by the demonstration of Gram-negative intracellular diplococci in smears; this technique is >95% sensitive and specific in males. Gram stain is less sensitive in women, and culture of cervical, urethral and rectal swabs is necessary for maximum sensitivity.

Gonorrhoea has become a rare disease in many industrialized countries, especially in northern Europe. In Sweden, the majority of reported cases are now acquired abroad. In the USA it remains the most common reportable infectious disease, although there is believed to be considerable underreporting; the reported incidence was approximately 200 per 100 000 total population in 1993 (Centers for Disease Control and Prevention, 1993). The incidence was similar in men and women, and 90% of reported cases occurred in young adults aged 15–34 years. Risk factors for gonorrhoea were similar to those for syphilis: low socio-economic status, minority ethnic group and illicit drug use. The incidence in whites was similar to that reported in England and Wales (50 per 100 000); the incidence in blacks was 1400 per 100 000.

The incidence of gonorrhoea is not accurately known in any developing country, since reporting is not systematic and many cases are treated outside the official health sector. Hospital-based studies in two African cities concluded that the incidence was 3000–15 000 per 100 000 total population (De Schryver & Meheus, 1990). Surveys among antenatal clinic attenders in African cities have generally found 5–10% to have gonorrhoea (De Schryver & Meheus, 1990), implying that 1.5–3% of infants are likely to acquire gonococcal ophthalmia neonatorum. In addition to being more common, gonorrhoea is also more difficult to treat in developing than in developed countries, due to the high and increasing level of antimicrobial resistance. In many countries in Africa and Asia, >50% of isolates produce β-lactamase, making them completely resistant to penicillin; plasmid-mediated tetracycline resistance is also widespread and quinolone resistance is becoming increasingly prevalent (Bogaerts *et al.*, 1993; West *et al.*, 1995a).

The virtual eradication of gonorrhoea from affluent populations in developed countries has shown that, given sufficient resources, it is possible to control the disease through the provision of accessible and effective treatment, combined with contact tracing. In developing countries the high prevalence of infection, much of which is asymptomatic, the absence of diagnostic facilities for the identification of infected women, the high cost of the newer therapeutic regimens which are now required and the difficulties of partner notification are all major obstacles. Moreover, and most importantly, STD control is not seen by policymakers as a high priority; there are many other calls on dwindling government health budgets. Under these circumstances, advocacy is of the utmost importance; gonorrhoea will not be controlled in developing countries until policymakers in health ministries and in the international donor community are persuaded that the burden of disease which could be averted in terms of infertility, ectopic pregnancy, blindness and increased rates of HIV transmission is worth the investment.

The prevention of ophthalmia neonatorum (ON) should be a simple matter. It was shown by Crede more than 100 years ago that the instillation of 1% silver nitrate drops into the eyes of infants at delivery prevented the disease. More recently, it was shown that 1% tetracycline ointment, which is cheap, widely available and easy to store, was equally effective (Laga *et al.*, 1988). Given the high incidence of ON, and its devastating consequences, this simple measure is one of the most cost-effective health interventions available. Yet there are very few developing countries in which ON prophylaxis is carried out on a systematic basis.

Chancroid

Chancroid is an ulcerative disease caused by the Gram-negative bacterium *Haemophilus ducreyi*. After an incubation period of 3–7 days, a papule arises at the site of inoculation, which rapidly ulcerates. Chancroidal ulcers are typically soft and painless, and may be multiple. Painful inguinal adenopathy, which may suppurate, is seen in approximately 50% of cases.

Several studies have shown that even experienced clinicians are not able to distinguish chancroid reliably from other causes of genital ulceration (Dangor *et al.*, 1990).

The diagnosis of chancroid depends on the isolation of *H. ducreyi* from an ulcer or from pus obtained from a lymph nodes. It is a fastidious and slow-growing organism, requiring enriched selective medium, and grows best at 33°C. Since a mixed growth is often obtained from genital ulcers even using selective media, the identification of *H. ducreyi* requires considerable experience, and laboratory diagnosis is not usually possible under the conditions prevailing in most developing countries. Recently, DNA amplification techniques have been used to identify *H. ducreyi* in clinical material (West *et al.*, 1995b), but these are not commercially available.

Chancroid is, more than any other STD, a disease of core groups. It is very uncommon in most industrialized countries, but several well-documented outbreaks have occurred in North America in recent years: 5000 cases were reported in the USA in 1987 but this had declined to 1000 by 1994. The epidemiological characteristics of these outbreaks have been similar: they have involved marginalized and socio-economically deprived populations, there has been a high male:female case ratio and many of the female cases have been commercial sex workers or have exchanged sex for drugs. The high male:female case ratio suggested that asymptomatic females might play an important role in the epidemiology of chancroid, but studies among high-risk women in Kenya and the Gambia have shown that, while asymptomatic carriage does occur, it is rare (Plummer *et al.*, 1983; Hawkes *et al.*, 1995). In Africa, studies in several countries have shown that chancroid is responsible for *c.* 60% of genital ulcers presenting to hospital. Mixed infections, with concomitant syphilis or Herpes simplex, are common (Trees & Morse, 1995).

Given the high incidence of genital ulcer disease (GUD) in developing countries, the high proportion of cases of GUD that is due to chancroid, and the greatly increased risk of HIV transmission in the presence of GUD, it is clear that the overlapping epidemics of chancroid and HIV infection among core groups in Africa have interacted in a disastrous manner; it is likely that a similar process is now under way in parts of Asia. The control of chancroid in developing countries is therefore of great public-health importance.

In view of the lack of laboratory facilities and the unreliability of clinical diagnosis, the World Health Organization recommends that patients with genital ulcers in developing countries should be treated for both chancroid and syphilis (Anon., 1993). Unfortunately strains of *H. ducreyi* resistant to the cheaper antimicrobials (e.g. trimethoprim/sulphamethoxazole) are now prevalent in Asia and in parts of East Africa (Trees & Morse, 1995). A 1-week course of oral erythromycin remains effective, but this is more expensive, and compliance may be a problem, given the frequency of adverse gastrointestinal side effects to erythromycin. A single dose of azithromycin has been shown to be effective (Tyndall *et al.*, 1994), but is extremely expensive and therefore not widely available in developing countries. Interventions which target core groups, e.g. sex workers, are particularly important for the control of chancroid: condom promotion and delivery should be combined with health education and the provision of accessible and effective medical care.

Lymphogranuloma venereum

Lymphogranuloma venereum (LGV) is caused by the LGV biovar of the obligate intracellular bacterium, *Chlamydia trachomatis*. After a variable and uncertain incubation period, a small, often painless and self-limiting ulcer appears at the site of inoculation. This is followed by painful swelling of the draining lymph nodes, often accompanied by malaise and fever. In homosexual men, LGV can cause a severe proctitis. If untreated, it can lead to destruction of the local lymphatics giving rise to lymphoedema or to rectal stricture.

The diagnosis of LGV is difficult and unsatisfactory. Clinically, it can easily be confused with other causes of genital ulceration and inguinal adenopathy, e.g. chancroid. In order to be certain of the diagnosis it is necessary to isolate *C. trachomatis* from the lesion (ulcer or lymph node), and to type it by microimmuno-fluorescence as one of the three serotypes of the LGV biovar. This is seldom possible, since this laborious procedure can only be undertaken in one or two reference laboratories worldwide. Serology can be helpful, but is not specific, since cross-reaction may

be seen with other (non-LGV) strains of *C. trachomatis* or even with the highly prevalent respiratory pathogen, *Chlamydia pneumoniae*, depending on which assay is used. Given the difficulty in diagnosing LGV, little can be said about its epidemiology, other than that it is rare in industrialized countries, but is sometimes seen in developed countries. The principles of control are as for other STDs: early and effective treatment of cases combined with partner notification. Treatment for 2 weeks with a tetracycline or with erythromycin is recommended.

Conclusion

The enormous differences in the incidence of bacterial STDs between industrialized and developing countries, and between affluent and deprived communities within industrialized countries, show conclusively that these are now diseases of poverty. Given sufficient resources, they could be controlled and perhaps even eradicated. We are faced by two major challenges. Firstly we need to persuade policymakers in government health departments and in the international donor community to make sufficient resources available. The recent study from Tanzania showing that improved STD services can significantly reduce HIV incidence (Grosskurth *et al.*, 1995), and the *World Development Report* (1993), which concluded that STD control was among the most cost-effective health interventions, provide useful ammunition for advocacy.

Secondly, we need to identify the most cost-effective ways to control STDs in developing countries. The developed country model, a vertical system of specialist STD clinics, is too expensive to transfer to the developing world. Clinical services will have to be integrated with existing primary health-care programmes (Latif *et al.*, 1986) and if they are to achieve any public-health benefit, treatment will have to be extremely cheap for the patients, or preferably free. It was shown in Nairobi that the introduction of user charges dramatically reduced the number of patients attending the main municipal STD clinic (Moses *et al.*, 1992). Given the high prevalence of asymptomatic STDs, and the lack of laboratory facilities in many developing countries, the development of simple, cheap screening tests should be given the highest priority. In the interim, imaginative alternative strategies, such as mass treatment of populations with high STD prevalences, should be evaluated.

References

Anon. (1993) *Recommendations for the Management of Sexually Transmitted Diseases.* WHO Advisory Group Meeting on Sexually Transmitted Disease Treatments. WHO/GPA/STD/ 93.1. WHO, Geneva.

Bogaerts, J., Tello, W.M., Akingeneye, J., Mukantabana, G., Van Dyck, E. & Piot, P. (1993) Effectiveness of norfloxacin and ofloxacin for treatment of gonorrhoea and decrease in *in vitro* susceptibility to quinolones over time in Rwanda. *Genitourinary Medicine,* **69**, 196–200.

Cameron, D.W., Simonsen, J.N., D'Costa, L.J. *et al.* (1989) Female to male transmission of human immunodeficiency virus type 1: risk factors for seroconversion in men. *Lancet,* **ii**, 403–407.

Centers for Disease Control and Prevention (1993) Surveillance for sexually transmitted disease. *Mortality Morbidity Weekly Record,* **42** (SS-3), 1–13.

Dangor, Y., Ballard, R.C., Exposito, F., Fehler, G., Miller, S.D. & Koornhof, H.J. (1990) Accuracy of clinical diagnosis of genital ulcer disease. *Sexually Transmitted Diseases,* **17**, 184–189.

De Schryver, A. & Meheus, A. (1990) Epidemiology of sexually transmitted diseases: the global picture. *Bulletin of the World Health Organization,* **68**, 639–654.

Grosskurth, H., Mosha, F., Todd, J. *et al.* (1995) Impact of improved treatment of sexually transmitted diseases on HIV infection in rural Tanzania: randomised controlled trial. *Lancet,* **346**, 530–536.

Grosskurth, H., Mayaud, P., Mosha, F. *et al.* (1996) Asymptomatic gonorrhoea and chlamydial infection in rural Tanzanian men. *British Medical Journal,* **312**, 277–280.

Hawkes, S., West, B., Wilson, S., Whittle, H. & Mabey, D. (1995) Asymptomatic carriage of *Haemophilus ducreyi* confirmed by polymerase chain reaction. *Genitourinary Medicine,* **71**, 224–227.

Hethcote, H.H. & Yorke, J.A. (1984) *Gonorrhea Transmission Dynamics and Control. Lecture Notes in Biomathematics 56.* Springer Verlag, New York.

Hira, S.K., Bhat, G.J., Chikamata, D.M. *et al.* (1990) Syphilis intervention in pregnancy: Zambian demonstration project. *Genitourinary Medicine,* **66**, 159–164.

Horton, R. (1996) The infected metropolis. *Lancet,* **347**, 134–135.

Hutchinson, J. (1887) *Syphilis.* Cassell, London.

Laga, M., Plummer, F.A., Piot, P. *et al.* (1988) Prophylaxis of gonococcal and chlamydial ophthalmia neonatorum. A comparison of silver nitrate and tetracycline. *New England Journal of Medicine,* **318**, 653–657.

Laga, M., Manoka, A., Kivuvu, M. *et al.* (1993) Non-ulcerative sexually transmitted diseases as risk factors for HIV-1 transmission in women: results from a cohort study. *AIDS,* **7**, 95–102.

Latif, A.S., Mbengeranwa, O.L., Marowa, E., Paraiwa, E. & Gutu, S. (1986) The decentralisation of the sexually transmitted disease service and its integration into primary health care. *African Journal of Sexually Transmitted Diseases,* **2**, 85–88.

Mabey, D.C.W. (1996) Sexually transmitted diseases in developing countries. *Transactions of the Royal Society of Tropical Medicine and Hygiene,* **90**, 97–99.

Meheus, A. & Antal, G.M. (1992) The endemic treponematoses: Not yet eradicated. *World Health Statistics Quarterly,* **454**, 228–231.

Moses, S., Manji, F., Bradley, J.E., Nagelkerke, N.J.D., Malisa, M.A. & Plummer, F.A. (1992) Impact of user fees on attendance at a referral centre for sexually transmitted diseases in Kenya. *Lancet,* **340**, 463–466.

Over, M. & Piot, P. (1991) Health sector priorities review: HIV infection and sexually transmitted diseases. In: *Disease Control Priorities in Developing Countries* (eds D. Jamison & W.H. Mosley). Oxford University Press, New York.

Plummer, F.A., D'Costa, L.J., Nsanze, H., Dylewski, J., Karasira, P. & Ronald, A.R. (1983) Epidemiology of chancroid and *Haemophilus ducreyi* in Nairobi, Kenya. *Lancet,* **ii**, 1293–1295.

Schulz, K.F., Cates, W. & O'Masra, P.R. (1987) Pregnancy loss, infant death, and suffering: legacy of syphilis and gonorrhoea in Africa. *Genitourinary Medicine,* **63**, 320–325.

Temmerman, M., Mohamed Ali, F. & Fransen, L. (1993) Syphilis prevention in pregnancy: an opportunity to improve reproductive and child health in Kenya. *Health Policy and Planning,* **8**, 122–127.

Trees, D.L. & Morse, S.A. (1995) Chancroid and *Haemophilus ducreyi*: an update. *Clinical Microbiology Review,* **8**, 357–375.

Tyndall, M.W., Agoki, E., Plummer, F.A., Malisa, W., Ndinya-Achola, J.O. & Ronald, A.R. (1994) Single dose azithromycin for the treatment of chancroid: a randomised comparison with erythromycin. *Sexually Transmitted Diseases,* **21**, 231–234.

West, B., Changalucha, J., Grosskurth, H. *et al.* (1995a) Antimicrobial susceptibility, auxotype and plasmid content of *Neisseria gonorrhoeae* in Northern Tanzania: emergence of high level plasmid mediated tetracycline resistance. *Genitourinary Medicine,* **71**, 9–12.

West, B., Wilson, S.M., Changalucha, J. *et al.* (1995b) A simplified polymerase chain reaction for the detection of *Haemophilus ducreyi* and the diagnosis of chancroid. *Journal of Clinical Microbiology,* **33**, 787–790.

World Development Report 1993: Investing in Health. Oxford University Press for the World Bank, New York.

Skin Mycobacterial Infections: Tuberculosis, Atypical Mycobacterial Infections and Leprosy

V. VINCENT

Tuberculosis

Tuberculosis is a human chronic infectious disease caused by *Mycobacterium tuberculosis*, which usually affects the lungs. Two other related bacteria, *M. bovis* and *M. africanum*, are agents of bovine tuberculosis, possibly transmitted to man, and human tuberculosis, mainly encountered in West African countries, respectively. Tuberculosis is transmitted by airborne droplet nuclei generated from patients with smear-positive pulmonary disease. The pulmonary form is a communicable disease which does not require close contacts for infection, whereas extrapulmonary forms are not contagious (Kubica & Wayne, 1984).

Cutaneous tuberculosis is a disease which can produce a wide variety of skin changes, including papules, nodules, abscesses, verrucous and vegetating plaques, tumours, ulcers and scars. These changes may be very ill-defined and non-specific; they are partially related to the age and health of the patient, mode and pattern of infection, individual immunity and association with concomitant tuberculous disease. The histological response is also varied and the typical tuberculous granuloma, characterized by granulomatous inflammation with caseous necrosis and Langerhans-type giant cells, is relatively rare (Noble *et al.*, 1989; European Society for Mycobacteriology, 1991). Exogenous as well as endogenous sources may be involved. In the case of an exogenous source, the cutaneous infection occurs during or after a traumatic event; it is usually limited and spread to regional lymph nodes is variable. Infection may develop from an endogenous source by autoinoculation or contiguous spread or may result from a haematogenous dissemination (Tomecki & Hall, 1987; Noble *et al.*, 1989).

The present WHO estimations indicate that in 1990 one-third of the world population was infected by the tubercle bacilli (Good, 1992; Sudre *et al.*, 1992). Each

year, from this huge reservoir, 8 million new cases occur and 3 million persons die of tuberculosis. Since the beginning of the century, the mortality rate and annual incidence steadily decreased in developed countries. The widespread use of effective chemotherapy, available in the 1950s, strengthened this downward trend and eradication was thought to be reached by the twenty-first century. In the USA, the case rate dropped from 53 to 9.3 per 100 000 population between 1953 and 1984. However, since 1985 marked changes occurred and the number of reported cases increased in the USA as well as in various European countries (Sudre *et al.*, 1992). The lack of a continuing fall is due to the deterioration of socio-economic conditions and to the increase of immunodeficient population, particularly due to the AIDS epidemic. The immunosuppressive effect of HIV infection can lead to activation of a dormant, primary infection or make the person highly susceptible to new infection.

Cutaneous tuberculosis is a rare disease throughout the world, representing 1% of total tuberculosis cases (Kubica & Wayne, 1984; Tomecki & Hall, 1987; Noble *et al.*, 1989; Society for Mycobacteriology, 1991). The intact skin provides a protective barrier against *M. tuberculosis* infection. Invasion of the skin may be due to an inoculation from an exogenous source in individuals who have no active tuberculosis or may result from the secondary spread of tubercle bacilli from an endogenous source or from haematogenous dissemination in tuberculous patients.

Cutaneous tuberculosis following inoculation from an exogenous source is rare and accounts for < 2% of all cases (Tomecki & Hall, 1987; Noble *et al.*, 1989). Tubercle bacilli usually infect skin during or after a traumatic event. Individuals at risk mainly include pathologists who perform autopsies on tuberculosis patients, employees in slaughterhouses and children with open fractures subsequently exposed to adults with tuberculosis. Cases have been reported following circumcision, injections with contaminated syringes or mouth-to-mouth resuscitation. The earliest lesion is a papule which indurates and enlarges to form an ulcer. This tuberculous chancre is usually associated with a regional lymphadenopathy and bacilli are numerous in both lesions.

Cutaneous tuberculosis due to autoinoculation from

a pre-existing internal source of tubercle bacilli is also very rare (Tomecki & Hall, 1987; Noble *et al.*, 1989). It occurs in elderly patients with visceral tuberculosis and reduced immunity and consists of the implantation of tubercle bacilli at mucocutaneous junctions.

The endogenous source may lead to cutaneous tuberculosis by contiguous spread. Skin lesions (scrofuloderma) thus result from the involvement and breakdown of the skin overlying a tuberculous focus, usually a lymph node, but sometimes an infected bone or joint. The typical presentation is cervical lymphadenitis with secondary extension to the skin, which affects more frequently children and young adults.

Haematogenous dissemination may lead to nodules and abscesses, arising independently of any clinically apparent tuberculous focus, usually a visceral site (Tomecki & Hall, 1987; Noble *et al.*, 1989). It occurs mainly in poorly nourished children. The severe forms of cutaneous tuberculosis due to haematogenous dissemination are miliary tuberculosis and lupus vulgaris. The miliary form primarily affects infants and children and is characterized by a scattered eruption of papules, nodules or plaques. The underlying disease may be cryptic and thus the skin lesions may be the presenting sign. The patient is often gravely ill, and mortality is high. By contrast, lupus vulgaris is a progressive form of cutaneous tuberculosis. It usually involves the face (nose, cheeks, lips) and the extremities. The characteristic lesion is a plaque of an 'apple-jelly colour' which extends peripherally while scarring occurs, causing considerable tissue destruction.

The treatment of cutaneous tuberculosis is achieved following the guidelines for pulmonary tuberculosis. In developed countries, the treatment used most consists of a 6-month therapy with isoniazid and rifampicin in combination with pyrazinamide and ethambutol for the first 2 months (World Health Organization, 1991). Resistance develops by mutation and selection. Combination of drugs practically eliminates selection of drug-resistant mutants and therefore the development of drug resistance.

Since skin tuberculosis is rare and shows considerable variability in its morphological features, reliable bacteriological tests are critical to confirm the diagnosis. Most forms of cutaneous tuberculosis are pauci-bacillary and acid-fast bacteria are rarely detected microscopically. Culture is currently the single test for the diagnosis but requires long delays, at least several weeks (Kubica *et al.*, 1984; European Society for Mycobacteriology, 1991). The polymerase chain reaction (PCR) could represent an attractive alternative as it is theoretically an exquisitely sensitive and rapid method for detection of microorganisms (Perronne & Vincent, 1995; Degitz, 1996). Several case reports indicated the usefulness of PCR in the diagnosis of lupus vulgaris, scrofuloderma, exogenous inoculation following trauma and autoinoculation cases (Penneys *et al.*, 1993; Serfling *et al.*, 1993; Steidl *et al.*, 1993; Taniguchi *et al.*, 1993; Nachbar *et al.*, 1996). However, technical pitfalls are frequent and may lead to false-positive as well as false-negative results. A cooperative, blind study led by WHO in seven laboratories demonstrated dramatic divergences in terms of sensitivity and specificity (Noordhoek *et al.*, 1994). The sensitivity of PCR compared to traditional culture techniques varied from 2 to 90% depending on the laboratory. The proportion of false negatives varied from 3 to 20%. Based on numerous evaluations, the specificity of tuberculosis PCR is rarely better than 97% so that the positive predictive value varies from 5 to 75%, depending on the incidence of tuberculosis in the tested population, from 0.2 to 10% (Raoult, 1994). Commercially available kits and standardized simplified techniques contribute to more reliable results (Ichiyama *et al.*, 1996; Wobester *et al.*, 1996). Amplification methods other than PCR have been developed and evaluated. However, quality controls will remain essential to validate the method in each laboratory (Perronne & Vincent, 1995). Consequently, current management strategies cannot be developed or changed solely on the grounds of PCR results (Centers for Disease Control and Prevention, 1993).

Specific probes used in PCR tests are diverse but the sequence encoding the 16S rRNA and the insertion sequence IS*6110* are the most widely used. Moreover, the repeated sequence IS*6110* represents a remarkable epidemiological marker, characteristic of a single strain, as both copy number and distribution within the genome vary from strain to strain (Van Embden *et al.*, 1993). This marker has been applied in numerous studies to trace outbreaks with fully sensitive or multidrug-resistant strains, to differentiate relapses from new infections, to identify false-positive cases due to the contamination of endoscopes or to laboratory contamination and to determine nosocomial cases. Using this marker, large national or regional surveys have allowed determination of the genetic diversity and spread of tubercle bacilli in communities (Vincent, 1996). However, all these reports were concerned with the transmission of pulmonary tuberculosis. Interest in the development of these techniques for the epidemiological study of cutaneous tuberculosis is poor.

Tuberculin skin testing is used to search for infected persons in populations (Kubica & Wayne, 1984; European Society for Mycobacteriology, 1991; Good, 1992). The tuberculins are purified proteins from the media in which tubercle bacilli were grown. The Mantoux test consists of the intradermal injection of the bioequivalent of 5 tuberculin units. An induration diameter of > 10 mm, developed 48–72 hours after injection, indicates a positive reaction. A negative result does not rule out tuberculosis as 20–30% of tuberculous individuals will be negative and develop a positive reaction later on during treatment. In non-vaccinated persons, a reaction of 6 mm suggests infection. Approximately 6 weeks after vaccination, BCG leads to a positive reaction.

BCG vaccination has been considered the main way to prevent tuberculosis (European Society for Mycobacteriology, 1991; Good, 1992). Nowadays, it is accepted that BCG cannot cut tuberculosis transmission and its utility is limited to prevent, in children, the severe forms like meningitis and miliary tuberculosis. As BCG is a live vaccine, some complications may follow vaccination. Millions of persons have received a BCG vaccination and complications are exceptional (Kubica & Wayne, 1984). Cutaneous BCG-induced mycobacteriosis is uncommon. However, scrofuloderma-like and lupus vulgaris-like reactions have been reported to occur at the site of vaccination (Kubica & Wayne, 1984; Tomecki & Hall, 1987; Noble *et al.*, 1989).

Leprosy

M. leprae, or Hansen bacillus, is the aetio-logical agent of leprosy. Since its description in 1873, tentative *in vitro* cultivation has never been successful. Two animal models for experimental infection are available: the mouse footpad and the nine-banded armadillo. These models allowed the study of the chemical components of the leprosy bacillus as well as the selection of appropriate drug treatments. *M. leprae* grows very slowly; in mouse footpad, the generation time is 14 days during the exponential phase of growth (versus 20 min for *Escherichia coli* in standard media). It is a strict intracellular parasite, able to reproduce only in macrophages and in Schwann cells (Kubica & Wayne, 1984; Shepard, 1986; European Society for Mycobacteriology, 1991).

Between 1960 and 1985, the prevalence of leprosy was estimated around 10–12 million patients. Then the use of the polychemotherapeutic treatment caused a dramatic decrease of cases, estimated in 1991 to be around 5.5 million. However, 2–3 million individuals considered as cured still suffer from mutilations and severe handicap due to leprosy lesions. About 50% of the world's cases occur in India and most of the remaining cases are found in other South-East Asia countries, in Brazil and in Africa, with 50% of the African cases in Nigeria. Although leprosy was endemic in Europe in the Middle Ages, nowadays only few cases are found in Ireland, Italy, Portugal, Spain and Turkey (Fine, 1982; Kubica & Wayne, 1984; Nordeen *et al.*, 1992; Leinhardt & Fine, 1994).

The incubation phase lasts for several years and leprosy bacilli may lie dormant in tissues for long periods. Thus, transmission mechanisms may not be established precisely but epidemiological data indicate that person-to-person transmission is the unique contamination mode. Multibacillary patients, who can excrete 10^7 viable bacilli in nasal excretions, present a risk of infection to their contacts two- to fivefold greater than that for the contacts of paucibacillary patients, and these have a risk twofold greater than the risk of the general population in an endemic area. The main mode of transmission is the respiratory route. Bacilli, present in the droplets generated from nasal discharge of lepromatous patients, pass through pulmonary alveoli with no generation of primary lesions and reach their nidation sites by haematogenous dissemination. Another possibility for transmission is via passage of bacilli to the surface of the body through broken skin or ulcers. For entry through the skin, repeated close skin-to-skin contact is important. Babies carried on the back of their mothers often develop lesions on the forehead, whereas babies carried on the hip may display the first lesion on the thigh. Furthermore, *M. leprae* has been found in secretions such as milk, sebum or semen of lepromatous patients. The low contagiosity of leprosy is not due to the low virulence of *M. leprae*, which is able to yield severe lesions, but is related to the immune response of some individuals who are not able to control the disease. Young children acquire the disease on briefer contact than adults (Kubica & Wayne, 1984; European Society for Mycobacteriology, 1991).

Leprosy is characterized by its chronic, slow progress leading to mutilating and disfiguring lesions. In the cutaneous form, large nodules (lepromas) are distributed widely and on the face they create the characteristic leonine appearance. In the neural form, parts of peripheral nerves are involved yielding localized patches of anaesthesia. Both forms may be present in the same patient. Clinical leprosy can display a large variety of manifestations, the clinical forms corresponding to different degrees of immunological responses. From the onset of the disease, there is unhampered multiplication of the bacilli in persons unable to develop immunity (lepromatous leprosy) whereas bacterial multiplication is checked in persons capable of developing immunity (tuberculoid leprosy). In tuberculoid lesions, bacilli are scanty and well-organized granuloma are formed. In contrast, in the lepromatous form, the disease is disseminated and granuloma are absent. Bacillaemia is common and bacilli may be detected in most tissues such as skin, nerves, liver, spleen, the capillary endothelium, muscle and bone marrow. Between these two polar forms, many intermediate stages exist that correspond to a gradual decrease of immunity. Moreover, shifts from one phase to another, with exacerbation and remission, are frequent (Kubica & Wayne, 1984; European Society for Microbacteriology, 1991; Leinhardt & Fine, 1994).

Diagnostic criteria are limited and essentially clinical. In advanced lepromatous forms, diagnosis is apparent at a glance. However, in early stage or in other leprosy forms, clinical manifestations may be subtle. Bacteriological diagnosis is achieved by detection of bacilli in scrapings from ulcerated lesions, or in fluid from super-ficial incisions over non-ulcerated lesions. Although acid-fast as with any *mycobacterium*, *M. leprae* bacilli are more sensitive to decolorization than other mycobacterial species. A slight decolorization solution must be used (1% hydrochloric acid in 70% ethanol instead of the standard 3% in 95%, respectively) to display the bacilli acid-fastness. The smear is then examined to determine both bacteriological (BI) and morphological index (MI). The BI reflects the density of bacilli including viable and non-viable bacilli whereas the MI distinguishes between evenly solid-stained (viable) and irregularly stained (non-viable) bacilli. A decrease in MI is a good indication of effective chemotherapy (Kubica & Wayne, 1984; European Society for Mycobacteriology, 1991).

The lepromin test is a skin test using as antigen a heat-killed suspension of leprosy bacilli (originally recovered from patient lesions, nowadays from armadillo-infected tissues). The test is positive if a Mitsuda reaction, i.e. the development of an induration at 21 days, is scored at the intradermal injection site. The test has no diagnostic value but it is useful in determining the prognosis and the phase of the disease, as tuberculoid patients are lepromin-positive and lepromatous patients are lepromin-negative. Moreover, in a community exposed to leprosy infection, individuals who are lepromin-negative are more likely to have the disease than those who are lepromin-positive (Kubica & Wayne, 1984; European Society for Mycobacteriology, 1991).

The serological test, using a specific antigen from *M. leprae* (the phenolic glycolipid, PGL-I), allows the diagnosis of lepromatous forms but shows a low sensitivity for the diagnosis of tuberculoid forms (Kubica & Wayne, 1984).

The treatment recommended by WHO consists of a combination of dapsone and rifampicin in the case of the tuberculoid form, with the addition of clofazimine in cases of the lepromatous form. Drugs have to be given for at least 2 years for patients with widespread lepromatous disease. Treatment results may be evaluated by counting the bacilli in serial biopsies and skin scrapings (World Health Organization, 1989, 1991).

The strategic fight against leprosy is based on chemotherapy to decrease the prevalence and the incidence. The two additional objectives for the control of the disease are the prevention of disabilities and the integration of patients into the social life of the community.

Atypical mycobacterial infections

Mycobacteria other than tubercle and leprosy bacilli are often referred to as 'atypical' mycobacteria. This designation is convenient for the inclusion of a large number of bacterial species, more than 60, but has no scientific justification. All these mycobacteria are truly genuine mycobacteria, sharing all the characteristics for their inclusion into the *Mycobacterium* genus. Most of these mycobacteria are frequently isolated in the environment and some may be agents for various diseases in man and animals. In HIV-seronegative patients, diseases due to these bacteria are mainly pulmonary infections, adenopathies and cutaneous infections whereas disseminated infections are rare. By contrast, in HIV-seropositive patients, digestive and disseminated infections are frequent, and caused principally by *M. avium*. Recent reports showed that *M. avium* infection is the most frequently disseminated infection diagnosed in AIDS patients. The precise incidence of these mycobacterial diseases is difficult to estimate as the diseases do not have to be declared. Estimation cannot rely on laboratory records only, since bacterial isolation is rarely clinically relevant (Kubica & Wayne, 1984; Collins, 1989; European Society for Mycobacteriology, 1991; Wayne & Sramek, 1992; Wolinsky, 1992; Falkinham, 1996).

In the absence of evidence of person-to-person transmission, it was proposed that the environment was the source of infection. Regional differences in the incidence of various mycobacterial pulmonary diseases are consistent with this hypothesis. Mycobacteria other than tubercle bacilli are free-living saprophytes which may be recovered from natural and tap water, soil, dust and aerosols. Thus, in contrast to tubercle bacilli, the history of infection due to other mycobacteria most likely involves interactions with the environment rather than infected patients. Mycobacteria present in tap water are not contaminants from another source: they are able to survive and growth herein. This ability is related to the resistance of mycobacteria to disinfection, a redoubtable property which has led to nosocomial infections via materials or solutions

improperly considered as sterile. Moreover, mycobacterial cell hydrophobicity is responsible for the formation of biofilms resulting in the persistence of the bacteria in water-delivery systems. It has been demonstrated that the skin of healthy individuals can be colonized by environmental mycobacteria, including potential pathogens such as *M. avium*, *M. fortuitum* and *M. simiae* as well as other saprophytic species. Clinicians should be aware that mycobacteria from the natural skin flora can be isolated from clinical specimens without having any clinical significance (Collins *et al.*, 1984; Salem *et al.*, 1989; Vincent Lévy-Frébault, 1991; Portaels, 1995). However, unlike all mycobacteria other than tubercle bacilli, *M. ulcerans*, *M. marinum* and *M. haemophilum* are not widespread in nature and their isolation from human samples is always clinically significant. These species along with the so-called '*fortuitum* complex' represent the main agents of mycobacterial cutaneous infections.

Skin ulcers due to *M. ulcerans* are the third most frequent mycobacterial disease diagnosed in HIV-seronegative patients after tuberculosis and leprosy. Most cases have been reported in tropical countries in Africa, in Central and South-East Asia and a few cases in Australia and Central America (Mexico, Guyana). *M. ulcerans* occupies a unique position among the agents of mycobacterial diseases. It has never been recovered from the environment but water is a possible source as cases are often clustered in swampy areas or river valleys. Moreover, *M. ulcerans* is the unique *Mycobacterium* species in synthesizing a toxin. Experimental infections in mice showed that injection of this fat-soluble substance causes tissue necrosis. It is suggested that the toxin is responsible for lesion extension (Kubica & Wayne, 1984; Portaels, 1989; European Society for Mycobacteriology, 1991; Wolinsky, 1992).

The disease first presents as a small subcutaneous nodule, usually located on the external face of arm or leg, which later invades the dermis. As the initial lesion enlarges, the skin over the centre ulcerates and there is necrosis of the subcutaneous fat. The ulcer remains indolent while deeply rooted, and often causes massive destruction of skin and subcutaneous tissue resulting in severe deforming lesions and effective loss of use of the limb involved. In children, lesions can occur on the face or on the trunk. The necrosis may extend into muscle and even bone. Unusually for mycobacteria other than tubercle bacilli, no case of *M. ulcerans* infection has been reported in AIDS patients.

The diagnosis is often obvious considering the characteristic aspect of the lesions. Moreover, extracellular acid-fast bacteria are found in large numbers in the necrotic areas on the edges of the ulcerated regions. The bacteriological diagnosis is usually hampered by the fastidious growth of *M. ulcerans* which may require up to several months to form colonies on solid medium.

Treatment involves the radical surgical excision of diseased tissues and may be sufficient at early stage of the lesions but has to be followed by skin grafts and plastic surgery at advanced stages. Medical treatment is usually disappointing; rifampicin may heal lesions, depending on their extent. Early diagnosis and treatment are essential for significantly reducing the disabilities that often result from delayed diagnosis (Kubica & Wayne, 1984; Portaels, 1989; European Society for Mycobacteriology, 1991).

M. marinum causes chronic granulomatous infection of the skin, clinically and histologically resembling tuberculosis. The organism is a fish pathogen and is found in water contaminated either by fish or humans, where it can proliferate to yield very large numbers of bacteria. Cases have thus been described in individuals frequenting swimming pools or bathing in natural waters (sea or river), in tropical fish aquarium enthusiasts and especially in persons with occupational hazards such as fishermen performing tasks during which the hands can be cut (Kubica & Wayne, 1984; European Society for Mycobacteriology, 1991).

Infection with *M. marinum* requires skin abrasion followed by exposure to the organism. The commonly affected sites are the hands and arms, usually related to fishing activities and elbows or knees for bathing activities. The initial lesion is an erythematous inflammatory nodule which develops within a few weeks after a minor trauma, enlarges to form a papule or a plaque, opens and drains a small amount of pus. At later stages of the disease, lesions may progress to an ulcer, limited to the skin and subcutaneous tissue. Lesions may be single or multiple. They may appear as a group of reddish-brown papules suggestive of lupus vulgaris. Sometimes further subcutaneous nodules develop in linear chains, extending up from the original lesion and mimicking sporotrichosis with lymphangitis. Regional lymph nodes are not involved and disseminated disease is very rare. *M. marinum* cutaneous infections evolving towards disseminated disease have been reported in AIDS patients.

Biopsy of a lesion shows non-specific inflammation in early stages while typical granulomas with the presence of acid-fast bacilli are often revealed in later stages. Histology and culture are essential for diagnosis confirmation. Unlike the scarce growth of *M. ulcerans*, *M. marinum* is characterized by easy and luxuriant growth; a positive culture can thus be obtained in 70% of cases.

In the case of localized infection, treatment may be unnecessary since lesions may resolve spontaneously. However, healing is slow and occurs with scarring, in 1–3 years. Surgery consisting of excision or curettage is the most effective treatment. If several lesions are present, with or without a sporotrichosis aspect, *M. marinum* usually respond to chemotherapy with tetracyclines (minocycline, tetracycline, doxycycline) or co-trimoxazole or clarithromycin (Kubica & Wayne, 1984; Wallace *et al.*, 1990; European Society for Mycobacteriology, 1991).

M. haemophilum is the agent of cutaneous lesions occurring mainly in immunodeficient patients, including persons on therapy to prevent a graft- versus-host reaction or AIDS patients. Cases of cervical adenitis have also been reported in immunocompetent children. Initial signs include multiple cutaneous ulcerating lesions, most frequently found on the extremities, often overlying joints. Only a few cases have been reported since *M. haemophilum* was first described as a human pathogen in 1978. This may be due to the special culture requirements of the species which cannot grow on standard Löwenstein–Jensen medium, but only in media supplemented with ferric ammonium citrate, haemin or haemoglobin and an optimal incubation temperature of 30°C. Similarly, antibiotic susceptibility testing cannot be done routinely. Much remains unknown about *M. haemophilum*, including its reservoir, its mode of transmission, the incidence of infection and the spectrum of disease associated with infection (Kubica & Wayne, 1984; European Society for Mycobacteriology, 1991).

The other main agents of mycobacterial skin infections are members of the so-called '*fortuitum* complex'.

The taxonomy of this group has changed dramatically in recent years and nowadays five different species are recognized, namely *M. fortuitum*, *M. peregrinum*, *M. chelonae*, *M. abscessus* and *M. mucogenicum*. Depending on the year of the report, some confusion concerning designation may be found in the literature.

Skin diseases involving these species mainly follow trauma (cuts, wounds), injections (with contaminated needles), transplantation or surgery. It is now well established that the epidemiology varies for each species. *M. fortuitum* is more frequently involved in postsurgical infections and wounds resulting from domestic or agricultural accidents whereas *M. chelonae* and *M. abscessus* are usually recovered from subcutaneous or intramuscular postinjection abscesses. This may be related to the fact that *M. fortuitum* is widespread in the environment and can be recovered from dust or soil whereas *M. chelonae* and *M. abscessus* are more frequently isolated from tap water. These latter bacteria are highly resistant to disinfection and may cause nosocomial or iatrogenic infections due to poor aseptic and antiseptic procedures. Such cases have been reported associated with the use of jet injectors, vaccination, drug injection and wound treatments, and often occur in outbreaks (Kubica & Wayne, 1984; European Society for Mycobacteriology, 1991; Vincent Lévy-Frébault, 1991; Portaels, 1995).

The abscesses due to these mycobacteria are indolent and often escape proper consideration and accurate diagnosis before chronic formation of fistulas is established. Affected patients are usually afebrile and asymptomatic. Following exposure to the organism, a cellulitis or non-descript subcutaneous abscess or nodule develops at the site of the wound. The lesion usually drains and may produce sinus formation. Disseminated diseases are rare in non-immunocompromised patients. Biopsy of the lesions is usually non-specific and culture is necessary both to ascertain the diagnosis and establish the antibiotic susceptibility.

Healing occurs with prominent scarring. As for *M. marinum* infections, localized lesions are suitably treated by excision. For extensive disease, debridement, incision and drainage followed by chemotherapy are necessary. However, unlike *M. marinum*, these species are usually resistant to chemotherapeutic agents, especially *M. abscessus*. Susceptibility testing is useful to determine the antibiotic therapy. Usually, strains are sensitive to amikacin, cefoxitin and macrolides, allowing use of multidrug regimens to prevent the development of drug resistance (Kubica & Wayne, 1984; Wallace *et al.*, 1990; European Society for Mycobacteriology, 1991).

References

Centers for Disease Control and Prevention (1993) Diagnosis of tuberculosis by nucleic acid amplification methods applied to clinical specimens. *Morbidity and Mortality Weekly Report*, **42**, 686.

Collins, F.M. (1989) Mycobacterial disease, immunosuppression, and acquired immunodeficiency syndrome. *Clinical Microbiology Review*, **2**, 360–377.

Collins, C.H., Grange, J.M. & Yates, M.D. (1984) Mycobacteria in water. *Journal of Applied Bacteriology*, **57**, 193–211.

Degitz, K. (1996) Detection of mycobacterial DNA in the skin. Etiologic insights and diagnostic perspectives. *Archives of Dermatology*, **132**, 71–75.

Down, J.A., O'Connell, M.A., Dey, M.S. *et al.* (1996) Detection of *Mycobacterium tuberculosis* in respiratory specimens by strand displacement amplification of DNA. *Journal of Clinical Microbiology*, **34**, 860–865.

European Society for Mycobacteriology (1991) *Manual of Diagnosis and Public Health Mycobacteriology*. Bureau of Hygiene and Tropical Diseases, London.

Falkinham, J.O. (1996) Epidemiology of infection by nontuberculous mycobacteria. *Clinical Microbiology Review*, **9**, 177–215.

Fine, P.E.M. (1982) Leprosy: the epidemiology of a slow bacterium. *Epidemiological Review*, **4**, 161–188.

Good, R.C. (1992) The genus *Mycobacterium*. In: *The Prokaryotes. A Handbook on the Biology of Bacteria: Ecophysiology, Isolation, Identification, Applications*, Vol. 2, pp. 1238–1270. Springer Verlag, New York.

Ichiyama, S., Iinuma, Y., Tawada, Y. *et al.* (1996) Evaluation of Gen-Probe amplified *Mycobacterium tuberculosis* direct test and Roche PCR-microwell plate hybridization method (Amplicor Mycobacterium) for direct detection of mycobacteria. *Journal of Clinical Microbiology*, **34**, 130–133.

Kubica, G.P. & Wayne, L.G. (1984) *The Mycobacteria. A Sourcebook*. Marcel Dekker, New York.

Leinhardt, C. & Fine, P.E.M. (1994) Type 1 reaction, neuritis and disability in leprosy. What is the current epidemiological situation? *Leprosy Review*, **65**, 9–33.

Nachbar, F., Classen, V., Meurer, M., Nachbar, T., Schirren, C.G. & Degitz, K. (1996) Orificial tuberculosis: detection by polymerase chain reaction. *British Journal of Dermatology*, **135**, 106–109.

Noble, W.C., Hay, R.J. & Stanford, J.L. (1989) Mycobacterial infections of the skin. In: *Biology of Mycobacteria*, Vol. 3, pp. 477–510. Academic Press, London.

Noordhoek, G., Kolk, A.H.J., Bjune, G. *et al.* (1994) Sensitivity and specificity of PCR for detection of *Mycobacterium tuberculosis*: a blind comparison study among seven laboratories. *Journal of Clinical Microbiology*, **32**, 277–284.

Nordeen, S.K., Lopez Bravo, L. & Sundaresan, T.K. (1992) Nombre estimatif de cas de lèpre dans le monde. *Bulletin de l'Organisation Mondiale de la Santé*, **70**, 161–164.

Penneys, N.S., Leonardi, C.L., Cook, S. *et al.* (1993) Identification of *Mycobacterium tuberculosis* DNA in five different types of cutaneous lesions by the polymerase chain reaction. *Archives of Dermatology*, **129**, 1594–1598.

Perronne, C. & Vincent, V. (1995) Diagnostic génétique des infections à mycobactéries atypiques par réaction de polymérisation en chaine (PCR). *Annales de Dermatologie et de Venereologie*, **122**, 213–215.

Pfyffer, G.E., Kissling, P., Jahn, E.M.I., Welscher, H.M., Salfinger, M. & Weber, R. (1996) Diagnostic performance of amplified *Mycobacterium tuberculosis* direct test with cerebrospinal fluid, other nonrespiratory, and respiratory specimens. *Journal of Clinical Microbiology*, **34**, 834–841.

Portaels, F. (1989) Epidémiologie des ulcères à *Mycobacterium ulcerans*. *Annales de la Societe Belge de Médecine Tropicale*, **69**, 91–103.

Portaels, F. (1995) Epidemiology of mycobacterial diseases. In: *Clinics in Dermatology*, Vol. 13, pp. 95–125. Elsevier, New York.

Raoult, D. (1994) Predictive value of PCR applied to clinical samples for *Mycobacterium tuberculosis* detection. *Journal of Clinical Microbiology*, **32**, 273–275.

Salem, J.I., Gontijo Filho, P., Lévy-Frébault, V. & David, H.L. (1989) Isolation and characterization of mycobacteria colonizing the healthy skin. *Acta Leprologica*, **7**, 18–20.

Serfling, U., Penneys, N.S. & Leonardi, C.L. (1993) Identification of *Mycobacterium tuberculosis* DNA in a case of lupus vulgaris. *Journal of the American Academy of Dermatology*, **28**, 318–322.

Shepard, C.C. (1986) Experimental leprosy. In: *Leprosy* (ed. R.C. Hastings), pp. 269–286. Churchill Livingstone, Edinburgh.

Steidl, M., Neubert, U., Volkkenandt, M., Chatelain, R. & Degitz, K. (1993) Lupus vulgaris confirmed by polymerase-chain reaction. *British Journal of Dermatology*, **129**, 314–318.

Sudre, P., Ten Dam, G. & Kochi, A. (1992) La tuberculose aujourd'hui dans le monde. *Bulletin de l'Organisation Mondiale de la Santé*, **70**, 297–308.

Taniguchi, S., Chanoki, M. & Hamada, T. (1993) Scrofuloderma: the DNA analysis of mycobacteria by polymerase chain reaction. *Archives of Dermatology*, **129**, 1618–1619.

Tomecki, K.J. & Hall, G.S. (1987) Tuberculosis of the skin. In: *Clinical Dermatology*, Vol. 3, pp. 1–26. Harper & Row, Philadelphia.

Van Embden, J.D.A., Cave, M.D., Crawford, J.T. *et al.* (1993) Strain identification of *Mycobacterium tuberculosis* by DNA fingerprinting: recommendations for a standardized methodology. *Journal of Clinical Microbiology*, **31**, 406–409.

Vincent, V. (1996) Typage moléculaire des bacilles de la tuberculose. *Revue d'Epidemiologie et de Santé Publique*, **44**, 63.

Vincent Lévy-Frébault, V. (1991) Ecologie des mycobactéries et mode de contamination humaine. *Médecine et Maladies Infectieuses*, **21**, 16–25.

Wallace, R.J. Jr, O'Brien, R., Glassroth, J. *et al.* (1990) Diagnosis and treatment of disease caused by nontuberculous mycobacteria. *American Review of Respiratory Diseases*, **142**, 940–953.

Wayne, L.G. & Sramek, H.A. (1992) Agents of newly recognized or infrequently encountered mycobacterial diseases. *Clinical Microbiology Review*, **5**, 1–25.

Wobester, W.L., Krajden, M., Conly, J. *et al.* (1996) Evaluation of Roche Amplicor PCR assay for *Mycobacterium tuberculosis*. *Journal of Clinical Microbiology*, **34**, 134–139.

Wolinsky, E. (1992) Mycobacterial diseases other than tuberculosis. *Clinical Infectious Diseases*, **15**, 1–12.

World Health Organization (1980) *Guide de la Lutte Antilépreuse*, 2nd edn. WHO, Geneva.

World Health Organization (1991) *Drugs Used in Mycobacterial Diseases*. WHO, Geneva.

Cutaneous Leishmaniasis

R. PRADINAUD, K. PALMA-LARGO AND H. DESPERRIÈRE

Leishmaniasis diseases are parasitic diseases caused by different species of *Leishmania* protozoa, transmitted by sandflies, that take four main clinical forms: visceral, cutaneous, mucocutaneous and diffuse cutaneous (Fig. 16.1).

• The visceral leishmaniasis (VL or kala-azar) can be severe in terms of mortality if not treated. It is characterized by fever, splenomegaly, hepatomegaly, loss of weight, lymphadenopathies and anaemia. This form can also be considered as an opportunist infection in HIV-infected patients. After recovery, patients may develop a chronic form called 'post-kala-azar dermal leishmaniasis' that requires long and expensive treatment.

• Cutaneous leishmaniasis produces skin ulcers which can result in disfiguring scars.

• Mucocutaneous leishmaniasis produces extensive destruction of oral, nasal and pharyngeal cavities with disfiguration (mutilation) of the face.

• Diffuse cutaneous leishmaniasis occurs in individuals with defective cell-mediated immune responses. Lesions resemble those of lepromatous leprosy, which never heal spontaneously and tend to relapse after treatment.

Control strategies and prevention methods should be based on knowledge of the epidemiological factors such as parasites, hosts, reservoirs, insect vectors and human susceptibility.

Geographical distribution

Knowledge of the geographical distribution of leishmaniasis has clearly improved in recent years. The WHO estimates a prevalence of 12 million cases worldwide with an annual incidence of 600 000 newly reported clinical cases. However, as declaration is obligatory in only 32 of the 88 countries affected by leishmaniasis, a substantial number of cases are never recorded (Table 16.5).

In the last two decades, leishmaniasis has become a growing public-health problem due to several factors: (i) the development of agroindustrial projects; (ii) the establishment of large non-immune populations in endemic zones (as happened in Nicaragua during the civil war and in French Guyana where there are training zones for European military forces (the foreign legion, for example), rangers and US marines, as well as research workers from various international institutes); and (iii) large-scale migration between countries, rapid and unplanned urban expansion, environmental changes caused by dams and irrigation and the reduction or termination of insecticide spraying for malaria control. The population at risk is estimated to be approximately 350 million; 90% of all cutaneous leishmaniasis cases occur in Afghanistan, Brazil, Iran, Peru, Saudi Arabia and Syria (Fig. 16.2).

Epidemiology

Parasites

Leishmaniasis is caused by a flagellate protozoan belonging to the genus *Leishmania*. It is transmitted via the bite of the female sandfly which belongs to the genus *Lutzomyia* in the New World and *Phlebotomus* in the Old World. Leishmania parasites can be found in different environments, at altitudes of 200–2000 m. They have a great capacity for adaptation to diverse climates because of their utilization of various types of reservoir and various species of sandfly.

The infection of the female sandfly by *Leishmania* is initiated when the sandfly takes a blood meal from an infected mammal. In the mammal, the parasite presents itself in the amastigote form, which becomes a promastigote in the mid-gut of the phlebotomine.

There are two subclasses of the parasite:
• Vianna, whose paramastigotes change to paramastigotes with a short flagellum which they insert into the digestive tube wall, near the pylorus; even so, some of the promastigotes can freely reach the oesophagus.
• Leishmania, whose promastigotes divide in the gut lumen. Some are hooked to the walls of the gut lumen in a different way and never in the pylorus.
In both cases, the parasite finally migrates in an anterior direction. After 4 days, infective forms of the parasite can be found in the mouthparts of the sandfly.

Classification of leishmaniasis takes into consideration their clinical manifestations and bio-ecological characteristics. Several species of *Leishmania* have been identified by their clinical forms, geographical distribution, epidemiological cycles, identification of vector species and animal reservoir hosts and immunological, biochemical and genomic characteristics.

Molecular techniques such as the polymerase chain reaction (PCR) and pulse field electrophoresis are tests commonly used to identify different species.

The DNA of *Leishmania* is identified by analysis of zymodem and <10 parasites are sufficient to amplify the specific DNA products. Some of the literature identifies leishmaniasis with initials like *L. infantum* MON and *L. infantum* LON, indicating the location of the laboratory that made the zymodem identification: MON indicates Montpellier (France) and LON indicates London, (UK).

Vectors

The insect vectors of leishmaniasis are dipteran Nematoceres of the Psychodidae family, and form the Phlebotominae subfamily. They can be found throughout the world's intertropical and temperate regions (Table 16.6).

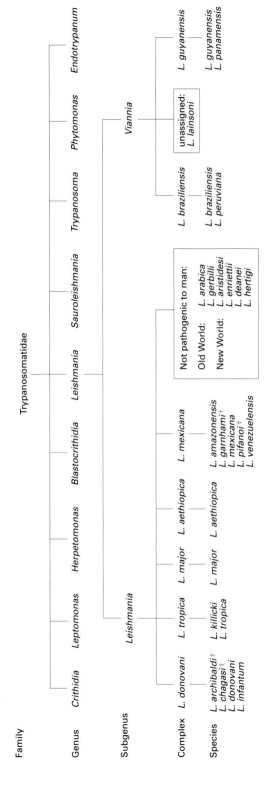

Fig. 16.1 Taxonomy of *Leishmania*. The classification of genera and subgenera is based on extrinsic characters, and that of the complexes mainly on intrinsic characters (isoenzymes). †Some workers do not consider these to be separate species. (Courtesy of WHO, 1990.)

Table 16.5 Cutaneous leishmaniasis: main areas of endemic foci.

Old World

Leishmania major	Kenya, Senegal, Islamic Republic of Iran, Israel, Jordan, Morocco, Saudi Arabia, Tunisia, USSR, India (Rajastan)
Leishmania tropica	Morocco, Saudi Arabia, USSR
Leishmania infantum	France, Spain, Italy, Algeria, Malta
Leishmania aethiopica	Ethiopia, Kenya

New World

Leishmania guyanensis	Brazil, Colombia, French Guyana, Surinam
Leishmania braziliensis	Brazil, Colombia, Bolivia
Leishmania amazonensis	Brazil (Amazon Basin), Colombia, French Guyana
Leishmania mexicana	Belize, southern Mexico
Leishmania panamensis	Colombia, Costa Rica, Panama

The larvae has four phases that can survive as long as 6 weeks in tropical zones. The female sandfly feeds all through the night but especially at dusk, afterwards laying her eggs in the burrows of certain rodents, in old trees, in ruined buildings, in cracks in house walls and in household rubbish.

The insect, which is the only vector of leishmaniasis, absorbs the parasite with the blood from an infected host. The parasite life cycle of the sandfly is 4–25 days, after which the parasite can be inoculated into another animal or human when the fly takes a new blood meal. During feeding, saliva is introduced into the host, one component of which is considered to be one of the most potent vasodilators ever discovered.

Other notable points include: sandflies are classified in the New World into three genera: *Warileya*, *Brumptomyia* and *Lutzomyia*; climatic factors as well as darkness affect the activity of sandflies; some species are known to be highly anthropophilic; certain observations suggest that males produce the pheromone on the host to attract females for courtship and mating; the host serves both as a food source and mating site.

Reservoirs

Cutaneous leishmaniasis depends on rodents, sloths, marsupials, hyraxes, primates and other mammals as the reservoir. A *Leishmania* species in a given area is usually maintained by a single reservoir host, even if other mammals may sometimes be infected. Secondary hosts may play some role in the maintenance of the system and may occasionally bring the parasite from its enzootic genus into close contact with man. Man is directly involved as a reservoir host in the cutaneous leishmaniasis caused by *L. tropica*. Dogs have been found to be infected by *L. braziliensis*, especially in suburban areas. The possible role of this animal and of donkeys, mules and horses as secondary reservoirs should not be overlooked.

In the New World, several species of sloth are important reservoir hosts of different leishmania. A lesser ant-eater (*Tamandua tetradactyla*), which has arboreal habits, plays an important role as the primary reservoir host in the transmission cycle of *L. guyanensis*. This nomadic animal could be responsible for dispersal of the parasites.

Two rodents, *Proechimys guyanensis* and *P. cuvrieri*, are incidental hosts of *L. guyanensis* and primary reservoir hosts of *L. amazonensis*. *Leishmania braziliensis* has been identified in two rodents in two states of Brazil: *Akoden articuloides* (Minas Gerais state) and *Rattus rattus frugiborus* (Ceara state). The primary host of *L. braziliensis* must be a terrestrial animal because all the known vectors only fly at low levels.

In the Old World, rodents and hyraxes are the animals mostly implicated as reservoirs of cutaneous leishmaniasis. *Psammomys obesus*, a reservoir of *L. major* in West Asia and North Africa, feeds on plants of the family Chenopodiaceae, which grows in salty ground and dry river valleys. Hence, the distribution of *P. obesus* is largely confined to these biotopes. *Meriones shawi* is involved in the transmission of *L. major*. In the Maghreb, it lives on cereals and vegetables but in sub-Saharan oases, the same species feeds on wastes of various kinds, including faeces. This peridomestic contact with man explains how serious epidemics have arisen in such areas.

Auricanthis spp. are suspected reservoir hosts of cutaneous leishmaniasis in Senegal and Sudan. Two species of hyrax are the reservoir hosts of *L. aethiopica* in East Africa and of an unnamed *Leishmania* species in Namibia.

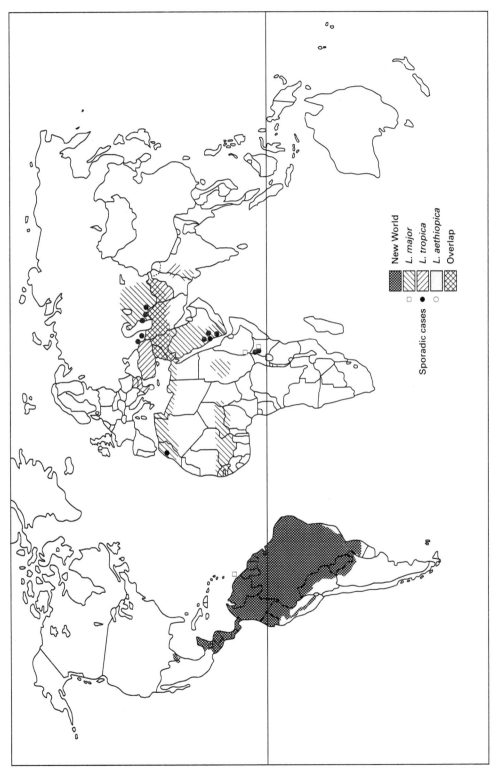

Fig. 16.2 Distribution of Old World and New World cutaneous leishmaniasis (1990). (Courtesy of Dr P. Desjeux; WHO, 1992.)

Table 16.6 Cutaneous leishmaniasis: parasites and proven vectors.

Old World *(Phlebotomus)*	
Leishmania major	*Phlebotomus duboscqi*
	Phlebotomus papatasi
	Phlebotomus salehi
Leishmania tropica	*Phlebotomus sergenti*
	Phlebotomus rossi
Leishmania infantum	*Phlebotomus ariasi*
	Phlebotomus erfiliewi
	Phlebotomus perniciosus
Leishmania aethiopica	*Phlebotomus longipes*
	Phlebotomus pedifer
New World *(Lutzomyia)*	
Leishmania guyanensis	*Lutzomyia anduzei*
	Lutzomyia umbratilis
	Lutzomyia whitmani
Leishmania braziliensis	*Lutzomyia whitmani*
	Lutzomyia carrerai carrerai
	Lutzomyia llanos martinsi
	Lutzomyia yucumensis
	Lutzomyia wellcomei
	Lutzomyia spinicrassa
Leishmania amazonensis	*Lutzomyia flaviscutellata*
Leishmania mexicana	*Lutzomyia olmeca olmeca*
Leishmania panamensis	*Lutzomyia trapidoi*
	Lutzomyia ylephiletor
	Lutzomyia gomezi

Human host

Patients with cutaneous leishmaniasis usually live in endemic zones of the disease. In the New World, however, the disease more frequently affects men, because of their leisure and professional activities in enzootic areas. When women participate in these activities, or if their residence is not far from the forest, there is no difference between the sexes.

As with any infectious disease, leishmaniasis results from the virulence of the agent, quantity of inoculum, promoting factors and the defending capacity of the host. Immunological mechanisms are of first importance in these host reactions.

Immunogenetic reaction of the host

Following inoculation via the skin, multiplication of *Leishmania* inside the macrophages leads to secretion of interferon-γ (INF-γ). In response to IFN-γ, the macrophage produces toxic oxygen and nitrogen radicals which are leishmanicidal. IFN-γ is produced both by the macrophages and by natural killer (NK) cells. *Leishmania* also induces macrophage production of tumour necrosis factor-α (TNF-α) which potentiates the action of IFN-γ and promotes macrophage activation and transforming growth factor-β (TGF-β), which is linked to inhibition of IFN-γ and macrophage deactivation.

At the same time, parasitized epidermal Langerhans cells (constitutively expressing major histocompatibility class (MHC) class II antigen) function as antigen-presenting cells (APCs). These cells transport *Leishmania* to the draining lymph nodes and induce the antigen-specific T-cell response mediated by CD8$^+$ cytotoxic T cells.

Two functional subsets of T lymphocyte CD4$^+$, T-helper 1 (Th$_1$) and T-helper 2 (Th$_2$), present with different profiles of cytokine secretion. Th$_1$ cells produce cytokines (interleukin-2, IFN-α and TNF-α) involved in cell-mediated immunity and macrophage activation, leading to *Leishmania* destruction.

Th$_2$ cells produce cytokines (the interleukins IL-4, IL-5, IL-6, IL-10) implicated in antibody production and macrophage deactivation and no *Leishmania* destruction.

The induction of the Th$_1$ or Th$_2$ response is of utmost importance in the course of the disease. A Th$_1$-predominant response seems to be linked with a favourable outcome, whereas a predominant Th$_2$ response is linked to a progressive and extensive disease.

In the network of cytokines, IL-12 (produced by the macrophage) is worth identification because it drives a Th$_1$ response and enhances IFN-γ production and cytotoxicity of T cells and NK cells.

Prevention

Restricted transmission

Prevention methods to restrict the transmission of the cutaneous leishmaniasis begin by following simple prophylactic recommendations to control the vector. These preventive measures can be handled at different levels.

Individual level

Personal protection involves using insect repellants applied to the skin and bed nets or curtains impregnated with residual insecticide of the pyrethrinoid family. These are currently being assessed for effectiveness. When the risk is occasional, wearing of appropriate clothing is recommended.

The treatment and control in human cases of cutaneous leishmaniasis is indicated prophylactically only in the rare zones where patients are identified as reservoirs of the disease:
• Wearing of an ultrasound machine could be useful for persons with occasional contact with vectors.
• Taking 500 mg to 1 g/day of vitamin B_1 covers the skin with of an odour that repels the insect vector and makes it uncomfortable to bite its victim.
• Although Pentacarinat has been used as a prophylactic drug for trypanosomiasis, it has never been used for leishmaniasis, but it could be studied in patients temporarily going to endemic zones.

Community level

The following can be recommended:
• The spraying of residual insecticides inside and around houses.
• Destruction of the sites (used for resting and breeding) or certain species of sandfly vectors.
• Deforestation must be of 300 m around villages in order to isolate the villages from parasite vectors and reservoirs.

Identification of the reservoir is a prerequisite for the selection and application of selective control methods. In the case of cutaneous leishmaniasis where rodents are the reservoirs, the control techniques are linked with agriculture activities: poisonous baits and anticoagulants should be placed in rodent burrows; the plants on which they feed should be eliminated.

Active case detection and treatment in domestic reservoir hosts, accompanied by measures for preventing re-infection, should reduce or eliminate the parasite load and reduce transmission. Surveillance of stray, feral and domestic dogs is required in endemic zones. Ideally, all symptomatic dogs should be destroyed or treated, followed with a close supervision for relapses.

Immunization

Old practice of 'leishmanization'

This primitive form of immunization used in the Ottoman Empire was still going on in at least three countries until recently. The process was to scratch a leishmaniasis sore with a needle, and then scratch someone who had not had the disease with the same needle, on some comestically unimportant part of the body, to transfer the pus. This produced a local lesion usually lasting up to a year after which the patient would be immune.

In the former USSR, individuals who had to go to highly endemic areas were given live virulent *L. major* promastigotes grown in culture, on their arms, 3 or 4 months before travel, after which it was felt that ulcers would be very small and heal quickly. In Israel, this was performed on soldiers serving in desert areas which are highly infected with reservoir host animals. In Iran, during the Iran–Iraq war, leishmanization was given to more than 2 million people over several years.

However, this is not a recommended method of vaccination and has been halted because not everyone who receives the inoculation this way heals within a year. Follow-up studies in Iran indicated that 2–3% would have a lesion for over a year, and half of them would not heal after many years (and would need treatment). An additional risk to take into consideration with this method is the transmission of other viruses such as herpes simplex, hepatitis B and C and HIV.

Vaccines

Cutaneous leishmaniasis produces a strong protective immune response and therefore the development of a vaccine has focused the attention of much work over the years. Vaccination probably presents the long-term hope for controlling the disease.

As a large number of antigens among leishmania species are cross-reacting, it is conceivable that a single vaccine with common antigens could induce protective immunity. In regard to the results of leishmanization, killed vaccines must be used to avoid the occurrence of many cases induced by vaccination.

All studies already conducted have used killed vaccine (sonicated or irradiated promastigotes, avirulent mutant clones). One study took place in Brazil, using a vaccine of whole sonicated promastigotes from five strains of *Leishmania*, administered intramuscularly, but it was inconclusive. It seems that an appropriate adjuvant is required to make the vaccine efficient. Bacterial adjuvants are tried, such as BCG, which is used in many different trials. *Salmonella* has been used as well and confers the advantage of an oral route for vaccination.

Another approach is the use of cytokine as adjuvant and studies with IL-12 are promising.

To ensure that any candidate vaccine would not induce exacerbation of the disease, single and purified antigenic preparations from promastigotes have been developed, particularly: lipophosphoglycan, a membrane antigen found in all leishmanial species; glycoprotein-63 (Gp-63), a major surface glycoprotein expressed on all leishmanial species; and Gp-46, a membrane glycoprotein detected on *L. amazonensis* and conferring a significant protection against *L. amazonensis*.

Many problems, however, remain in the search for an efficient vaccine. The immunity obtained with a single antigen is not enough and additional antigens are required for active certain immunity. Lack of knowledge of the immunogenic components is one of the most important failings. Also, the route of vaccine administration is critical and studies have shown that intravenous administration seems superior to other routes.

Further reading

Alfonso, L.C., Scharton, T.M., Vieira, L.Q., Wysocka, M., Trinchieri, G. & Scott, P. (1994) The adjuvant effect of interleukin-12 in a vaccine against *Leishmania major*. *Science*, **263**, 235–237.

Barral-Netto, M., Machado, P. & Barral, A. (1995) Human cutaneous leishmaniasis: recent advances in physiopathology and treatment. *European Journal of Dermatology*, **5**, 104–113.

Carrada-Bravo, T. (1993) Cellular immunity and vaccination against cutaneous leishmaniasis. Recent progress and prospects. *Revista Alergia*, **40**, 98–105.

Castes, M., Blackwell, J., Trujillo, D. *et al.* (1994) Immune response in healthy volunteers vaccinated with killed leishmanial promastigotes plus BCG. I. Skin-test reactivity, T-cell proliferation and interferon-gamma production. *Vaccine*, **12**, 1041–1054.

Combemalle, P., Deruaz, D., Villanova, D. & Guillaumont, P. (1992) Les insectifuges ou les répellents. *Annales de Dermatologie et de Venereologie*, **119**, 411–434.

Dedet, J.P., Esterre, P. & Pradinaud, R. (1987) Individual clothing prophylaxis of cutaneous leishmaniasis in the Amazonian area. *Transactions of the Royal Society of Tropical Medicine and Hygiene*, **81**, 748.

Dedet, J.P., Pradinaud, R. & Gray, F. (1989) Epidemiological aspects of human cutaneous leishmaniasis in French Guyana. *Transactions of the Royal Society of Tropical Medicine and Hygiene*, **83**, 616–620.

Desjeux, P. (1992) Human leishmaniases: Epidemiology and public health aspects. *World Health Statistics Quarterly*, **45**(2–3), 267–275.

Grimaldi, G. Jr, Tesh, R.B. & McMahon-Pratt, D. (1989) A review of the geographic distribution and epidemiology of leishmaniasis in the New World. *American Journal of Tropical Medicine and Hygiene*, **41**, 687–725.

Hashigochi, Y. (1985) A review of leishmaniasis in the New World with special reference to its transmission mode and epidemiology. *Japanese Journal of Tropical Medicine and Hygiene*, **13**, 205–243.

Peters, W. (1992) Leishmaniases. In: *A Colour Atlas of Arthropods in Clinical Medicine*, pp. 115–134. World Publishing.

Rabinovitch, M. & Veras, P. (1995) Leishmanies: biologie. *Encycl. Méd. Chir., Maladies infectieuses*, 8-506-A-10. Elsevier, Paris.

Raccurt, C., Pratlong, F., Moreau, B., Pradinaud, R. & Dedet, J.P. (1995) French Guyana must be recognised as an endemic area of *Leishmania (Vianna) braziliensis* in South America. *Transactions of the Royal Society of Tropical Medicine and Hygiene*, **89**, 372.

Ranque, J., Quilici, M. & Dunan, S. (1975) Les leishmanioses du Sud-Est de la France. Ecologie–epidémiologie–prophylaxie. *Acta Tropica*, **32**, 371–380. Assemblée Soc. Franç. Parasit.

Ridel, P.R., Esterre, P., Dedet, J.P., Pradinaud, R., Santoro, F. & Capron, A. (1988) Killer cells in human cutaneous leishmaniasis. *Transactions of the Royal Society of Tropical Medicine and Hygiene*, **82**, 223–226.

Walton, B.C. (1987) American cutaneous leishmaniasis.

In: *The leishmaniases in Biology and Medicine* (eds P.W. Killick-Kendrick & R. Killick-Kendrick), Vol. 1 pp. 637–664. Academic Press, London.

WHO (1990) *Control of the Leishmaniases:report of a WHO Expert Committee*. Technical Report Series No. 793. World Health Organization, Geneva.

WHO (1992) Human leishmaniases: Epidemiology and public health aspects. *Rapport Trimestriel de Statistiques Sanitaires Mondiales*, **45**, No. 2/3. World Health Organization, Geneva.

17
Disorders due to Drugs and Chemical Agents

Prevention of Allergic Contact Dermatitis

J.M. LACHAPELLE

The prevention of allergic contact dermatitis has been approached in several reviews, including Adams (1990) and Rycroft *et al.* (1995). It is very often divided into two parts: general and individual measures of prevention. It is intended here to discuss the problem in a rather different way, i.e. in terms of primary, secondary and tertiary prevention. This approach permits a better evaluation of the problems encountered in daily life. It is particularly important for preventing and/or controlling outbreaks of allergic contact dermatitis that occur in various fields such as, for example, dermatocosmetology or occupational dermatology.

Primary, secondary and tertiary prevention

Outline of principles

Authorities involved in public-health services are well aware of the urgent need for better organization of preventive measures in all fields of medicine. Many of them consider that this commitment is the highest priority and the main goal to reach at the turn of the century. Prevention of allergic contact dermatitis (Lachapelle, 1995; Flyvholm, 1996) can be divided into primary, secondary and tertiary prevention. It is surprising that this concept and the terms themselves have escaped the attention of authors of recent textbooks in environmental dermatology (Adams, 1990; Rycroft *et al.*, 1995).

- *Primary prevention* of allergic contact dermatitis focuses on induction of contact sensitization and controlling the exposure which eventually leads to contact sensitization.
- *Secondary prevention* focuses on elicitation of allergic contact dermatitis.
- *Tertiary prevention* is related to all measures used when the disease becomes a clear-cut reality and a distressing impairment to the quality of life.

The measures for primary and secondary prevention can differ in some respects, but in several instances exposure assessment made for secondary prevention provides the knowledge necessary for initiation of measures for primary prevention, and the measures for primary prevention may constitute the secondary prevention by preventing new outbreaks of eczema in sensitized subjects.

A survey of general and individual measures

Preventing allergic contact dermatitis is the cornerstone of all current projects. It is crucial that over the next few years the number of cases has to be dramatically reduced. Two types of considerations must be borne in mind: individual aspects (for instance, in occupational dermatology, some workers are disabled by many interruptions to their activities in the course of a year) and socio-economic aspects. Prevention is a difficult task, including both general and individual measures of protection; unavoidably, it also implies a wide range of treatment procedures.

There is one general principle: general measures of prevention and protection are more effective than individual measures, since the latter depend upon the personal will and constant application of each

Table 17.1 Primary prevention of allergic contact dermatitis.

Use of potent haptens in closed systems

Replacement of strongly haptenic chemicals by chemicals of weak or no haptenic potential

Reduction of hapten content in industrial products (e.g. addition of iron (ferrous) sulphate to cement to reduce the amount of free chromate salts)

Hapten (or allergen) removal, e.g. in topical drugs and/or cosmetic formulations (monitoring of drugs and cosmetics)

Measurement of atmospheric pollution to reduce the amount of aeroallergens

Specific measures in the work environment, e.g. automation, ventilation, medico-technical supervision in the workplace, entrapment of allergic chemicals

Initiatives to improve current knowledge of the chemical composition of end products

Protective clothing (with special attention to gloves)

'Barrier' creams and/or gels

Labelling of cosmetics and end products in industry

Medical education of consumers and workers by means of posters, teaching sessions for people at risk and courses on prevention of skin disorders and skin protection

Medical guidelines related to the vocational choice of a profession (mainly for atopics)

Table 17.2 Secondary prevention of allergic contact dermatitis.

Early detection of the incipient clinical signs of allergic contact dermatitis

Careful investigation of anamnestic data leading to the possibility (or not) of a direct link between environmental conditions and clinical signs

Building up of diagnostic procedures in order to confirm (or refute) aetiological factors (patch tests, prick tests, open tests, repeated open application tests, RAST tests)

In the case of positive allergic reactions, determination of the relevance (or the non-relevance) of positive reactions

Information systems: product labelling, leaflets on product types or occupations, databases

Protective clothing (with special attention to gloves)

Use of appropriate 'barrier' creams and/or gels, with all the limitations linked to the insufficient protective effect of such items

Skin cleaners of low irritant potential

Discussion and conclusions leading to the removal or the reduction of contact with the offending agent(s)

individual person (Tucker, 1988; Lachapelle, 1995). A list of procedures used in preventive dermatology for eradication of allergic contact dermatitis is presented in Tables 17.1 to 17.3. We have attempted to classify measures in terms of primary prevention (Table 17.1), secondary prevention (Table 17.2) and tertiary prevention (Table 17.3).

A practical example to illustrate the measures: allergic contact dermatitis to acrylates in dental surgeons

Occupational allergic contact dermatitis in dental surgeons due to the use of acrylic resins in composite materials provides a good example to illustrate the various facets of such a prevention programme. Finger-tip dermatitis is the most common clinical symptom,

but as exposure continues, the sides and the backs of the fingers also become involved (Kanerva *et al.*, 1994).

The most commonly used acrylates are ethylene glycol dimethacrylate (EGDMA), diethyleneglycol dimethacrylate (DEGDMA) and trimethylpropane trimethacrylate (TMPTMA). Most of the dental composite resin materials are 'diluted' with less-viscous 'difunctional' acrylates. These are the methacrylic monomers of which EGDMA, DEGDMA, triethyleneglycol dimethacrylate (TREGDMA) and 1,4-butanedioldimethacrylate (BUDMA) are the most extensively used.

As regards prevention against acrylics, many problems have not been satisfactorily solved. When considering *primary prevention*, it has been suggested (Kanerva *et al.*, 1995) that dental products containing acrylics should be delivered in bottles/packings such that no-touch techniques could be used when handling acrylics, but currently this is not the case. Another approach is therefore needed: it consists of repeated teaching of dentists about the risks encountered in

Table 17.3 Tertiary prevention of allergic contact dermatitis.

Diagnosis of disabling allergic contact dermatitis

Careful investigation of anamnestic data leading to the probability of a direct link between environmental conditions and clinical signs

Building up of diagnostic procedures in order to confirm the aetiological factors (patch tests, prick tests, open tests, repeated open application tests, RAST tests)

Determination of the relevance of the positive reaction

Removal of the allergenic culprit(s)

When removal is utopian, building up of an individual strategy based on reduction of contact and wearing of protective clothes

Treatment of allergic contact dermatitis (topical and/or systemic)

In occupational dermatology, registration of the side effects and application of legal measures (which may differ from one country to another)

Alleviation of potential conflicts in the industrial environment

Psycho-social (global) approach to solve the problems

---

touching dental composite resins and dentin primers without wearing gloves.

Secondary prevention is exclusively related to the use of appropriate gloves. Rubber gloves are readily penetrated by acrylics (Pegum & Medhurst, 1971). Polyvinylchloride, polyethylene, polyvinylacetate and polyvinylalcohol plastic gloves are also inadequate. A new glove material, 4-H glove®, a laminate made of five layers of polyethylene–ethylenevinylalcohol copolymer–polyethylene (PE/EVOH/PE), with a thickness of 0.065 mm has been introduced and shown to inhibit the penetration of various acrylates (Roed-Petersen, 1989). Nevertheless, the 4-H glove® is not of good anatomical fit for delicate tasks. It has been therefore suggested that a fingerpiece of the 4-H glove® under a disposable glove may be used by dental personnel. Another possibility is to use the fingerpiece on the disposable latex or vinyl glove (Kanerva *et al.*, 1991).

In practice, when manipulations are of short duration, the use of a nitrile glove (i.e. N-Dex® Best glove)

is quite convenient, despite the fact that such a glove is theoretically penetrated by acrylics.

Tertiary prevention is in the present case very similar to secondary prevention. In some rare instances, fingertip dermatitis does not heal completely, and requires long-term topical therapy, including corticosteroid and emollient preparations.

Specific points of current interest in prevention

Some specific aspects in the prevention of allergic contact dermatitis deserve special attention.

Removal of allergens

Is removal of allergen(s) needed in all cases of allergic contact dermatitis? Removal of the responsible allergen has been advocated in most cases of allergic contact dermatitis and is considered to be the only efficacious measure to obtain complete healing of active lesions. This general principle remains valuable in the vast majority of cases but can be tempered in some circumstances.

Chromate allergy related to cement or concrete in building-industry workers

Workers in the building industry who become allergic to chromates present in traces in cement and/or concrete are often forced to withdraw from their job. Nevertheless, the addition of ferrous sulphate to cement immediately before mixing reduces the hexavalent chromium to the trivalent state and may thus prevent dermatitis (Avnstorp, 1992). In some countries, ferrous sulphate is available (in sacks) to be added to cement (Mesalt®).

The follow-up of workers in order to evaluate the efficacy of such prevention measures (Avnstorp, 1989) has shown an interest in adding ferrous sulphate, but it is nonetheless difficult to evaluate its precise impact, since automation has also played an important role in reducing the number of affected workers. The practical implication of this discussion is the fact that, contrary to set ideas, it is possible to envisage that workers allergic to chromates may not necessarily be removed from the workplace. In other words, each individual worker is submitted to an objective (re) evaluation, on a regular basis. Each individual decision concerning withdrawal from work is weighed up, taking into consideration medical and social aspects.

Hairdressers

Allergic contact dermatitis to hair dyes in hairdressers

It is very problematical to prevent hair-dye dermatitis in susceptible hairdressers, since they work without wearing gloves. Young hairdressers becoming allergic to hair dyes (paraphenylenediamine or derivatives) are forced to move to another job. Wearing gloves seems impractical; moreover, dyed hair still contains allergens in minute amounts; the contact of fingers with hair is sufficient to worsen hand dermatitis in allergic hairdressers. In this particular example, removal of the allergen(s) seems therefore unavoidable (Holness & Nethercott, 1990).

Allergic contact dermatitis to permanent-wave allergens

Glyceryl monothioglycolate, a waving agent used in acid permanent waving products, sensitizes the occasional consumer, but is usually an occupational hazard for the hairdresser (Storrs, 1984). Some manufacturers of waving agents provide kits including polyethylene gloves which are impermeable to thioglycolates, therefore offering a good protection. Wearing such gloves allows young hairdressers allergic to glycerylmonothioglycolate to perform permanent waving without any further skin problems (secondary and tertiary prevention). Improved education of apprentices about the risk of allergic contact dermatitis remains of course the best approach, as it is a classical example of primary prevention (Matsunaga *et al.*, 1988).

The Kathon CG® biocide story

The biocide Kathon CG® has provoked outbreaks of allergic contact dermatitis among consumers of cosmetic products in which Kathon CG® had been introduced in the 1980s and early 1990s. Most cases occurred when Kathon CG® was incorporated on a large scale into 'leave-on' formulations, at a concentration of 15 ppm. Removal of the biocide was necessary, due to many complaints from consumers on one hand, and the concern of dermatologists on the other. After repeated discussions, it has been decided to maintain Kathon CG® as a biocide in 'rinse-off' formulations, such as shampoos, at a concentration of 7.5 ppm. This decision proved useful, since such shampoos are well tolerated in patients who had previously experienced allergic problems from 'leave-on' preparations containing Kathon CG® at a 15 ppm concentration. In this example, the risk-analysis process for a microbiocide with broad applications as well as varied human exposure patterns involves assiduous planning along with development and implementation of appropriate action to monitor and reduce risk levels. The cooperation of industry and the dermatology community was instrumental in achieving the goals of the programme (Moss, 1994).

Use of protective gloves in prevention

The use of protective gloves is one of several possibilities to avoid developing a contact dermatitis or a relapse (Wahlberg & Maibach, 1994). When the use of gloves at work is practically possible, they can provide good protection in some patients allergic to a defined allergen. A classical example is provided by epoxy resin allergic contact dermatitis which can be suppressed or reduced by wearing PE/EVOH/PE gloves (Roed-Petersen, 1989) Enthusiasm must be tempered by drawbacks related to wearing of gloves, such as reduction of ductility (mainly when finger-tips play a crucial role in occupational skill, as for example in surgeons' activities), irritation due to occlusion, inadequacy of ill-fitted gloves and penetration of allergens through gloves (Mellström *et al.*, 1994).

Use of barrier creams and/or gels

'Active' barrier creams have in the past been very popular in some European countries. The term 'active' applies to creams containing active ingredients that are supposed to work by trapping or transforming allergens (ascorbic acid, glutathione, cysteine, ion exchangers). It has been claimed in recent reviews that they can be considered as ineffective (Lachapelle, 1996). Indeed, this opinion is broadly expressed by practising dermatologists. Nevertheless, some recent publications have entertained doubts about this clear-cut view.

Studies are two-sided: (a) application of creams or gels before applying the allergens in a patch test system on the skin of sensitive subjects and evaluation of the reducing effect of the cream or gel on the positive patch test reaction at 24, 48 or 72 hours; (b) 'use tests' mimicking real conditions of skin contact with the allergen. For instance, beneficial results were reported in some chromate-sensitive construction workers using a barrier cream composed of silicone, tartaric acid, glycine and other ingredients. The tartaric acid and glycine apparently chelate chromate and reduce chrome(VI) to chrome(III), which is less allergenic (Romaguera *et al.*, 1985).

On the other hand, some compounds offer potential for use in the prophylaxis of nickel dermatitis (Gawkrodger *et al.*, 1995). Chelating agents and other substances can be used to bind nickel or reduce its penetration through the skin, and hence to reduce the symptoms in subjects with nickel sensitivity. The most effective ligand for nickel so far described is 5-chloro-7-iodoquinolin-8-ol. Although normally regarded as safe, its use in some situations may be limited by concerns about its toxicity. Other ligands with demonstrable effect include ethylenediamine tetraacetic acid (EDTA) in various forms, diphenyl-glyoxime and dimethylglyoxime. Cation-exchange resins can effectively bind nickel and work both *in vitro* and *in vivo*. Propyleneglycol, petrolatum and lanolin reduce absorption of nickel through the skin. In a recent study (Fullerton & Menné, 1995), application of a Carbopol gel with 10% $CaNa_2$-EDTA beneath a nickel disc completely abrogated the allergic contact response in 21/21 (100%) nickel-sensitive patients. A Carbopol gel without $CaNa_2$-EDTA was less effective, inhibiting the response in 15/21 patients (71.4%). Further studies are being conducted in this direction (Menné, 1995).

Poison ivy/oak (*Toxicodendron*) dermatitis is the most common allergic contact dermatitis in the United States. The allergen is 3-pentadecylcatechol. Related dermatoses are *Lithrea* dermatitis, commonly encountered in some countries of South America, and lacquer tree dermatitis frequently described mainly in Japan, but also in several countries of South-East Asia. Until recently, despite extensive research, the use of topical barrier preparations to prevent *Toxicodendron* dermatitis has been only minimally successful.

A very extensive study has been conducted in the United States, in order to find 'active' protective creams and reduce the disability of this quite common skin problem (Grevelink *et al.*, 1992). The results of this study indicate that some barrier creams (Stokogard®, Hollister Moisture Barrier® and Hydrope®) are able to reduce — to a certain extent — the skin symptoms in sensitive subjects. Even more promising is the very recent use of a new topical lotion containing 5% quaternium-18 bentonite (Marks *et al.*, 1995).

All these trials indicate that new approaches are under current evaluation, but there is still no real consensus in this difficult and controversial field of research.

References

Adams, R.M. (1990) *Occupational Skin Disease*, 2nd edn. W.B. Saunders, Philadelphia.

Avnstorp, C. (1989) Follow-up of workers from the pre-fabricated concrete industry after the addition of ferrous sulphate to Danish cement. *Contact Dermatitis*, **20**, 365–371.

Avnstorp, C. (1992) Cement eczema. An epidemiological intervention study. *Acta Dermato-Venereologica (Stockholm)*, **72** (Suppl 179), 1–22.

Flyvholm, M.A. (1996) Prevention by exposure assessment. In: *Prevention of Contact Dermatitis* (eds P. Elsner, J.M. Lachapelle, J. Wahlberg & H.I. Maibach), pp. 97–105. Karger, Basel.

Fullerton, A. & Menné, T. (1995) *In vitro* and *in vivo* evaluation of the effect of barrier gels in nickel contact allergy. *Contact Dermatitis*, **32**, 100–106.

Gawkrodger, D.J., Healy, J. & Howe, A.M. (1995) The prevention of nickel contact dermatitis. A review of the use of binding agents and barrier creams. *Contact Dermatitis*, **32**, 257–265.

Grevelink, S.A., Murrell, D.F. & Olsen, E.A. (1992) Effectiveness of various barrier preparations in preventing and/or ameliorating experimentally produced *Toxicodendron* dermatitis. *Journal of the American Academy of Dermatology*, **27**, 182–188.

Holness, D.L. & Nethercott, J.R. (1990) Dermatitis in hairdressers. *Dermatologic Clinics*, **8**, 119–126.

Kanerva, L., Turjanmaa, K., Estlander, T. & Jolanki, R. (1991) Occupational allergic contact dermatitis from 2-hydroxyethyl methacrylate (2-HEMA) in a new dentin adhesive. *American Journal of Contact Dermatitis*, **2**, 24–30.

Kanerva, L., Henriks-Eckerman, M.L., Estlander, T. *et al.* (1994) Occupational allergic contact dermatitis and composition of acrylates in dentin bonding systems. *Journal of the European Academy of Dermatology and Venereology*, **3**, 157–168.

Kanerva, L., Estlander, T., Jolanki, R. & Tarvainen, K. (1995) Statistics on allergic patch test reactions caused by acrylic compounds, including data on ethyl methacrylate. *American Journal of Contact Dermatitis*, **6**, 1–4.

Lachapelle, J.M. (1995) Principles of prevention and protection in contact dermatitis (with special reference to occupational dermatology) In: *Textbook of Contact Dermatitis* (eds R.J.G. Rycroft, T. Menné & P.J. Frosch), 2nd edn, pp. 695–702. Springer-Verlag, Berlin.

Lachapelle, J.M. (1996) The efficacy of protective creams and/or gels. In: *Prevention of Contact Dermatitis* (eds P. Elsner, J.M. Lachapelle, J. Wahlberg & H.I. Maibach), pp. 182–192. Karger, Basel.

Marks, J.G., Fowler, J.F., Sherertz, E. & Rietschel, R.L. (1995) Prevention of poison ivy/oak allergic contact dermatitis by quaternium-18 bentonite. *Allergologie*, **18**, 452.

Matsunaga, K., Hosokawa, K., Suzuki, M. *et al.* (1988) Occupational allergic contact dermatitis in beauticians. *Contact Dermatitis*, **18**, 94–96.

Mellström, G.A., Carlsson, B. & Boman, A.S. (1994) Testing of protective effect against liquid chemicals. In: *Protective Gloves for Occupational Use* (eds G.A. Mellström, J.E. Wahlberg & H.I. Maibach), pp. 53–77. CRC Press, Boca Raton.

Menné, T. (1995) Prevention of nickel dermatitis. *Allergologie*, **18**, 447.

Moss, J.N. (1994) Reconciling clinical data with risk: the Kathon® biocide story. In: *Occupational Skin Disease*: *State of the Art Reviews* (ed. J.R. Nethercott), Vol. 9, pp. 113–119. Hanley and Belfus, Philadelphia.

Pegum, J.S. & Medhurst, F.A. (1971) Contact dermatitis from penetration of rubber gloves by acrylic monomer. *British Medical Journal*, **ii**, 141.

Roed-Petersen, J. (1989) A new glove material protective against epoxy and acrylate monomer. In: *Current Topics in Contact Dermatitis* (eds P. Frosch, A. Dooms-Goossens, J.M. Lachapelle & R.J.G. Rycroft), pp. 603–606. Springer-Verlag, Berlin.

Romaguera, C., Grimalt, F., Vilaplana, J. *et al.* (1985) Formulation of a barrier cream against chromate. *Contact Dermatitis*, **12**, 49–52.

Rycroft, R.J.G., Menné, T. & Frosch, P.J. (1995) *Textbook of Contact Dermatitis*, 2nd edn. Springer-Verlag, Berlin.

Storrs, F. (1984) Permanent wave contact dermatitis: contact allergy to glycerylmonothioglycolate. *Journal of the American Academy of Dermatology*, **11**, 74–85.

Tucker, S.B. (1988) Prevention of occupational skin disease. *Dermatologic Clinics*, **6**, 87–96.

Wahlberg, J.E. & Maibach, H.I. (1994) Prevention of contact dermatitis. In: *Protective Gloves for Occupational Use* (eds G.A. Mellström, J.E. Wahlberg & H.I. Maibach), pp. 7–9. CRC Press, Boca Raton.

Drug-Induced Skin Reactions

J.-C. ROUJEAU

Skin is the organ which is the most frequently affected by adverse drug reactions (ADRs) (Zürcher & Krebs, 1992). Most of these reactions are idiosyncratic, i.e. non-predictable and occurring in a minority of treated patients. Knowledge of the epidemiology of skin ADRs is hampered by the lack of generally accepted definitions and classification criteria. These reactions are frequent nevertheless. Many drugs in current use induce skin rashes in 1–3% of users. Adverse skin reactions to drugs affect 2-3% of hospitalized patients (Zürcher & Krebs, 1992). Severe cutaneous drug reactions affect about 1 per 1000 hospitalized patients (Roujeau & Stern, 1994).

Quantification of risk

Premarketing clinical trials

Because of the limited number of subjects exposed to a drug, the size of premarketing clinical trials is insufficient to detect severe effects. Moreover, even the more frequent mild effects are underestimated in these clinical trials (Coles *et al.*, 1983). Among the many factors concurring to lower the rates of ADRs in clinical trials are: strict inclusion criteria usually resulting in non-inclusion of patients at increased risk; strict definition of the indication for drug use; restricted exposure to other risk factors (e.g. sunlight, simultaneous utilization of other drugs). Premarketing clinical trials, however, generally allow prediction of the side-effect profile of a new drug.

Spontaneous reports

After marketing of a drug, the bulk of the information

on ADRs is provided by the collection of spontaneous reports (pharmacovigilance). Pharmacovigilance has proved very efficient in the generation of 'signals', i.e. early detection of severe and rare side effects (Moore *et al.*, 1985). However, it does not allow a correct quantification of risk for the following reasons:

• Even in countries like France where the report of ADRs is a legal obligation for physicians, underreporting is massive (Bégaud *et al.*, 1994). It was estimated that no more than 1 in 1000 reactions were reported when they were both mild and well known. Even for life-threatening reactions like toxic epidermal necrolysis (TEN), no more than half of the cases are reported to the organisation Pharmacovigilance in France.

• Another important limitation inherent to spontaneous reporting is the unknown size of the population at risk. Indirect calculations are often done from the total volume of drug sales (Roujeau *et al.*, 1990; Schöpf *et al.*, 1991). Total sales are usually expressed as number of defined daily doses (DDDs), the average dose for one day of treatment. Such indirect calculations provide only a very rough estimate of the number of exposed patients. For example, 365 DDDs may correspond to a single patient for drugs used in the long term, like antihypertensive agents, and to 365 patients in the case of drugs used in the very short term, like analgesics.

Cohorts

When feasible, studies of cohorts of patients receiving a drug provide the best estimates of ADR rates. They proved useful for frequent/mild ADRs (Bigby *et al.*, 1986) but are not appropriate for rare events. For example an accurate quantification of the risk of Stevens–Johnson syndrome (SJS) or TEN would need a cohort of more than 1 million users, which is obviously not feasible.

Registries

Registries deal with rare diseases. When based on an active detection network, they usually collect cases much more efficiently than spontaneous reporting systems. In addition, they allow a good ascertainment of cases (Rzany *et al.*, 1996). They can therefore provide good

estimates of the overall incidence of the reaction in a population. The limitation is the unknown size of what part of that population has been exposed to the risk. This can only be derived from DDDs, with the same bias as for systems collecting spontaneous reports.

Database linkage

Database linkage has been used for years in epidemiological studies looking for associations between diseases. For example, evidence of association between dermatomyositis and cancer was provided by linking a Swedish cancer database and a national registry collecting information about people who were hospitalized (Sigurgeirsson *et al.*, 1992). In the field of ADRs, database linkage can be used when drug utilization is recorded in a database (Strom *et al.*, 1987; Coopman *et al.*, 1993). This is the case in most health maintenance organizations. Advantages are well-defined population size and quantification of exposure to prescription drugs (exposure to 'over-the-counter' drugs is not evaluated). The size of the database is not always large enough for the rarest side effects. The major limitation of databases is a poor ascertainment of cases. This is a problem with skin reactions which are too often incorrectly labelled by general physicians.

Case-control studies

For rare reactions such as SJS or TEN, case-control studies are the most accurate way to quantify the risks linked to drug use (Kaufman, 1994). They allow a good ascertainment of cases and can evaluate the risks of any type of exposure (over-the-counter as well as prescription-only drugs). Limitations are the need for a very large population base to collect enough cases of rare diseases and the difficulty in getting appropriate controls. For these reasons, case-control studies need considerable time, manpower and expense.

Clinical types of skin ADRs (Table 17.4)

It is traditional to state that every kind of skin disease can be induced, aggravated or mimicked by drug reactions (Bruinsma, 1987; Zürcher & Krebs, 1992). Some kinds of reaction are frequent while many are much rarer. Because it is mainly based on hospital series or a collection of spontaneous reports, information on the relative frequency of different types of reactions is biased toward overestimation of severe or unusual reactions. From available data (Kauppinen & Stubb, 1984; GISED, 1991; Zürcher & Krebs, 1992) it is nevertheless clear that so-called maculopapular eruptions ('drug rash', morbilliform eruptions) are the most frequent pattern (30–40% of notifications), followed by urticaria and pruritus (both accounting for about 20% of notifications. Fixed drug eruptions are frequent in some countries, e.g. India and Finland, where this pattern is second in frequency in hospital series (Kauppinen & Stubb, 1984; Arora *et al.*, 1989), while it is an uncommon reaction in many other countries (<5% of notifications). Contact dermatitis is not commonly notified but the figures are probably biased by major underreporting. Photosensitivity reactions are infrequent or infrequently reported (*c.* 3% of notifications).

Taken together, severe reactions, including angioedema and anaphylaxis, vasculitis, exfoliative dermatitis, 'hypersensitivity syndrome', anticoagulant skin necrosis, SJS and TEN account for nearly 10% of skin ADRs in hospital series (Kauppinen & Stubb, 1984) and in the database of spontaneous reporting systems. A figure of 2% is probably a more accurate estimate of the real proportion of skin ADRs which are severe (Roujeau & Stern, 1994).

There is no general agreement on the definitions of these severe drug-induced reactions. A good example of the confusion is the term 'hypersensitivity syndrome'. Most skin ADRs are considered to result from some kind of immunological reaction and could therefore be labelled as 'hypersensitivity reactions'. The name 'hypersensitivity syndrome' has anyhow been progressively linked to a subtype of reaction characterized by the severity and persistence of the cutaneous lesions and their association to visceral and biological alterations (Shear & Spielberg, 1988; Roujeau & Stern, 1994). Systemic manifestations frequently include lymph-node enlargement and hepatitis and less frequently interstitial pneumonitis, nephritis or myocarditis. Blood eosinophilia is usual, often >1500 eosinophils/μl, and probably contributes to visceral lesions involving the same target organs than during eosinophilia of other causes. Atypical lymphocytosis is often associated, as well as serological disturbances suggesting a polyclonal activation of the immune response. Such a constellation of systemic and biological alterations probably results from a peculiar pathway of cytokine activation and release. It is noteworthy that eosinophilia and atypical lymphocytosis are not observed in SJS and TEN. In TEN, the commonest blood-count alterations are lymphopenia and neutropenia. Eosinophilia is not present in the initial course of TEN (Bombal *et al.*, 1983).

Rates of mild reactions

The overall incidence of 'maculopapular eruptions' is not known. Several cohorts of in-patients and clinical trials have demonstrated that 'rashes' can occur in $\leqslant 1\%$ of patients receiving placebo (Zürcher & Krebs, 1992) and in 1–5% of those receiving active drugs. The Boston Collaborative Drug Surveillance Program has surveyed 15 438 consecutive in-patients (Bigby *et al.*, 1986). In that study, patients administered antibacterial agents developed 'maculopapular eruptions' with rates varying from 0.4% with gentamicin to 3.4% with co-trimoxazole and 5.1% for amoxycillin. A similar study in Bern, Switzerland, observed similar rates of reactions: 2.8% with co-trimoxazole and 8% for aminopenicillins (Sonntag *et al.*, 1986). Some drugs are associated with higher rates of skin ADRs. Captopril, radiocontrast media, anticonvulsants and β-lactam antibiotics all induce 'rashes' in >3% users (Pollack *et al.*, 1979; Zürcher & Krebs, 1992). The rates are often >10% for many drugs used as 'disease modifiers' in the management of rheumatoid arthritis (gold salts, *d*-penicillamine, tiopronine, sulphasalazine) (Zürcher & Krebs, 1992). On the other hand, for many drugs the risks of skin ADRs are very low and possibly not higher than for placebos. The Boston Collaborative Drug Surveillance Program found reaction rates <0.3% for digoxin, antacids, acetaminophen (paracetamol), aminophylline, isosorbide dinitrate and many other drugs in current use (Bigby *et al.*, 1986).

Rates of severe reactions

Incidence figures are not available for most types of severe cutaneous reactions.

Table 17.4 Main types of drug-induced skin reactions.

Condition	Definition/clinical pattern	Incidence	Percentage drug-induced	Percentage fatal
Mild forms				
Maculopapular eruptions	Morbilliform or papular erythema, often pruritic	1–10% with many drugs*	70 (adults)	0
Urticaria	Pruritic evanescent wheals	0.5–3%*	10	0
Severe forms				
Angioedema/anaphylaxis	Acute non-pruritic deep oedema, wheezing, hypotension	0.001–0.01%*	50	1–6
Anticoagulant skin necrosis	Escarrotic necrosis on fatty areas	0.01%*	100	>10
Acute generalized exanthematic pustulosis	Acute pustular eruption, fever, neutrophilia ± eosinophilia	Unknown 1–3 per 10^6?†	80–100	<5
Exfoliative dermatitis	Erythema and scale involving all skin surface. Can be part of 'hypersensitivity syndrome'	Unknown	20	5
Hypersensitivity syndrome	Widespread infiltrated eruption, frequent facial oedema, systemic lesions (nodes, liver, lung, kidney), eosinophilia, lymphocytosis	Unknown 1–3 per 10^6?†	80–100	10
Vasculitis	Purpura ± systemic lesions (gastrointestinal tract, arthritis, kidney)	Unknown	10	<5
Stevens–Johnson syndrome	Blisters arising on purple macules. Widespread but limited confluence. Mucosal erosions	1–1.5 per 10^6†	>80	5
Toxic epidermal necrolysis	Similar to Stevens–Johnson syndrome with confluent blisters and extensive detachment of epidermis. Mucosal erosions	1–1.5 per 10^6†	>80	30

* Range among persons exposed to a treatment.
† Yearly incidence in population (exposed and new exposure).

Angioedema and anaphylaxis

These are the most severe forms of IgE-mediated immediate reactions. With many drugs, similar reactions result from direct release of inflammatory mediators without production of specific IgE ('anaphylactoid reactions'). Angioedema occurs in about 1 per 10 000 courses of penicillin and probably more often (2–10 per 10 000) in new users of angiotensin-converting enzyme (ACE) inhibitors (Hedner *et al.*, 1992; Roujeau & Stern, 1994). Other drugs associated with angioedema are iodinated contrast media, drugs used in anaesthesia, blood products and β-lactam antibiotics.

Stevens–Johnson syndrome (SJS) and toxic epidermal necrolysis (TEN)

The incidence of TEN is 1–1.5 per million per year in France (Roujeau *et al.*, 1990), Italy (Naldi *et al.*, 1990), USA (Chan *et al.*, 1990), Germany (Schöpf *et al.*, 1991) and Singapore (Chan, 1995). The incidence of SJS is about the same as that for TEN (1 per million per year) when using disease definitions which distinguish drug-induced SJS from infection-related erythema multiforme major (Schöpf *et al.*, 1991). A North American study where erythema multiforme major and SJS were not separated found an incidence figure of 2–4 per million per year (Chan *et al.*, 1990). It was recently proposed considering SJS and TEN as severity variants of the same drug-induced disease (Bastuji-Garin *et al.*, 1993a). The overall incidence of this disease can be estimated at 1.5–3 per million per year, without important variations in different countries. Antibacterial sulphonamides, anticonvulsants, oxicam and pyrazolone non-steroidal anti-inflammatory drugs, allopurinol and chlormezanone are the drugs associated with the higher risks of developing SJS or TEN. Higher estimates of the risks obtained from indirect calculations were 1–3 per 100 000 users for co-trimoxazole, 10 per 100 000 for Fansidar (a long-acting combination of sulphadoxine and pyrimethamine) (Miller *et al.*, 1986) and 14 per 100 000 for carbamazepine (Askmark & Wiholm, 1990). An international case-control study of SJS and TEN found relative risks between 50 and 172 for new users (treatment duration of less than 2 months) of the above-mentioned drugs

and also for corticosteroids (Roujeau *et al.*, 1995). In that study, excess risks for associated drug were in the range 1–4.5 per million users per week. SJS and TEN typically begin 10–14 days after the introduction of a new drug (Guillaume *et al.*, 1987) and sometimes a few days after the drug has been withdrawn.

The incidence of other types of severe cutaneous reactions has never been evaluated by formal studies. From comparisons of the numbers of cases observed by hospital teams, it can be estimated that the incidence of acute generalized exanthemic pustulosis and hypersensitivity syndrome is probably of the same magnitude as that of SJS and TEN (1–3 per million per year for each condition). The incidence of drug-induced vasculitis is probably lower.

'Hypersensitivity syndrome' (HSS)

This is essentially associated with the same drugs as SJS and TEN. Antibacterial sulphonamides (Rieder *et al.*, 1989) and anticonvulsants (Shear & Spielberg, 1988) are the most frequent cause of HSS with an estimated incidence of 1 per 5000 patients. These reactions are probably more frequent among black people. Pyrazolone non-steroidal anti-inflammatory drugs, allopurinol, gold salts, sorbinil, ACE inhibitors and several antibiotics have also been associated with the syndrome. The reaction typically occurs later than other skin ADRs, 2–6 weeks after a drug is first used, and may persist for weeks.

Acute generalized exanthematic pustulosis (AGEP)

This is characterized by a very acute pustular eruption often predominating in intertriginous areas and associated with fever and leucocytosis (Roujeau *et al.*, 1991). Aminopenicillins, macrolides and calcium-channel antagonists are the most frequent causes. The reaction typically occurs within 2 days after the beginning of treatment. A substantial proportion of patients with AGEP have a history of contact dermatitis to the same or to similar antibiotics. Such history and the timing of the reaction suggest that AGEP could be some recall reaction in highly sensitized patients.

Risk factors for skin ADRs

Age

Skin ADRs are observed at any age. Rates of reactions and specially of the more severe ones are higher in the elderly (Schöpf *et al.*, 1991; Bastuji-Garin *et al.*, 1993b). This is explained in part by an increased consumption of drugs. For many drugs, the risk of skin reactions among exposed persons nevertheless increases with age. This may be explained by poly-medications, impaired detoxification resulting from decreased liver or kidney functions and altered immune response.

Gender

In Western countries, women are slightly more at risk of developing cutaneous ADRs. The sex ratio is about 1.5:1 for many types of reactions. This probably results only from a higher consumption of medications by women and from the unbalanced sex ratio observed in elderly populations. In developing countries, skin ADRs are more often reported in men, who may have easier access to health care (and drugs) than women.

Race

Some types of drug reactions (SJS and TEN, for example) occur with a similar frequency in all countries, without any racial predisposition. Fixed-drug eruption appears to be much more frequent in India and Africa than in western European countries. It is also more prevalent in Scandinavia. Maculopapular eruptions provoked by sulphonamides in patients with AIDS have been reported to occur more frequently in white persons than black persons (Colebunders *et al.*, 1987). Conversely, 'hypersensitivity syndrome' is more frequent in black patients (Roujeau & Stern, 1994). These racial variations may be explained by some genetic predisposition to skin ADRs.

Genetic background

Familial aggregations of cases of SJS (Fisher & Shigeoka, 1983) and of cases of fixed-drug eruptions (Pellicano *et al.*, 1992) have been reported. Because of the rarity of these conditions these associations cannot be explained by chance only, and suggest the existence of a genetic predisposition to these ADRs.

The first candidates are the genes of the major histocompatibility complex which are known to control immunological reactivity to many antigens. Several studies have demonstrated that some human leucocyte antigens (HLA) phenotypes were associated with an increased risk of drug reactions. Drug-induced lupus erythematosus is more frequent in patients expressing HLA DR4. SJS and TEN are associated with HLA B12 (Roujeau *et al.*, 1987). Fixed-drug eruption has been linked to HLA B22 (Pellicano & Ciavarella, 1994). The risk of skin reaction to allopurinol is increased in patients with HLA B17 (Chan & Tan, 1989). In all instances, the relative risks are not very high (2–3) and these associations need to be confirmed by other studies.

Other candidates are the genes controlling the metabolism of drugs and other xenobiotics. Drugs are metabolized by phase I enzymes (cytochrome P450 oxidoreductase, flavine monooxygenase) and by phase II enzymes (epoxide hydrolase, glutathione *S*-transferase, *N*-acetyl transferase) leading to toxic or non-toxic metabolites. The biotransformation by P450 oxidoreductase and a defect in detoxication leads to the generation and accumulation of reactive drug metabolites, which are more toxic than the parent compounds. The major metabolic pathway for sulphonamides is *N*-acetylation by *N*-acetyl transferase 1 and/or *N*-acetyl transferase 2, and *N*-acetyl transferase 2 is responsible for the *in vivo* acetylation polymorphism (Cribb *et al.*, 1993). Both sulphonamides and anticonvulsants are oxidized by cytochrome P450 oxidoreductase into chemically reactive metabolites that need to be actively detoxified (Shear *et al.*, 1988; Rieder *et al.*, 1989). This detoxication could involve conjugation with glutathione by glutathione *S*-transferase. *N*-acetyl transferase 2 and glutathione *S*-transferase have a genetic polymorphism that could modulate the toxicity of these drugs. For example, half of the Caucasian population expresses a phenotype of fast acetylation and the other half a phenotype of slow acetylation. The slow acetylation phenotype increases the risk of 'hypersensitivity syndrome', SJS or TEN in relation to antibacterial sulphonamides (Shear *et al.*, 1986; Rieder *et al.*, 1991). For example,

17 of 18 patients with sulphonamide-related SJS or TEN had a slow acetylator genotype compared to 10 of 20 healthy volunteers ($P = 0.003$; odds ratio, 17; 95% confidence interval, 1.9–153.3) (Wolkenstein et al., 1995). Slow metabolism of aromatic anticonvulsants (barbiturates, phenytoin and carbamazepine) has also been demonstrated to be a risk factor for adverse reactions to these drugs (Spielberg et al., 1981).

Smoking habits

Because tobacco can impair drug metabolism, smoking can be expected to alter the rates of drug reactions. A single study suggested that smoking increased the risk of adverse skin reactions to gold salts in the treatment of rheumatoid arthritis (Kay & Jayson, 1987). In a case-control study, smoking was not found to be a risk factor for the occurrence of drug-induced SJS or TEN (SCAR Study Group, unpublished data).

Malignancies and bone-marrow transplantation

Increased rates of reactions to ampicillin have been reported in patients with chronic lymphocytic leukaemia (Cameron & Richmond, 1971) and with non-lymphocytic leukaemias (Verhagen et al., 1987). Anticonvulsant-related hypersensitivity syndromes and SJS may occur more frequently than expected in patients treated with brain irradiation for CNS malignancies (Janinis et al., 1993).

In a case-control study of risk factors of SJS and TEN, recent radiotherapy was more frequent among cases than controls (Roujeau et al., 1995).

Patients undergoing bone-marrow transplantation have a very high rate of skin rashes. In this context, it is usually very difficult to distinguish drug eruptions from viral rashes and from cutaneous manifestations of acute graft-versus-host disease. TEN, for example, may occur as part of severe acute graft-versus-host disease and as a drug reaction (VIllada et al., 1990).

Viral infections

An unexpectedly high frequency of cutaneous rashes has been reported among patients with infectious mononucleosis treated with ampicillin (Patel, 1967; Pullen et al., 1967). The risk is high (80–100%) but limited in time to the acute phase of Epstein–Barr virus (EBV) infection. Later on, the risk decreases to the background of 3–5% of reactions observed in the general population (Lund & Bergan, 1975). Increased rates of rashes were also observed with other drugs and with other lymphotropic viral infections such as cytomegalovirus (Klemola, 1970) and mainly HIV.

Increased risk of skin ADRs in HIV-infected subjects

Up to 60% of AIDS patients may develop a rash during treatment of *Pneumocystis carinii* pneumonitis with high doses of sulphamethoxazole–trimethoprim (SMX–TMP) (Jaffe et al., 1983; Kovacs et al., 1984). The risk appeared lower when the same treatment was administered to patients suffering from *Pneumocystis carinii* pneumonitis in the context of other kinds of immunosuppression (Kovacs et al., 1984). When SMX–TMP is used at lower doses, skin reactions occur in 10–30% in HIV-infected subjects in contrast to 3–5% of reactions in non-HIV-infected subjects.

Many other drugs have been shown to induce unusually frequent skin reactions in HIV-infected subjects, including sulphadiazine (30–50% reactions), aminopenicillins (10–20%), dapsone plus pyrimethamine (10%) and pyrimethamine alone (8%).

More than two-thirds of these reactions are mild eruptions which disappear in a few days even when the inducing drug is not withdrawn (Table 17.5). Most physicians in charge of AIDS patients consider that withdrawing a suspect drug is not mandatory and that they can 'treat through' mild rashes.

Unfortunately, several types of severe skin reactions including exfoliative dermatitis, SJS and TEN also occur much more frequently than expected in association with HIV infection (Porteous & Berger, 1991). The incidence of TEN among AIDS patients has been estimated to be 1 per 1000 per year, versus 1 per million per year in the general population (Saiag et al., 1992; Rzany et al., 1993). In a recent large series from a referral centre for TEN, HIV infection was present in 20% of cases (Correia et al., 1993). In a case-control study of SJS and TEN, HIV infection was the most strongly associated non-drug factor with a relative risk of 45 (Roujeau et al., 1995). In developing

Table 17.5 Drug-induced skin reactions in HIV-infected subjects. Clinical types of 117 consecutive reactions.

Reaction	Percentage
Maculopapular eruptions	73
Exfoliative dermatitis	11
Stevens–Johnson syndrome/toxic epidermal necrolysis	10
Urticaria	6

countries, the treatment of AIDS-associated tuberculosis with thiacetazone resulted in large numbers of life-threatening skin reactions (Marfatia, 1994).

The frequent occurrence of drug rashes in AIDS patients is not explained by an increased exposure to unusually high doses of 'high-risk' drugs such as antibacterial sulphonamides. With the same dosage of the same drug, the risk is definitely higher in HIV-infected subjects (Kovacs *et al.*, 1984). The rate of reactions per treatment course increases with the progression of the disease (Coopman *et al.*, 1993). It has been suggested that the risk increased in inverse proportion to the blood level of CD4 T lymphocytes and decreased again in the ultimate stage of disease progression when there was < 25 CD4 T lymphocytes/µl (Battegay *et al.*, 1989; Carr *et al.*, 1993). These findings need confirmation and may not apply to all types of reactions. Most cases of SJS or TEN in patients with AIDS occur as a complication of central nervous system (CNS) toxoplasmosis treated with sulphadiazine. Because CNS toxoplasmosis is a late complication of HIV infection, the blood level of CD4 T lymphocytes in these patients is usually < 100/µl and often < 25/µl.

The frequent occurrence of drug reactions in association with HIV-induced immune suppression has not yet been explained. An imbalance between T-helper Th_1 and Th_2 types of immune response could only increase the risk of reactions mediated through a Th_2 type of reaction (i.e. related to IGE or other classes of antibodies, and/or associated with eosinophilia). The most frequent reactions in HIV-infected subjects are not associated with drug-specific antibodies and do not behave as immediate IgE-related reactions. Because 'hypersensitivity reactions' to sulphonamides had been previously linked to abnormal metabolism of these drugs and because these drugs are frequently

the cause of drug rashes in HIV-infected subjects, the hypothesis of an abnormal metabolism has been generally accepted as the most probable explanation of the high rate of drug reactions (Van der Ven *et al.*, 1991). Sulphonamides are mostly inactivated by acetylation in the liver. Oxidation also occurs through cytochrome P450 leading to a reactive hydroxylamine. This reactive metabolite is detoxified by glutathione conjugation, an usual way of cell protection towards free radicals and reactive metabolites. It has been shown that 90% of patients with reactions to sulphonamides (both HIV-infected or not infected) were slow acetylators (Lee *et al.*, 1993) in contrast to the usual 50% in Caucasian populations. In addition, the hydroxylamine derivative of sulphamethoxazole has been shown to be more toxic *in vitro* for lymphocytes of patients with hypersensitivity reactions than for control lymphocytes, suggesting a defect in the detoxification mechanisms. Plasma glutathione levels are decreased in HIV-infected subjects (Buhl *et al.*, 1989). Slow acetylation phenotypes might be more frequent than expected in HIV-infected patients (Carr *et al.*, 1994). This might result from interaction of virus, other medications or poor general condition with drug pharmacokinetics (Chang *et al.*, 1978). The metabolic hypothesis does not, however, explain high reaction rates to drugs which are not metabolized through acetylation. It does not explain also the timing of reactions: 9–12 days after first exposure and 1–3 days in cases of positive rechallenge. The hypothesis that these rashes might be drug-enhanced viral eruption has been proposed (Chosidow *et al.*, 1994).

Effect of duration of therapy

Clinicians have noticed for some time that most skin reactions to drugs occurred quite soon after initiation of therapy. Maculopapular eruptions usually begin within two weeks (mean 7–10 days). The characteristic timings are shorter for uricaria/angioedema (minutes to hours), fixed-drug eruptions (within 2 days) and AGEP (within 2 days). Hypersensitivity syndrome typically begins later: 2–6 weeks after onset of treatment.

Long-term treatments are associated with a much lower risk. For example, the risk of allopurinol-related SJS or TEN is not constant over time. In a case-control study, the relative risk for any use was 5.5, a mixture of higher risk during the first 2 months of therapy (52) and no risk later on (0.5) (Roujeau *et al.*, 1995). A drug eruption can occur after the drug has been withdrawn. This has been mainly observed with drugs with long elimination half-lives. It is probably true that a drug may initiate the reaction as long as it is present in the body. When a drug is withdrawn after a steady-state concentration has been obtained, total elimination from the body requires fivefold the elimination half-live. For drugs with elimination half-lives of >48 h (e.g. barbiturates or oxicam non-steroidal anti-inflammatory drugs), a drug reaction may begin 10 days or more after withdrawal (Roujeau *et al.*, 1995).

Conclusion

Severe skin reactions to drugs are unlikely to be detected in premarketing clinical trials. High risks associated with new drugs can be identified only if clinicians report such reactions to regulatory authorities or drug companies. More sophisticated investigations will then be needed to quantify that risk and decide whether it requires that the drug should be relabelled or withdrawn from the market.

References

Arora, P.N., Aggarwal, S.K., Ramakrishnan, K.R. & Chattopadhyay, S.P. (1989) Drug eruptions: a series of 148 cases. *Indian Journal of Dermatology*, **34**, 75–80.

Askmark, H. & Wiholm, B-E. (1990) Epidemiology of adverse reactions to carbamazepine as seen in a spontaneous reporting system. *Acta Neurologica Scandinavica*, **81**, 131–140.

Bastuji-Garin, S., Rzany, B., Stern, R.S., Shear, N.H., Naldi, L. & Roujeau, J-C. (1993a) A clinical classification of cases of toxic epidermal necrolysis, Stevens-Johnson syndrome and erythema multiforme. *Archives of Dermatology*, **129**, 92–96.

Bastuji-Garin, S., Zahedi, M., Guillaume, J.C. & Roujeau, J-C. (1993b) Toxic epidermal necrolysis (Lyell syndrome) in 77 elderly patients. *Age and Ageing*, **22**, 450–456.

Battegay, M., Opravil, M., Wüthrich, B. & Lüthy, R. (1989) Rash with amoxycillin–clavulanate therapy in HIV-infected patients. *Lancet*, **334**, 1100.

Bégaud, B., Haramburu, F., Moride, Y. *et al.* (1994) Assessment of reporting and underreporting in pharmacovigilance. In: *European Medicine Research: Perspective in Pharmacotoxicology and Pharmacovigilance* (ed. G.N. Fracchia), pp. 276–283. IOS Press, Amsterdam.

Bigby, M., Jick, S., Jick, H. & Arndt, K. (1986) Drug-induced cutaneous reactions: a report from the Boston Collaborative Drug Surveillance Program on 15438 consecutive in-patients, 1975 to 1982. *Journal of the American Medical Association*, **256**, 3358–3363.

Bombal, C., Roujeau, J-C., Kuentz, M., Revuz, J. & Touraine, R. (1983) Anomalies hématologiques au cours du syndrome de Lyell. *Annales de Dermatologie et de Venereologie*, **110**, 113–119.

Bruinsma, W. (1987) *A Guide to Drug Eruptions*. De Zwaluw, Oosthuizen, The Netherlands.

Buhl, R., Jaffe, H.A., Holroyd, K.J. *et al.* (1989) Systemic glutathione deficiency in symptom-free HIV-seropositive individuals. *Lancet*, **334**, 1294–1298.

Cameron, S.J. & Richmond, J. (1971) Ampicillin hypersensitivity in lymphatic leukaemia. *Scottish Medical Journal*, **16**, 425–427.

Carr, A., Swanson, C., Pennys, R. & Cooper, D.A. (1993) Clinical and laboratory markers of hypersensitivity to trimethoprim–sulfamethoxazole in patients with *Pneumocystis carinii* pneumonia and AIDS. *Journal of Infectious Diseases*, **167**, 180–185.

Carr, A., Gross, A., Hoskins, J., Penny, R. & Cooper, D.A. (1994) Acetylation phenotype and hypersensitivity to trimethoprim–sulphamethoxazole in HIV-infected patients. *AIDS*, **8**, 333–337.

Chan, H.L. (1995) Toxic epidermal necrolysis in Singapore, 1989 through 1993: incidence and antecedent drug exposure. *Archives of Dermatology*, **131**, 1212.

Chan, H.L., Stern, R.S., Arndt, K.A. *et al.* (1990) The incidence of erythema multiforme, Stevens–Johnson syndrome and toxic epidermal necrolysis, a population-based study with particular reference to reactions caused by drugs among outpatients. *Archives of Dermatology*, **126**, 43–47.

Chan, S.H. & Tan, T. (1989) HLA and allopurinol drug eruption. *Dermatologica*, **179**, 32–33.

Chang, K.C., Lauer, B.A., Bell, T.D. & Chai, H. (1978) Altered theophylline pharmacokinetics during acute respiratory viral illness. *Lancet*, **311**, 1132–1133.

Chosidow, O., Bourgault-Villada, I. & Roujeau, J-C. (1994) Drug rashes: what are the targets of cell-mediated cytotoxicity? *Archives of Dermatology*, **130**, 627–629.

Colebunders, R., Izaley, L., Bila, K. *et al.* (1987) Cutaneous reactions to trimethoprim–sulfamethoxazole in African patients with the acquired immunodeficiency syndrome. *Annals of Internal Medicine*, **107**, 599–600.

Coles, L.S., Fries, J.F. & Kraines, R.G. (1983) From experiment to experience: side effects of nonsteroidal anti-inflammatory drugs. *American Journal of Medicine*, **74**, 820–828.

Coopman, S.A., Johnson, R.A., Platt, R. & Stern, R.S. (1993) Cutaneous disease and drug reactions in HIV infection.

New England Journal of Medicine, **328**, 1670–1674.

Correia, O., Chosidow, O., Saiag, P., Bastuji-Garin, S., Revuz, J. & Roujeau, J-C. (1993) Evolving pattern of drug-induced toxic epidermal necrolysis. *Dermatology*, **186**, 32–37.

Cribb, A.E., Nakamura, H., Grant, D.M., Miller, M.A. & Spielberg, S.P. (1993) Role of polymorphic and monomorphic human arylamine *N*-acetyltransferases in determining sulfamethoxazole metabolism. *Biochemical Pharmacology*, **45**, 1277–1282.

Fisher, P.R. & Shigeoka, A.O. (1983) Familial occurrence of Stevens–Johnson syndrome. *American Journal of Diseases of Children*, **137**, 914–916.

GISED (Gruppo Italiano Studi Epidemiologici in Dermatologia) (1991) Spontaneous monitoring of adverse reactions to drugs by Italian dermatologists: a pilot study. *Dermatologica*, **182**, 12–17.

Guillaume, J-C., Roujeau, J-C., Penso, D. *et al.* (1987) The culprit drugs in 87 cases of toxic epidermal necrolysis (Lyell's syndrome). *Archives of Dermatology*, **123**, 1166–1170.

Hedner, T., Samuelsson, O., Lunde, H., Lindholm, L., Andrén, L. & Wiholm, B.E. (1992) Angio-oedema in relation to treatment with angiotensin converting enzyme inhibitors. *British Medical Journal*, **304**, 941–945.

Jaffe, H.S., Ammann, A.J., Abrams, D.I., Lewis, B.J. & Golden, J.A. (1983) Complication of cotrimoxazole in treatment of AIDS associated *Pneumocystis carinii* pneumonia in homosexual men. *Lancet*, **ii**, 1109–1111.

Janinis, J., Panagos, G., Panousaki, A. *et al.* (1993) Stevens–Johnson syndrome and epidermal necrolysis after administration of sodium phenytoin with cranial irradiation. *European Journal of Cancer*, **29A**, 478–479.

Kaufman, D.W. (1994) Epidemiologic approaches to the study of toxic epidermal necrolysis. *Journal of Investigative Dermatology*, **102**, 31S–33S.

Kauppinen, K. & Stubb, S. (1984) Drug eruptions: causative agents and clinical types. *Acta Dermato-Venereologica*, **64**, 320–324.

Kay, E.A. & Jayson, M.I.V. (1987) Risk factors that may influence development of side effects of gold sodium thiomalate. *Scandinavian Journal of Rheumatology*, **16**, 241–245.

Klemola, E. (1970) Hypersensitivity reactions to ampicillin in cytomegalovirus mononucleosis. *Scandinavian Journal of Infectious Diseases*, **2**, 29–31.

Kovacs, J.A., Hiemenz, J.W., Macher, A.M. *et al.* (1984) *Pneumocystis carinii* pneumonia: a comparison between patients with acquired immunodeficiency syndrome and patients with other immunodeficiencies. *Annals of Internal Medicine*, **100**, 663–671.

Lee, B.L., Wong, D., Benowitz, N.L. & Sullam, P.M. (1993) Altered patterns of drug metabolism in patients with acquired immunodeficiency syndrome. *Clinical Pharmacology and Therapeutics*, **53**, 529–535.

Lund, B.M.A. & Bergan, T. (1975) Temporary skin reactions to penicillins during the acute stage of infectious mononucleosis. *Scandinavian Journal of Infectious Diseases*, **7**, 21–28.

Marfatia, Y.S. (1994) Stevens–Johnson syndrome and toxic epidermal necrolysis. *Archives of Dermatology*, **130**, 1073–1074.

Miller, K.D., Lobel, H.O., Satriale, R.F. *et al.* (1986) Severe cutaneous reactions among American travelers using pyrimethamine–sulfadoxine (Fansidar) for malaria prophylaxis. *American Journal of Tropical Medicine and Hygiene*, **35**, 451–458.

Moore, N., Paux, G., Begaud, B., Biour, M., Loupi, E. & Boismare, F. (1985) Adverse drug reaction monitoring: Doing it the French way. *Lancet*, **ii**, 1056–1058.

Naldi, L., Locatti, F., Marchesi, I. *et al.* (1990) Incidence of toxic epidermal necrolysis in Italy. *Archives of Dermatology*, **126**, 1103–1104.

Patel, B.M. (1967) Skin rash with infectious mononucleosis and ampicillin. *Pediatrics*, **40**, 910–911.

Pellicano, R. & Ciavarella, G. (1994) Genetic susceptibility to fixed drug eruption: evidence of a link with HLA B22. *Journal of the American Academy of Dermatology*, **30**, 52–54.

Pellicano, R., Silvestris, A., Iannantuono, M., Ciavarella, G. & Lomuto, M. (1992) Familial occurrence of fixed drug eruption. *Acta Dermato-Venereologica (Stockholm)*, **72**, 292–293.

Pollack, M.A., Burk, P.G. & Nathanson, G. (1979) Mucocutaneous eruptions due to antiepileptic drug therapy in children. *Annals of Neurology*, **5**, 262–267.

Porteous, D.M. & Berger, T.G. (1991) Severe cutaneous drug reactions (Stevens–Johnson syndrome and toxic epidermal necrolysis) in human immunodeficiency virus infection. *Archives of Dermatology*, **197**, 740–741.

Pullen, H., Wright, N. & Murdoch, J.M.C. (1967) Hypersensitivity reactions to antibacterial drugs in infectious mononucleosis. *Lancet*, **290**, 1176–1178.

Rieder, M.J., Uetrecht, J., Shear, N.H., Cannon, M., Miller, M. & Spielberg, S.P. (1989) Diagnosis of sulfonamide hypersensitivity reactions by *in vitro* rechallenge with hydroxylamine metabolites. *Annals of Internal Medicine*, **110**, 286–289.

Rieder, M.J., Shear, N.H., Kanee, A. & Tang, B.K. (1991) Prominence of slow acetylator phenotype among patients with sulfonamide hypersensitivity reactions. *Clinical Pharmacology and Therapeutics*, **49**, 13–17.

Roujeau, J-C. & Stern, R.S. (1994) Severe cutaneous adverse reactions to drugs. *New England Journal of Medicine*, **331**, 1272–1285.

Roujeau, J-C., Huynh, T.N., Bracq, C., Guillaume, J.C., Revuz, J. & Touraine, R. (1987) Genetic susceptibility to toxic epidermal necrolysis. *Archives of Dermatology*, **123**, 1171–1173.

Roujeau, J-C., Guillaume, J.-C., Fabre, J.-P. *et al.* (1990) Toxic epidermal necrolysis (Lyell syndrome) incidence and drug etiology in France, 1981–1985. *Archives of Dermatology*, **126**, 37–42.

Roujeau, J-C., Bioulac-Sage, P., Bourseau, C. *et al.* (1991) Acute generalized exanthematous pustulosis: analysis of 63 cases. *Archives of Dermatology*, **127**, 1333–1338.

Roujeau, J-C., Kelly, J.P., Naldi, L. *et al.* (1995) Medication use and the risk of Stevens–Johnson syndrome or toxic epidermal necrolysis. *New England Journal of Medicine*, **333**, 1600–1607.

Rzany, B., Mockenhaupt, M., Stocker, U., Hamouda, O. & Schöpf, E. (1993) Incidence of Stevens–Johnson syndrome and toxic epidermal necrolysis in patients with the acquired immunodeficiency syndrome in Germany. *Archives of Dermatology*, **129**, 1059.

Rzany, B., Mockenhaupt, M., Baur, S. *et al.* (1996) Epidemiology of erythema exsudativum multiforme majus (EEMM), Stevens–Johnson syndrome (SJS) and toxic epidermal necrolysis in Germany; structure and results of a population based registry (1990–1992). *Journal of Clinical Epidemiology*, **49**, 769–773.

Saiag, P., Caumes, E., Chosidow, O., Revuz, J. & Roujeau, J-C. (1992) Drug-induced toxic epidermal necrolysis (Lyell syndrome) in patients with the human immunodeficiency virus. *Journal of the American Academy of Dermatology*, **26**, 567–574.

Schöpf, E., Stühmer, A., Rzany, B., Victor, N., Zentgraf, R. & Kapp, J.F. (1991) Toxic epidermal necrolysis and Stevens–Johnson syndrome; an epidemiologic study from West Germany. Archives of Dermatology, **127**, 839–842.

Shear, N.H. & Spielberg, S.P. (1988) Anticonvulsant hypersensitivity syndrome. *Journal of Clinical Investigation*, **82**, 1826–1832.

Shear, N.H., Spielberg, S.P., Grant, D.M., Tang, B.K. & Kalow, W. (1986) Differences in metabolism of sulfonamides predisposing to idiosyncratic toxicity. *Annals of Internal Medicine*, **105**, 179–184.

Sigurgeirsson, B., Lindelöf, B., Edhag, O. & Allander, E. (1992) Risk of cancer in patients with dermatomyositis or polymyositis; a population based study. *New England Journal of Medicine*, **326**, 363–367.

Sonntag, M.R., Zoppi, M., Fritschy, D. *et al.* (1986) Exantheme unter häufig angewandten Antibiotika und antibakteriellen Chemotherapeutika (Penicillin, speziell Aminopenicilline, Cephalosporine und Cotrimoxazol) sowie Allopurinol. *Schweiz Medizinische Wochenschrift*, **116**, 142–145.

Spielberg, S.P., Gordon, G.B., Blake, D.A. *et al.* (1981) Predisposition to phenytoin hepatotoxicity assessed *in vitro*. *New England Journal of Medicine*, **305**, 722–727.

Strom, B.L., Carson, J.L., Morse, M.L., West, S.L. & Soper, K.A. (1987) The effect of indication on hypersensitivity reactions associated with zomepirac sodium and other nonsteroidal antiinflammatory drugs. *Arthritis and Rheumatism*, **30**, 1142–1148.

Van der Ven, A.J.A.M., Koopmans, P.P., Vree, T.B. & Van Der Meer, J.W.M. (1991) Adverse reactions to co-trimoxazole in HIV infection. *Lancet*, **338**, 431–433.

Verhagen, C., Stalpers, L.J.A., de Pauw, B.E. & Haanen, C. (1987) Drug-induced skin reactions in patients with acute non-lymphocytic leukaemia. *European Journal of Haematology*, **38**, 225–230.

Villada, G., Roujeau, J.-C., Cordonier, C. *et al.* (1990) Toxic epidermal necrolysis following bone marrow transplantation; study of nine cases. *Journal of the American Academy of Dermatology*, **23**, 870–875.

Wolkenstein, P., Charue, D., Laurent, P., Revuz, J. Roujeau, J-C. & Bagot, M. (1995) Metabolic predisposition to cutaneous adverse drug reactions: role in toxic epidermal necrolysis caused by sulfonamides and anticonvulsants. *Archives of Dermatology*, **131**, 544–548.

Zürcher, K. & Krebs, A. (1992) *Cutaneous Drug Reactions; An Integrated Synopsis of Today's Systemic Drugs*. Karger, Basel.

18
Other Inflammatory Dermatoses

Acquired Autoimmune Bullous Skin Diseases

S. BASTUJI-GARIN

The autoimmune bullous disorders, although relatively uncommon, are of major clinical importance. The bullous diseases are life-threatening with high mortality and morbidity. The main disorders are pemphigus and subepidermal bullous diseases.

Pemphigus

Pemphigus is characterized by a loss of epidermal cell-to-cell adhesion provoked by autoantibodies directed against antigens of the cell surface of keratinocytes (Stanley, 1993). Pemphigus is a severe disorder; the use of corticosteroids dramatically improves the prognosis with a mortality rate of about 10% (Hietanen & Salo, 1982), but the morbidity remains rather high. Few studies have been dedicated to the epidemiology of pemphigus, but the incidence rates, clinical features and demographic characteristics vary greatly among countries, which lead to the suspicion of different risk factors.

Descriptive epidemiological data

Most cases of pemphigus occur sporadically throughout the world. The incidence rates have been estimated from 0.8 to 34 new cases per million inhabitants per year (Table 18.1). In a small population of the United States, the incidence rate has been estimated to 4.2 cases per million inhabitants (95% confidence interval 2.2–7.3) and 2.9 for non-Jewish residents (Simon et al., 1980). In Europe, the estimated rates were c.

1–2 cases per million inhabitants per year (Hietanen & Salo 1982; Bastuji-Garin et al., 1995). In these populations, the prevalent sex ratio was close to 1, and the disease was more frequent after the fourth decade. Pemphigus vulgaris (PV) was observed in c. 80% of series of patients with pemphigus (Ryan, 1971; Krain, 1974; Rosenberg et al., 1976; Hietanen & Salo, 1982). In France, the incidence rate of PV (1.3 cases per million inhabitants; 95% confidence interval 1.0–1.6) was significantly higher than the incidence rate of pemphigus foliaceus (PF) (0.5 cases per million inhabitants; 95% confidence interval 0.3–0.7) (Bastuji-Garin et al., 1995). Both incidences increased with age, in keeping with published series from several countries (Ryan, 1971; Krain, 1974; Rosenberg et al., 1976; Hietanen & Salo, 1982). In the United States survey, the incidence rate among the Jewish residents was about 32 cases per million inhabitants per year (95% confidence interval 9–83) (Simon et al., 1980). In the same way, among the Jewish residents of Jerusalem area, the incidence rate of PV was about 16.2 per million inhabitants (Pisanti et al., 1974).

In South America, pemphigus is considered endemic. The estimate of incidence was c. 5–7 new cases per million inhabitants per year, but reached 34 cases in endemic areas of Brazil (Diaz et al., 1989a). In contrast with North America, Europe and Israel, the cases were almost exclusively PF (95–99%) called fogo selvagem (Diaz et al., 1989a; Empinotti et al., 1990), which is clinically and immunologically similar to PF observed in Europe and North America (Diaz et al., 1989b, Stanley et al., 1986). Prevalent sex ratio was close to 1, but fogo selvagem occurred essentially in young patients with a peak incidence in the second and third decade.

Table 18.1 Incidence rates of pemphigus.

Region (reference)	Population (*n*)	Cases (*n*)	Survey period	Cases/10/year (*n*)*
Connecticut (Simon *et al.*, 1980)†	757 800	12	1972–77	4.2 (2–7)
Non-Jewish population	727 175	8		2.9 (1–6)
Jewish population	30 625	4		32 (9–83)
Finland (Hietanen & Salo, 1982)†	4 760 000	36	1969–78	1
Ile-de-France (Bastuji-Garin *et al.*, 1995)†	8 355 960	87	1985–90	1.7 (1–2)
Jerusalem (Pisanti *et al.*, 1974)**	4 720 497	76	1952–72	16
Ashkenazian population	2 259 259	61		27
Non-Ashkenazian population	2 461 238	15		6
Malaysia (Adam, 1992)**	2 858 320	84	1976–90	2
Tunisia (Bastuji-Garin *et al.*, 1995)††	4 909 449	198	1986–91	6.7 (6–8)
Goias, Brazil (Diaz *et al.*, 1989a)††	4 441 482	2700	1952–70	30

* 95% confidence interval in parentheses.
** Data concerning exclusively pemphigus vulgaris.
† Predominance of pemphigus vulgaris.
†† Predominance of pemphigus foliaceus.

In a small area of Tunisia, the incidence rate of pemphigus was estimated to be about 4 new cases per million inhabitants per year (Morini *et al.*, 1993). In a recent study conducted in Tunisia as a whole, the incidence rate was 6.7 new cases per million inhabitants per year (95% confidence interval 5.8–7.7) (Bastuji-Garin *et al.*, 1995), which is the same figure as the incidence rate in the whole of Brazil, and significantly higher than the rate observed in France. As in Brazil, in all series, PF was the more frequent type (60–87%) (Zahaf *et al.*, 1988). In Tunisia, the incidence rate of PF (3.9 cases per million inhabitants; 95% confidence interval 3.2–4.7) was significantly higher than the incidence rate of PV (2.5 cases per million inhabitants; 95% confidence interval 1.7–2.8) (Bastuji-Garin *et al.*, 1995). In men, the incidence rates of PF and PV were similar. The incidence of PV was remarkable in women, with a peak that reached 15.5 cases per million inhabitants per year (95% confidence interval 11.6–20.0) among the 25–34-year-old age group. Pemphigus was reported in all regions of Tunisia with significantly variable incidence rates. For women aged 25–34 years, the incidence rates were > 50 cases per million inhabitants per year in some regions located in the centre of Tunisia and in the southern desertic area (Bastuji-Garin *et al.*, 1995).

Risk factors of pemphigus

The causes of all forms of pemphigus are unknown, but several risk factors have been incriminated.

Genetic risk factors

The increased incidence of PV in a number of populations, specially among the Jewish Ashkenazian population, suggested the role of genetic risk factors. In the same way, a high frequency of familial cases (18–27%), particularly among genetically related members (93%; 187 families), was observed in Brazilian PF (Diaz *et al.*, 1989a). In contrast, in Tunisia, no case of pemphi-gus was reported among genetically related members (Bastuji-Garin *et al.*, 1995). Ahmed *et al.* (1993) demonstrated that low levels of the PV antibodies were present in 48% of a total of 120 asymptomatic relatives of 31 PV patients, suggesting that disease appears in susceptible individuals with a low level of antibody when a second factor, either environmental or genetic, induces high levels. Susceptibility to pemphigus is strongly associated with serologically defined gene products of the HLA-D region. PV is associated with two kinds of HLA-DR4: DQ8 haplotypes dominantly distributed among Jewish patients; and these plus DR6,

DQ5 haplotypes in non-Jewish patients. In both Jewish and non-Jewish patients, it was demonstrated that the association with DRw4 and DRw6 haplotypes concerned the DQβ region, in particular with either the DQw1 or DRw6 alleles (Szafer *et al.*, 1987). The association with DRw6 haplotype was due to the substitution of one amino acid on the β-chain of the DQ molecule (Sinha *et al.*, 1988). Genotyping of HLA-DQA1, -DQB1 and -DRB1 was performed for 32 Japanese PV patients (Niizeki *et al.*, 1994). A significant association of either DQB1*0503 or DRB1*1405 with PV, and a negative association of either DQA1*0103 or DQB1*0601 was found. Moares *et al.* (1991) reported that DRB1*0102 was associated with susceptibility, and DQB1*0201 with resistance, to PF in a Brazilian population. In a particular population (Xavante Indians), known as having neither DRB1*0202 nor DQB1*0201, a significant association was observed with DRB1*0404 (Cerna *et al.*, 1993). Thus, the strong association of the class II genes with pemphigus may indicate that these genes play a role in the pathogenesis of the disease, but the susceptibility alleles vary according to the type of pemphigus and the populations.

Drug risk factors

Many drugs have been reported to induce pemphigus. The drugs usually incriminated were thiol drugs. These drugs may be either drugs that contain thiol groups in their molecule (penicillamine, captopril), or drugs with disulphide bonds (pyritinol) or with a sulphur-containing cycle (piroxicam) (Ruocco & Sacerdoti, 1991). Penicillamine was frequently reported as a risk factor (Mutasim *et al.*, 1993); it is estimated that 7% of patients who take penicillamine for more than 6 months develop pemphigus or pemphigus-like lesions (Marsden *et al.*, 1976). The other thiol drugs incriminated (captopril, pyritinol, thiopronine, piroxicam and thiamazole) induced pemphigus very rarely with regard to their widespread use (Ruocco & Sacerdoti, 1991; Mutasim *et al.*, 1993). In the same way, at least ten cases of pemphigus have been attributed to penicillin and its derivatives (Ruocco & Sacerdoti, 1991). Few cases of pemphigus have been attributed to other drugs: rifampicin, pyrazolone compounds, beta-blockers and other miscellaneous drugs (Mutasim

et al., 1993). Nevertheless, no comparative study has been performed to determine the role of these drug risk factors. The potential role of sunburns (Kaplan *et al.*, 1983), cutaneous thermal burns (Hogan, 1992), X-rays (Ryan, 1971; Delaporte *et al.*, 1991), professional exposures (Krain, 1974) and cosmetic procedures (Kaplan *et al.*, 1993), which have been incriminated, has never been estimated.

Environmental risk factors

Environmental risk factors were also incriminated in Brazilian pemphigus. In a large series, 90% of patients were farmers living in rural areas, in close proximity to rivers where a blackfly, *Simulium pruinosum*, was highly prevalent (Diaz *et al.*, 1989a). Furthermore, the prevalence of the disease decreased after urbanization. A recent case-control study found a significant association between pemphigus and frequent exposure to the blackfly (odds ratio = 4.7, $P < 0.001$) (Lombardi *et al.*, 1992). This blackfly may be the vector of a transmissible agent that precipitates the disease. In Tunisia, high rates of PF among young people living in rural areas are reminiscent of Brazilian pemphigus. Nevertheless, the absence of cases among household members and the large predominance of women contrasts with Brazilian pemphigus. The higher incidence rates observed among young women and in desertic areas suggests a potential role of hormonal and/or environmental risk factors, but the role of these potential risk factors has never been investigated.

Subepidermal autoimmune bullous skin diseases

These bullous diseases are characterized by the histological presence of subepidermal cleavage, and *in vivo* deposition of immunoglobulins and/or complement at the basement membrane zone of the epidermis. Several entities with distinct clinical, immuno-electron microscopic and serological features are included: bullous pemphigoid, cicatricial pemphigoid, pemphigoid gestationis, linear IgA dermatosis, epidermolysis bullosa acquisita and vesiculobullous systemic lupus erythematosus. Epidemiological data concerning these diseases are very rare. Nevertheless, two prospective studies were recently published; the first one was conducted in three French regions (population base of 3 550 000 inhabitants) (Bernard *et al.*, 1995a), and the second one in a region of central Germany (population base of 1 700 000 inhabitants) (Zillikens *et al.*, 1995). The overall incidence rate in France was estimated to be about ten new cases per million inhabitants per year (Bernard *et al.*, 1995a).

Bullous pemphigoid

Descriptive epidemiological data

Bullous pemphigoid (BP) is the most frequent disorder. No racial or geographical predilection is recognized. Despite some conflicting data, BP is a potentially fatal disease, with a poor prognosis. The mortality rate after 1 year of treatment varies between 10 and 40%. A recent study of 78 consecutive patients showed that 38% of patients died during the first year of treatment, with 22% in the first 3 months (Bernard *et al.*, 1995b). From retrospective series, the incidence of BP among the general population varied from 1.2 in Malaysia (Adam, 1992), 10 in the UK (Grattan, 1985) to 30 new cases per million per year in Switzerland (Masouyé *et al.*, 1989). In the French prospective study, the estimate was seven new cases per million per year (Bernard *et al.*, 1995a) and 6.6 new cases per million per year in the German study (Zillikens *et al.*, 1995). Bullous pemphigoid occurs most frequently in the elderly population with the vast majority of patients being >60 years old. The mean age of onset varies from 65 to 80 years (Laskaris *et al.*, 1982; Grattan, 1985; Zillikens *et al.*, 1995; Bernard *et al.*, 1995a). From the data of the French study, considering that BP occurs in the elderly population, we estimated that the incidence among people ≥ 65 years was 50 new cases per million inhabitants per year. Men and women are equally affected.

Risk factors of bullous pemphigoid

The risk factors of BP are not well established. Despite numerous reports of malignancy associated with BP, it remains controversial whether BP and malignant disease are truly associated, or whether their concurrence is merely a reflection of the fact that both diseases are most common in the elderly. There has

been only two case-control studies. The first concluded that there was no higher incidence of malignant disease in BP patients than in age- and sex-matched controls (11% vs. 14%) (Stone & Schroeter, 1975). In contrast, the second reported a higher rate of cancer in BP patients than in the control group (11% vs. 5%) (Venning & Wojnarowska, 1990). However, the incidence of malignancy in the BP series being *c.* 11% (Lim *et al.*, 1968; Stone & Schoeter, 1975; Chorzelski *et al.*, 1978; Hodge *et al.*, 1981; Venencie *et al.*, 1984; Lindelöf *et al.*, 1990), the association described by Venning and Wojnarowska (1990) merely reflects an underestimation of the rate of cancer in the control group. In a literature review, an association was found in five studies (Person & Rogers, 1977; Chorzelski *et al.*, 1978; Hodge *et al.*, 1981; Venencie *et al.*, 1984; Morioka *et al.*, 1994) of ten studies (Lim *et al.*, 1968; Paslin, 1973; Ahmed *et al.*, 1977; Moss & Hanelin, 1977; Lindelöf *et al.*, 1990), but the expected incidence of malignancy was often low. In a retrospective study of 1113 BP cases, the prevalence of internal malignancies was estimated as *c.* 6% while it was estimated to be about 0.6% in the general population (Morioka *et al.*, 1994). The other recent study comparing the number of malignancies observed in a large series of BP (497 cases) to the expected number calculated on the basis of the age- and sex-standardized incidence data of the Swedish Cancer registry concluded that BP was not statistically associated with malignancies (61 vs. 83) (Lindelöf *et al.*, 1990). These data support the conclusion that BP is not significantly associated with cancer. There are many case reports of BP in association with a variety of autoimmune disorders. A case-control study found neither increase in the frequency of autoimmune disorders, nor particular associated haplotype (Taylor *et al.*, 1993). The occurrence of BP in several patients with multiple sclerosis suggested an association but epidemiological proof has never been established (Simjee *et al.*, 1985; Masouyé *et al.*, 1989). An association between BP and psoriasis has been suggested. There are several reports of BP arising during the treatment of psoriasis, usually following exposure to ultraviolet light, but a retrospective analysis of 62 BP cases and 62 matched controls suggested a significant association with psoriasis but not with the treatment (Grattan, 1985). Few cases of BP have been attributed to drugs. D-Penicillamine

(Velthuis *et al.*, 1985; Brown & Dubin, 1987; Yamaguchi *et al.*, 1989), captopril (Mallet *et al.*, 1989), frusemide (Fellner & Kat, 1976; Castel *et al.*, 1981; Halevy *et al.*, 1984), penicillins (Alcalay *et al.*, 1988; Hodak *et al.*, 1989), ibuprofen (Laing *et al.*, 1988) and phenacetin (Kashihara *et al.*, 1984) were the implicated agents. In a series of 48 BP cases and 48 matched controls, diuretics and amiodarone were more frequently used among cases as compared to controls (Doukan *et al.*, 1988). In a recent multicentre case-control study comparing the drugs used by 116 incident BP cases and 216 matched controls (Bastuji-Garin *et al.*, 1996), no significant association was observed with antibiotics, sulphydryl-containing drugs (D-penicillamine, captopril) and antiarrhythmics (including amiodarone which was twofold more frequent among the cases). Nevertheless, a significant association was observed between BP and aldosterone antagonists (odds ratio = 3.1; 95% confidence interval 1.4–7.1). Aldosterone antagonists could be a risk factor of BP, but since this drug has rarely been suspected to induce autoimmune disorders, this association should be further investigated.

Cicatricial pemphigoid

The incidence rate of cicatricial pemphigoid was estimated to be 1.2 new cases per million inhabitants per year in France (Bernard *et al.*, 1995a), and 0.9 new cases per million inhabitants per year in Germany (Zillikens *et al.*, 1995), but no other incidence data are yet available. Cicatricial pemphigoid is a disease of middle age and elderly patients, although it has been observed in all age group. The mean age of onset is about 70 years (Laskaris *et al.*, 1982; Zillikens *et al.*, 1995; Bernard *et al.*, 1995a). The female:male sex ratio was 1.5 in the Greek survey (Laskaris *et al.*, 1982), 7 in the German study (Zillikens *et al.*, 1995) and 0.3 in the French one (Bernard *et al.*, 1995a). These various figures could be expected by the small number of cases. There is no appearent racial or geographical predilection. The aetiology of this disorder is unknown.

Pemphigoid gestationis

Considering the whole population, the incidence rate

of pemphigoid gestationis was estimated to be 0.4 new cases per million inhabitants per year in France (Bernard *et al.*, 1995a), and 0.5 new cases per million inhabitants per year in Germany (Zillikens *et al.*, 1995). Nevertheless, pemphigoid gestationis is a disorder of women of child-bearing age; considering only pregnancies, the estimates varied from 1 in 50 000 pregnancies in the United States (Shornick *et al.*, 1993), to 1 in 7000 in Switzerland (Zurn *et al.*, 1992) and 1 in 1700 pregnancies in France (Roger *et al.*, 1994). The last may have been overestimated by a recruitment bias.

Linear IgA dermatosis

The incidence rate of linear IgA dermatosis was estimated to be about 0.5 new cases per million inhabitants per year in France, and 0.2 in Germany; no other incidence data are yet available. Linear IgA dermatosis may occur throughout adult life; patients are younger than BP patients, even though the peak incidence is after 60 years of age (Leonard *et al.*, 1982). In the French study, mean age was 61.8 ± 24.4 years (Bernard *et al.*, 1995a). There is a slight female preponderance (female:male sex ratio = 1.5) (Leonard *et al.*, 1982; Bernard *et al.*, 1995a). The aetiology of linear IgA dermatosis is unknown. There have been several case reports suggesting an association with malignancy and a 8.5-year follow-up of 70 linear IgA dermatosis patients found a significant excess of malignancies (Godfrey *et al.*, 1990). Nevertheless, all these studies are subject to investigative bias. Drug risk factors were suspected after several cases of drug-induced linear IgA dermatosis were reported. The drug most often implicated was vancomycin (Baden *et al.*, 1988; Carpenter *et al.*, 1992; Kuelchle *et al.*, 1994). The other drugs incriminated were lithium, cephamandole, captopril and diclofenac (Kuelchle *et al.*, 1994). However, it is difficult to determine how often the drug is coincidental and how often it is causal.

Other autoimmune subepidermal bullous disorders

The other autoimmune subepidermal bullous disorders are very rare. The incidence rates estimated per million inhabitants per year were 0.2 for epidermolysis bullosa acquisita and vesiculobullous systemic lupus erythematosus (Bernard *et al.*, 1995a; Zillikens *et al.*, 1995). Epidermolysis bullosa acquisita has been reported throughout the world, in all ethnic groups and both sexes, but its geographical distribution has not been well studied.

The very similar numbers for the incidence rates of autoimmune subepidermal blistering diseases in France and Germany suggest that the incidence of these disorders may be similar in different parts of Western Europe.

Conclusion

All autoimmune subepidermal bullous disorders may be a serious debilitating disease that results in significant morbidity and severe complications. The aetiology of these disorders is unknown, but several drugs and/or malignancies are suspected to be risk factors. Considering the rarity of epidemiological studies, it is not known if this is a chance occurrence or whether it is causal. All these associations have to be confirmed by formal epidemiological studies. The low incidence of these disorders precludes cohort studies; however, case-control studies could be performed. In terms of prevention, when a patient is exposed to a previously suspected drug, it could be suitable to change the treatment.

References

Adam, B.A. (1992) Bullous diseases in Malaysia: epidemiology and natural history. *International Journal of Dermatology*, **31**, 42–45.

Ahmed, A.R., Ming Chu, T. & Provost, TT. (1977) Bullous pemphigoid: clinical and serologic evaluation for associated malignant neoplasms. *Archives of Dermatology*, **113**, 1043–1046

Ahmed, A.R., Mohinen, A., Yunis, E.J. *et al* (1993) Linkage of pemphigus vulgaris antibody to the major histocompatibility complex in healthy relatives of patients. *Journal of Experimental Medicine*, **177**, 419–424.

Alcalay, J., David, M., Ingber, A., Hazaz, B. & Sandbank, M. (1988) Bullous pemphigoid mimicking bullous erythema multiforme: an untoward side effect of penicillins. *Journal of the American Academy of Dermatology*, **18**, 345–349.

Baden, L.A., Apovian, C., Imber, J.M. *et al.* (1988) Vancomycin-induced linear IgA bullous dermatosis. *Archives of Dermatology*, **124**, 1186–1188.

Bastuji-Garin, S., Souissi, R., Blum, L. *et al.* (1995) Comparative epidemiology of pemphigus in Tunisia and France: unusual incidence of pemphigus foliaceus in young Tunisian women. *Journal of Investigative Dermatology*, **104**, 302–305.

Bastuji-Garin, S., Joly, P., Picard-Dahan, C. *et al.* (1996) Drugs associated with bullous pemphigoid: a case control study. *Archives of Dermatology*, **132**, 272–276.

Bernard, P., Vaillant, L., Labeille, B. *et al.* (1995a) Incidence and distribution of subepidermal autoimmune bullous skin diseases in three French regions. *Archives of Dermatology*, **131**, 48–52.

Bernard, P., Enginger, V., Venot, J., Bedane, C., Bonnetblanc, J.M. (1995b) Pronostic vital de la pemphigoïde. Analyse d'une cohorte de 78 malades. *Annales de Dermatologie et de Vénéréologie*, **122**, 751–757.

Brown, M.D. & Dubin, H.V. (1987) Penicillamine-induced bullous pemphigoid-like eruption. *Archives of Dermatology*, **123**, 1119–1120.

Carpenter, S., Berg, D., Sidhu-Malik, N. *et al.* (1992) Vancomycin-associated linear IgA dermatosis. *Journal of the American Academy of Dermatology*, **26**, 45–48.

Castel, T., Gratarcos, R., Castro, S., Bergrada, E., Lecha, M. & Mascaro, J.M. (1981) Bullous pemphigoid induced by furosemide. *Clinical and Experimental Dermatology*, **6**, 635–638.

Cerna, M., Fernandez-Vina, M. & Friedman, H. (1993) Genetic markers for susceptibility to endemic Brazilian pemphigus foliaceus (fogo selvagem) in Xavante indians. *Tissue Antigens*, **42**, 138–140.

Chorzelski, T.P., Jablonska, S., Maciejowska, E., Beutner, E.H. & Wronkowski, L. (1978) Coexistence of malignancies with bullous pemphigoid. *Archives of Dermatology*, **114**, 964.

Delaporte, E., Piette, F. & Bergoend, H. (1991) Pemphigus vulgaire induit par radiothérapie. *Annales de Dermatologie et de Vénéréologie*, **118**, 447–451.

Diaz, L.A., Sampaio, S.A.P., Rivitti. E.A. *et al.* (1989a) Endemic pemphigus foliaceus (fogo salvagem). II. Current and historic epidemiologic studies. *Journal of Investigative Dermatology*, **92**, 4–12.

Diaz, L.A., Sampaio, S.A.P., Rivitti, E.A. *et al.* (1989b) Endemic pemphigus foliaceus (fogo salvagem). I. Clinical features and immunopathology. *Journal of the American Academy of Dermatology*, **20**, 657–669.

Doukan, S., Roujeau, J-C., Roudot-Thoraval, F. & Touraine, R. (1988) Pemphigoïde bulleuse et médicaments. *Annales de Dermatologie et de Vénéréologie*, **115**, 646. (Abstract.)

Empinotti, J.C., Diaz, L.A., Martins, C.R. *et al.* (1990) Endemic pemphigus foliaceus in western Parana, Brazil (1976–1988). *British Journal of Dermatology*, **123**, 431–437.

Fellner, M.J. & Kat, J.M. (1976) Occurrence of bullous pemphigoid after furosemide therapy. *Archives of Dermatology*, **122**, 75–77.

Godfrey, K., Wojnarowska, F. & Leonard, J. (1990) Linear

IgA disease of adults: association with lymphoproliferative malignancy and possible role of other triggering factors. *British Journal of Dermatology*, **123**, 447–452.

Grattan, C.E.H. (1985) Evidence of an association between bullous pemphigoid and psoriasis. *British Journal of Dermatology*, **113**, 281–283.

Halevy, S., Levni, E. & Sandbank, M. (1984) Bullous pemphigoid associated with furosemide. *Harefuah*, **106**, 125–126.

Hietanen, J. & Salo, O.P. (1982) Pemphigus: an epidemiological study of patients treated in Finnish hospitals between 1969 and 1978. *Acta Dermato-Venerologica (Stockholm)*, **62**, 491–496.

Hodak, E. & Ben-Shetrit, A., Ingber, A. & Sandbank, M. (1989) Bullous pemphigoid—an adverse effect of ampicillin. *Clinical and Experimental Dermatology*, **15**, 50–52.

Hodge, L., Marsden, R.A., Black, M.M., Bhogal, B. & Corbett, M.F. (1981) Bullous pemphigoid: the frequency of mucosal involvement and concurrent malignancy related to indirect immunofluorescence findings. *British Journal of Dermatology*, **105**, 65–69.

Hogan, P. (1992) Pemphigus vulgaris following a cutaneous thermal burn. *International Journal of Dermatology*, **31**, 46–49.

Kaplan, R.P. & Callen, J.P. (1983) Pemphigus associated disease and induced pemphigus. *Clinical Dermatology*, **1**, 42–71.

Kaplan, R.P., Detwiler, S.P. & Saperstein, H.W. (1993) Physically induced pemphigus after cosmetic procedures. *International Journal of Dermatology*, **32**, 100–103.

Kashihara, M., Danno, K., Miyachi, Y., Horiguchi, Y. & Imamura, S. (1984) Bullous pemphigoid-like lesions induced by phenacetin. *Archives of Dermatology*, **120**, 1196–1199.

Krain, L.S. (1974) Pemphigus — epidemiologic and survival characteristics of 59 patients, 1959–1973. *Archives of Dermatology*, **110**, 862–865.

Kuechle, M.K., Stegemeir, E., Maynard, B., Gibson, L.E., Leiferman, K.M. & Peters, M.S. (1994) Drug-induced linear IgA bullous dermatosis: report of six cases and review of the literature. *Journal of the American Academy of Dermatology*, **30**, 187–192.

Laing, V.B., Sherertz, E.F. & Flowers, F.P. (1988) Pemphigoid-like bullous eruption related to ibuprofen. *Journal of the American Academy of Dermatology*, **19**, 91–94.

Laskaris, G., Sklavounou, A. & Stratigos, J. (1982) Bullous pemphigoid, cicatricial pemphigoid, and pemphigus vulgaris. A comparative clinical survey of 278 cases. *Oral Surgery*, **54**, 656–662.

Leonard, J.N., Haffenden, G.P., Ring, N.P. et al. (1982) Linear IgA disease in adults. *British Journal of Dermatology*, **107**, 301–316.

Lim, C.C., McDonald, R.H. & Rook, A.J. (1968) Pemphigoid

eruption in the elderly. *Transactions of the St Johns Hospital Dermatology Society*, **54**, 148–151.

Lindelöf, B., Islam, N., Eklund, G. & Arfors, L. (1990) Pemphigoid and cancer. *Archives of Dermatology*, **126**, 66–68.

Lombardi, C., Borges, P.C., Chaul, A. et al. (1992) Environmental risk factors in endemic pemphigus foliaceus (fogo selvagem). *Journal of Investigative Dermatology*, **98**, 847–850.

Mallet, L., Cooper, J.W. & Thomas, J. (1989) Bullous pemphigoid associated with captopril. *Drug Intelligence and Clinical Pharmacology*, **23**, 63.

Marsden, R.A., Ryan, T.J., VanHegan, R.I. et al. (1976) Pemphigus foliaceus induced by penicillamine. *British Medical Journal*, **iv**, 1423.

Masouyé, I., Schmied, E., Didierjean, L., Abba, Z. & Saurat, J.H. (1989) Bullous pemphigoid and multiple sclerosis: more than a coincidence? *Journal of the American Academy of Dermatology*, **21**, 63–68.

Moares, J.R., Moares, M.B., Fernandez-Vina, M. et al. (1991) HLA antigens and risk for development of pemphigus foliaceus (fogo selvagem) in endemic areas of Brazil. *Immunogenetics*, **33**, 388–391.

Morini, J.P., Jomaa, B., Gorgi, Y. et al. (1993) Pemphigus foliaceus in young women. An endemic focus in the Sousse area of Tunisia. *Archives of Dermatology*, **129**, 69–73.

Morioka, S., Sauma, M. & Ogawa, H. (1994) The incidence of internal malignancies in autoimmune blistering diseases: pemphigus and bullous pemphigoid in Japan. *Dermatology*, **189**, 82–84.

Moss, A.A. & Hanelin, L.G. (1977) Occult malignant tumors in dermatologic diseases. *Radiology*, **123**, 69–71.

Mutasim, D.F., Pelc, N.J. & Anhalt, G.J. (1993) Drug-induced pemphigus. *Dermatologic Clinics*, **3**, 463–471.

Niizeki, H., Inoko, H., Mizuki, N. et al. (1994) HLA-DQA1, -DQB1 genotyping in Japanese pemphigus vulgaris patients by the PCR–RFLP method. *Tissue Antigens*, **44**, 248–251.

Paslin, D.A. (1973) Bullous pemphigoid and hypernephroma: a critical review of bullous pemphigoid and malignancy. *Cutis*, **12**, 554–555.

Person, J. & Rogers, E. (1977) Bullous and cicatricial pemphigoid: clinical, histopathologic and immuno-pathologic correlations. *Mayo Clinic Proceedings*, **52**, 54–66.

Pisanti, S., Sharav, Y., Kaufman, E. & Posner, L.N. (1974) Pemphigus vulgaris: incidence in Jews of different ethnic groups according to age, sex and initial lesion. *Oral Surgery*, **38**, 382–387.

Roger, D., Vaillant, L., Fignon, A. et al. (1994) Specific pruritic diseases of pregnancy. A prospective study of 3192 pregnant women. *Archives of Dermatology*, **130**, 734–739.

Rosenberg, F.R., Sanders, S. & Nelson, C.T. (1976) Pemphigus: a 20-year review of 107 patients treated with corticosteroids. *Archives of Dermatology*, **112**, 962–970.

Ruocco, V. & Sacerdoti, G. (1991) Pemphigus and bullous pemphigoid due to drugs. *International Journal of Dermatology*, **30**, 307–312.

Ryan, J.G. (1971) Pemphigus. A 20-year survey of experience with 70 cases. *Archives of Dermatology*, **104**, 14–20.

Shornick, J.K., Bangert, J.L., Freeman, R.G. & Gilliam, J.N. (1993) Herpes gestationis: clinical and histologic features of twenty-eight cases. *Journal of the American Academy of Dermatology*, **8**, 214–224.

Simjee, S., Konqui, A. & Ahmed, A.R. (1985) Multiple sclerosis and bullous pemphigoid. *Dermatologica*, **170**, 86–89.

Simon, D.G., Krutchkoff, D., Kaslow, R.A. & Zarbo, R. (1980) Pemphigus in Hartford County, Connecticut, from 1972 to 1977. *Archives of Dermatology*, **116**, 1035–1037.

Sinha, A.A., Brautbar, C. & Szafer, F. (1988) A newly characterized HLA DQ beta allele associated with pemphigus vulgaris. *Science*, **239**, 1026–1029.

Stanley, J.R. (1993) Cell adhesion molecules as targets of autoantibodies in pemphigus and pemphigoid, bullous diseases due to defective epidermal cell adhesion. *Advances in Immunology*, **53**, 291–325.

Stanley, J.R., Klaus-Kovtun, V. & Sampiao, S.A.P. (1986) Antigenic specificity of fogo selvagem autoantibodies is similar to North American pemphigus and distinct from pemphigus vulgaris autoantibodies. *Journal of Investigative Dermatology*, **87**, 197–201.

Stone, S.P. & Schroeter, A.L. (1975) Bullous pemphigoid and associated malignant neoplasm. *Archives of Dermatology*, **111**, 991–994.

Szafer, F., Brautbar, C., Tsfoni, E. *et al.* (1987) Detection of disease-specific restriction fragment length polymorphisms in pemphigus vulgaris linked to the Dqw1 and Dqw3 alleles of the HLA-D region. *Proceedings of the National Academy of Sciences (USA)*, **84**, 6542–6545.

Taylor, G., Venning, V., Wojnarowska, F. & Welch, K. (1993) Bullous pemphigoid and autoimmunity. *Journal of the American Academy of Dermatology*, **29**, 181–184.

Velthuis, P.J., Hendrikse, J.C. & Nefkens, J.J. (1985) Combined features of pemphigus and pemphigoid induced by penicillamine. *British Journal of Dermatology*, **112**, 615.

Venencie, P.Y., Rogers, R.S. & Schoeter, A.L. (1984) Bullous pemphigoid and malignancy: relationship to indirect immunofluorescent findings. *Acta Dermato-Venereologica*, **64**, 316–319.

Venning, V.A. & Wojnarowska, F. (1990) The association of bullous pemphigoid and malignant disease: a case control study. *British Journal of Dermatology*, **123**, 439–445.

Yamaguchi, R., Oryu, F. & Hidano, A. (1989) A case of bullous pemphigoid induced by tiobutarit (D-penicillamine analogue). *Journal of Dermatology*, **16**, 308–311.

Zahaf, A., Baklouti, A. & Doukali, M. (1988) Le pemphigus dans le Sud Tunisien (à propos de 22 cas). *Nouvelles Dermatologiques*, **7**, 369–372.

Zillikens, D., Wever, S., Weidenthaler-Barth, B., Hashimoto, T. & Bröcker, E.B. (1995) Incidence of autoimmune subepidermal blistering dermatoses in a region of central Germany. *Archives of Dermatology*, **131**, 957–958.

Zurn, A., Celebi, C.R., Bernard, P., Didierjean, L. & Saurat, J.H. (1992) A prospective immunofluorescence study of 111 cases of pruritic dermatoses of pregnancy: IgM anti-basement membrane zone antibodies as a novel finding. *British Journal of Dermatology*, **126**, 474–478.

Systemic Lupus Erythematosus

D. LE THI HUONG AND C. FRANCES

Systemic lupus erythematosus (SLE) is a disease of unknown origin, characterized by the presence of autoantibodies. Antinuclear antibodies are present in >95% of SLE patients but are not specific for SLE. Antibodies to double-stranded (ds) DNA and to Sm are relatively specific. Initial presentation of SLE may be limited to the involvement of only one organ, with additional manifestations occurring later, or may be multisystemic. The most common symptoms are, besides fever and fatigue, cutaneous (of which the malar 'butterfly' rash is typical), musculoskeletal, renal and nervous system. The presence of multisystemic involvement distinguishes cutaneous lupus of a benign course from systemic lupus of poorer prognosis.

Knowledge about the epidemiology of SLE is based on numerous epidemiological and clinical studies conducted worldwide, especially in United States and the UK.

Prevalence and incidence

Several studies have been conducted to estimate prevalence and incidence rates of SLE in various countries (Table 18.2). A recent study from Birmingham, UK, suggests the existence of a substantial number of undiagnosed cases of SLE. In this study, a ten-item questionnaire was completed by a search for antinuclear antibody and a rheumatologist consultation. Three cases of undiagnosed SLE and four priorly diagnosed SLE were picked up. The prevalence rate of SLE revealed by this survey was 200 per 100 000 women whereas the prevalence of diagnosed SLE was 54 per 100 000 women in the 18–65-year age group. Hence, all the following data are probably underestimated (Johnson *et al.*, 1996).

In Europe, prevalence rate varies from 12.5 cases per 100 000 females in England (Hochberg, 1987b) to 42 per 100 000 population of both sexes in Sweden (Jonsson *et al.*, 1989). However, the average annual incidence of SLE is remarkably similar in Sweden (Jonsson *et al.*, 1989), Iceland (Gudmusson & Steinsson, 1990) and the UK (Johnson *et al.*, 1995), ranging between 3.3 and 4 per 100 000 population. In France, the only data available come from an epidemiological study in Paris and the suburbs, and concern childhood SLE. Incidence was 0.22 (0.36 in girls and 0.08 in boys) per 100 000 children, i.e. 120 new cases in 3 years (Lévy *et al.*, 1989). Annual SLE incidence seems temporally stable since a similar incidence was observed for the 1971–75 period and the 1981–82 period in Sweden (Nived *et al.*, 1985).

In the United States, the overall prevalence of SLE ranges between 14.6 (Siegel & Lee, 1973) and 50.8 cases per 100 000 population (Fessel, 1974). Prevalence of SLE seems higher in black, Hispanic and Oriental people. The respective prevalence of SLE in males and females is similar in the different studies in black, Hispanic and Oriental people. Annual incidence

rate varies between 1.8 (Michet *et al.*, 1985) and 7.6 cases (Fessel, 1974) per 100 000 population. This variability depends on different methods of case ascertainment, including use of general practice diagnostic registries, hospital-discharge records, out-patient clinic records or combinations thereof, and the racial composition of the population. The hypothesis that there is a geographical cluster of SLE in the United States seems not to be valid (Wallace & Quismorio, 1995). When compiling the data obtained from surveys available in 1989, the National Arthritis Data Workgroup estimated that there were 131 000 cases of SLE in the United States. SLE was considered to be present in 74 000 Caucasian women, 43 000 Afro-American women, 7000 Caucasian men and 7000 Afro-American men. These data correspond to a prevalence rate of SLE as high as 1 in 245 women and as low as 1 in 30 000 in Caucasian men. These data were admitted to be underestimated since they did not include estimates for Hispanic and Oriental people in whom SLE prevalence is considered to be higher compared with Caucasians (Lawrence *et al.*, 1989). A temporal trend in the incidence among white females was observed in Rochester. Incidence increased by a factor of 2.5 from the 1950–54 period to the 1975–79 period. In contrast, the annual incidence rate of SLE remained stable over the 1985–90 period in Pittsburgh (McCarty *et al*, 1995).

Table 18.2 Incidence rate of systemic lupus erythematosus per 100 000 population in selected epidemiological studies.

Authors	Location	Survey period	Prevalence rate per 100 000	Annual incidence rate per 100 000
Siegel *et al.*	New York, USA	1956–65	14.6	2.0
Michet *et al.*	Rochester, USA	1950–79	40.0	1.8
Fessel	San Francisco, USA	1963–73	50.8	7.6
Hochberg	Baltimore, USA	1970–77		4.6
Gudmundsson & Steinsson	Iceland	1975–84	34.6	3.3
Jonsson *et al.*	Sweden	1981–86	42	4.0
Samanta *et al.*	Leicester, UK	1989	26.1	
Hopkinson *et al.*	Nottingham, UK	1989–90	24	3.7
Nossent	Curaçao	1980–89	47	4.6
Johnson *et al.*	Birmingham, UK	1991	24	3.8
McCarty *et al.*	Pittsburg, USA	1985–90	27.7	2.4

Effects of age and gender on morbidity rates

SLE is observed at all ages. Age of diagnosis peaks between 20 and 50 years, with a median of 40 years. Clinical studies demonstrated a female predominance approaching 90% of SLE cases. This excess in females is noteworthy in the 15–65-year age group where sex-specific incidence rates are six- to tenfold that observed in males. This excess is lower at <15 years and >65 years (Siegel & Lee, 1973; Michet *et al.*, 1985; Nived *et al.*, 1985). These differences are attributed to hormonal changes during puberty and the child-bearing period.

Age-specific prevalence rates were estimated to be 1 and 4 per 1000 females for white and black females in the United States aged 15–64 years, respectively (Fessel, 1974). Similar rates were reported in Sweden with 0.99 per 1000 women (Nived *et al.*, 1985).

Among Caucasian females, annual age-specific incidence rate is highest in the 15–44-year age group with 3.8 per 100 000 population. It is 6.3 in the 25–44-year age group and 7.0 in the 35–54-year age group (Siegel & Lee, 1973). In Caucasian males, age-specific incidence is difficult to establish because of the small numbers of cases in these studies. SLE seems to develop later in Caucasian males than in Caucasian females. In Caucasian men, annual age-specific rate peaks in the age group >65 years with 4.5 and 0.9 per 100 000 population in New York (Siegel & Lee, 1973) and Rochester (Michet *et al.*, 1985).

Effects of race on morbidity rates

A greater SLE incidence and prevalence were found among American black people compared with American Caucasians. Studies in New York (Siegel & Lee, 1973), San Francisco (Fessel, 1974), Baltimore (Hochberg, 1985) and in Pittsburgh (McCarty *et al.*, 1995) found a three- to fourfold greater prevalence in black females aged 15–64 years. In black females, age-specific incidence was greatest in the 15–44-year age group in New York (Siegel & Lee, 1973) and the 25–34-year age group in Baltimore (Hochberg, 1985), exceeding 20 per 100 000 females per year. In black males, age-specific incidence rate peaks in the 45–65-year age group with 5 per 200 000 males. Average

annual incidence rate was a twofold increase in incidence among Afro-American males compared with Caucasian males (McCarty *et al.*, 1995). In Baltimore, the mean age at SLE diagnosis in black females was 35.5 years compared with 41.7 years in Caucasian females. This corresponded with an earlier peak age of diagnosis in the 25–34-year age group compared with the 35–54-year age group, respectively (Hochberg, 1985). In Pittsburgh, the mean age at SLE diagnosis in black females was 35.2 years compared with 49.8 years in Caucasian females. The reasons for the excess morbidity from SLE in American black people may be related to differences in exposure to environmental factors rather than differences in genetic predisposition. A possible role for natural selection in explaining the difference between black people and Caucasians has been also suggested.

SLE prevalence is also higher in Afro-Caribbean subjects. Mean age at diagnosis was 31 years and age of diagnosis peaked in the 21–30-year age group in Jamaican black SLE patients (Wilson & Hughes, 1979). In Birmingham, UK, the Afro-Caribbean age-standardized incidence rate was fourfold (22.8 compared with 4.5) and the prevalence rate fivefold (111.8 compared with 20.7) the rates observed in Caucasians. Afro-Caribbean females were younger than Caucasian female patients. Prevalence peaks were in the 30–39-year age group in Afro-Caribbean females, compared with a peak prevalence in the 40–49-year age group in Caucasian females. No influence between ethnic prevalence rates by place of birth was observed (Johnson *et al.*, 1995).

Controversial data exist about the prevalence rate of SLE among Orientals as compared to Caucasians. In Hawaii, the age-adjusted prevalence estimate was 5.8 per 100 000 Caucasians compared with 17.0 per 100 000 in Orientals in the 1970–75 period (Serdula & Rhoads, 1979). In Auckland, SLE age-adjusted prevalence rates were 14.6 in Caucasians and 50.6 in Polynesians, respectively (Hart *et al.*, 1983). Higher SLE frequency among Asians than in white people was also observed in Malaysia (Frank, 1980) and in China (Woo *et al.*, 1987). In Leicester, England, a higher prevalence of SLE was found in Asian Indians than among white people (Samanta *et al.*, 1991). In China, a population survey found a prevalence of SLE of 40–70 per 100 000 persons (Nal-Cheng, 1983).

However, a comparative study between Chinese and Caucasians did not find a significant difference in San Francisco but the estimate among Asians was based on only eight cases and had wide confidence intervals (Fessel, 1974). A survey in Taiwan found also only one case of SLE among 1836 residents and no case among 2000 student women (Chou *et al.*, 1986).

SLE prevalence seems also higher among North American Indians compared with whites (Morton *et al.*, 1976; Atkins *et al.*, 1988). Incidence of hospitalized SLE in 72 of 75 participating tribes ranged between 0 and 6.9 per 100 000 patients. A noteworthy higher incidence was observed in the Crow (27.1 per 100 000), the Arapaho (24.3 per 100 000) and the Sioux (16.6 per 100 000) (Morton *et al.*, 1976). However, the small size of tribes leads to wide confidence intervals. SLE incidence rates among Puerto Rican females and males were found to be intermediate between rates in Afro-Americans and whites (Siegel & Lee, 1973). Clinical reports from Kenya (Hall, 1966), Nigeria (Greenwood, 1968), South Africa (Rovers & Coovadia, 1979), Uganda (Shaper, 1961) and Zimbabwe (Taylor & Stein, 1986) noted that SLE is rare.

Mortality data, causes of death and prognosis indicators

In Europe, nationwide studies have estimated the annual mortality rate from SLE to be 4.7 per million in Finland (Helve, 1985) and 2.5 per million in England & Wales. In the latter, a fourfold greater rate of mortality was observed in females compared with males (Hochberg, 1987a). However, gender does not appear as a significant predictor when differences in age distribution between the genders are considered. Age at SLE diagnosis appears also to have little influence on survivorship.

In the United States, data from the National Center for Health Statistics estimated that 3614 deaths may be primary attributed to SLE for the 1968–1972 period: 2096 in white females, 561 in white males, 772 in black females and 106 in black males. The overall annual mortality rate was 6.3 per million in females (5.2 in whites and 14.8 in blacks), i.e. fourfold that for males at 1.6 per million (1.5 in whites and 2.2 in blacks). The overall annual mortality rate was 2.6-fold for blacks. Age-specific mortality rates rise earlier in females than in males. Mortality rate increased with age in whites whereas an accentuation and decline during early and middle adult ages were noted in blacks. Gender and race appeared to act synergistically to increase the mortality rate in black women. Interaction of age during the child-bearing period appeared to account for much of the disproportionate risk to the black females (Kaslow & Masi, 1978). Compiled data from 12 states having 88% of US residents of Asian descent showed that annual mortality rates were threefold higher among blacks (8.4 per million) and twofold higher among Asians (6.8 per million) as compared with whites (2.8 per million) (Kaslow, 1982). The age-adjusted annual mortality rate was 7.5 per million in Chinese, 6.8 in Japanese and 5.1 in Filipinos. A higher mortality rate was observed in Puerto Ricans in New York (Siegel & Lee, 1973), but not confirmed in a study conducted both in Puerto Rico and in five south-western states (Lopez-Acuna *et al.*, 1982).

A temporal trend in mortality rate was observed in developed countries. Age-adjusted annual mortality rate declined during the 1968–78 period for all gender and race groups in the United States (Lopez-Acuna *et al.*, 1982) and during the 1974–83 period in England (Hochberg, 1987a). During the 1979–91 period, mortality rates for white women in the United States displayed little change. In contrast, black women experienced an overt jump in mortality from 1978 to 1980: the mean annual rate increased from 14.2 per million to 18.9, a 33% increase. During the 1979–91 period, an upward trend was also observed, but less significant (Walsh *et al.*, 1995). Controversy persists about the relationship between race and socio-economic status in SLE. Two studies found that the effect of black race resulting in lower survival rates disappeared when socio-economic status and disease severity were taken into account (Ginzler *et al.*, 1982; Ward *et al.*, 1995b). Four other studies were unable to show a significant correlation between socio-economic status, race and disease severity (Studenski *et al.*, 1987; Esdaile *et al.*, 1988; Reveille *et al.*, 1990; Petri *et al.*, 1991). The components of the socio-economic status such as education, stability of insurance status, income, employment status, occupational prestige and private insurance/Medicare were carefully analysed. Higher education and private insurance were associated with less disease activity at diagnosis. Health insurance, income and employment status appeared unstable measures of socio-economic status. This may explain the variability in conclusions of studies on the role of socio-economic factors in SLE (Karlson *et al.*, 1995).

Decrease in mortality was essentially the effect of lower mortality among white females <45 years despite increasing mortality among those beyond the age of 55 years. Clinical studies attributed these improvements to early diagnosis of SLE, better management via use of antibiotics, corticosteroids and immunosuppressive therapy, dialysis and antihypertensive drugs. Whereas clinical studies suggested a survival of only 50% at 5 years in the 1950s, the most recent studies showed a 10-year cumulative survival rate approaching or exceeding 80% (Table 18.3). However, prolonged survival in younger white females shifted SLE mortality to older women. Effect of improved therapy has not been to cure SLE but to postpone death from SLE, allowing death from other causes. During the 1960–70 period, deaths were considered directly attributable to SLE in 67.9% of the cases. Nephritis was present in half of the SLE-related deaths. Infection represented 16.9% and myocardial infarction 3.7% of the cases. No case of neoplasm was reported (Estes & Christian, 1971). During the period 1965–78, SLE became the primary cause of death in 31% of the patients. Infection was the primary cause of death in 33% of the patients

and its occurrence was significantly related to the highest-dosage corticosteroid therapy. Cardiovascular complications (such as stroke, myocardial infarction, presumed cardiac sudden death) represented 8.1% of the causes of death. No case of neoplasm was observed (Rosner *et al.*, 1982). During the 1969–83 period, active SLE represented a stable part of the causes of death (34%), whereas infection tended to decline (22%) and cardiovascular complications (22%) and neoplasm (6%) to increase (Ward *et al.*, 1995a).

Effect of specific organ involved on SLE outcome was analysed in clinical series. In the 1960s, renal and central nervous system manifestations had an adverse effect on survival (Estes & Christian, 1971). However, in multivariate analysis, seizures and organic brain syndrome did not appear as independent predictors of survival. Seizures may result from the effect of active nephritis and renal dysfunction rather than from lupus cerebritis. Patients with high serum creatinine level at study entry had the lowest survival rates. Haematocrit, degree of proteinuria, number of American Rheumatism Association criteria for SLE and type of medical care at study entry also appeared as independent indicators but less significant than initial renal failure (Ginzler *et al.*, 1982). Prognosis indicators in SLE nephritis have been extensively analysed. Nephrotic syndrome (Wallace *et al.*, 1981), high serum creatinine level (Esdaile *et al.*, 1989; McLaughlin *et al.*, 1994), hypocomplementaemia (Esdaile *et al.*, 1989), elevated blood pressure (Cameron *et al.*, 1979; Wallace *et al.*, 1982; Esdaile *et al.*, 1989;

Table 18.3 Survival rates at 5 and 10 years in selected clinical studies.

Reference	Location	Survival rate at:	
		5 years	10 years
Merill & Shulman (1955)	Baltimore, USA	51%	
Kellum & Haserick (1964)	Cleveland, USA	70%	53%
Estes & Christian (1971)	New York, USA	77%	59%
Feinglass *et al.* (1976)	Baltimore, USA	94%	82%
Godeau *et al.* (1977)	Paris	88%	79%
Hochberg *et al.* (1981)	Baltimore, USA	97%	90%
Wallace *et al.* (1981)	Los Angeles, USA	88%	79%
Ginzler *et al.* (1982)	USA	88%	71%
Swaak *et al.* (1989)	The Netherlands	94%	87%
Jonsson *et al.* (1989)	Sweden	95%	
Ward *et al.* (1995b)	Durham, USA	82%	71%

Reveille *et al.*, 1990; Ginzler *et al.*, 1993), high SLE activity (McLaughlin *et al.*, 1994), presence of proliferative lesions and glomerulonephritis on initial renal biopsy (Appel *et al.*, 1987; McLaughlin *et al.*, 1991) and chronicity index (Esdaile *et al.*, 1989; McLaughlin *et al.*, 1991) appeared as the strongest indicators for survivorship. However, the interest of renal biopsy remains controversial. Results of histological examination of renal biopsy enhanced the prediction of clinical data in some studies (Austin *et al.*, 1983; McLaughlin *et al.*, 1991) unlike others (Cameron *et al.*, 1979; Esdaile *et al.*, 1989; Ward & Studenski, 1992). Transformation of nephritis pattern and improvement in the prognosis for the more severe forms of SLE nephritis have probably eroded the precision of the prognosis given by the initial renal biopsy. In recent studies, influence of lupus nephritis in survivorship has considerably diminished. Survival rate at 10 years for patients with SLE nephritis who underwent renal biopsy in the 1970–84 period was 74% (McLaughlin *et al.*, 1994). Hence, renal survival (Ward & Studenski, 1992; Ginzler *et al.*, 1993) or doubling serum creatinine (Austin *et al.*, 1994; Ginzler *et al.*, 1993) have become the most frequently studied outcome variables. Elevated serum creatinine (Goulet *et al.*, 1993; Austin *et al.*,1994; Esdaile *et al.*, 1994), high degree proteinuria (Goulet *et al.*, 1993; Esdaile *et al.*, 1994), duration of prior renal disease (Goulet *et al.*, 1993; Esdaile *et al.*, 1994), low haematocrit (Austin *et al.*, 1994), raised anti-dsDNA antibodies (Esdaile *et al.*, 1994), hypocomplementaemia (Esdaile *et al.*, 1994), thrombocytopenia (Esdaile *et al.*, 1994), black race (Austin *et al.*, 1994), high SLE activity score (Goulet *et al.*, 1993; Esdaile *et al.*, 1994), co-morbidity index (Esdaile *et al.*, 1994), hypertension (Ward & Studenski, 1992), smoking (Ward & Studenski, 1992) appeared as strongest prognosis indicators of renal outcome in multivariate analyses. The strongest biopsy prognosis factors seem to be activity (Esdaile *et al.*, 1994) and chronicity index (Austin *et al.*, 1983; Esdaile *et al.*, 1994), cellular crescents (Austin *et al.*, 1994), interstitial fibrosis (Austin *et al.*, 1994) and subendothelial deposits (Esdaile *et al.*, 1994).

References

Appel, G.B., Cohen, D.J., Pirani, C.L., Meltzer, J.I. & Estes, D. (1987) Long-term followup of patients with lupus nephritis. A study based on the classification of the World Health Organization. *American Journal of Medicine*, **83**, 877–885.

Atkins, C., Rueffel, L., Roddy, J., Platts, M., Robinson, H. & Ward, R. (1988) Rheumatic disease in the Nuu-Chah-Nulth native Indians of the Pacific Northwest. *Journal of Rheumatology*, **15**, 684–690.

Austin, H.A., Boumpas, D.T., Vaughan, E.M. & Balow, J.E. (1994) Predicting renal outcomes in severe lupus nephritis: contributions of clinical and histologic data. *Kidney International*, **45**, 544–550.

Austin, H.A., Muenz, L.R., Joyce, K.M. *et al.* (1983) Prognostic factors in lupus nephritis. Contribution of renal histologic data. *American Journal of Medicine*, **75**, 382–391.

Cameron, J.S., Turner, D.R., Ogg, C. *et al.* (1979) Systemic lupus erythematosus with nephritis: a long-term study. *Quarterly Journal of Medicine*, **48**, 1–24.

Chou, C., Lee, F. & Schumacher, H. (1986) Modification of a screening technique to evaluate systemic lupus erythematosus in a Chinese population in Taiwan. *Journal of Rheumatology*, **13**, 806–809.

Esdaile, J.M., Sampalis, J.S., Lacaille, D. & Danoff, D. (1988) The relationship of socioeconomic status to subsequent health status in systemic lupus erythematosus. *Arthritis and Rheumatism*, **31**, 423–427.

Esdaile, J.M., Levinton, C., Federgreen, W., Hayslett, J.P. & Kaskgarian, M. (1989) The clinical and renal biopsy predictors of long-term outcome in lupus nephritis: a study of 87 patients and review of the literature. *Quarterly Journal of Medicine*, **72**, 779–833.

Esdaile, J.M., Abrahamowicz, M., McKenzie, T., Hayslett, J.P. & Kaskgarian, M. (1994) The time-dependence of long-term prediction in lupus nephritis. *Arthritis and Rheumatism*, **37**, 359–368.

Estes, D. & Christian, C.L. (1971) The natural history of systemic lupus erythematosus by prospective analysis. *Medicine*, **50**, 85–94.

Feinglass, E.J., Arnett, F.C., Dorsch, C.A., Zizic, T.M. & Stevens, M.B. (1976) Neuropsychiatric manifestations of systemic lupus erythematosus; diagnosis, clinical spectrum, and relationship to other features of the disease. *Medicine*, **55**, 323–339.

Fessel, W. (1974) Systemic lupus erythematosus in the community: incidence, prevalence, outcome, and first symptoms; the high prevalence in black women. *Archives of Internal Medicine*, **134**, 1027–1035.

Frank, A. (1980) Apparent predisposition to systemic lupus erythematosus in Chinese patients in West Malaysia. *Annals of Rheumatic Diseases*, **39**, 266–269.

Ginzler, E.M., Diamond, H.S., Weiner, M. *et al.* (1982) A multicenter study of outcome in systemic lupus erythematosus: I. Entry variables as predictors of prognosis. *Arthritis and Rheumatism*, **25**, 601–611.

Ginzler, E.M., Felson, D.T., Anthony, J.M. & Anderson, J.J. (1993) Hypertension increases the risk of renal deterioration in systemic lupus erythematosus. *Journal of Rheumatology*, **20**, 1694–1700.

Godeau, P., Betourné, C., Piette, J.C., Herreman, G., Wechsler, B. & Lévy, R. (1977) Evolution et pronostic à long terme du lupus érythémateux. *Annales de Médicine Interne*, **128**, 17–30.

Goulet, J.R., Mackenzie, T., Levinton, C., Hayslett, J.P., Ciampi, A. & Esdaile, J.M. (1993) The longterm prognosis of lupus nephritis. The impact of the disease activity. *Journal of Rheumatology*, **20**, 59–65.

Greenwood, B. M. (1968) Autoimmune disease and parasitic infections in Nigerians. *Lancet* **ii**, 380–382.

Gudmundsson, S. & Steinsson, K. (1990) Systemic lupus erythematosus in Iceland 1975 through 1984: a nationwide epidemiological study in an unselected population. *Journal of Rheumatology*, **17**, 1162–1167.

Hall, L. (1966) Polyarthritis in Kenya. *East African Medical Journal*, **43**, 161–170.

Hart, H.H., Grigor, R.R. & Caughey, D.E. (1983) Ethnic difference in the prevalence of systemic lupus erythematosus. *Annals of Rheumatic Diseases*, **42**, 529–532.

Helve, T. (1985) Prevalence and mortality rates of systemic lupus erythematosus and causes of death in SLE patients in Finland. *Journal of Rheumatology*, **14**, 43–46.

Hochberg, M.C. (1985) The incidence of systemic lupus erythematosus in Baltimore, Maryland, 1970–1977. *Arthritis and Rheumatism*, **28**, 80–86.

Hochberg, M.C. (1987a) Mortality from systemic lupus erythematosus in England and Wales, 1974–1983. *British Journal of Rheumatology*, **26**, 437–441.

Hochberg, M.C. (1987b) Prevalence of systemic lupus erythematosus in England and Wales, 1981–1982. *Annals of Rheumatic Diseases*, **46**, 664–666.

Hochberg, M.C., Dorsch, C.A., Feinglass, E.J. & Stevens, M.B. (1981). Survivorship in systemic lupus erythematosus. Effect of antibody to extractable nuclear antigen. *Arthritis and Rheumatism*, **24**, 54–59.

Hopkinson, N.D., Dopherty, M. & Powell, R.J. (1993) The prevalence and incidence of systemic lupus erythematosus in Nottingham, UK, 1989–1990. *British Journal of Rheumatology*, **50**, 490–492.

Johnson, A.E., Gordon, C., Palmer, R.G. & Bacon, P.A. (1995) The prevalence and incidence of systemic lupus erythematosus in Birmingham, England. Relationship to ethnicity and country of birth. *Arthritis and Rheumatism*, **38**, 551–558.

Johnson, A.E., Gordon, C., Hobbs, F.D.R. & Bacon, P.A. (1996) Undiagnosed systemic lupus erythematosus in the community. *Lancet*, **347**, 367–369.

Jonsson, H., Nived, O. & Sturfelt, G. (1989) Outcome in systemic lupus erythematosus: a prospective study of patients from a defined population. *Medicine*, **68**, 141–150.

Karlson, E.W., Daltroy, L.H., Lew, R.A. *et al.* (1995) The independence and stability of socioeconomic predictors of morbidity in systemic lupus erythematosus. *Arthritis and Rheumatism*, **38**, 267–273.

Kaslow, R.A. (1982) High rate of death caused by systemic lupus erythematosus among U.S. residents of Asian descent. *Arthritis and Rheumatism*, **25**, 414–416.

Kaslow, R.A. & Masi, A.T. (1978) Age, sex, and race effects on mortality from systemic lupus erythematosus in the United States. *Arthritis and Rheumatism*, **21**, 473–479.

Kellum, R. & Haserick, J. (1964) Systemic lupus erythematosus. A statistical evaluation of mortality based on a consecutive series of 299 patients. *Archives of Internal Medicine*, **113**, 200–207.

Lawrence, R.C., Hochberg, M.C., Kelsey, J.L. *et al.* (1989) Estimates of the prevalence of selected arthritis and musculoskeletal diseases in the United States. *Journal of Rheumatology* **16**, 427–441.

Lévy, M., Montes de Oca, M. & Babron, J.C. (1989) Incidence du lupus érythémateux disséminé de l'enfant en région parisienne. *Presse Medicale*, **18**, 2022.

Lopez-Acuna, D., Hochberg, M.C. & Gittelsohn, A.M. (1982) Do persons of Spanish-heritage have an increased mortality from systemic lupus erythematosus compared to other Caucasians? *Arthritis and Rheumatism*, **25** (Suppl), S67.

McCarty, D.J., Manzi, S., Medsger, T.A., Ramsey-Goldman, R., La Porte, R. & Kwok, C.K. (1995). Incidence of systemic lupus erythematosus. Race and gender defferences. *Arthritis and Rheumatism*, **38**, 1260–1270.

McLaughlin, J., Gladman, D.D., Urowitz, M.B., Bombardier, C., Farewell, V.T. & Cole, E. (1991) Kidney biopsy in systemic lupus erythematosus. II. Survival analyses according to biopsy results. *Arthritis and Rheumatism*, **34**, 1268–1273.

McLaughlin, J., Bombardier, C., Farewell, V.T., Gladman, D.D. & Urowitz, M.B. (1994) Kidney biopsy in systemic lupus erythematosus. III. Survival analysis controlling for clinical and laboratory variables. *Arthritis and Rheumatism*, **37**, 559–567.

Merill, M. & Shulman, L.E. (1955) Determination of prognosis in chronic disease, illustrated by systemic lupus erythematosus. *Journal of Chronic Diseases*, **1**, 12–32.

Michet, C.J., McKenna, C.H., Eveback, L.R., Kaslow, R.A. & Kurland, L.T. (1985) Epidemiology of systemic lupus erythematosus and other connective tissue disease in Rochester, Minnesota, 1950 through 1979. *Mayo Clinic Proceedings*, **60**, 105–113.

Morton, R.O., Gershwin, M.E., Brady, C. & Steinberg, A.D. (1976) The incidence of systemic lupus erythematosus in North American Indians. *Journal of Rheumatology*, **3**, 186–190.

Nai-Cheng, C. (1983) Rheumatic disease in China. *Journal of Rheumatology*, **10**, 41–45.

Nived, O., Sturfelt, G. & Wollheim, F. (1985) Systemic lupus erythematosus in an adult population in southern Sweden: incidence, prevalence and validity of ARA revised classification criteria. *British Journal of Rheumatology*, **24**, 147.

Nossent, J.C. (1992) Systemic lupus erythematosus on the Caribbean island of Curaçao: an epidemiological investigation. *Annals of Rheumatic Diseases*, **51**, 1197–1201.

Petri, M., Perez-Gutthann, S. & Longenecker, J.C. (1991) Morbidity of systemic lupus erythematosus: role of race and socioeconomic status. *American Journal of Medicine*, **91**, 345–353.

Reveille, J.D., Bartolucci, A. & Alarcon, G.S. (1990) Prognosis in systemic lupus erythematosus. Negative impact of increasing age at onset, black race, and thrombocytopenia, as well as causes of death. *Arthritis and Rheumatology*, **33**, 37–48.

Rosner, S., Ginzler, E.M., Diamond, H.S. *et al.* (1982) A multicenter study of outcome in systemic lupus erythematosus. II. Causes of death. *Arthritis and Rheumatisms*, **25**, 612–617.

Rovers, M. & Coovadia, H. (1981) Systemic lupus erythematosus in children: a report of 3 cases. *South African Medical Journal*, **60**, 711–713.

Samanta, A., Feehally, J., Roy, S., Nichol, F.E., Sheldon, P.J. & Walls, J. (1991) High prevalence of systemic disease and mortality in Asian subjects with systemic lupus erythematosus. *Annals of Rheumatic Diseases*, **50**, 490–492.

Serdula, M.K. & Rhoads, G.G. (1979) Frequency of systemic lupus erythematosus in different ethnic groups in Hawaii. *Arthritis and Rheumatism*, **22**, 328–333.

Shaper, A. (1961) Systemic lupus erythematosus: a review of the disorder as seen in African patients in Uganda. *East African Medical Journal*, **38**, 135–144.

Siegel, M. & Lee, SL. (1973) The epidemiology of systemic lupus erythematosus. *Seminars in Arthritis and Rheumatism*, **3**, 1–54.

Siegel, M., Holley, H. & Lee, S.L. (1970) Epidemiologic studies on systemic lupus erythematosus, comparative data for New York City and Jefferson County, AL, 1956–1965. *Arthritis and Rheumatism*, **13**, 802–811.

Studenski, S., Allen, N.B., Caldwell, D.S., Rice, J.R. & Polisson, R.P. (1987) Survival in systemic lupus erythematosus: a multivariate analysis of demographic factors. *Arthritis and Rheumatism*, **30**, 1326–1332.

Swaak, A.J., Nossent, J.C., Bronsveld, W. *et al.* (1989) Systemic lupus erythematosus. I. Outcome and survival. Dutch experience with 110 patients studied prospectively. *Annals of Rheumatic Diseases*, **48**, 447–454.

Taylor, H. & Stein, C. (1986) Systemic lupus erythematosus in Zimbabwe. *Annals of Rheumatic Diseases*, **45**, 645–648.

Wallace, D.J. & Quismorio, F.P. (1995) The elusive search for geographic clusters of systemic lupus erythematosus. *Arthritis and Rheumatism*, **38**, 1564–1567.

Wallace, D.J., Podell, T.E., Weiner, J.M. (1982) Lupus nephritis. Experience with 230 patients in a private practice from 1950 to 1980. *American Journal of Medicine*, **72**, 209–220.

Wallace, D.J., Podell, T., Weiner, J., Klinenberg, J.R., Forouzesh, S. & Dubois, E.L. (1981) Systemic lupus erythematosus: survival patterns. Experience of 609 patients. *Journal of the American Medical Association*, **245**, 934–938.

Walsh, S.J., Algert, C., Gregorio, D.I., Reisine, S.T. & Rothfield, N.F. (1995) Divergent racial trends in mortality from systemic lupus erythematosus. *Journal of Rheumatology*, **22**, 1663–1668.

Ward, M. & Studenski, S. (1992) Clinical prognostic factors in lupus nephritis. The importance of hypertension and smoking. *Archives of Internal Medicine*, **152**, 2082–2088.

Ward, M.M., Pyun, E. & Studenski, S. (1995a) Causes of death in systemic lupus erythematosus. Long-term follow-up of an inception cohort. *Arthritis and Rheumatism*, **38**, 1492–1499.

Ward, M.M., Pyun, E. & Studenski, S. (1995b) Long-term survival in systemic lupus erythematosus. Patient characteristics associated with poorer outcomes. *Arthritis and Rheumatism*, **38**, 274–283.

Wilson, W.A. & Hughes, G.R.V. (1979) Rheumatic disease in Jamaica. *Annals of Rheumatic Diseases*, **38**, 20.

Woo, J., Wong, R., Wang, S. & Woo, P. (1987) Patterns of rheumatoid arthritis and systemic lupus erythematosus in Hong Kong. *Annals of Rheumatic Diseases*, **46**, 644–646.

Vascular Skin Disorders

L. NALDI

The term 'vascular skin disorders' is very general and non-specific. Traditionally, included under this heading are vascular leg ulcers and an array of other conditions such as Raynaud's phenomenon, acrocyanosis, livedo reticularis, chilblains and erythromelalgia. These disorders are heterogeneous in terms of aetiology, clinical importance and prognosis, which raises the question of whether it is advisable to group them all together. Many of the foregoing conditions do not represent diseases *per se* but are rather signs of more general derangements in circulation which may involve organs other than the skin. In addition, the diagnosis and the treatment of vascular skin disorders may vary according to country and local health organization. This clearly affects the representativeness of any clinically-based series of patients. The general lack of diagnostic criteria to be employed in epidemiological studies further complicates the issue.

Venous and arterial leg ulcers

Disease definition and occurrence

A skin ulcer has been defined as a loss of dermis and epidermis produced by sloughing of necrotic tissue. Ulcers persisting for 4 weeks or more have been rather arbitrarily classified as chronic ulcers in a number of studies (Baker *et al.*, 1991). Still others have failed to provide any criteria at all. Venous and arterial leg ulcers are recognized as the most common chronic wounds in Western populations.

Reliable information on the occurrence of venous and arterial leg ulcers can be obtained by screening a large population for chronic ulceration and by further examining a representative sample to identify those with venous or arterial abnormalities. Table 18.4 presents some recent estimates of the prevalence of leg ulcers in the general population. Point prevalence estimates, which take into account active ulcers at a definite time, provide lower values compared to life-time prevalence estimates which consider the presence of an ulcer at any time during the subject's life. Moreover, studies restricted to the older age groups have provided higher estimates compared to those considering the whole population. The criteria adopted for the diagnosis of the disease, including ulcer location and modalities of assessment (questionnaires or direct inspection), vary greatly from one study to another.

Surprisingly few studies have attempted to separate the more prevalent varieties of chronic leg ulcers. Once again, diagnostic criteria vary from one study to another. In the Lothian and Forth Valley Health District Survey, a sample of 600 patients reporting leg and foot ulcers on a postal questionnaire were examined and venous disease was clinically diagnosed in 76% of cases while evidence of arterial impairment was observed in 21% of cases (Callam *et al.*, 1985). In another study (Cornwall *et al.*, 1986) based on a health district population, all patients with a leg ulcer were identified by contacting general practitioners, wards, nursing homes, old people's homes and residential homes within the district. A sample of 100 patients was examined by ultrasound and photoplethysmography to assess venous and arterial circulation. A venous origin was diagnosed in 81% of cases; 38% of cases had evidence of deep-vein involvement and 43% had superficial vein incompetence. An ischaemic element was present either in isolation (9%) or combined with venous disease (22%) in a total of 31% of cases. In another study, patients suffering from leg and foot ulcers in a metropolitan population were recruited by contacting health professionals and institutions in the study area and by self-referral facilitated by publication of an article in local newspapers. The recruited patients were examined by ultrasound and photoplethys-mography. A venous ulcer was diagnosed in 57% of cases (Baker *et al.*, 1991). Finally, in a cross-sectional population survey, a sample of 382 patients with leg ulcers was examined with bidirectional Doppler ultrasonography. Venous insufficiency was documented in 72% of cases. Some element of arterial disease was

Table 18.4 Some recent estimates of the prevalence of leg ulcers (any cause).

Reference	Age group (years)	Measure*	Estimate (%)
Widmer *et al.* (1978)	40–65	LT	1
Callam *et al.* (1985)	All ages	PT	0.15
Cornwall *et al.* (1986)	All ages	PT	0.18
Baker *et al.* (1991)	All ages	PT	0.1
Nelzén *et al.* (1991a)	All ages	PT	0.3
Lindholm *et al.* (1992)	All ages	PT	0.1
Andersson *et al.* (1993)	>65	PT	1.0

* PT, Point prevalence; LT, lifetime prevalence.
† Foot ulcers are included.

observed in 40% of cases and ischaemia was judged to represent the main factor in 18% of cases (Nelzén *et al.*, 1991b). The variations in the ratio of venous to arterial ulcers may represent true variations among different populations or may reflect problems with entry criteria and disease definition. Interestingly, in a study of leg and foot ulcers involving medical doctors and nurses in the city of Malmö, Sweden, the aetiology of the ulcers was considered to be unknown in 36% of the leg ulcer patients and in 22% of the foot ulcer patients. This might reflect an overall uncertainty about the underlying cause and is a clear indication to improve the standardization of diagnostic criteria (Lindholm *et al.*, 1992). There have been recent suggestions that there has been a change in the aetiology of leg ulcers towards arterial and mixed ulcers (Philips *et al.*, 1994). However, no clear evidence emerges from the available data.

Risk factors

Venous and arterial leg ulcers are the consequence of multifactorial processes. The ulcer point prevalence increases considerably with age. Prevalence figures reflect both incidence and chronicity. In fact, in the Lothian and Forth Valley study where an increased prevalence with age was documented, 22% of patients had their first episode before the age 40 years and 40% before the age of 50 years (Callam *et al.*, 1985). Sex variations with a male to female ratio lower than one have been documented in most studies. However, in the older age groups there is a female predominance and when prevalence figures according to age and sex were taken into consideration, no impressive differences between sexes were documented (Baker *et al.*, 1991). An inverse relation of leg ulcer prevalence with socio-economic status has been suggested but remains unproven.

Venous ulcers are the end result of superficial or deep venous insufficiency (Biland & Widmer, 1988). Deep-vein thrombosis represents a major determinant of deep-vein insufficiency which in turn leads to venous thrombosis. It has been quoted that deep-vein reflux is documented in *c*. 50% of cases of venous ulcer (Douglas & Simpson, 1995). Additional risk factors for venous ulcers include a positive family history and varicose veins (Andersson *et al.*, 1993).

Arterial ulcerations may be regarded as a multi-step process, starting, in general, with a systemic vascular derangement such as atherosclerosis. Most of the evidence linking risk factors to atherosclerotic disorders deals with the major and most life-threatening manifestation, namely coronary heart disease. Although the same risk factors do in general apply to other atherosclerotic events such as occlusive peripheral arterial diseases, some important differences exist. In the Framingham Study, cigarette smoking was the strongest contributor to peripheral vascular disorders in men, followed by hypertension and diabetes (Kannel, 1988). These data have been confirmed by a recent cohort study conducted in Israel (Bowlin *et al.*, 1994). Notably, ex-smokers had an elevated risk for developing intermittent claudication in 5 years.

An area which has been largely neglected is the analysis of risk factors for venous and arterial ulcers of early onset.

Prognosis and public-health issues

Surveys in the general population point to the less than satisfactory prognosis of leg ulcers in terms of healing and recurrence. In the Lothian and Forth Valley survey, out of 827 ulcers in 600 patients, 20% had not healed in over 2 years and 8% in 5 years (Callam *et al.*, 1985). The majority of patients had had recurrences, 66% having had episodes of ulceration for more than 5 years. In a large-scale clinical study, the healing time of leg ulcers varied according to the dimension of the ulcers, their duration and the mobility of the patients (Moffatt *et al.*, 1992). Morbidity and mortality in ulcer patients may be higher than in the general population. In a follow-up study of patients attending a dermatology/department for leg ulcers, the mortality rate for ischaemic heart disease was twice as high for both men and women as in the same age groups of the general population (Hansson *et al.*, 1987). An increased risk for squamous-cell carcinoma has been clinically suggested in patients with chronic ulcers and a recent record-linkage study in Sweden has provided some epidemiological evidence for it (Baldursson *et al.*, 1993). The quality of life of ulcer patients may be severely affected. In a survey conducted in Boston, 42% of patients with leg ulcers who were not working at the time of the interview stated that their ulcer was a factor in their decision to stop work. The same group in Boston has documented social isolation, depression and negative self-image associated with ulcers in a high percentage of patients (Philips *et al.*, 1994). A number of studies point to the less than satisfactory management of ulcer patients in the community including the lack of any clinical assessment leading to long periods of ineffective or inappropriate treatment and delay in instituting effective pain-relieving strategies. This problem emerges more clearly when an epidemiological perspective rather than a clinical view of selected patients on a short-term basis is adopted (Cornwall *et al.*, 1986; Callam *et al.*, 1987).

The economic cost of chronic non-healing wounds is enormous. It has been calculated that in Sweden the annual ulcer-care costs amount to about $25 million (Phillips, 1993) while the annual cost in the UK has been estimated at about $300 million (Douglas & Simpson, 1995). The evaluation of interventional programmes aimed at optimizing resources and improving the effectiveness of the treatment and the quality of life of patients is highly desirable. Interestingly, ulcer clinics in vascular surgical services in the UK proved to offer advantages over home treatment (Moffat *et al.*, 1992). The overwhelming rates of recurrence clearly suggest that more attention should be paid to prevention and correction of underlying aetiological factors. The identification of individuals at higher risk for deep-vein thrombosis and adoption of effective prophylactic measures for thrombosis may serve to reduce the incidence of venous ulceration. No data, however, are available on the effectiveness of any preventive measure.

Raynaud's phenomenon

Definition and occurrence

Raynaud's phenomenon refers to the sequence of digital blanching, cyanosis and erythema, frequently accompanied by numbness or pain, occurring in response to cold or emotional stimuli. It usually involves the fingers, sometimes the toes, and very occasionally the nose, tongue or ears. The diagnosis of Raynaud's phenomenon should be based on anamnestic enquiry since it is difficult to reproduce an attack of Raynaud's phenomenon in the laboratory and functional assessments, including measurements of baseline digital flow and determination of cold-induced changes in finger systolic blood pressure or blood flow, do not reliably differentiate between normal and pathological status (Maricq & Weinrich, 1988). The reliability of anamnestic enquiry depends on the patient's ability to properly understand the physician's question and accurately describe in unambiguous terms the signs and symptoms. An attempt to improve standardization was made by Maricq and Weinrich (1988) from South Carolina. They combined a simple standardized questionnaire with colour charts consisting of a 12-point colour scale and a series of photographs illustrating blanching and cyanosis. In a preliminary trial they demonstrated a good identification of blanching on colour charts but less reliable reporting of cyanosis. Criteria were limited to blanching. The diagnostic per-formance of the instrument was judged as satisfactory in a study involving 294 subjects with known Raynaud's phenomenon status. The diagnostic instrument was used in a population survey involving a probability sample of households that yielded 5246 adults in South Carolina (Weinrich *et al.*, 1990).

Table 18.5 Prevalence estimates of Raynaud's phenomenon. (After Weinrich *et al.*, 1990).

Reference	Region	Age (years)	Prevalence estimates(%) Women	Men
Olsen & Nielsen (1978)	Denmark	–	22.0	–
Heslop *et al.* (1983)	England	20–59	10.4	5.0
Maricq *et al.* (1986)	South Carolina	18–84	4.9	3.8
Leppert *et al.* (1987)	Sweden	18–59	15.6	–
Weinrich *et al.* (1990)	South Carolina	18–86	4.3	2.6

Table 18.5 presents some recent estimates of the prevalence of Raynaud's phenomenon. If the differences are real, they may be explained by climatic conditions (higher rates in cooler countries), regional lifestyles and possibly genetic characteristics. However, disease definitions varied from one study to another and some studies, although aimed at estimating the prevalence in the general population, were based on selected groups of subjects, such as physiotherapists (Olsen & Nielsen, 1978) and patients in general practice (Heslop *et al.*, 1983). As an aside, when asking about the occurrence of Raynaud's phenomenon, it is advisable to specify a period of time and prevalence estimates over the same period of time should be compared. Unfortunately, most studies have assessed symptoms over a loosely defined period of time.

Risk factors

Raynaud's phenomenon is more frequent in women than in men. In the South Carolina study, the prevalence adjusted to the US population was 4.33 in women and 2.67 in men (Weinrich *et al.*, 1990). Moreover, a higher prevalence in Blacks compared to Whites was documented in the same study. Interestingly, a higher prevalence of systemic sclerosis has also been reported in Blacks (Medsger & Masi, 1971). Several factors have been associated with Raynaud's phenomenon, including drugs, e.g. ergotamine, beta-blockers and oral contraceptives, and occupational factors, i.e. vibrating tools and exposure to vinyl chloride. Assessment of their role in quantitative terms is, however, largely lacking. Recently, an association with reduced fertility prior to disease presentation was documented in women, pointing to the potential role of reproductive factors (Kahl *et al.*, 1990). Since Raynaud's phenomenon is associated with systemic sclerosis, the analysis of risk factors for Raynaud's phenomenon may throw some light on risk factors for the latter.

Prognosis and public-health issues

The natural history of Raynaud's phenomenon is largely unknown. In a study conducted in an outpatient department of internal medicine in The Netherlands, the rate of development of systemic sclerosis in patients suffering from Raynaud's phenomenon was estimated to be about 25% after 5 years (Kallenberg *et al.*, 1988). It has also been stated that 'between 5 and 15% of patients with Raynaud's phenomenon will develop overt scleroderma' (Grigg & Wolfe, 1991). If we apply these figures to the prevalence estimates for Raynaud's phenomenon, even the most conservative, obtained in population surveys, we can conclude that the cumulative lifetime incidence of systemic sclerosis associated with Raynaud's phenomenon is not lower than 1 in 1000 of the total population. In fact, the annual incidence rate of systemic sclerosis has been estimated at around 1–10 per million per year (Silman & Hochberg, 1993). Clinical experience and epidemiological evidence seem to diverge to some extent and this underlines the need for formal prognostic studies. In a clinical series it has been noted that the presence of antinuclear antibodies detected by immunoblotting has a discriminative power for the future development of connective-tissue diseases and that the antigenic specificities of the antinuclear antibodies are indicative of the clinical entity that will develop (Kallenberg *et al.*, 1988).

Livedo reticularis and other vascular skin disorders

The difficulties we have pointed to in relation to vascular ulcers and Raynaud's phenomenon also apply to other vascular skin disorders. Epidemiological data are almost completely lacking for conditions like livedo reticularis, acrocyanosis, chilblains and erythromelalgia. That these manifestations escape epidemiological interest is not surprising. Given their functional nature, they are difficult to define and ascertain. Livedo reticularis, for example, waxes and wanes and, to some extent, may be considered as a variation in the 'norm'. With the possible exception of chilblains and erythromelalgia, they cause only a slight discomfort, representing, in some cases, no more than an annoying cosmetic problem. As a consequence, their interest in terms of public health appears rather low. On the other hand, some conditions may represent clues to underlying systemic disorders and might have a prognostic value. The use of epidemiological methods to document the existence of coalitions of signs and symptoms may help to clarify pathogenetic processes and may have clinical implications. In a number of studies, for example, livedo reticularis has been associated with antiphospholipid antibodies (Weinstein *et al.*, 1987; Naldi *et al.*, 1993). In our study (Naldi *et al.*, 1993), all the patients who were referred for the first time to the coagulation service of a general hospital for their first determination of antiphospholipid antibodies were eligible. Patients referred by dermatologists were excluded, as were patients who were diagnosed as suffering from systemic lupus erythematosus at any time during the study period. All patients were examined by two dermatologists blind to the results of the serological investigations. Strict criteria were defined for the physical examination. The study was analysed as a case-control study, cases and controls being defined according to the results of antiphospholipid antibody tests. Acrocyanosis and Raynaud's phenomenon, besides livedo reticularis, appeared to be associated with antiphospholipid antibodies. The study suggests that these cutaneous manifestations are rather specific and appear early in the development of the antiphospholipid syndrome.

Conclusion

Vascular skin disorders are a neglected area. Obvious concerns for the future must be the development of standardized diagnostic criteria (including severity grading), the definition of adequate sampling strategies and the use of more formal study designs in the evaluation of aetiology and prognosis.

References

Andersson, E., Hansson, C. & Swanbeck, G. (1993) Leg and foot ulcer prevalence and investigation of the peripheral arterial and venous circulation in a randomized elderly population. An epidemiology survey and clinical investigation. *Acta Dermato-Venereologica*, **73**, 57–61.

Baker, S.R., Stacey, M.C., Jopp-MacKay, A.G., Hoskin, S.E. & Thompson, P.J. (1991) Epidemiology of chronic venous ulcers. *British Journal of Surgery*, **78**, 864–867.

Baldursson, B., Sigurgeirsson, B. & Lindelöf, B. (1993) Leg ulcers and squamous cell carcinoma. *Acta Dermato-Venereologica*, **73**, 171–174.

Biland, L. & Widmer, L.K. (1988) Varicose veins and chronic venous insufficiency. Medical and socio-economic aspects. Basle Study. *Acta Chirurgica Scandinavica*, **544** (Suppl), 9–11.

Bowlin, S.J., Medalie, J.H., Flocke, S.A., Zyzanski, S.J. & Goldbourt, U. (1994) Epidemiology of intermittent claudication in middle-aged men. *American Journal of Epidemiology*, **140**, 418–430.

Callam, M.J., Ruckley, C.V., Harper, D.R. & Dale, J.J. (1985) Chronic ulceration of the leg. Extent of the problem and provision of care. *British Medical Journal*, **290**, 1855–1856.

Callam, M.J., Harper, D.R., Dale, J.J. & Ruckley, C.V. (1987) Chronic ulcer of the leg: clinical history. *British Medical Journal*, **294**, 1389–1391.

Cornwall, J.V., Dore, C.J. & Lewis, J.D. (1986) Leg ulcers. Epidemiology and aetiology. *British Journal of Surgery*, **73**, 693–696.

Douglas, W.S. & Simpson, N.B. (1995) Workshop Report. Guidelines for the management of chronic venous leg ulceration. Report of a multidisciplinary workshop. *British Journal of Dermatology*, **132**, 446–452.

Grigg, M.H. & Wolfe, J.H.N. (1991) ABC of vascular diseases, Raynaud's phenomenon and similar conditions. *British Medical Journal*, **303**, 913–916.

Hallböök, T. (1988) Leg ulcer epidemiology. *Acta Chirurgica Scandinavica*, **544** (Suppl), 17–20.

Hansson, C., Andersson, E. & Swanbeck, G. (1987) A follow-up study of leg and foot ulcer patients. *Acta Dermato-Venereologica*, **67**, 496–500.

Heslop, J., Coggon, D. & Acheson, E.D. (1983) The prevalence of intermittent digital ischemia (Raynaud's phenomenon) in a general practice. *Journal of the Royal College of General Practitioners*, **33**, 85–89.

Kahl, L.E., Blair, C., Ramsey-Goldman, R. & Steen, V.D. (1990) Pregnancy outcomes in women with primary Raynaud's phenomenon. *Arthritis and Rheumatism*, **33**, 1249–1255.

Kallenberg, C.G.M., Wouda, A.A., Hoet, M.H. & Van Venrooij, W. (1988) Development of connective tissue disease in patients presenting with Raynaud's phenomenon: a six year follow up with emphasis on the predictive value of antinuclear antibodies as detected by immunoblotting. *Annals of Rheumatic Diseases*, **47**, 634–641.

Kannel, W.B. (1988) An overview of the risk factors for cardiovascular disease. In: *The Challenge of Epidemiology. Issues and Selected Readings* (eds. C. Buck, A. Llopis, E. Nájera & M. Terris), pp. 699–718. Pan American Health Organization, Washington, DC.

Leppert, J., Aberg, H., Ringqvist, I. & Sorensson, S. (1987) Raynaud's phenomenon in a female population: prevalence and association with other conditions. *Angiology*, **38**, 871–877.

Lindholm, C., Bjellerup, M., Christensen, O.B. & Zederfeldt, B. (1992) A demographic survey of leg and foot ulcer patients in a defined population. *Acta Dermato-Venereologica*, **72**, 227–230.

Maricq, H.R., Weinrich, M.C., Keil, J.E. & LeRoy, E.C. (1986) Prevalence of Raynaud phenomenon in the general population. A preliminary study by questionnaire. *Journal of Chronic Diseases*, **39**, 423–427.

Maricq, H.R. & Weinrich, J. (1988) Diagnosis of Raynaud's phenomenon assisted by color charts. *Journal of Rheumatology*, **15**, 454–459.

Medsger, T.A. & Masi, A.T. (1971) Epidemiology of systemic sclerosis (scleroderma). *Annals of Internal Medicine*, **74**, 714–721.

Moffatt, C.J., Franks, P.J., Olroyd, M. *et al.* (1992) Community clinics for leg ulcers and impact on healing. *British Medical Journal*, **305**, 1389–1392.

Naldi, L., Locati, F., Marchesi, L. *et al.* (1993) Cutaneous manifestations associated with antiphospholipid antibodies in patients without systemic lupus erythematosus: a case-control study. *Annals of Rheumatic Diseases*, **52**, 219–222.

Nelzén, O., Bergqvist, D. & Lindhagen, A. (1991a) Leg ulcer etiology. A cross-sectional population survey. *Journal of Vascular Surgery*, **14**, 557–564.

Nelzén, O., Bergqvist, D., Lindhagen, A. & Hallbrook, T. (1991b) Chronic leg ulcers. An underestimated problem in primary health care among elderly patients. *Journal of Epidemiology and Community Health*, **45**, 184–187.

Olsen, N. & Nielsen, S.L. (1978) Prevalence of primary Raynaud phenomena in young females. *Scandinavian Journal of Clinical and Laboratory Investigation*, **37**, 761–764.

Phillips, T.J. (1993) Chronic cutaneous ulcers: etiology and epidemiology. *Journal of Investigative Dermatology*, **102**, 38S–41S.

Phillips, T.J., Stanton, B., Provan, A. & Lew, R. (1994) A study of the impact of leg ulcers on quality of life: financial, social and psychologic implications. *Journal of the American Academy of Dermatology*, **31**, 49–53.

Silman, A.J. & Hochberg, M.C. (1993) Scleroderma. In: *Epidemiology of the Rheumatic Diseases* (eds A.J. Silman & M.C. Hochberg), pp. 192–219. Oxford University Press, Oxford.

Thromboembolic Risk Factors (THRIFT) Consensus Group (1992) Risk of and prophylaxis for venous thrombo-embolism in hospital patients. *British Medical Journal*, **305**, 567–574.

Weinrich, M.C., Maricq, H.R., Keil, J.E., McGregor, A.R. & Diat, F. (1990) Prevalence of Raynaud's phenomenon in the adult population of South Carolina. *Journal of Clinical Epidemiology*, **43**, 1343–1349.

Weinstein, C., Miller, M.H., Axtens, R., Buchanan, R. & Littlejohn, G.O. (1987) Livedo reticularis associated with increased titers of anticardiolipin antibodies in systemic lupus erythematosus. *Archives of Dermatology*, **123**, 596–600.

Widmer, L.K. (1978) *Peripheral Venous Disorders. Prevalence and Sociomedical Importance*, pp. 43–50. Hans Huber, Bern.

Acne

R. STERN

Introduction

In 1991, there were more than 6 million visits to office-based physicians for acne in the United States. Acne is one of the most common reasons for visits by persons aged 15–35 years to physicians and accounts for *c.* 20% of visits to dermatologists (Stern & Nelson, 1993). In the United States, the cost of caring for acne almost certainly exceeds $500 000 000 per year.

Most adolescents will develop acne to some degree. Yet data that describe the incidence or prevalence of acne of varying clinical severities or the impact of this disease on affected individuals are quite limited. Data on the duration of acne and factors that predict the development or persistence of more severe forms are even more limited. Here, current knowledge about the descriptive epidemiology of acne is reviewed. In addition, the contributions of epidemiological studies to our understanding of the treatment of acne and the risks of therapy are discussed.

Prevalence of acne

Although acne to some degree is an almost universal experience among young adults, concern about the appropriateness of use of oral isotretinoin in women led to a contentious debate about the frequency of severe or cystic acne (Stern, 1992). Some individuals claim that severe or cystic acne is rare in women. Based on these claims, they alleged that rates of utilization of isotretinoin in this group are far beyond those clinically justified.

Between 1971 and 1974, as part of the National Health and Nutrition Examination Survey, a population-based examination study of the health of nearly 21 000 US residents, data on the prevalence of acne of varying severities were collected. Dermatological residents utilized standardized techniques to examine these persons. This study provided an estimated prevalence of acne conglobata (grade 4 acne) among women aged 15–44 years in the United States of 250 000 (Stern, 1992). For men in this age group, approximately 600 000 were similarly affected. An estimated additional 582 000 women and 749 000 men had moderate acne which included cysts or scars. Therefore, about 800 000 women and 1 300 000 men aged 15–44 years had moderate or severe acne which included cysts or scars (Stern, 1992). In contrast to claims that severe, cystic or scarring acne was rare among women, these data demonstrated that severe acne is not rare in women. This study also indicated that males were about 1.6-fold more likely to have moderate acne that included cysts or scarring or severe acne compared to females of the same age. This point prevalence study indicated that, at the time of examination, nearly 2% of women and 3% of men aged 15–44 years have substantial acne involvement (Stern, 1992).

Even this well-designed and executed point prevalence study left unanswered many questions about acne. Further, the precision of these estimates must be questioned for a number of reasons. First, the degree to which ratings of acne were standardized among observers is subject to question. There was wide variability in the prevalence of acne of varying degrees at different examination sites. Second, many patients with acne were under treatment at the time of their examination. Therefore, the true prevalence of more severe types of acne independent of therapy is likely to be underestimated. Third, patients who agreed to participate might not be representative of the general population. This point prevalence study did not collected data on the duration of acne of varying degrees. Therefore, information on the incidence of acne of a given severity was not provided.

Studies of the prevalence of acne in other populations provide a wide range of estimates of disease frequency. A 1980 study of Swedish students aged 12–16 years revealed an overall prevalence of acne that was nearly identical among males and females (38% and 35%, respectively) (Larsson & Liden, 1980). This prevalence of acne increased with age, from 27% among 12-year olds to 47% among 16-year olds, the oldest age group studied. Unfortunately, this study was restricted to quite young individuals and did not report the prevalence of acne of varying severities.

A study in the UK demonstrated that acne was common among adolescents and young adults. This study indicated that for women, this disease continued into their fourth decade and even beyond (Cunliffe & Gould, 1979). Ten years later, however, publishing in the same journal, another group from Scotland suggested that, although acne was almost universal at the age of 16 years (95% of males and 83% of females), at least among school children aged 12–17 years, <2% of boys and <0.1% of girls had clinically substantial acne (Rademaker *et al.*, 1989).

More recent results from a genetically similar population living in a very different climate suggest that severe acne is far more prevalent than the earlier Scottish study suggested. In a New Zealand study, acne of some degree was nearly universally noted in a sample of senior high-school students. Severe acne was present in 1% of the young women and 7% of males examined (Lello *et al.*, 1995).

Differences in the prevalence of acne as determined from comparisons of cross studies are likely to reflect genetic factors as well as criteria used in scoring acne severity. Among the most important factors accounting for differences in the results of these studies are the differences in the populations studied. The prevalence of severe acne varies with age. Although milder forms of acne are extremely common among children aged 12–17 years, recent community-based studies that estimate the prevalence of more severe types of acne among older persons (i.e. >17 years) are lacking. Since severe acne often first develops in persons >17 years, studies of younger persons (i.e. 12–17 years) are likely to underestimate the prevalence of more severe forms of acne.

The estimated prevalence of severe acne in a population will also vary with the treatment this population is utilizing. For example, if three groups with equal prevalence of acne at a given point in time were compared again 1 year later with one group receiving isotretinoin, a second group no therapy and the third group treatment with topical antibiotics, one would expect these initially indistinguishable groups to have very different prevalences of acne of varying severities when examined 1 year later. Further, in deciding on treatment, it would be desirable to not only consider the severity of acne at the time of presentation but the expected duration of disease. In fact, without robust estimates of the duration of this chronic disease, it is not possible to estimate the proportion of individuals who in the absence of treatment would be affected by severe acne sometime during their lifetime.

In spite of its nearly universal occurrence among young and middle-aged subjects, precise and current information on the duration or incidence of acne is lacking. Also lacking is knowledge about what patient characteristics are associated with the development or persistence of more severe forms of acne. Clearly, these issues are amenable to epidemiological analysis. Given the resources devoted to the care of acne and its importance to dermatological practice, such studies would seem justified.

Epidemiology of acne therapy

Although studies that determine the prevalence, duration, incidence and impact of acne in populations are largely lacking, epidemiology has played an important role in the evaluation of the risks of the most effective treatment for severe acne, isotretinoin. A variety of types of epidemiological studies have helped to identify and quantitate the risks associated with isotretinoin, especially its teratogenic hazards.

The teratogenic effects of isotretinoin were well documented in animals prior to its initial marketing in the United States in 1982. In spite of warnings about its use in women who might become pregnant, a speciality-based reporting system, the American Academy of Dermatology's Adverse Drug Reaction Reporting System working together with the Food and Drug Administration, identified 10 cases of birth defects in women exposed to isotretinoin who were born within 18 months of its marketing in the United States (Stern *et al.*, 1984). This study helped to define the spectrum of birth defects associated with intrauterine exposure to this drug. A subsequent cohort study of exposed pregnancies documented the outcomes of exposed pregnancies and the high relative risk of these specific malformations among these exposed pregnancies (Lammer *et al.*, 1985). Additional postmarketing surveillance confirmed that even brief exposure during pregnancy was associated with a high risk of fetal malformations (Dai *et al.*, 1992).

Based on knowledge from animals and about the mechanism of isotretinoin-associated teratogenesis one would expect that pregnancies beginning more than a few days after the discontinuation of isotretinoin should not have a higher risk of congenital malformations. In a study of women who reported conception after discontinuation of isotretinoin treatment, no increased risk of fetal malformations was detected (Dai *et al.*, 1989). This finding helps assure clinicians and patients that the teratogenic risk of this drug, which has been used by more than 1 million women worldwide, is limited to the period of its use.

Because of its teratogenic potential, in the United States there is a comprehensive programme meant to prevent pregnancy among users and to ensure that only appropriate candidates for therapy receive isotretinoin (Mitchell *et al.*, 1995). To evaluate the effectiveness of this 'Pregnancy Prevention Program' and to better document the characteristics and outcomes among women treated with isotretinoin, in 1989 a postmarketing survey was undertaken that attempts to enroll all women beginning isotretinoin in the United States and follows them until outcomes of any exposed pregnancies could be determined (Mitchell *et al.*, 1995). Patients are recruited through prescribing physicians, with an enrolment form included with the medication's packaging and with a toll-free telephone line. Between January 1989 and December 1993, 177 216 eligible women enrolled in this survey. This survey demonstrated very low pregnancy rates (< 1 per 1000 population per year drug use) and that most women (72%) who became pregnant during treatment with isotretinoin had elective abortions. Further, of the remaining pregnancies, over half had spontaneous abortions and only 8% of exposed pregnancies were documented as leading to live births. Therefore, only about 1 in 4000 women who used isotretinoin and who enrolled in the study was known to have delivered a live infant who was reported to be exposed to this highly teratogenic drug (Mitchell *et al.*, 1995).

These results demonstrate that at least among the women who enrolled in the survey and were followed, the occurrence of congenital malformations as a consequence of the use of this drug is infrequent relative to the number of women prescribed this medication. Unfortunately, this study cannot determine to what extent the female isotretinoin users who do not enroll in the study may have had better, worse or the same outcomes compared to the >100 000 women who enrolled in the study. Clearly, determining the extent to which a study population is representative of the entire population of users of this drug is crucial for a complete understanding of the risks of this treatment in the general population. Identifying and quantifying potential biases in ascertainment is a continuing and prime issue in determining the generalizability of he results of this and many other epidemiological studies.

The most helpful studies concerning the epidemiology of acne have been related to the safety of drugs used in its treatment, especially the identification and quantification of the teratogenic risks of isotretinoin. Although feasible and of substantial potential benefit to clinical decision-making, epidemiological studies of duration, prognosis and predictors of severity of this common chronic disease are largely lacking.

References

Cunliffe, W.J. & Gould, D.J. (1979) Prevalence of facial acne vulgaris in late adolescence and in adults. *British Medical Journal*, **i**, 1109–1110.

Dai, W.S., Hsu, M.A. & Itri, L.M. (1989) Safety of pregnancy after discontinuation of isotretinoin. *Archives of Dermatology*, (1992) **125**, 362–365.

Dai, W.S., La Braico, J.M. & Stern, R.S. (1992) Epidemiology of isotretinoin exposure during pregnancy. *Journal of the American Academy of Dermatology*, **26**, 599–606.

Lammer, E.J., Chen, D.T. Hoar, R.M. *et al.* (1985) Retinoic acid embryopathy. *New England Journal of Medicine*, **313**, 837–841.

Larsson, P.A. & Liden, S. (1980) Prevalence of skin diseases among adolescents 12–16 years of age. *Acta Dermato-Venereologica (Stockholm)*, **60**, 415–423.

Lello, J., Pearl, A., Arroll, B., Yallop, J. & Birchall, N.M. (1995) Prevalence of acne vulgaris in Auckland senior high school students. *New Zealand Medical Journal*, **108**, 287–289.

Mitchell, A.A., Van Bennekom, C.M. & Louik, C. (1995) A pregnancy-prevention program in women of childbearing age receiving isotretinoin. *New England Journal of Medicine*, **333**, 101–106.

Rademaker, M., Garioch, J.J. & Simpson, N.B. (1989) Acne in schoolchildren: no longer a concern for dermatologists. *British Medical Journal*, **298**, 1217–1219.

Stern, R.S. (1992) The prevalence of acne on the basis of physical examination. *Journal of the American Academy of Dermatology*, **26**, 931–935.

Stern, R.S. & Nelson, C. (1993) The diminishing role of the dermatologist in the office-based care of cutaneous diseases. *Journal of the American Academy of Dermatology*, **29**, 773–777.

Stern, R.S., Rosa, F. & Baum, C. (1984) Isotretinoin and pregnancy. *Journal of the American Academy of Dermatology*, **10**, 851–854.

Index